Environmental Physiology of Animals

ENVIRONMENTAL PHYSIOLOGY OF ANIMALS

EDITORS

J. BLIGH BSc, PhD
Institute of Animal Physiology
Babraham, Cambridge

J. L. CLOUDSLEY-THOMPSON PhD, DSc
Professor of Zoology
Birkbeck College, London

A. G. MACDONALD BSc, PhD
Physiology Department
University of Aberdeen

A HALSTED PRESS BOOK

JOHN WILEY & SONS
NEW YORK

Osney Mead, Oxford,
8 John Street, London, WC1
9 Forrest Road, Edinburgh,
P.O. Box 9, North Balwyn, Victoria, Australia.

First published 1976

Distributed in the United States of America by
Halsted Press, a Division of
John Wiley & Sons, Inc, New York

Library of Congress Cataloging in Publication Data
Main entry under title:

Environmental physiology of animals.

Includes index.
1. Adaptation (Physiology). 2. Bioclimatology.
3. Evolution. I. Bligh, J. II. Cloudsley-Thompson, J. L. III. MacDonald, Alister Gordon.
QP82.E59 1976 591.5 76-25459
ISBN 0-470-98923-8
ISBN 0-470-98925-4 pbk.

Printed in Great Britain

Contents

PART IV · ACQUIRED ADAPTATIONS

PART V · IMMEDIATE HOMEOSTATIC OR SENSORY RESPONSES

PART VI

APPENDICES

Contributors

J. BLIGH, A.R.C. Institute of Animal Physiology, Babraham, Cambridge CB2 4AT

P. J. BUTLER, Department of Zoology, University of Birmingham, P.O. Box 363, Birmingham B15 2TT

A. G. CAIRNS-SMITH, Department of Chemistry, University of Glasgow, Glasgow G12 8QQ

J. L. CLOUDSLEY-THOMPSON, Department of Zoology, Birkbeck College, Malet Street, London WC1E 7HX

P. C. CROGHAN, School of Biological Sciences, University of East Anglia, Norwich NR4 7TJ

E. EDNEY, Laboratory of Nuclear Medicine & Radiation Biology, University of California, Los Angeles, California, U.S.A.

LESLEY GOODMAN, Department of Zoology, Queen Mary College, Mile End Road, London E1 4NS

R. D. HARKNESS, Department of Physiology, University College London, Gower Street, London WC1E 6BT

H. E. HINTON, Department of Zoology, University of Bristol, Bristol BS8 1TH

A. G. MACDONALD, Physiology Department, Marischal College, University of Aberdeen, Aberdeen AB9 1AS

C. MONGE, Universidad Peruana Cayetano Heredia, Avenida Honorio Delgado No. 932, Lima, Peru.

K. NAGY, Laboratory of Nuclear Medicine & Radiation Biology, University of California, Los Angeles, California, U.S.A.

J. PATTERSON, Centre for Overseas Pest Research, College House, Wrights Lane, London W8 5SJ

H. POHL, Max-Planck-Institut für Verhaltenphysiologie, 8131 Erling-Andechs, West Germany.

P. TYTLER, School of Biological Sciences, University of Stirling, Stirling FK9 4LA

M. SMITH, A.R.C. Institute of Animal Physiology, Babraham, Cambridge CB2 4AT

M. WHITFIELD, Marine Biological Association, The Laboratory, Citadel Hill, Plymouth PL1 2PB

J. WHITTEMBURY, Universidad Peruana Cayetano Heredia, Avenida Honorio Delgado No. 932, Lima, Peru.

PART I

INTRODUCTION

Chapter 1
Introduction

1.1 ENVIRONMENTAL PHYSIOLOGY

The main preoccupation of the physiologist is to study what goes on inside an organism. In the words of the distinguished Argentinian physiologist B.A. Houssay 'Physiology is the science that studies the phenomena occurring in living organisms and endeavours to establish their laws'. An understanding of function brings with it the realization that life is a dynamic system which involves continual interchanges between organism and environment. The Russian physiologist K. Bykov defines our subject thus: 'Physiology of man and animals is the study of function of human and animal organisms in their interaction with the environment'. Bykov's broader definition of physiology makes the title of this book somewhat redundant but, to avoid ambiguity and as a concession to common usage, we have used the term 'environmental physiology'. It is our view that the functions of an organism are only really meaningful when studied in the context of the environment with which the organism is interacting. This book will provide abundant evidence to support that assertion.

1.2 THE COMMON DENOMINATOR

In their cells all organisms share many features. Genetic laws are a good example; indeed, Mendel established the basic rules of heredity, which are applicable to man and fruit-fly alike, by cross-breeding peas in a Moravian monastery garden. Subsequent detailed studies of cellular physiology have amply confirmed that the other functions of living cells, both plant and animal, have a great deal in common particularly in respect of their metabolic and regulatory processes.

At the same time, differences between species depend on differences in the genetic code and these differences are made manifest by the structure and function of individual cells.

1.3 THE BASIS OF EVOLUTIONARY CHANGE

That evolution is based on random changes in the genetic constituents of cells is now well established, and there is no reason to dispute that mutations succeed or fail according to whether the individual which possesses a unique variation in its structure or function is thereby afforded, at some time and in some particular circumstances, marginally improved survival. Only in this way can an organism pass on to future generations improved genetic fitness to live and reproduce *in the particular environmental circumstances in which this fitness has been put to the test.*

If this is substantially the way organisms evolve, then it follows that every variation in form and function must have come about through a long series of natural selections of random changes, each of which gave an individual organism some small advantage in particular environmental circumstances. Thus, it may reasonably be claimed, it is the physical environment, together with biotic factors, that have shaped each species and its particular physiology. It also follows that the forms and functions of organisms are expressions of the relations between these organisms and their environments *at some time* in their evolution. In other words, every variation in form or function has a historical environmental significance, but not necessarily a contemporary environmental significance.

1.4 THE AUTONOMY OF THE CELL AS THE UNIT OF LIFE

Life can be imagined to have started during some phase in the geological history of the Earth as it cooled, which favoured the formation of particular complex molecules or complexes of molecules (Chapter 2). These early transitory unstable structures would have existed dynamically, by constant formation and destruction, and this dynamic feature is still characteristic of living things.

At some relatively late stage their persistence in a changing environment was favoured by the formation of a bounding membrane which protected the molecules from the external environment and provided them with a buffered, local environment. Thus, it may be speculated, a primitive cell membrane constituted an early adaptive structure which protected the 'embryonic chemistry of life' from the harmful effects of environmental changes. By their active processes the membranes of all contemporary cells perform this essential function of sustaining the stability of the intracellular environment despite its difference from, and despite changes in, the extracellular environment.

Life is believed to have existed on earth for approximately 3×10^9 years, but it is quite impossible to say for what part of this period life was exclusively unicellular. What is abundantly clear, however, is that all the basic machinery of cellular life had become established, and largely irrevocably so, before life radiated into the myriad unicellular and multicellular forms that constitute the contemporary array of the fauna and flora.

The great variation in the form and function of unicellular organisms, and the ability of unicellular organisms to become adapted to environmental changes, is ample evidence that all the machinery of genotypic adaptation, and probably also of phenotypic adaptation, is invested in the individual cell. Every cell, whether free-living or a member of a multi-cellular structure, retains a large degree of autonomy within its local environment. The integrative functions of multicellular organisms are to be explained in terms of the interaction of individual cells with their local environments. This, at any rate, is a reasonable reductionist view held by most physiologists. A cell can influence other cells by what it removes from or discharges into a common aqueous medium. A cell may respond to the presence of substances released by other cells (or to other environmental influences). As a consequence of mutations, cells vary in these two properties. Functionally specialized members of a multicellular complex thus contribute blindly to the greater unit of the whole organism.

Consider, for example, a simple neuronally operated reflex response to an externally applied stimulus. A cell, or rather part of the membrane of a cell, is specifically responsive to the particular environmental change (e.g. in light, temperature, pressure or the concentration of a chemical constituent of the environment). This disturbance sets up a change in the ionic permeability of the cell membrane which sweeps across the surface of the axon. When this progressive wave of change in the membrane permeability reaches the end of the nerve axon it causes the discharge of a particular substance into the extracellular environment. This substance acts on a specialized part of another nerve-cell membrane which is specifically sensitive to it. A similar sequence of events is thus activated in the other cell and this has the effect of passing on a message if it is an interneurone, or of responding to the message if it is an effector cell. A functional and apparently purposeful reflex response of the whole organism to an environmental stimulus is thus achieved by a succession of responses of individual cells to changes in their local environments. The ability of millions of cells to act in consonance as a macro-unit of life resides in the differences in the ways in which cells interact with their immediate surroundings. The macro-differences between species are an expression of the micro-differences in the functional specializations of member cells, and of the influences one cell exerts on another as a component of the environment of the other cell.

Thus it is the restraining influences of other cells which 'discipline' the individual cells in acting as integral components of a higher order of unit, the multicellular organism. Each cell, however, remains an entity which lives or dies according to the constitution of the chemical matrix in which it is bathed, and according to its ability to respond to changes in its environment so as to maintain its internal processes of life.

Much the same can be said of the whole multicellular organism. It can only survive as a member of a population. As an individual it is bathed in a fluid matrix which may be aqueous or gaseous. Survival depends on the constitution of its local environment, and on the ability of the organism to maintain the integrity of its internal environment within which its constituent cells are bathed, and on its ability to reproduce its kind.

1.5 TIME SCALES OF ADAPTIVE PROCESSES

Adaptive processes occur on 3 major time scales. The first of these is that of the adaptation of life over a period of 3×10^9 years to the different environments of the earth's crust. This is the time scale of *genotypic adaptations* based on the natural selections of chance mutations.

The second scale concerns the periodic adaptations of animals to the regular (cyclic) environmental changes imposed by the movements of the solar system. This time scale has three sub-divisions: the annual cycle of seasons governed by the movement of the earth round the sun; the monthly cycle governed by the movement of the moon round the earth, and the nychthemeral (or 24-hourly) cycle governed by the rotation of the earth on its axis.

The third major time scale is a very short one, and covers the rapid responses to changes in the immediate environment of an organism such as the presence of a prey or of a predator. This category includes sensory physiology, motor control and the physiology of other effectors.

This book is divided into sections which more or less consider these three time scales of adaptation to the environment. There is no rigid division that makes it easy, or even desirable, to consider only one of these time scales when discussing a representative facet of environmental physiology. Genotypic adaptations of physiological functions, which have been established over the longest time scale, are expressed in the qualitative and quantitative nature of the rapid reflex or slower acclimatory responses. For example, the ability of one species of mammal to sweat and of another to pant during heat stress are genotypic adaptations to particular environmental circumstances. The activation of sweating or panting is a rapid reflex response to heat stress. However, the improvement in the effectiveness of either of these processes that may occur during prolonged heat stress is a phenotypic acclimatory change in the function or capacity of a process and exemplifies what may happen naturally in response to seasonal changes in the climate. Contributors have not, therefore, been asked to limit their treatments to the time scale which the section of the book in which their chapters appear is most concerned.

1.6 CONCLUSION

Because all life depends on the responsiveness of individual cells to their immediate environments, because all the manifestations of life are the consequence of interactions between cells and their environments, and because the whole organism is in a state of continual change in response to environmental changes, it is legitimate to argue that *all physiology is environmental physiology*. On the same premisses some would argue that *all physiology is cellular physiology*. But this view would be unacceptable to many who hold that the physiology of multicellular organisms is to do with the properties which arise from the interactions between specialized component cells and particular environmental changes. To whichever point in the spectrum of reductionist-holistic thinking the reader is inclined, there can be no escaping the validity of Bykov's statement that physiology is the study of organisms in their interactions with the environment. The principal purpose of this book is to amplify that statement.

Progress in the understanding of the functions of living organisms has resulted from countless careful and detailed investigations of particular tissues or systems under controlled laboratory conditions. Thus physiology, like all other sciences, relies in the first instance, on the breaking down of complex concurrent and interacting functions into component parts. The resultant crumbs of biological knowledge are quite useless unless and until they are brought together and used to indicate how a whole organism, or even a whole ecosystem operates. This book is concerned with the overall, dynamic pattern of animal life. Because of the magnitude of the subject it cannot be comprehensive. Instead, considerable selection has been exercised on the items which have been included to illustrate the theme. The contributors and editors have tried to present them in a way which will help the student of biology to synthesize an understanding of the phenomena of life and its absolute dependence on the environment in which it occurs. Unless the student seeks to achieve this wider concept of biology he will fall short of achieving scientific maturity, and become someone who may know everything about his subject except its ultimate significance.

PART II

THE ORIGIN OF LIFE

Chapter 2
The origin and early evolution of organisms

A.G.CAIRNS-SMITH

2.1 INTRODUCTION

'But if (and oh what a big if) we could conceive of some warm little pond, with all sorts of ammonia and phosphate salts,—light, heat, electricity etc., present, that a protein compound was chemically formed, ready to undergo still more complex changes . . .'

Darwin made these remarks in a letter written to Hooker in 1871 [19]. His attitude was properly tentative—as ours should still be when considering the subject matter of this chapter. We do not know how life first appeared on earth, nor do we have much clear evidence bearing on its very early evolution—by which I will mean the evolution of the fundamental biochemical machinery that is now shared by all life on earth. But there are several important respects in which we should have an advantage over Darwin in thinking about this problem. We know more biochemistry; we can make better informed guesses as to when and under what general circumstances life on earth might have arisen; we have a much better grasp of the innate capacities of atoms and molecules; and we should have a better understanding of the minimum requirements for any system able to evolve under natural selection. We should indeed be able to mimic, using our intelligence a synthesis that nature achieved at least once by chance. The initial conceptual difficulty is to try to see which if any of the characteristics that we now associate with life had to be there from the start.

2.1.1 Cells, metabolism and genes

Some thinkers place particular emphasis on the cell as the central unit of life now and see some kind of cellular organization as having been essential for the initiation of any true evolutionary process. According to this view particular importance may be attached to cell-like structures that form spontaneously in purely physico-chemical systems. For others metabolism is the key phenomenon and the possibility that complex transformations of organic molecules might have taken place on the primitive earth is seen as particularly significant. Such processes might have occurred more or less diffusely in extended zones of molecules adsorbed on minerals (Bernal's 'subvital regions' [6]). Even whole primitive oceans have been thought of as 'metabolising' (according to Ycas [73]). Then again the gene has been seen as the true basis of life [46, 47] and a number of biologists have suggested that the initial organisms that we seek are in effect 'naked genes'. We will return to these points of view later.

2.1.2 Chemical evolution

A currently popular line of thought on a somewhat different tack starts from the common sense notion of original biochemical similarity—that whatever else may be said about them, early organisms used at least some of the sorts of molecules that are now universal to life, amino acids, sugars and so on; that a major intermediate goal is thus to understand how such 'molecules of life' might have been put together under primitive conditions before life itself arose.

It is suggested that biological evolution was preceded by an extended period of 'chemical evolution' during which small molecules arose and then, through their further organized reactions, larger molecules of the kinds now typical of modern organisms. This was pure 'chemical evolution' but it gave way gradually, through the eventual appearance of reproducing systems based on nucleic acid-like and protein-like molecules, to a true biological evolution [15, 37, 50].

An attractive feature of the doctrine of the continuity of a chemical and early biological evolution is that it appears to be accessible to a piecemeal experimental verification. Our problem can be broken into separate questions: 'Can typical biochemical units, such as amino acids, form under the kinds of conditions that might have been present on the primitive earth?' 'Could these have reacted further to give, for example, protein-like polymers?' 'Can cell-like structures form mixtures of such molecules?' and so on. The answers to these particular questions is probably 'yes', which has convinced many that a solution to the problem of the origin of life along these lines is only a matter of time.

2.2 THEORY AND EXPERIMENT

2.2.1 The Oparin–Haldane hypothesis

The germinal idea of the modern doctrine of chemical evolution was due to Oparin [48] and Haldane [28] who, in the 1920s, realized that organic molecules could probably have formed and accumulated on a primitive earth that was devoid of oxygen and of pre-existing micro-organisms. There would have been sources of energy, such as solar radiation, lightning and local hot regions that might have helped to form high energy substances, like aldehydes. These could have further reacted to give more complex products. Thus organic molecules would have been common in the primitive oceans. This whole idea was helped considerably by the suggestion that the primitive atmosphere was perhaps not only devoid of oxygen, but indeed strongly reducing—dominated by hydrogen—with the hydrides of the non-metals, in particular methane and ammonia, as important constituents. Under these circumstances the energy of formation of complex organic molecules should be relatively low [65].

2.2.2 Miller's experiment

As discussed in Chapter 3, a reducing early atmosphere would probably not have lasted for very long and there is as yet no clear agreement as to whether the atmosphere was strongly reducing when life first arose [17, 18, 37, 50]—it may have been CO_2-dominated like the present atmospheres of Venus and Mars. But the assumption of initial reducing conditions is by no means excluded on present knowledge and this formed the basis of a famous experiment by Stanley Miller [43]. Miller took a mixture of hydrogen, methane, ammonia and water vapour at below 100°C and passed electric sparks through it so as to simulate a primordial thunderstorm, allowing the immediate products to accumulate and react away from the sparks—thus further simulating plausible primordial conditions. Among the products found after a few days were glycine, alanine, aspartic acid and glutamic acid.

Subsequent experiments, using different mixtures of starting gases and different energy sources, have greatly increased the number of 'biochemicals' that could apparently have been formed on the primitive earth through processes as natural as the weather [15, 37, 39, 50, 63].

It may be significant, however, that there are often diverse ways in which the same 'biochemicals' can be formed. For example many protein amino acids are produced from reducing mixtures of simple gases not only with electric discharges [58], but with long-wave ultraviolet radiation [60], ionizing radiation [54], heating to 1000°C with silica catalysts [29, 30] or by heating mixtures of carbon monoxide, heavy hydrogen and deuterated ammonia with Nickel-alumina or clay catalysts [32]. Shock waves too have been found to be a particularly effective synthetic energy source [3, 4]. Then again amino acids can be produced by heating aqueous ammonia and formaldehyde [25], or by refluxing hexamethylene tetramine with hydrochloric acid [71].

Formaldehyde and cyanide are small molecule intermediates frequently detected in these syntheses. Formaldehyde itself has long been known as a starting material for a particularly facile sugar synthesis. Butlerow in 1861 made, in effect, the first 'chemical evolution' experiment showing that a sugary product 'formose' is obtained on mixing formaldehyde and lime [8]. Other mineral catalysts are also effective [13, 26, 57] in producing this very complicated and variable mixture of mono-saccarides.

Adenine is the most accessible of the nucleic acid bases. It has been formed in small yields by electron beam irradiation of a CH_4, NH_3, H_2O mixture [56] and, with guanine and cytosine, by heating a CO, NH_3, H_2 mixture at 600°C with Bi—Fe catalysts [72]. Adenine forms easily from cyanide: from aqueous ammonium cyanide [51], from cyanide in liquid ammonia [68], and with guanine by ultraviolet irradiation of aqueous HCN [55]. A yield of 40–50% of adenine has been obtained by heating formamide in a sealed vessel at 120°C with $POCl_3$ [45]. Uracil and cytosine have been formed from CO_2, NH_3 and kaolin [31].

Organic molecules have been detected in interstellar media—these are often of the small reactive intermediate class—for example, formaldehyde and cyanide [7, 66]. Organic constituents of meteorites are helpful too in compiling a list of common molecules of the universe [38]. Here particularly 'biochemicals' are common, although typically at least 70% of the organic material is only partly analysed polymeric material and most of the smaller molecules are not 'biochemicals' [58, 1, 70].

The general conclusion to be drawn from all these researches on the non-biological formation of typically biological molecules is that organisms now use molecules that belong to classes that are fairly easy to make [64]—often in a variety of different ways. This is certainly consistent with the idea of original biochemical similarity but it by no means proves it. This general conclusion is not really surprising enough to indicate what historical significance, if any, it has for the origin of our life system [11]. In any case one might expect organisms to have settled down eventually to using molecular parts that are not too troublesome to make. But when was the particular set of easily made parts that we now use decided on? It seems unlikely that the entire set was determined before life started: some at least would surely have been brought in in response to later evolutionary pressures. Perhaps they all were.

2.2.3 Macromolecules

Given the necessary small organic molecules then, according to currently favoured ideas, the next stages would have been their polymerization into molecules like proteins and nucleic acids. A difficulty here is that under aqueous conditions the processes of forming all the main biopolymers from their units is energetically uphill. Fox has shown that baking a mixture of dry amino acids containing an excess of glutamic and aspartic acids provides a clean way of eliminating water and produces a material, 'proteinoid', on subsequent treatment with water [22, 24]. Calvin has suggested that small high-energy molecules like cyanamide might have acted as primordial coupling agents [15]. Schwartz has considered in detail how phosphorylation might have been possible under primitive conditions [61].

2.3 MODELS FOR PRIMITIVE SYSTEMS

2.3.1 Multimolecular structures

If molecules are to become organized further into higher order systems there must be (at least) some coherence mechanism—some means of holding the molecules together. For Ycas [73] an ocean was the 'reaction vessel'. Darwin's pond, referred to in the opening quotation, was perhaps a similar idea. Some other suggestions (summarized in Table 2.1) will now be considered briefly.

Coacervates

Oparin saw in the phenomenon of coacervation the key to the stage in biogenesis following the formation of suitable molecules [49]. According to his view, macromolecules in the primordial ocean would have tended to form discrete associations—gummy droplets separating from the general solution. Effects of this kind are well known from laboratory studies of suitable mixtures. These coacervates would have been in a kind of simple competition with each other in the sense that the more stable ones would have survived for longer. And reactions would have tended to take place within them characteristic of the individual droplets in so far as they might have particular kinds of catalyst particles present within them. There would thus have been selection, too, on the basis of the kinds of reactions that were going on inside the droplets: some reactions, using molecules diffusing in from the surrounding medium, would tend to increase the amount of material in a droplet so that it would grow at the expense of others and perhaps through some mechanical effect such as a breaking wave it would be split into pieces that would continue to grow in a characteristic way.

Thus gradually, from the simplest selection of the most stable coacervates, through selection of the most dynamically effective and then to those that could reproduce, would the first true organisms have arisen—that is the first systems fully subject to natural selection.

Microspheres

Cell-like objects, microspheres, are formed when the proteinoid polymer produced by baking suitable amino acid mixtures comes in contact with water. It is claimed that budding and fission can be observed among the myriads of microspheres and Fox places great importance on these structures in his theory of molecular and cellular origins [22, 23, 24].

Micelles and monolayers

Micelles derived from amphiphobic molecules like soaps are among the most readily formed higher order molecular structures. Although the formation of lipid-like molecules have featured less prominently in pre-biotic simulation experiments, a number of authors have suggested that structures such as cell membranes could have been formed through purely physico-chemical processes. Some of these ideas are discussed by Calvin [15]. For example, it has been proposed that the collapse of suitable monolayers on water surfaces through the action of wind would have produced membrane enclosed droplets [27].

Organo-clay complexes

As pointed out particularly by Bernal [5, 6], mineral crystals could have provided organizing and catalytic surfaces for pre-biotic organic molecules—encouraging further reactions to give more complex products. Bernal stressed particularly a possible role for clays. This class of minerals have very small particles, and hence a large relative surface area, as well as a known specific affinity for a number of significant types of organic molecules [67].

A typical clay particle consists of a stack of negatively charged silicate platelets that are held together by counterions such as sodium or potassium. The counterions can often be replaced by organic molecules, for example N-alkyl ammonium ions, but uncharged organic molecules of a variety of types can also be taken up within the regions between the silicate layers. The edges of clay platelets often carry a positive charge and tend preferentially to bind negative species—for example carboxylic acids or pyrophosphates [67]. Given also the catalytic powers of clays, these minerals provide very interesting sites for possibly significant pre-biotic organic chemistry. The work of Paecht-Horowitz and her collaborators on the formation of polypeptides in clays is of particular interest [53] as are the studies of Degens and his school [20].

An extension of the possible role of clays in the origin of life is to see them as having provided not only a factory for making suitable 'biochemicals' but a niche within which 'sub-vital' metabolic processes started [6]. My own view is that clay, or some other microcrystalline inorganic mineral, took a still more active part in biogenesis: that the initial organisms virtually *were* growing mineral crystals [9, 10]. I will return to this idea later.

Jeewanu

Cell-like structures formed through irradiation with light of solutions of suitable inorganic components—containing, for example, molybdic acid—have been studied for many years by Bahadur and his associates [2]. These he calls 'jeewanu' meaning 'particles of life'. It is claimed that jeewanu show enzyme-like properties and that in the presence of simple feed molecules 'biochemicals' such as amino acids and nucleotide bases are formed within them.

Table 2.1. Multimolecular structures of possible relevance to the origin of life.

Type	Description	References
Coacervates	Microscopic organic macromolecular associations entraining other organic and inorganic small molecules and ions	[49]
Microspheres	Microscopic spherical bags of proteinoid	[22, 23, 24]
Micelles	Submicroscopic clusters of amphiphobic (soap-like) molecules	[15, 27]
Organo-clay complexes	Intracrystalline associations between organic molecules and clays	[5–10]
Jeewanu	Precipitates consisting of microscopic particles of inorganic materials, with associated organic molecules, and formed by the action of light on suitable solutions	[2]
Calcerous structures	Inorganic–organic precipitates from supersaturated solutions of calcium salts containing also organic molecules	[16]

Calcerous structures

Quasi-crystalline microscopic calcium rich structures have been observed from time to time in sterilized media—for example blood sera. On account of their life-like appearance they were even considered to be evidence in favour of spontaneous generation. Cinatl has studied these again more recently and has suggested that some such 'calcerous structures' might have had a role in the origins of life [16].

2.3.2 Open systems

The kinds of models that we have been discussing so far owe their appeal in many cases to their physical resemblance to modern cells or organelles. But the modern cell is evidently the product of a prolonged evolutionary process: there is little guarantee that the original ancestral systems were indeed at all structurally similar to modern organisms. Another approach is to try to think of models that contain analogies to more abstract and perhaps more fundamental aspects of living things. A flame is an ancient example of such a model—or a whirlpool. These objects are very much part of the ordinary physico-chemical world, yet they contain an essentially life-like feature: they 'metabolize' in the sense that they are maintained through a continual exchange of matter and energy. Like organisms they are metastable—yet they may persist for a long time. Sherrington saw an organism as a kind of self-maintaining eddy system in an energy stream, and evolution as a progressive increase in the complexity and self-maintaining powers of such systems [62]. According to this view the organism is not only to be seen as necessarily part of the environment, but is only able to arise and flourish in a certain kind of environment—one that is in some sense a stream. The organism is a complicatedly dynamic part of what must be in any case a dynamic environment. On the earth now this point is somewhat concealed by the remoteness, now, of the connection between the fundamental environmental flows that maintain life—mainly the flow of photons from the sun—and the activities of particular organisms that we may happen to be thinking about, such as the higher animals. But perhaps this remoteness is an evolutionary consequence. Perhaps the first life forms were more literally like eddies in some real environmental stream.

2.3.3 Primitive genes

Another more abstract approach has been to suppose that life arose from some class of replicating gene-like structures that were produced spontaneously from an initially purely physico-chemical milieu. Such systems could be immediately subject to natural selection within a suitable situation. Early ideas along these lines, for example that suggested in 1924 by C. B. Lipman, tended to be rather vague about possible structures and appealed to remote accidents for the initial system (reference [49], p. 96). With the discovery of the genetic role of nucleic acid in modern organisms there have been a number of proposals that our original ancestor was some primitive kind of nucleic acid molecule [34, 36, 42].

The work of Speigelmann and his school on replicating RNA molecules has illustrated vividly the essential correctness of the supposition that replicating molecules can evolve—given suitable selection pressures [40, 44]. Eigen [21] has developed a theoretical model for the evolution of accurate from inaccurate nucleic acid replication.

But there are difficulties in the idea that evolution started from a nucleic acid molecule. One lucky accidental synthesis of a starter molecule would not have been nearly enough. There would have had to exist suitable conditions for its repeated replication. In Speigelman's experiments this included an enzyme. But even if an accurate enough non-enzymic mechanism operated to begin with, or could have evolved sufficient accuracy sufficiently quickly, there would have been another even tougher requirement for that early environment: it would have had to provide a supply of the necessary units for replicative synthesis—activated nucleotides—and it would have had to continue to do so until the evolving life system had learned to make these units for itself. Pre-biotic simulations have, to my mind, failed to produce convincing evidence that activated nucleotides could have been consistently supplied by a non-biological environment over the very long periods that would presumably have been required for metabolic machinery of the necessary sophistication to have evolved. As any organic chemist will tell you, activated nucleotides are difficult molecules to make—and our metabolic system seems to find them quite hard to come by too [12].

We may agree that the nucleotide bases, particularly adenine, might well have been present on the primitive earth. But so would many other similar molecules. Ribose and deoxyribose too might well have been there—but again usually grossly contaminated with other sugars, decomposition products etc. Nucleotides would have been much rarer achievements—and they would have been still more contaminated with many of the now very large number of possible molecules of that kind of complexity. We should remember that even our system with its amazing capacities of molecular recognition can nevertheless be confused by molecules ('antimetabolites') that are similar to its central components. But even an environmental supply (over millions of years) of correct nucleotides would still have been inadequate. The nucleotides would have had to be activated (ATP, GTP, etc., or their equivalents) and this, even if achieved, leads to further problems created by the number of possible side reactions between such molecules and each other and the even larger number of reactions possibly with the multifarious components of a 'soup'.

As if this was not enough these difficulties are still further compounded by the general situation that is so often said to have been necessary for the origin of life, in which organic reactions were particularly prolific because conditions were reducing and there were strong energy sources available. The ultraviolet flux from the sun would have been particularly trying for nucleic acids. A modern bacterium would last on average for less than 0·3 seconds in its glare [59]. Perhaps the first organisms were confined to dark niches. It might have been possible to have hidden from the primordial sun, but it would have been much more difficult to hide from the products of its activities, particularly those small easily diffusible reactive molecules like cyanide and formaldehyde. Such molecules would have made organized organic chemistry very difficult and dark resinous substances the almost invariable products.

2.3.4 The 'gene in a stream' model

The above objections are not to the idea that life arose from primitive gene structures, but to the idea that these were nucleic acid molecules. Some kind of initial gene structures seem indeed to have been necessary in so far as we seek the origins of a Darwinian evolutionary process. Such a process depends on heredity and heredity depends on stable replicable structures [10, 46].

We can combine the idea that living organisms are necessarily open systems with the idea that they must necessarily contain stable genetic structures in an extension of Sherrington's model. An organism is like an eddy pattern produced by a stone of a particular shape placed in a stream. The stream is the environment, the stone's shape is the (static) genotype which produces by interaction with the (dynamic) environment a particular dynamic pattern of eddies—the phenotype.

To be more realistic we would have to try to imagine some system in which the 'stone' was replicable and the 'eddies' able to assist the replication process. We should not, I think, be prejudiced about the kinds of materials that might have been involved in the first place or of the kinds of replication assisting 'eddies' that might have been most effective for the most primitive life systems. In particular we should not assume that any of the modern 'biochemicals' were necessarily involved or that early phenotypes had any obvious cell-like characteristics.

2.4 A CASE FOR AN ALIEN ANCESTRY?

2.4.1. Matching a genetic material to an environment

We can see the phenotype of a modern organism as a specific disturbance in the environment produced by a set of DNA base sequences. The special problem of the origin of life arises because DNA, at least in our present environment, requires an exceedingly elaborate pre-existing disturbance not only to replicate efficiently but to replicate at all. In this sense DNA is badly matched to our general environments. It is like a traveller from an alien world who must carry with him essential and complex life support systems. And herein lies the paradox of the origin of life: how did the support systems arise in the first place? The usual way of trying to resolve this paradox is by supposing that there was a situation on earth in the remote past when DNA or something like it, was more at home—where the support systems were not initially required. It is supposed that there *used to be* a non-biological matched environment for DNA.

As indicated in the earlier discussion I am inclined to think that there was never a non-biological matched environment for any nucleic acid-like molecules, that these are essentially sophisticated genetic materials: like magnetic tape, they can be a very efficient means of handling information but they are necessarily committed to pre-existing complex machinery: in nature they are matched only to an environment that consists of the interior of a well-equipped cell.

It is a commonplace observation in considering man-made mechanisms that optimal structures, materials, methods of construction and even principles of operation change with changes in the surrounding technology. Given a sophisticated technology new ways of doing things emerge: stone tablets were replaced with papyrus then paper. Pirie has used similar arguments against the necessity of proteins in early organisms (reference [5], p. 71).

When we look at the higher levels of the organization of organisms we can see how new ways of doing things have emerged during evolution. Vertebrate limbs evolved from fins; our speech mechanism depends on a pair of bellows devised for aerial respiration, and so on. Never was there any forethought—it just turned out that given certain pre-existing inventions other inventions became possible. Is it not likely that very early evolution, concerned with the creation and perfection of the exceedingly ingenious central biochemical machine, was similarly devious and opportunist: that the way it started was not at all the way it turned out?

According to this line of thought our original ancestors were 'alien' in the sense that their biochemistry was not based on anything like the now universal nucleic acid/protein mechanisms [12]. (They may have been alien also or instead in the sense that they arrived from some other part of the universe, but we are choosing to ignore this possibility.) We seek, then, a matched genetic material-environment pair by thinking not only about primitive environments that might have been different from ours, but also about primitive genetic materials that might have been very different.

While there may well be organic molecules that could have replicated within simpler environments than are needed for nucleic acids, I am doubtful whether any would have been effective in a wholely non-biological milieu: as discussed earlier organic reactions, unless carefully controlled, tend too easily to yield tarry mixtures. Crystallization processes, on the other hand, can be far more accurately self-controlled and there are several possible modes of pattern replication that can take place during crystallization [9].

2.4.2 Crystals as primitive genes?

I have suggested that the central genetic machinery of primitive organisms might have consisted of the spontaneous continuous crystallization of a suitable mineral on the primitive earth, a mica-type clay being a particularly attractive possibility [9, 10]. Such clays can form spontaneously from solutions produced by the weathering of rocks.

In mica-type clays the minute crystallites each consist of a stack of very thin (~ 1 nm) silicate sheets piled on top of each other. The negative charges result from substitution in their structure, the most significant of these being substitutions of aluminium atoms for a proportion of the silicon atoms. The sheets are held together through sandwiched cations such as sodium or potassium.

The negative charge pattern on the silicate layers is a variable feature that might be inheritable during a layer-on-layer growth process—and there is now some direct evidence of such an inheritance [69]. In addition to being replicable there is good reason to suppose that charge patterns could affect simple properties of clays such as rheology. These could, in particular situations, affect the chances of clays containing particular patterns being preserved.

I have pursued this speculation at greater length elsewhere [10]. The point to be made here is that one can envisage a population of mineral crystallites under a simple kind of natural selection. Once we have a natural selection operating efficiently on a genetic material which has a large potential information capacity—and layer silicates have—then at least in principle highly biologically organized systems might be brought into being. This organization would be written in the form of certain prevalent genetic patterns, but as we know from our present-day life, the means to this apparently straightforward end could be exceedingly indirect. (Who would have guessed that the elephant would be a good way of propagating DNA sequences?) For example, clay crystal growth might be interfered with by some ion present in an environment. Only clays that could somehow remove the effect of this ion would be able to flourish in this environment. Perhaps this could be done by catalysing the synthesis of a certain general class of organic molecules as chelating agents. Then there would be a selection pressure to make these molecules more efficiently. Having done this, deeper inroads into even less clement environments might be possible, with now new selection pressures for the evolution of further adaptations. Perhaps some of these would find that the machinery for making those chelating molecules could be used also for making a slightly different kind that could function in other ways, for example as a glue for holding the replicating crystallite population in a fast flowing stream particularly rich in silica and alumina 'nutrients'.

Thus, gradually, charge patterns might have come into being with increasingly sophisticated means of controlling their environments—from controlling rheology to controlling in a broad way the adsorption of organic molecules perhaps, then more specific adsorption, then unspecific catalysis, then increasingly specific catalysis and the evolution of metabolic pathways [12, 14].

However it happened the origin and early evolution of life would have required two things of its environment. First that there should be at least one easy niche where a spontaneously forming genetic material could replicate without having to contain any clever genetic information. Then there must be other progressively more difficult niches to provide selection pressures for the elaboration of more complex modes of survival and propagation. (In such a complicated heterogeneous and changeable place as the surface of the earth the second of these requirements does not seem too difficult given the first.)

2.4.3 Genetic metamorphosis—assisted take-off of secondary genetic systems

But how could such a Darwinian evolution based on a primitive alien genetic system have helped towards the discovery of a 'high technology system' like ours? The quick answer is 'by creating a new set of environments'. These new environments would have been the phenotypes of the now well-evolved primitive life form. They would constitute new, much more reliable and cleaner sources of particular organic molecules. Consider the earth now. It contains a rich variety of chemical factories—particularly in the secondary metabolisms of the plants. Now imagine the earth as it might have been following the extensive evolution of some alien primitive life form. The earth would have been transformed from a situation in which organic molecules were present mainly as more or less grossly impure tars and 'gunks', into a set of more or less discrete factories producing 'fine chemicals'.

Not only could an evolved primitive life form have thus provided 'food' for secondary systems, but also 'shelter' and 'jobs'. Someone else's phenotype can be an easy place to live. A new kind of genetic material being formed by accident within an evolved phenotype would have a much better chance of catching on than a similar event in a tarry soup. From the point of view of the alien primitive organism, the new genetic molecules would be something like viral infections. The ideal situation would be where the 'virus' was a symbiote: where its presence gave some marginal advantage to the host. And this is not too difficult to envisage. We imagine that the alien life form had evolved to the point where it could make regular polymers—molecules like cellulose for example—and it would most probably be a co-polymer related to one of these that would first acquire a measure of replicability—through synthesis of new polymer taking place preferentially on pre-existing polymer. The first of the new genes, that is, would be made of material very similar to stuff that the host found useful anyway. Given a symbiotic relationship—however minor the role of the new partner—the system as a whole would now tend to evolve in such a way as to encourage the effective replication of *both* the genetic systems now present.

Whereas the choice of primitive genetic systems would have depended on which materials available on the primitive earth could have held and printed effective information in the absence of an on-going biochemistry, the choice of secondary materials would have depended on fitting a rather different set of specifications: effectiveness in a chemically civilized milieu would now be the criterion. In the early days of a new genetic material it would not have been at all clear whether it would be more than a trivial optional extra. That would have depended on what happened next. Perhaps we can see why a primitive nucleic acid-like molecule was eventually to prove a winner: it discovered how to make protein. Eventually we must suppose, there was somewhere in some population of organisms a complete take-over by the new system, this system having gradually, step by step, taken over control of all the biochemical reactions needed for the synthesis of its components. With the original alien genetic material now gone there was left the seemingly paradoxical situation in which a complicated system *needs* that complicated system to work at all.

2.5 THE STYLE OF EARLY BIOCHEMICAL EVOLUTION

2.5.1 'Backwards' or 'forwards'?

So far we have considered two general explanations for the origin of our genetic control system. Each of these was based on the idea that our genetic system evolved from nucleic acid-like molecules, but they differed in their account of how these molecules arose and under what circumstances they subsequently evolved. We may ask some other general questions about the likely style of early metabolic evolution. We may ask, for example, if it took place 'forwards' towards complex metabolites, like nucleotides, from simple atom sources, or 'backwards' from an initial external supply of key complex foods. A 'backwards' mechanism was proposed by Horowitz [33] along the following lines. Suppose that there exists now some train of reactions within an organism, for example:

$$A \rightarrow B \rightarrow C \rightarrow D$$

where D is some vital component. This indicates that at one time D was available in the environment, then as the supplies of it ran out there was a selection pressure to make D from C which was still abundant. As C ran out catalysts to make it from B evolved—and so on. This seems to be the most generally favoured mechanism for very early metabolic evolution, but it involves serious difficulties in that the primitive environment would have had to supply often quite unstable intermediates [12].

Lipmann [41] proposed a 'forward' mechanism for our metabolism starting from carbon dioxide through sugars, acetate, lipids, and then amino acids and after that nucleotides. This is certainly a very direct way of reading the metabolic charts, but it becomes possible, I think, only if one presupposes an earlier gene-catalyst system [12].

2.5.2 Complication or simplification?

It seems likely that early metabolic processes would have used unspecific catalysts and hence that the early pathways would have been exceedingly complicated —as for example the production of sugars from formaldehyde using simple inorganic catalysts is an exceedingly complicated process. On this view early evolution would have been largely concerned with refining catalytic specificity and hence simplifying reaction networks rather than with step-by-step construction of pathways [14].

2.5.3 Methane or carbon dioxide?

As discussed earlier, a reduced primitive atmosphere containing plenty of methane etc. would have made organized organic chemistry rather difficult— a more inert environment would have been preferable. An attractive feature of the primitive mineral gene idea is that it does not need a primordial soup: life could have started from a CO or CO_2 carbon source and evolved gradually ('forwards'). That formaldehyde at least could have been produced locally by solar radiation in association with minerals under such an atmosphere is strongly suggested by experiments on the production of organic molecules under simulated Martian conditions. It was found that UV radiation of the kind that would reach the Martian surface produced simple organic molecules, including formaldehyde, from carbon monoxide and water in the presence of silicates [35]. (A predominantly carbon dioxide atmosphere would contain some carbon monoxide through atmospheric UV photolysis of carbon dioxide.) The first clumsy organic phenotypes were perhaps formose-like mixtures of sugars produced by somewhat unspecific effects of early mineral genes [13, 12]. There would be selection pressures on such organisms to become more accurate in their specification of metabolic processes and also to discover ways of photoreducing the more available carbon dioxide.

Table 2.2. Some questions on the origin and early evolution of life and some tentative answers consistent with two doctrines. In each case a genetic view of life is taken and organisms considered to be systems subject indefinitely to natural selection.

	CHEMICAL EVOLUTION	GENETIC METAMORPHOSIS
What were the main initial 'foods'?	Complex products of chemical evolution as well as H_2O and other small molecules and ions—i.e. a 'primordial soup'.	Rock weathering products particularly SiO_2 and Al_2O_3 and inorganic ions. H_2O and atmospheric CO.
What were the next 'foods'?	A 'soup' becoming depleted of some of the key constituents.	As above, but with CO_2 in place of CO and then also inorganic nitrogen.
How did most of our 'biochemicals' first arise in organisms?	They were picked up from a primitive (reducing) environment, i.e. discovered externally.	They were 'discovered' internally during the metabolic evolution of a primitive life that did not initially need them, i.e. they need never have been in the environment.
What was the principle mode of evolution of primary metabolic pathways?	'Backwards' towards simpler foods.	'Forwards' towards more elaborate metabolites.
What can we say of the sequence of incorporation of the main classes of 'biochemicals'?	First, at least 2 nucleotides. Then, probably, prevalent environmental types favoured with amino acids among these.	First, non-nitrogenous classes—sugars, lipids, Krebs acids, then amino acids and after that nucleotides.
What was the main factor driving the transition to the modern arrangement of genetic and metabolic systems?	Final disappearance of reducing conditions. This left CO_2 and inorganic nitrogen as C and N sources. Metabolic routes had to be established from these.	Final takeover by previously symbiotic secondary genetic system of the metabolic routes required to make its components. Disappearance of mineral genes.

2.5.4 An early or late entry for nitrogen?

If we suppose that the first organisms used the same sort of genetic system as modern organisms then these first organisms needed nitrogen. With primitive mineral genetic systems, however, nitrogen need only have come in at a much later stage after a well-organized non-nitrogenous metabolism had been established. This is in accordance with Lipmann's proposed sequence of metabolic evolution and with the central position of the extensive non-nitrogenous part of our metabolic pathways.

2.5.5 Chemical evolution or genetic metamorphosis?

It is possible to formulate schemes for the origin and early evolution of life that involve both the doctrine of chemical evolution—that early organisms needed sophisticated non-biologically produced foods, and that of genetic metamorphosis—that early evolution proceeded through a radical change in genetic materials. A silicate-based early life for example might have required a 'soup' as its original source of organic molecules. Yet on the basis of present knowledge these doctrines can be seen as alternatives: neither really needs the other. This is illustrated by the series of questions and alternative answers given in Table 2.2.

2.6 REFERENCES

1 Anders E., Hayatsu R. & Studier M.H. (1973) Organic compounds in meteorites. *Science* **182,** 781–90.

2 Bahadur K. (1970) The photochemical formation of self-sustaining coacervates. *J. Brit. Interplanetary Soc.* **23,** 813–29.

3 Bar-Nun A., Bar-Nun N., Bauer S.H. & Sagan C. (1970) Shock synthesis of amino acids in simulated primitive environments. *Science* **168,** 470–2.

4 Bar-Nun A., Bar-Nun N., Bauer S.H. & Sagan C. (1971) Shock synthesis of amino acids in simulated primitive environments. In *Molecular Evolution I: Chemical Evolution and the Origin of Life* (eds R. Buvet & C. Ponnamperuma) pp. 114–22. North Holland, Amsterdam.

5 Bernal J.D. (1951) *The Physical Basis of Life.* Routledge & Kegan Paul, London.

6 Bernal J.D. (1967) *The Origin of Life.* Weidenfeld & Nicolson, London.

7 Buhl D. (1974) Galactic clouds of organic molecules. *Origins of Life* **5.** Also in ref. [74], Vol. I, pp. 29–40.

8 Butlerow A. (1861) Bildung einer zuckerartigen Substanz durch Synthese. *Ann.* **120,** 295–8.

9 Cairns-Smith A.G. (1966) The origin of life and the nature of the primitive gene. *J. theor. Biol.* **10,** 53–88.

10 Cairns-Smith A.G. (1971) *The Life Puzzle: on crystals and organisms and on the possibility of a crystal as an ancestor.* Oliver & Boyd, Edinburgh.

11 Cairns-Smith A.G. (1974) Ambiguity in the interpretation of abiotic syntheses. *Origins of Life* **6,** 265–7. Also in ref. [74], Vol. II, pp. 265–7.

12 Cairns-Smith A.G. (1975) A case for an alien ancestry. *Proc. Roy. Soc. Lond. B.* **189,** 249–74.

13 Cairns-Smith A.G., Ingram P. & Walker G. (1972) Formose production by minerals: possible relevance to the origin of life. *J. Theor. Biol.* **35,** 601–4.

14 Cairns-Smith A.G. & Walker G.L. (1974) Primitive metabolism. *Biosystems* **5,** 173–86.

15 Calvin M. (1969) *Chemical Evolution: Molecular Evolution Towards the Origin of Living Systems on the Earth and Elsewhere*. Clarendon Press, Oxford.

16 Cinatl J. (1969) Inorganic–organic multimolecular complexes of salt solutions, culture media and biological fluids and their possible significance for the origin of life. *J. theor. Biol.* **23,** 1–10.

17 Cloud P.E. (1968) Atmospheric and hydrospheric evolution on the primitive earth. *Science* **160,** 729–36.

18 Cloud P.E. (1969) Prepaleozoic sediments and their significance for organic geochemistry. In *Organic Geochemistry* (eds G. Eglinton & M. T. J. Murphy), pp. 727–36. Longman, London.

19 Darwin F. (1887) *Life and Letters of Charles Darwin*, Vol. 3, p. 18. London (Quoted in ref. [6], p. 4 and ref. [48], p. 79).

20 Degens E.T. & Matheja J. (1968) Origin, development and diagenesis of biogeochemical compounds. *J. Brit. Interplanetary Soc.* **21,** 52–82.

21 Eigen M. (1971) Selforganisation of matter and the evolution of biological macromolecules. *Naturwiss.* **58,** 465–523.

22 Fox S.W. (1964) Thermal polymerisation of amino acids and production of formed microparticles on Lava. *Nature* **201,** 336–7.

23 Fox S.W. (1965) A theory of macromolecular and cellular origins. *Nature* **205,** 328–40.

24 Fox S.W. & Dose K. (1972) *Molecular Evolution and the Origin of Life*. Freeman, San Francisco.

25 Fox S.W. & Windsor C.R. (1970) Synthesis of amino acids by the heating of formaldehyde and ammonia. *Science* **170,** 984–95.

26 Gabel N.W. & Ponnamperuma C. (1967) Model for origin of monosaccharides. *Nature* **216,** 453–5.

27 Goldacre R.J. (1958) Surface films, their collapse on compression, the shapes and sizes of cells and the origin of life. *Surface Phenomena in Chemistry and Biology*, pp. 278–98. Pergamon Press, Oxford.

28 Haldane J.B.S. (1929) The origin of life. *Rationalist Annual 3*. (Reprinted in Bernal J.D. *The Origin of Life*, pp. 242–9. Weidenfeld & Nicolson, London.)

29 Harada K. & Fox S.W. (1964) Thermal synthesis of natural amino acids from a postulated primitive terrestrial atmosphere. *Nature* **201,** 335–6.

30 Harada K. & Fox S.W. (1965) The thermal synthesis of amino acids from a hypothetically primitive terrestrial atmosphere. In *The Origins of Prebiological Systems* (ed. S. W. Fox), pp. 187–201. Academic Press, New York & London.

31 Harvey G.R., Degens E.T. & Mopper K. (1971) Synthesis of nitrogen heterocycles on kaolinite from CO_2 and NH_3. *Naturwiss.* **58,** 624–5.

32 Hayatsu R., Studier M.H. & Anders E. (1971) Origin of organic matter in early solar system—IV. Amino acids: confirmation of catalytic synthesis by mass spectrometry. *Geochim. Cosmochim. Acta* **35,** 939–51.

33 Horowitz N.H. (1945) On the evolution of biochemical syntheses. *Proc. Nat. Acad. Sci. U.S.A.* **31,** 153–7.

34 Horowitz N.H. (1959) On defining life. In *The Origin of Life on the Earth* (eds F. Clark & R. L. M. Synge), pp. 106–7. Pergamon Press, Oxford.

35 Hubbard J.S., Hardy J.P. & Horowitz N.H. (1971) Photocatalytic production of organic compounds from CO and H_2O in a simulated Martian Atmosphere. *Proc. Nat. Acad. Sci. U.S.A.* **68,** 574–8.

36 Huxley J. (1963) *Evolution: The Modern Synthesis*. Allen & Unwin, London.

37 Kenyon D.H. & Steinman G. (1969) *Biochemical Predestination*. McGraw Hill, New York.

38 Kvenvolden K.A. (1974) Natural evidence for chemical and early biological evolution. *Origins of Life* **5.** Also in ref. [74], Vol. I, pp. 71–86.

39 Lemmon R.M. (1970) *Chemical Evolution. Chem. Rev.* **70,** 95–109.

40 Levisohn R. & Spiegelman S. (1968) The cloning of a self-replicating RNA molecule. *Proc. Nat. Acad. Sci. U.S.A.* **60,** 866–72.

41 Lipmann F. (1965) Projecting backward from the present state of evolution of biosynthesis. In *The Origins of Prebiological Systems* (ed. S. W. Fox), pp. 259–80. Academic Press, New York & London.
42 Maynard Smith J. (1966) *The Theory of Evolution*, p. 96. Penguin Books, Harmondsworth.
43 Miller S.L. (1953) A production of amino acids under possible primitive earth conditions. *Science* **117,** 528–9.
44 Mills D.R., Kramer F.R. & Spiegelman S. (1973) Complete nucleotide sequence of a replicating RNA molecule. *Science* **180,** 916–27.
45 Morita K., Ochiai O. & Marumoto R. (1968) A convenient one step synthesis of adenine. *Chem. and Ind.* p. 1117.
46 Muller H.J. (1947) *The Gene. Proc. Roy. Soc.* **134**B, 1–37.
47 Muller H.J. (1955) *Life. Science* **121,** 1–9.
48 Oparin A.I. (1924) *The Origin of Life.* (Translated from the Russian and reprinted in Bernal, J.D. *The Origin of Life*, pp. 199–241. Weidenfeld & Nicolson, London.)
49 Oparin A.I. (1957) *The Origin of Life on the Earth.* Oliver & Boyd, Edinburgh.
50 Orgel L.E. (1973) *The Origins of Life: Molecules and Natural Selection.* Chapman & Hall, London.
51 Oro J. (1960) Synthesis of adenine from ammonium cyanide. *Biochem. Biophys. Res. Communs.* **2,** 407–12.
52 Oro J., Miller S.L., Ponnamperuma C. & Young R.S. (eds) (1974) *Cosmochemical Evolution and the Origins of Life* (Proceedings of the fourth international conference on the origin of life and the first meeting of the international society for the study of the origin of life, Barcelona, June 1973) Reidel, Dordrecht and Boston. These papers also published in *Origins of Life*, Vols 5 and 6.
53 Paecht-Horowitz M., Berger J. & Katchalski A. (1970) Prebiotic synthesis of polypeptides by heterogeneous polycondensation of amino acid adenylates. *Nature* **228,** 636–9.
54 Palm C. & Calvin M. (1962) Primordial organic chemistry. I. Compounds resulting from irradiation of $C^{14}H_4$. *J. Am. Chem. Soc.* **84,** 2115–21.
55 Ponnamperuma C. (1965) A biological synthesis of some nucleic acid constituents. In *The Origins of Prebiological Systems* (ed. S. W. Fox), pp. 221–42. Academic Press, New York & London.
56 Ponnamperuma C., Lemmon R.M., Mariner R. & Calvin M. (1963) Formation of adenine by electron irradiation of methane, ammonia and water. *Proc. Nat. Acad. Sci. U.S.A.* **49,** 737–40.
57 Reid C. & Orgel L.E. (1967) Synthesis of sugars in potentially prebiotic conditions. *Nature* **216,** 455.
58 Ring D., Wolman Y., Friedman N. & Miller S.L. (1972) Prebiotic syntheses of hydrophobic and protein amino acids. *Proc. Nat. Acad. Sci. U.S.A.* **69,** 765–8.
59 Sagan C. (1973) Ultraviolet selection pressures on the earliest organisms. *J. theor. Biol.* **39,** 195.
60 Sagan C. & Khare B.N. (1971) Long wavelength ultra-violet production of amino acids. *Science* **173,** 417–22.
61 Schwartz A.W. (1974) An evolutionary model for prebiotic phosphorylation. In *The Origin of Life and Evolutionary Biochemistry* (eds K. Dose, S. W. Fox, G. A. Deborin & T. E. Pavlovskaya), pp. 435–43. Plenum Press, New York & London.
62 Sherrington C. (1940) *Man on His Nature* (1937 Gifford Lectures), p. 88. Cambridge University Press, London.
63 Stephen-Sherwood E. & Oro J. (1973) Chemical evolution: recent synthesis of bioorganic molecules. *Space Life Sci.* **4,** 5–31.
64 Studier M. (1969) Origin of organic matter in meteorites. In *Extra-terrestrial Matter* (ed. C. A. Randall) pp. 25–56. Northern Illinois University Press, DeKalb, Illinois.
65 Toupance G., Raulin F. & Buvet R. (1971) Primary transformation processes under the influence of energy for models of primordial atmospheres in thermodynamic equilibrium.

In *Molecular Evolution I: Chemical Evolution and the Origin of Life* (eds. R. Buvet & C. Ponnamperuma), pp. 83–95. North Holland, Amsterdam.
66 Turner B.E. (1973) Interstellar molecules. *Sci. Amer.* **228,** No. 3, 50–69.
67 Van Olphen H. (1963) *An Introduction to Clay Colloid Chemistry.* Wiley Interscience, New York.
68 Wakakatsu H., Yamasa Y., Sato T., Kumashiro I. & Takenishi T. (1966) Synthesis of adenine by oligomerisation of hydrogen cyanide. *J. Org. Chem.* **31,** 2035–6.
69 Weiss A. (1976) In preparation.
70 Wolman Y., Haverland W.J. & Miller S.L. (1972) Non-protein amino acids from spark discharges and their comparison with Murchison meteorite amino acids. *Proc. Nat. Acad. Sci. U.S.A.* **69,** 809–11.
71 Wolman Y., Miller S.L., Ibanez J. & Oro J. (1971) Formaldehyde and ammonia as precursors to prebiotic amino acids. *Science* **174,** 1039.
72 Yang C.C. & Oro J. (1971) Synthesis of adenine, guanine, cytosine, and other nitrogen organic compounds by a Fischer-Tropsch-like process. In *Molecular Evolution I: Chemical Evolution and the Origin of Life* (eds R. Buvet & C. Ponnamperuma), pp. 152–67. North Holland, Amsterdam.
73 Ycas M. (1955) A note of the origin of life. *Proc. natl. Acad. Sci. U.S.A.* **41,** 714–16.

Chapter 3
The evolution of the oceans and the atmosphere

M. WHITFIELD

3.1 INTRODUCTION

The evolution of life has proceeded quite slowly against a background of relentless geological activity [10].* If the whole of the earth's history (4·8 By†) were compressed into a single day the scene on the earth's surface would be one of frantic activity with the continental land masses fusing together and pulling apart in fluid patterns. The present spate of continental drifting was initiated some 270 My† ago. This time span is equivalent to only one and a half hours of the 'earth-day'. The remnants of older continental plates attest to the existence of earlier sequences of continental drift. Throughout this hectic day the waters in the oceans would be completely renewed every second, and each hour the accumulated sediment on the ocean floors would be removed under the edges of the roving continental plates. These sediments would in turn be lithified and uplifted as continental rocks for re-erosion. The rate of erosion is very rapid. At its present intensity it would require only three minutes of the 'earth-day' to reduce the existing continents to sea level. This is compatible with a complete erosion of the available sedimentary rocks every four hours of the 'earth-day'. Throughout the last few hours of the day the oxygen content of the atmosphere

* Readers might find Appendix 2 (p. 444) helpful.
† My = 10^6 years; 1 By = 10^3My.

would be renewed every second and the carbon dioxide content thirty times every second.

In contrast, the first hint of complex life in the form of individual procaryotic cells does not appear until eight o'clock in the morning. Firm evidence for the evolution of eucaryotic cells is found at eight o'clock at night (Fig. 3.3). By nine o'clock metazoa have evolved and a sudden outburst of multicellular life is underway. At ten o'clock the colonization of land begins which leads, by thirty-five minutes to midnight to the appearance of mammals on land. This pattern of slow initial development followed by rapid diversification is intimately linked with the evolution of the atmosphere and the oceans—in particular with the development of an oxygenic atmosphere.

3.2 THE PRIMORDIAL ANOXIC ATMOSPHERE AND OCEANS (4·8 By to 3·2 By ago)

3.2.1 Atmosphere

The earth probably grew by the cold agglomeration of material in a jet stream of dust caught in orbit around the sun. According to the simplest model the

Table 3.1. Tentative models of ancient atmospheres.

	Proposed composition (partial pressure, atm)‡			
Component	Stage 1 4 By ago [18]	Stage 2 3 By ago [18]	[17]	Present day
H_2	10^{-2} (?)	—	$10^{-0\cdot11}$	—
CH_4	10^{-2}	10^{-4}	$10^{-4\cdot39}$	—
CO_2*	—	10^{-2}–10^{-4}†	$10^{-1\cdot2}$	$10^{-3\cdot5}$
N_2	10^{-2}–10^{-4}	10^{-2}	$10^{-0\cdot108}$	$10^{-0\cdot11}$
NH_3	10^{-2}–10^{-4}	10^{-4} (?)	$10^{-6\cdot95}$	—
H_2O	10^{-2}–10^{-4}	10^{-2}–10^{-4}		—
H_2S	10^{-2}–10^{-4}	10^{-4} (?)†	$10^{-8\cdot34}$	—
SO_2	—	10^{-4} (?)		10^{-6}
He	10^{-4}	10^{-4}	—	$10^{-5\cdot3}$
Ar	10^{-2}–10^{-4}	10^{-2}–10^{-4}	—	$10^{-2\cdot0}$
O_2	—	—	—	$10^{-0\cdot68}$

* CO rather than CO_2 has also been considered as the oxidized form [1].

† Partial pressures in the range 10^{-1}–10^{-2} atm have also been suggested [19].

‡ The composition is given in relative rather than absolute units since estimates of the pressure exerted by the early atmosphere vary by several orders of magnitude. The absolute pressure of the Stage 1 atmosphere, for example, would depend largely on the quantity of hydrogen released by the primordial degassing.

primordial atmosphere and oceans were formed by the outgassing of the accreting material because of localized heating during the final stages of the growth of the planet [2, 14]. The process was essentially completed 4·5 By ago. The element-by-element composition of the primary gases and vapours released from the earth can be estimated from the volatile materials that are found today in the earth's ocean, atmosphere and crust. However, it is not so easy to decide on the actual chemical compounds that would be present.

The contemporary terrestrial atmosphere represents a pinpoint of oxidation in a reducing universe and the primordial dust cloud would certainly have accumulated in a reducing atmosphere. The growing mineral grains would contain elements such as iron and phosphorus in a reduced form and reduced gases such as H_2, CH_4 and NH_3 would be occluded within the crystals. The resulting reducing conditions on the primitive earth were an essential prerequisite for the formation of organic compounds from inorganic ingredients by abiological processes. The primary anoxic atmosphere possibly evolved in two stages [18]. At high partial pressures of hydrogen (Stage 1, Table 3·1) carbon would be mainly present as methane, nitrogen as ammonia and sulphur as hydrogen sulphide. In such an atmosphere, hydrogen sulphide would replace carbon

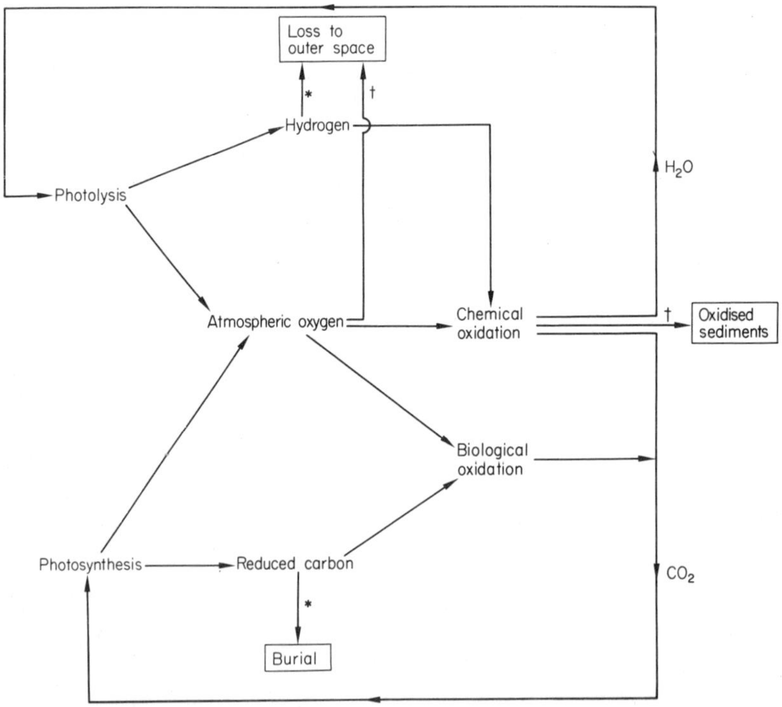

Fig. 3.1. Components of the oxygen balance. The upper half of the diagram indicates factors dominant until the evolution of oxygen-producing photosynthetic organisms. Processes in the lower half of the diagram are now dominant. The link with the carbon dioxide system is clearly shown (* Net sources of oxygen; † net sinks of oxygen).

dioxide as the major recyclable weathering agent [19]. This atmosphere would be transitory. The volatile hydrides are sensitive to photolysis by ultraviolet light, releasing the free element and hydrogen, which would eventually escape into outer space (Fig. 3.1). Some of the atmospheric gas components would be oxidized by small quantities of oxygen released by the photolysis of water vapour. The net effect would be to replace ammonia in the atmosphere by nitrogen and methane by carbon monoxide and, eventually, carbon dioxide (Stage 2, Table 3.1). This process would probably be completed shortly after the formation of the primordial atmosphere [1]. Certainly in the oldest sedimentary rocks (formed 3·2 By ago) the presence of carbonate minerals suggests that CO_2 and not CH_4 was the dominant form of carbon in the atmosphere and the presence of substantial quantities of chemically precipitated silica indicates that ammonia, if present, was not sufficiently abundant to elevate the oceanic pH appreciably [8]. Equilibrium models describing interactions between the atmospheric gases and the weathered rocks can be used to estimate the composition of the atmosphere at this stage (Table 3.1, Stage 2).

3.2.2 Oceans

Aqueous solutions of the primordial volatile acids (HCl and CO_2) would have reacted rapidly with the primordial basaltic rocks [16] to yield a mildly alkaline

Table 3.2. Composition of ancient anoxic oceans.

	Sea water composition (moles/Kg H_2O)				
	Anoxic oceans (3 By ago)				Present-day
Component	1.	2.	3.	4.	sea water
Na^+	0·24	0·30	0·47	0·47	0·47
K^+	0·03	0·07	0·01	1×10^{-3}	0·01
Ca^{2+}	0·10	0·09	0·01	0·013	0·01
Mg^{2+}	0·14	0·08	0·03	0·005	0·06
Fe^{2+}	—	—	$10^{-4·1}$	—	—
Cl^-	0·60	0·57	0·55	0·478	0·55
SO_4^{2-}	—	—	$10^{-10·4}$	—	0·03
HS^-	—	—	$10^{-5·4}$	0·03	—
HCO_3^-	—	—	0·0094	0·007	0·002
SiO_2	—	—	0·002	—	2×10^{-5}
pH	—	—	6·68	6·17	8·2

1. Cation balance based on detailed reconstruction of weathering pattern from sedimentary record. Adjusted to 35‰ salinity and charge balanced by Cl^- [25].
2. As for 1 [13].
3. Based on equilibration of ocean and atmosphere with selected ferrous minerals, calcite and silica [17].
4. Based on equilibrium reaction between basic igneous rocks and acid volatiles in the absence of oxygen [21]. Salinity adjusted to 35‰

ocean containing the most abundant and soluble cations (Na^+, K^+, Mg^{2+}, Ca^{2+}). It is unlikely that the total salt content of the oceans, even at this time, was very different from that observed today. However, estimates of the cation composition vary according to the geological clues used in constructing the model ocean (Table 3.2). These models certainly cannot be used to give support to the hypothesis that the present-day cationic composition of the body fluids of animals can be related to the oceanic composition at the time of their evolution. The chloride anion, in contrast, has probably been constant throughout the history of the oceans, and there also seems to be some agreement that the pH of the ancient oceans was much lower than its present-day level. (See also the section on the Oceans, p. 39 *et seq.*) An anoxic ocean in equilibrium with a range of ferrous minerals ($FeCO_3$, $FeSiO_3$, FeS_2) and with calcite, dolomite and amorphous silica [17] is characterized by the presence of bisulphide rather than sulphate ions, by high concentrations of ferrous iron, silica and bicarbonate and by its low pH.

3.3 TRANSITION TO AN OXYGENIC ATMOSPHERE (3·2 to 0·7 By ago)

The elimination of the volatile hydrides from the atmosphere represented the first stage in the development of the modern oxygenic atmosphere [3]. In the absence of life, oxygen was introduced by the photolysis of water vapour (Fig. 3.1). When photosynthetic blue-green algae evolved, a new source of oxygen became available. The net production of oxygen *via* photosynthesis is achieved by the burial of a certain proportion of the reduced organic carbon produced before it can be re-oxidized by chemical or microbiological processes (Fig. 3.1). Burial would be rapid initially when the oxygen partial pressure was low but would become less efficient as oxygen partial pressures increased (Fig. 3.2). The re-oxidation of reduced carbon would also be enhanced as organisms developed respiratory mechanisms to take advantage of the efficient energy conversions resulting from the use of molecular oxygen.

Initially any oxygen produced would be used up in the oxidation of reduced components in the primordial atmosphere and oceans and in rock debris revealed by weathering (Fig. 3.2). The transition to an oxygenic atmosphere could only occur after the rate of oxygen production exceeded the rate of oxygen utilization. It is difficult to estimate the relative rates of these processes during the earth's history. For example calculations of the steady-state oxygen level that could be achieved by the photolytic process range from 0·01% [3] to 25% [4] of the present atmospheric level (abbreviated to PAL). Consequently no reliable quantitative models can be prepared and the probable state of oxidation of the earth's atmosphere and oceans must be deduced from the sedimentary record (Fig. 3.3).

The photosynthetic evolution of oxygen probably began about 3 By ago.

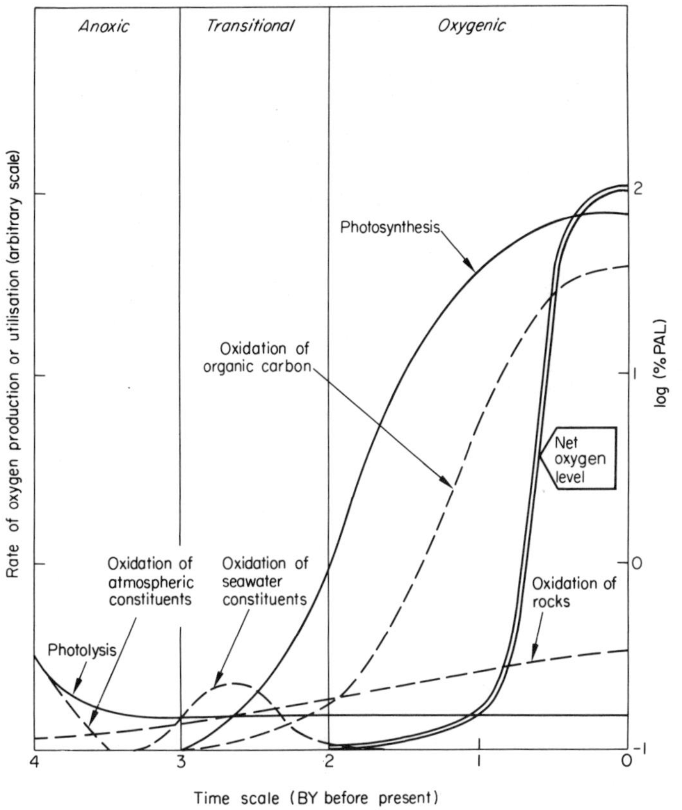

Fig. 3.2. A schematic picture of the sequence of events accompanying the transition from an anoxic to an oxygenic atmosphere. Solid lines indicate oxygen generating processes and broken lines oxygen utilizing processes (left-hand scale). The double line represents the resulting accumulation of oxygen in the atmosphere (right-hand scale) according to the Berkner–Marshall hypothesis [3].

Sedimentary rocks of this age contain microfossils that closely resemble the oxygen producing photosynthetic blue-green algae (cyanophyta). Large fossilized colonies of cyanophyta (known as stromatolites) made their appearance in the sedimentary record about 2·8 By ago [12, 28]. The fairly abundant occurrence of stromatolites in younger sediments and their wide geographical range suggest that photosynthetic oxygen evolution was proceeding quite rapidly by the beginning of the Proterozoic era [15]. This is reflected in the distribution of stable carbon isotopes in organic matter in sedimentary rocks [16, 23]. When carbon is fixed photosynthetically the lighter ^{12}C atoms are taken up in preference to ^{13}C atoms so that the resulting organic compounds are enriched in ^{12}C relative to the inorganic carbon source. The carbon isotope distribution in the earliest rocks (3 to 3·4 By old) is comparable with that of the carbonaceous meteorites, suggesting an inorganic origin. By 1·5 By ago, an enrichment of ^{12}C typical of that observed throughout the last 0·6 By is found, indicating that some

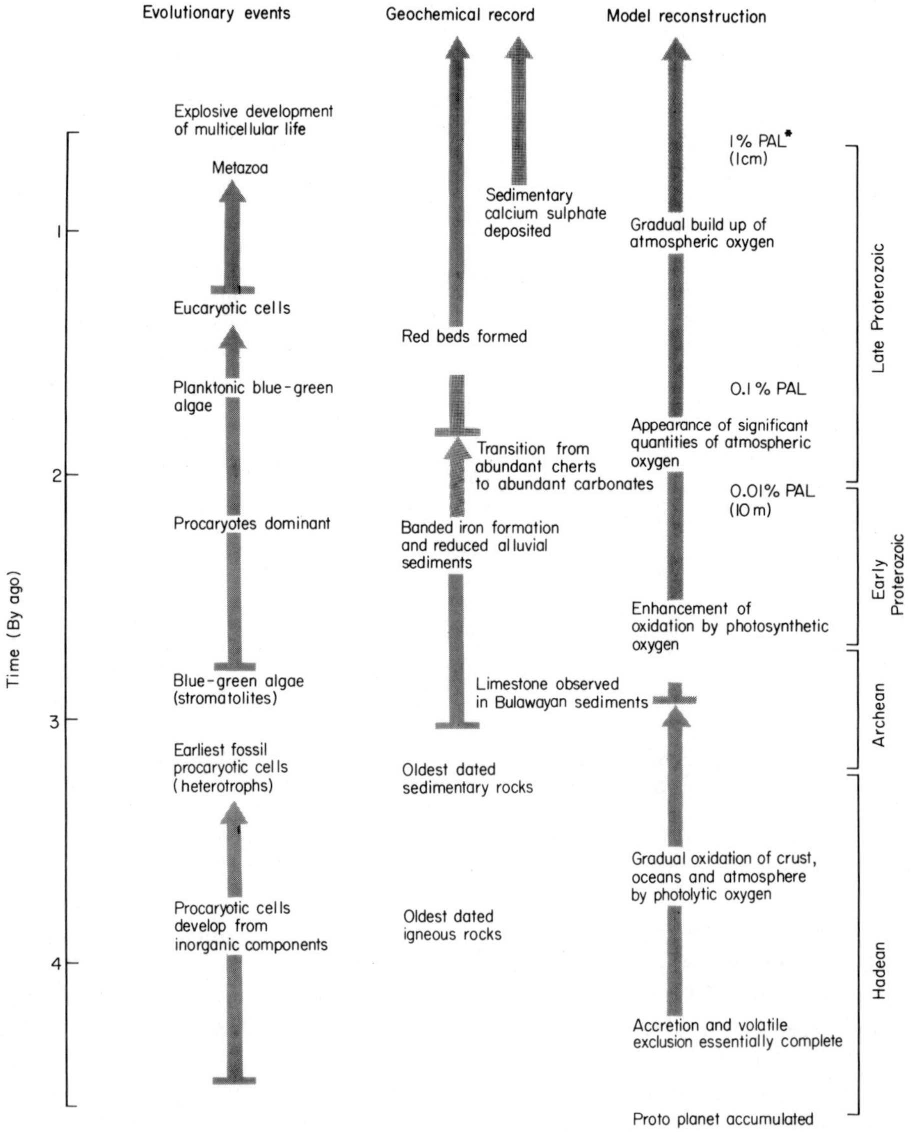

Fig. 3.3. Chronological appearance of life forms and the threads of evidence for the development of an oxygenic atmosphere [3, 11]. (* Oxygen levels suggested by the Berkner–Marshall (B–M) hypothesis [3]. Numbers in brackets indicate the depth of penetration of UV radiation in water. The B–M hypothesis probably underestimates the oxygen levels attained at each stage.)

biochemical mechanism capable of fractionating carbon (such as photosynthesis) had begun to make an important contribution to the cycling of carbon in the interim.

A number of geochemical features of the early sedimentary record (Fig. 3.3) indicate that the atmosphere remained largely anoxic until 2 By ago [26]. The presence of detrital uraninite (UO_2) grains in sedimentary material more than 2 By old suggests that these mineral fragments were weathered, transported and deposited in an atmosphere containing only traces of oxygen [8, 18]. The sands in which these inclusions occur also include ferrous minerals such as pyrites (FeS_2) and ilmenite ($Fe\ TiO_3$) as major constituents, contrasting markedly with silica and magnetite sands formed under an oxygenic atmosphere [26].

Some 3·2 By ago, extensive banded iron formations appeared in which the layers of iron-rich deposits alternate in a regular manner with layers of iron-poor cherts [8]. Reducing conditions would be required to transport the vast quantities of iron involved, as Fe(II). These deposits could no longer be formed when the atmospheric oxygen level had become high enough to trap iron as ferric hydroxide in the weathering profile. At this time (1·8 By ago) banded iron formations are replaced by red beds as the dominant form of iron deposits [8, 16]. These deposits (familiar as red sandstones) consist of fine-grained quartz sediments coated with a hydrous ferric oxide. The period from 2·0 By to 1·5 By ago also marks the transition from the characteristic pattern of early Proterozoic sediments with abundant chert and frequent inclusions of minerals in the reduced state to the modern pattern with abundant carbonate and oxidized inclusions [8].

Before significant increases in atmospheric oxygen could occur the bisulphide ion in the oceans would have been replaced by sulphate as the major sulphur species and ferrous iron would have been swept away by the photosynthetically produced oxygen (Fig. 3.2). By the end of the Proterozoic era the surface layer of the ocean would probably contain about 10% of the present level of dissolved oxygen [24]. Extensive areas of the ocean basin would remain anoxic, as they do even today, thus facilitating the burial of organic carbon and helping the net evasion of oxygen into the atmosphere. As the atmospheric carbon dioxide content decreased because of photosynthetic carbon fixation the pH of the surface layers of the ocean would begin to rise towards its present value. The rise in oceanic pH would favour the deposition of calcium carbonate from the oceans thereby slightly reducing the calcium ion concentration [11].

The development of eucaryotic cells, and later of the metazoa, probably reflects the rise in atmospheric oxygen levels following the transition to an oxygenic atmosphere 2 By ago [27]. All living unicellular eucaryotes are either obligate aerobes or are dependent on obligate aerobes. They are equipped to take advantage of the increase in metabolic efficiency that accompanies the transition from a fermentative to a respiratory metabolism which becomes feasible at oxygen levels exceeding 0·1% PAL. However, because of their intricate structure eucaryotic cells are much more susceptible to damage by ultraviolet (UV) radiation than are the more primitive procaryotic cells. The continued rise in the level of atmospheric oxygen would result in the formation of an ozone layer which would give progressively more effective protection to the earth's surface from UV radiation. As the shielding became more effective, eucaryotic organisms would be able to diversify to take advantage of the wider range of available habitats. This suggested correlation between the level of atmospheric oxygen and the extent of biological diversification is known as the Berkner–Marshall hypothesis (ref. [3]; Figs. 3.2, 3.3).

Once the *general* atmospheric concentrations had risen to 1% PAL the extent of UV shielding would be sufficient to restrict the penetration of damaging ultraviolet light to the first few centimeters of the water column [3]. This would greatly increase the range of environments available for planktonic algae and would consequently accelerate the evasion of oxygen from the ocean into the atmosphere. The earliest definite evidence for the existence of eucaryotic cells is found in the fossils which were deposited some 900 million years ago. The first multicellular organisms (metazoa) made their appearance at the end of the Proterozoic era (0·7 By ago, Fig. 3.3; refs. [9, 12]). These organisms required a sustained oxygen level of at least 3–10% PAL to support their respiratory metabolism [31] and so their presence suggests a minimum date for the attainment of this oxygen level (Fig. 3.2).

3.4 THE OXYGENIC SYSTEM AT STEADY STATE (0·7 By ago to the present day)

3.4.1 Atmosphere

At the beginning of the Phanerozoic era (0·6 By ago) the composition of the atmosphere was changing in response to the rapid acceleration in biological activity within the seas. The UV radiation penetrating the tenuous ozone layer in the atmosphere still made the land surface a hostile habitat. During the Phanerozoic era the continued build up of oxygen strengthened the protective screen provided by the ozone layer until, by the end of the Silurian period (0·42 By ago), radiation levels were low enough to permit the colonization of the land. It is likely that an oxygen concentration of at least 10% PAL would be required to provide this degree of shielding [3, 12]. Over the next few hundred million years the accumulation of atmospheric oxygen to the present level probably resulted from a net imbalance in the photosynthesis–respiration cycle. This cycle (Fig. 3.1) forges intimate links between the biota and the atmosphere on one hand and the geological weathering cycle and long-term climatic cycles on the other. Carbon dioxide tension influences the rate of weathering of continental rock by controlling the acidity of the rain and it influences the temperature of the earth's surface by trapping outgoing infra-red radiation. It also controls, in the short term at least, the oceanic pH. Oxygen tension has a controlling influence on the metabolism of metazoa and metaphyta and its presence in the atmosphere also provides a vital protective umbrella against the destructive influence of ultraviolet radiation.

Since the beginning of the Phanerozoic era the build up of oxygen in the atmosphere has progressed, if erratically, and the carbon dioxide content has never been too low ($<10^{-4}$ atm) nor too high ($>0{\cdot}3$ atm) for efficient photosynthesis. The feedback loops in the system of interactions have therefore worked surprisingly well [31]. However, in such a complex system it is inevitable that some link in the network will occasionally become overtaxed and thereby pull the whole system *temporarily* away from a steady state. Environmental conditions on the earth's surface have shown signs of such instability several times since the beginning of the Cambrian period. Going back to the 'earth-day' analogy, major ecosystem collapses occur every three quarters of an hour over the last three hours of the day.

The interplay of forces at work is nicely illustrated by the following hypothesis erected [30, 32] to explain the ecological collapse observed at the end of the Cretaceous period (28 My ago). Conditions in the Jurassic period apparently favoured the evolution of calcareous algae [24]. The resulting algal bloom depleted the atmosphere of carbon dioxide and the sea of calcium and carbonate ions. In the deep sea a zone of calcium carbonate undersaturation developed which migrated to the surface during the late Cretaceous period, decimating the phytoplankton population (and hence triggering off the ecological collapse) and producing a 1 My gap in the calcareous sedimentary record. The removal of large quantities of carbon dioxide from the atmosphere by the algal bloom resulted in a fall in the atmospheric and oceanic temperature thus enhancing the solubility of both carbon dioxide and calcium carbonate in the ocean waters and accentuating the downward spiral. The balance was gradually redressed as the combined effects of a lower oceanic pH and a drastically reduced rate of photosynthetic carbon dioxide fixation became apparent.

3.4.2 Oceans

The vigorous progress of the weathering and sedimentation cycles has resulted in a world ocean with a remarkably uniform composition of the major dissolved components with slight local changes in total concentration caused by the addition of fresh water from rivers, or from rain, and by the removal of water by evaporation. To simplify the discussion we can consider the world oceans as a bucket (Fig. 3.4). Although the quantity of material flowing through the oceans is large compared with the carrying capacity of the bucket (Fig. 3.4), the system has, by an intricate network of chemical reactions, been able to adjust itself to a steady state for many elements with material input matching material outfall [16, 29]. The extent to which a particular element accumulates in the water in the bucket will depend on the nature of the balance achieved (Fig. 3.5). The mean time that an element spends in the bulk of the ocean is known as its residence time (ref. [7], Fig. 3.5). Elements that enter and leave the system trapped within mineral particles without any chance of reacting with the aqueous phase will

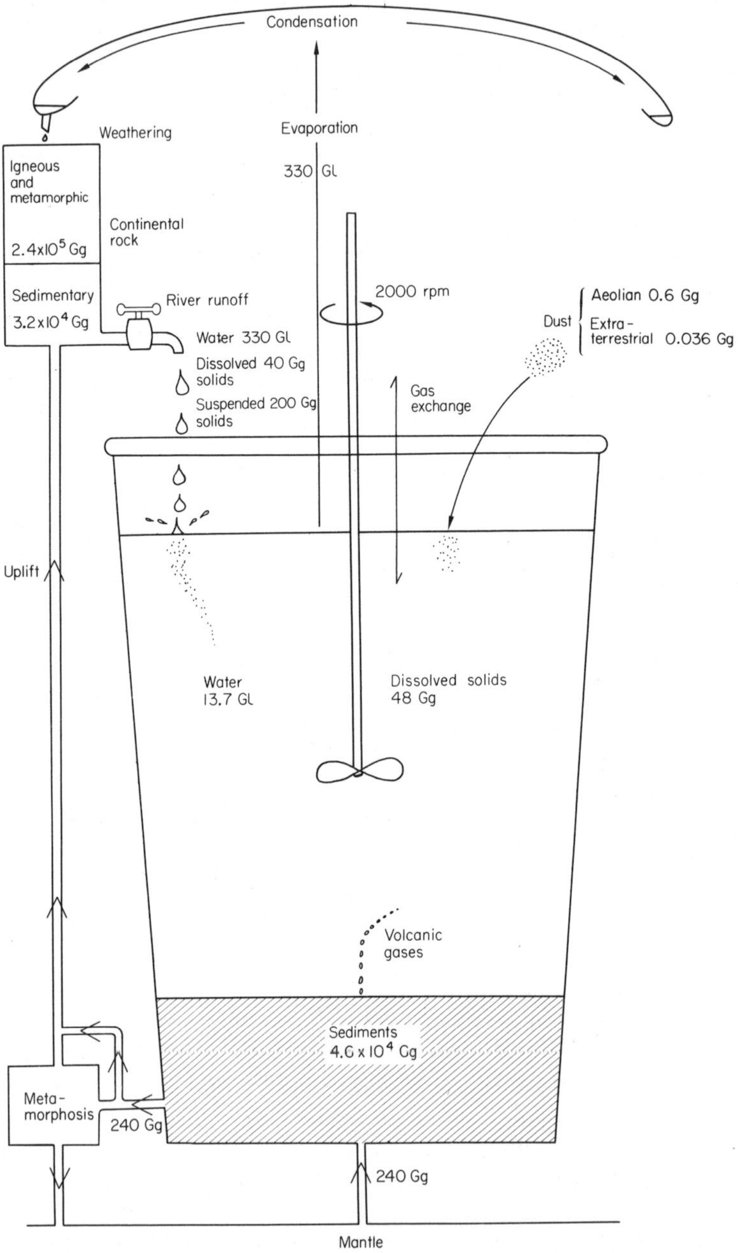

Fig. 3.4. The ocean as a bucket showing fluxes over a 1 My period (equivalent to 18 seconds of the 'earth-day'). The residence time of water in the ocean depths is approximately 1600 years corresponding to a stirring rate of 2000 rpm in the bucket model on the 'earth-day' time scale. 'Geo' units are used, 1 Gg = 10^{20} g and 1 Gl = 10^{20} l. A 46 Km (30 mile) cube of water has a mass of 1 Gg.

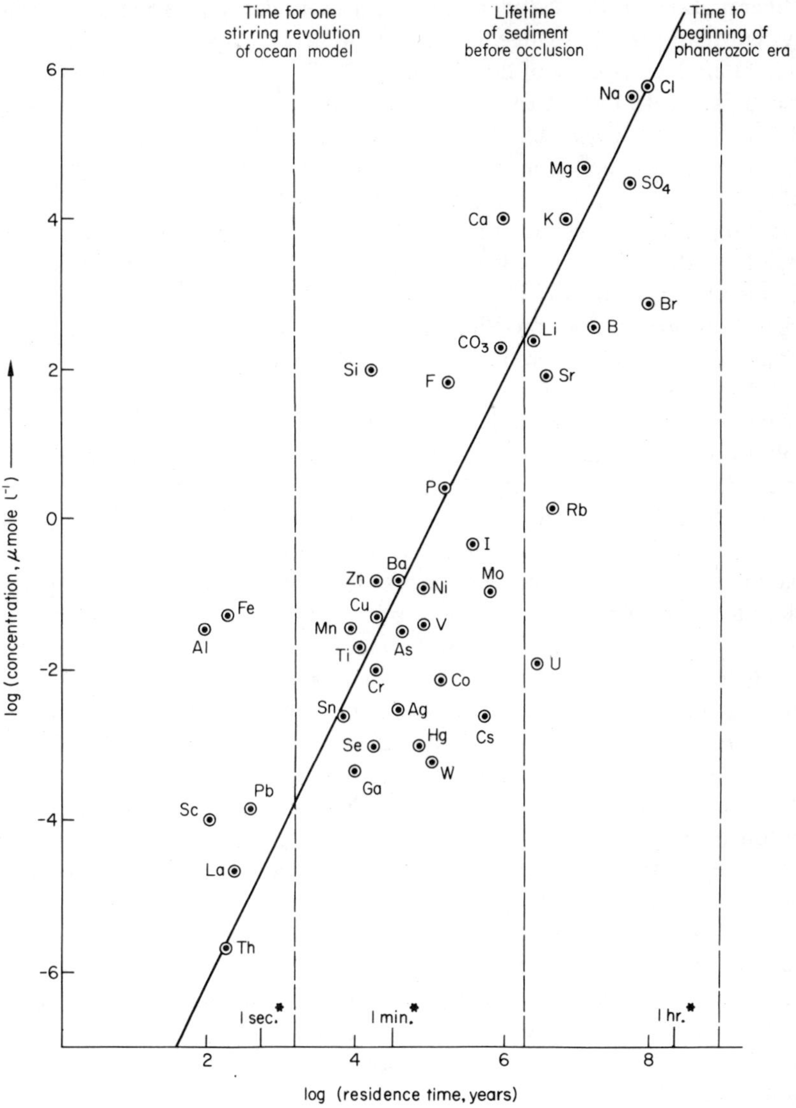

Fig. 3.5. Relationship between residence time [39] and concentration for sea water components illustrating a moderately linear steady-state correlation. Time intervals marked * relate to the 'earth-day' analogy.

have very short residence times. These elements are in short supply in the ocean and are apparently removed before the water in the bucket can complete a single stirring cycle (Fig. 3.5). Elements that form very soluble salts and are not preferentially incorporated either in mineral particles or in the cells of living organisms will tend to accumulate in the water and form the bulk of the sea salt. These elements will be removed largely by the trapping of sea water between mineral grains in the sediment and are a more permanent feature of the ocean system than are the sediments underlying it (Fig. 3.5). Between these two extremes are the majority of the elements (Fig. 3.5) which either have intermediate reactivities with respect to the minerals entering the sea or are in considerable demand as building blocks for the growth of plants and animals. Since there is no evidence of major changes in either the rate of throughput or the composition of material entering and leaving the oceans over the last 2 By [16] it is likely that the composition of the major sea water components has changed little during the last half of its history. Circumstantial evidence for this contention may be gleaned from a number of sources.

At various times in the Phanerozoic era, large quantities of sea water have evaporated in shallow ocean basins leaving behind, as layered salt formations (evaporite deposits), a fossil record of their composition. These evaporites are characterized by a regular initial sequence of deposition (carbonate minerals followed by sulphate and then chloride phases) which is identical to that observed in modern deposits. The ubiquity of this sequence, together with the solubility characteristics of the component salts suggest that concentrations of calcium, bicarbonate and sulphate ions are unlikely to have differed by more than a factor of two from the present values since late Proterozoic times [20]. Other clues tend to confirm this picture. Large shifts in the ratio of the stable sulphur isotopes, S^{34} and S^{32}, observed in Permian evaporites also indicate a maximum sulphate concentration some 45% higher than the present value [6, 16]. The uranium to calcium ratio in the matrix of well-preserved Miocene corals indicates that the calcium content of sea water at this time was no more than 1·4 times its present value [5, 6]. The uniformity of the boron content of illites during the Phanerozoic and Proterozoic eras also indicates a corresponding constancy in the boron content of sea water over the last 2·7 By [16]. This constancy can be attributed to the sheer inertia of the system because of the long residence times of the major components (Fig. 3.5).

The mechanisms responsible for the maintenance of the particular oceanic balance of anions and cations are not clearly understood. Possibly the cation composition and the oceanic pH are controlled by equilibrium reactions between detrital clays and dissolved cations within the sea. Carbon dioxide released by this reverse weathering process would also provide a buffer for the control of the atmospheric CO_2 content. Convincing mass balance equations show that such mechanisms are consistent with the known composition of the dissolved and particulate material brought down by the rivers and with the composition of the sediments formed [22]. The mineral reactions themselves, however, have not been unequivocally identified within the oceans nor have the modified clays been observed in any quantity within the sediments. It is more likely that the cation composition is maintained, not through a series of equilibrium reactions, but by a dynamic balance between addition and removal processes [5, 6].

The chloride and sulphate content of the oceans is largely dictated by the chance geological balance between the rate of formation of marine evaporites and the rate at which ancient deposits are exposed. A probable lower limit on the chloride content is set by the extensive withdrawal of salt from the oceans in the late Permian which could have produced a 5‰ drop in salinity if the salt was removed from a relatively thin oceanic surface layer. The continuity of modern faunal assemblages of echinoderms from the Ordovician period also suggests a fairly conservative range of oceanic salinity. An upper limit may be set by the consequences of the dissolution of existing evaporite deposits. It would take only 7% of the present deposits to saturate the oceans with respect to gypsum while increasing the salinity by only a few parts per thousand. Since there are no recorded open ocean gypsum deposits it is unlikely that the oceans have ever been much more saline than they are today.

Since more than three quarters of the available sulphate is locked up in evaporite deposits the concentration of sulphate in the ocean is likely to be somewhat less stable than that of chloride. It is not possible at the present time to prepare a balanced sulphur budget and the sulphate concentration of the oceans appears to be increasing at a rate that will double the present concentration within the next 14 million years.

The more reactive elements with the shorter residence times (Fig. 3.5) are more likely to be affected by short-term variations in the rate of supply of material to the oceans or in the rate of removal from the oceans. These elements exhibit large spatial and temporal variations in their absolute and relative concentrations in the contemporary oceans. Particularly variable are the biologically active elements such as phosphorus, nitrogen and silicon which show marked seasonal fluctuations in the surface waters. The elements which are in greatest biological demand are therefore subject to the greatest variability in concentration. A pattern of feedback loops can be devised to endow the system of nutrient supply with a certain flexibility in the face of changing conditions [5, 6]. This may be illustrated by considering the cycling of phosphorus in the deep sea. At present 95% of the phosphorus available in the surface waters is used by organisms and eventually sinks, as detrital particles into the deep ocean. One part of this phosphorus ultimately finds its way into the sediment and the remaining 94 parts are oxidized by biological action to produce inorganic phosphate which is eventually returned to the surface by upwelling currents. The particulate phosphate lost to the sediment is matched by new material fed into the system at the surface and the system is in a steady state. The rate of outfall of phosphorus to the sediment is directly related to the oxygen tension at depth. If the phosphorus input at the surface were suddenly increased the consequent rise in the organic fixation rate of phosphorus would be reflected in an enhanced downfall of detrital material. This would in turn result in a more rapid utilization of oxygen in the deep ocean and eventually to a sedimentation rate of phosphorus that matched the new input. The oxygen and carbon dioxide cycles are intimately linked with this network. Our state of ignorance is such that we cannot quantify any of these feedback systems but it is important to realize that ocean, biosphere, atmosphere and geosphere are closely interrelated and that variations in the chemistry of one section will be felt throughout the system.

3.5 REFERENCES

1 Abelson P.H. (1966) Chemical events on the primitive earth. *Proc. Natl. Acad. Sci. U.S.A.* **55,** 1365–72.

2 Arrhenius G., De B.R. & Alfvén H. (1974) Origin of the ocean. In *The Sea,* Vol. 5 (ed. E. Goldberg) pp. 839–61. Wiley Interscience, New York.

3 Berkner L.V. & Marshall L.C. (1965) On the origin and rise of oxygen concentration in the earth's atmosphere. *J. Atm. Sci.* **22,** 225–61.

4 Brinkmann R.T. (1969) Dissociation of water vapour and evolution of oxygen in the terrestrial atmosphere. *J. Geophys. Res.* **74,** 5355–68.

5 Broecker W.S. (1971) A kinetic model for the chemical composition of sea water. *Quaternary Res.* **1,** 188–207.

6 Broecker W.S. (1974) *Chemical Oceanography,* 214 pp. Harcourt, Brace Jovanovich, New York.

7 Carritt D.E. (1971) Oceanic residence time and geobiochemical interactions. In *Impingement of Man on the Oceans* (ed. D. W. Hood) pp. 191–9. Wiley Interscience, New York.

8 Cloud P.E. Jr. (1968) Atmospheric and hydrospheric evolution on the primitive earth. *Science* **160,** 729–36.

9 Cloud P.E. Jr. (1968) Pre-metazoan evolution and the origins of the metazoa. In *Evolution and Environment* (ed. E. T. Drake) pp. 1–72. Yale University Press.

10 Cloud P. (ed.) (1971) *Adventures in Earth History.* Freeman, San Francisco.

11 Cloud P. (1972) A working model of the primitive earth. *Am. J. Sci.* **272,** 537–48.

12 Cloud P.E. (1974) Evolution of ecosystems. *Am. Scientist.* **62,** 54–66.

13 Conway E.J. (1943) The chemical evolution of the ocean. *Proc. Roy. Irish Acad.* **B48,** 161–212.

14 Fanale F.P. (1971) A case for catastrophic early degassing of the earth. *Chem. Geol.* **8,** 79–105.

15 Fischer A.G. (1965) Fossils, early life and atmospheric history. *Proc. Natl. Acad. Sci. U.S.A.* **53,** 1205–15.

16 Garrels R.M. & MacKenzie F.T. (1971) *Evolution of Sedimentary Rocks.* Norton, New York.

17 Garrels R.M. & Perry E.A. Jr. (1974) Cycling of carbon, sulphur and oxygen through geological time. In *The Sea,* Vol. 5 (ed. E. D. Goldberg) pp. 303–36. Wiley Interscience, New York.

18 Holland H.D. (1962) Model for the evolution of the earth's atmosphere. In *Petrological Studies: A volume to honor A. F. Buddington* (eds Engel, James and Leonard) pp. 447–77. Geological Society of America, New York.

19 Holland H.D. (1974) Aspects of the geologic history of sea water. *Origins of Life* **5,** 87–91.

20 Holland H.D. (1974) Marine evaporites and the composition of sea water during the Phanerozoic. In *Studies in Paleo-oceanography* (ed. W. W. Hay) pp. 187–92. Soc. Econ. Paleontologists and Mineralogists Spec. Publ. No. 20. Tulsa, Okl. U.S.A.

21 Lafon G.M. & MacKenzie F.T. (1974) Early evolution of the oceans—a weathering model. In *Studies in Paleo-oceanography* (ed. W. W. Hay) pp. 205–18. Soc. Econ. Paleontologists and Mineralogists Spec. Publ. No. 20. Tulsa, Okl. U.S.A.

22 MacKenzie F.T. & Garrels R.M. (1966) Chemical mass balance between rivers and oceans. *Am. J. Sci.* **264,** 507–25.

23 Oehler D.Z., Schopf J.W. & Kvenvolder K.A. (1972) Carbon isotope studies of organic matter in Precambrian Rocks. *Science,* **175,** 1246–8.

24 Rhoads, D.C. & Morse, J.W. (1971) Evolutionary and ecological significance of oxygen deficient marine basins. *Lethaia* **4,** 413–28.

25 Ronov, A.B. (1968) Probable changes in the composition of sea water during the course of geological time. *Sedimentology* **10,** 25–43.

26 Rutten, M.G. (1962) *Geological Aspects of the Origin of Life on Earth*. Elsevier, Amsterdam, London & New York.

27 Sagan, L. (1967) On the origin of mitosing cells. *J. Theoret. Biol.* **14,** 225–74.

28 Schopf, J.W. (1970) Precambrian microorganisms and evolutionary events prior to the origin of vascular plants. *Biol. Rev.* **45,** 319–52.

29 Siever, R. (1974) The steady state of the earth's crust, atmosphere and oceans. *Scient. Am.* **230** (6), 72–9.

30 Tappan, H. (1968) Primary production, isotopes, extinctions and the atmosphere. *Palaeogeography, Palaeoclimatology and Palaeoecology* **4,** 187–210.

31 Weyl P.K. (1966) Environmental stability of the earth's surface; chemical considerations. *Geochim. Cosmochim. Acta.* **30,** 663–79.

32 Worsley T. (1974) The Cretaceous-Tertiary boundary event in the ocean. In *Studies in Paleo-oceanography* (ed. W. W. Hay) pp. 94–125. Soc. Econ. Paleontologists and Mineralogists. Spec. Publ. No. 20, Tulsa, Okl. U.S.A.

PART III
EVOLUTIONARY ASPECT

Chapter 4
Aquatic environments

A.G.MACDONALD

4.1 INTRODUCTION

The evolutionary significance of aquatic environments has dominated comparative and environmental physiology for many years, and for very good reasons. The chemical composition of the sea, which is the largest of environments, has not changed a great deal over the past 700×10^6 years (0·7 By) during which evolution has occurred (Chapter 3). Such changes in the ionic composition of seawater which it is generally agreed have taken place, the increase in pH for example, are difficult to assess physiologically. The gradual increase in pO_2 which occurred from 600×10^6 years (0·6 By) ago, and the other changes generated by the increase in the marine biomass are probably as important as any 'geochemical' change. It is important to understand the fact that organisms, 'biochemicals' and 'chemicals' are part of a cycle, the steady state of which give us the familiar standing stock of biomass and the characteristic concentrations of solutes. The organisms themselves have to be seen in dynamic equilibrium, both physiologically (individually) and ecologically (as a population) with their environment. Environmental physiologists take on the task of investigating the mechanisms by which organisms attain their equilibrium or 'adapted' state on the grand evolutionary scale, and how they regulate and tolerate the relatively minor seasonal and nychthemeral changes in their environment.

4.2 PHYSICAL DESCRIPTION OF AQUATIC ENVIRONMENTS

A practical problem in promoting a discussion of the distinctive features of biological environments is to decide on the appropriate way of describing their physical properties. Here the approach is to list the physical components of the environment in a way which makes physical-chemical sense, and then to evaluate the physiological significance of each variable. From the ecological viewpoint this procedure is probably simplistic but physiologically it is rigorous. Table 4.1 shows that temperature and hydrostatic pressure head the list, because these are prime thermodynamic variables, which determine the state of a substance and rate of chemical change.

Table 4.1 Physical and chemical factors in aquatic environments.

Temperature	
Pressure	
Radiation	
Magnetic field strength	
Gravity	
Bulk properties of water	
Solvent properties of water	—colligative properties
	—atmospheric gases
	—electrolytes
	—organic solutes
	—suspended material

4.2.1 Temperature

The forces which determine protein conformation, the state of lipoproteins and lipid bilayers are temperature dependent. In chemical reactions, small temperature increases achieve disproportionately large effects on reaction rates because of the fundamental nature of chemical reactions. The relation between environmental temperature and enzyme activity and its control raises many questions central to kinetic and protein chemistry [7]. The marine environment is generally a low temperature one. Spectacular examples of the ability to maintain a high body temperature are to be found in sea birds and marine mammals, and at the other end of the physiological temperature range we find fish and invertebrates living actively at environmental and tissue temperatures as low as $-1{\cdot}8$°C by virtue of specialized antifreeze mechanisms [4, 14]. Between these extremes, there exists a number of different solutions to particular thermal problems presented by various environments [12] (Chapters 20, 15, 13).

4.2.2 Hydrostatic pressure

Pressure affects equilibria and rate constants in a way related to the molar volume changes of the reactants and catalysts involved. Pressure increases by 1 atm or 101·3 kN m^{-2} with each 10 m of water depth. Deep sea pressures are undoubtedly sufficient to influence the conformation of macromolecules, the state of lipid phases and the molecular interactions which occur in enzymic reactions. Animals in general are always in equilibrium with the ambient pressure and do not regulate against it in a manner analogous to the way some animals regulate their temperature. An exception is the special case of certain cephelapods which maintain a limited pressure differential across the wall of their buoyancy shell (Chapter 18). However, toleration of the ambient high hydrostatic pressure in the deep sea is more apparent than real for, at the molecular level, adaptations are thought to exist which confer pressure stability on what otherwise would be pressure labile molecules. Deep sea pressures are sufficient to exert a very slight effect on the composition of seawater, and on its density, in a manner comparable to the naturally-occurring temperature variation in the sea. In contrast to temperature, hydrostatic pressure is a less well understood physical-chemical variable in the environment and is not one of the subjects chosen for special and representative discussion in this book. For further reading in high pressure physiology see [9, 17, 20].

4.2.3 Radiation

Radiation, and the visible part of the spectrum in particular, is an environmental factor of considerable biological significance as is evident from Chapters 2 and 3. Visible light is reflected from the surface of natural water, and that fraction which enters the water is attenuated by absorption and scattering as it passes down the water column. Both absorption and scattering are dependent on the frequency of the radiation. In general, open ocean water, which has few solid particles in suspension, transmits light to about 1000 m, at which depth its intensity is 10^{-15} that of the surface value, i.e. at the limit of the sensitivity of the human retina [2].

The peak frequency in the transmission spectrum of light in clear ocean water is between 400–500 nm, and consequently the colour of deep seawater is blue-green. In the turbid waters in lakes and coastal regions of the sea, light is absorbed by up to a million times more than in clear conditions, and the peak of its frequency spectrum is in the longer, more yellow-red wavelengths. In such waters naturally occurring substances also tend to colour the water yellow.

4.2.4 Magnetic field strength

Magnetic field strength is of interest to sensory physiologists and those involved in animal navigation studies but, so far as we know, it is not an environmental factor that has exerted an influence on animal evolution on a scale anywhere approaching that of light and temperature [13].

4.2.5 Gravity

Gravity, conversely, is undoubtedly an environmental force which has influenced the evolution of animal (and plant) physiology although, for most organisms it is an environmental constant. Space flight is creating human physiological problems and is opening up experimental possibilities for the study of the effects of earth's constant gravitational pull on living systems [18]. The density of water enables many animals to attain buoyancy, thereby offsetting some of the energy cost of countering gravity. This unique feature of aquatic environments is discussed in Chapter 18.

4.2.6 Water

In the lower part of Table 4.1 water is listed under two headings; bulk physical properties and solvent properties [5]. The most important bulk properties of pure water are its very large heat capacity and thermal conductance, its relatively high density and its low compressibility. The anomalous density maximum at 3·98°C and the low density of ice are also extremely important properties as they reduce temperature fluctuations in water masses. The diffusion of molecules through water as, for example, in the case of oxygen from the atmosphere, is extremely slow and in natural waters dissolved materials are distributed by flow and mixing, processes which involve the bulk properties of water. Vertical water movement is brought about by a density difference which arises from temperature variations or differences in salinity. Horizontal movement is generated in large water masses by wind and, in rivers, by gravity. Generally, no large aquatic environment is stagnant, although restricted pockets of still water do occur and, in these, anoxic conditions may prevail. The slow, ceaseless movement of the oceanic water masses, or the seasonal turnover in fresh water lakes, ensures the recycling of organic material and influences both the gross 'metabolism' of the ecosystem and the density of colonization of the living space. Animals occupy all known aquatic habits with the exception of hot brines in the depths of the Red Sea [3], and the hottest of the subterranean waters (Table 4.2).

The diffusion of gases in water influences numerous respiratory processes (Chapter 9) and, together with the bulk properties of water, influences much of the functional design strategies of gas exchange processes both within organisms and between organisms and their environments.

Obviously, the solvent and other molecular properties of water have determined much of the chemical basis of life (see Chapters 2, and 3), and it is the colligative properties of aqueous solutions which are of chief environmental significance (Chapter 5). The osmotic pressure of sea water at atmosphere pressure, 4°C and 33‰ salinity, is 23 atm. The freezing point is about −1·9°C. Typical fresh water has a relatively minute osmotic pressure corresponding to a freezing point of almost 0°C.

The partial pressure of dissolved atmospheric gases at the surface of a water mass will tend towards equilibrium with the atmospheric partial pressures. At equilibrium the amount of dissolved gas is determined by the product of the partial pressure and the solubility of the particular gas (Henry's law). In natural water masses, biological processes frequently influence the steady state levels of dissolved gases; but it is worth noting that gas solubility is reduced by an increase in temperature, hydrostatic pressure and solute concentration. Supersaturation of atmospheric gases can arise in natural waters by purely physical means (for example, wave action) or in the case of oxygen by the biological process of photosynthesis.

The electrolyte composition of oceanic seawater is very constant (Tables 3.2, 5.1), whereas in estuaries and other marginal areas of the sea it varies greatly. Similarly, the concentration of organic solutes is more predictable in the open ocean than inshore or in fresh waters. Suspended material likewise is distributed in a relatively constant fashion well away from land and in high concentrations and more variably inshore. The physiological consequences of these facts are mentioned in the next section.

Now we must progress from the simple list of physical variables to a consideration of how they integrate as a whole in natural conditions. Before doing so, however, it is instructive to compare an idealized aquatic environment with a terrestrial one. First it is a three dimensional, bulk environment. Its temperature is relatively low and constant (compared to that of the air) and it can absorb heat readily from bodies warmer than itself (for example, warm-blooded animals). Its density offers resistance to locomotion but provides buoyancy and favours smooth, fluent modes of progression; highly stressed skeletons are not required (Chapter 8). Although visible radiation is attenuated by the combined effect of water and suspended particles vision is an important sensory mode for aquatic animals, but it has a very limited range. Sound and vibrations are propagated very efficiently and so are chemical signals, but extremely slowly. Both sound receptor and chemoreceptor physiology are well developed in aquatic animals [6, 8, 10, 16, 19]. As a chemical medium, bulk aquatic environments may be either concentrated or dilute solutions of electrolytes, whose relative composition fluctuates only slowly [11, 15] (Chapters 3, 5). Dissolved oxygen is normally at a partial pressure with which the gas exchange mechanisms of most animals are able to cope. Bulk aquatic environments are, by definition, large and three dimensional. Animals occupying them always have to contend with a marked vertical gradient of pressure and light, and a milder and more variable vertical gradient of temperature and solutes. Small-scale aquatic environments take on terrestrial-like features, having a larger range of temperatures, but not of pressures, and are generally more variable in all other respects.

4.3 CLASSIFICATION OF AQUATIC HABITS

Table 4.2 summarizes the distinctive features of the main aquatic habitats. The details are not complete but the omissions will not influence the argument. The deep sea is distinctive in being a high-pressure environment, without sunlight

Table 4.2. The main types of aquatic habitats

LARGE	
Deep ocean	Low constant temperature 0–4°C. High pressure 100–1000 atm (i.e. 10–100 MNm^{-2}). No sunlight, no light rhythms, constant salinity, slow currents, enormous three-dimensional living space.
Shallow ocean	Temperature ranges 25–4°C and varies seasonally. 1–100 atm pressure (i.e. 100 kN – 10 MNm^{-2}). Vertical gradient of light, diurnal and seasonal rhythm, slow currents, enormous three dimensional living space.
Coastal seas	Similar temperature range to oceans. 1–20 atm pressure (i.e. 100 kN – 2 MNm^{-2}). Marked seasonal and vertical variation in temperature and light, salinity variable, slow currents, relatively restricted living space.
MARGINAL	
Estuaries	Large temperature range. 1–5 atm pressure (i.e. 100–500 kNm^{-2}). Salinity and the exposure of the substrate to air fluctuate predictably, turbid water, currents and turbulence significant, relatively small living space.
Sea shore	Large temperature and salinity range. 1–5 atm pressure (i.e. 100–500 kNm^{-2}). Exposure to air and radiation, much turbulence, very small living space.
RESTRICTED	
Lakes	Marked seasonal temperature range. Typically pressure no more than 10 atm (i.e. 1 MNm^{-2}). Light variable, low osmotic pressure, currents slow, restricted living space, many are transient on geological time scale.
Rivers and streams	As for lakes but more restricted and turbulent.
Underground waters	Relatively constant in temperature and absence of light, but a highly restricted living space.
Hot springs, streams	Low pressure, high temperatures, few support animals, algae and bacteria present.
Oil well brines	High pressure, high temperature, no animals, but bacteria reported.

or seasonal rhythms. It therefore differs fundamentally from coastal waters and the shallow ocean, which, although more subject to seasonal changes in physical conditions than the deep sea, are free from the violent variations in temperature and radiation experienced by animals which live in estuaries or on the sea shore. Lakes and rivers are distinctive in frequently being short-lived on a geological time scale, and they impose osmotic conditions quite different to those of the marine environment. It is worth considering whether some aquatic environments have more in common with certain terrestrial habitats than with the open ocean.

4.4 AQUATIC ENVIRONMENTAL PHYSIOLOGY

The range of aquatic environmental physiology is enormous, so some comments are necessary on the selection of chapters which come under the heading. Two types of contribution discuss phenomena on the evolutionary time scale. Chapters 2 and 3 deal with the early evolution of life and with the primeval environment. The inclusion of chemical and geochemical considerations is highly significant for, not only does it recognize the intrinsic importance of these factors in the matter of the origin of life, and the nature of the early environment, but it emphasizes the significance of early evolution in environmental physiology. We should not overlook the fact that biological environments are also the subject of study for oceanographers, geochemists, climatologists, soil scientists and many other non-biological scientists.

Contributions of the second type, which deal with evolutionary-scale aspects of aquatic physiology are to be found in Chapters 5 and 12. These contain rigorous treatments of ionic and osmoregulatory phenomena in marginal and restricted environments. The evolution of the cell membrane must have been an early and decisive event in the origin of organisms. In contemporary biology, the structure and function of membranes constitute a major field of research in the front line of regulatory physiology and biophysics. More complex regulatory organs and the strategies adopted by whole organisms are the levels of analysis dealt with in these two chapters and, additionally, the fundamental question of the energy-cost of regulation is discussed.

Adaptations relating to aquatic physiology, which manifest themselves in the life-time of organisms, are to be found in Chapters 12 and 18. The seasonal or migratory changes which take place in the frog skin or the fish gill provide fascinating examples of the 'regulation of regulation'.

If there is one piece of physiology which reflects the distinctive nature of 'ideal' or pure aquatic environments, it is, perhaps, the physiology of buoyancy (Chapter 18). Buoyancy mechanisms also illustrate the opportunist nature of evolution. Fish swimbladders probably arose from selective pressure to improve gas-exchange processes. The 'main-line' of evolution proceeded to form lungs, but here we focus on the 'side-line' which virtually liberated a whole class of animals from gravity. Having exploited morphology to create a buoyancy gas-chamber, evolution proceeded to elaborate the swimbladder. This is a most ingenious piece of chemical engineering capable of pumping gases to partial pressures of many hundreds of atmospheres. The counter-current rete of the fish swimbladder is the most fully understood example of active transport although admittedly a special case. The emphasis of Chapter 18 is on the day-to-day effector role of the swimbladder and other buoyancy devices.

The gas exchange role of gills (Chapter 9) is another distinctive case of homeostasis in an aquatic environment. To understand clearly the respiratory role of gills we have to understand their physics, physiology in the classical sense, comparative morphology and much else besides. Gills and buoyancy mechanisms share with other complicated physiological machinery a very important feature; they are not particularly amenable to the familiar reductionist analysis; tissues-cells-molecules. Gills and swimbladders, are not only to be analysed in terms of their cellular and molecular parts. The absolute size of a swimbladder rete, for example, is crucial to its proper functioning and there is no molecular model for counter-current multiplication in the rete or counter-current exchange in gills. Physical analogues, however, do provide valuable insights, so the analytical reduction of some aspects of these organs can often proceed straight to the level of physics which bypasses the cellular level of analysis. The swimbladder, and gills, and many other examples which come to mind, contrast in this respect with the cellular and biochemical systems of adaptation mentioned earlier, and provide examples of the different levels of analysis which environmental physiologists must learn to handle. In addition to those chapters which have been mentioned, aquatic physiology is touched on in many other chapters (see, for instance, Chapters 8 and 10) simply because life is an aqueous phenomenon.

One important area of physiology which we have not attempted to include in this book is human physiology. Rapid advances are being made in human underwater physiology, of which the reader should at least be aware. Environmental physiology, in the sense used here, certainly includes human physiology and only limitations of space have prevented its specific inclusion. Furthermore, the adaptation or survival of human beings in specific environments often provides very interesting examples. This is certainly the case in human underwater physiology [1]. The properties of idealized aquatic environments (see p. 53) may be shown to apply to the human diver; to his locomotion, thermal balance, sensory physiology and to the underlying molecular mechanisms responsible for the satisfactory working of his cellular machinery.

4.5 REFERENCES

1 Bennett P.B. & Elliot D.H. (1975) *The Physiology and medicine of diving and compressed air work*, pp. 566. Baillière Tindall, London.

2 Clarke G.L. & Denton E.J. (1962) Light and animal life. In *The Sea*, Vol. I (ed. M. N. Hill) pp. 456–68. Wiley Interscience, New York & London.

3 Degens E.T. & Ross D.A. (1970) The Red Sea Hot Brines. *Scient. Am.* **222,** April: 32–42.

4 DeVries A.L. (1974) Survival at freezing temperatures. In Biochemical and Biophysical Perspectives. In *Marine Biology*, Vol. 1 (eds D. C. Malins & J. R. Sargent) 289–330. Academic Press, New York & London.

5 Fogg G.E. (ed.) (1965) Symposium of the Society for experimental biology **19.** The state and movement of water in living organisms, pp. 432. Cambridge University Press, London.

6 Hersey J.B. & Backus R.H. (1962) Sound scattering by marine organisms. In *The Sea*, Vol. 1 (ed. M. N. Hill) pp. 498–539. Wiley Interscience, New York.

7 Hochachka P.W. & Somero G.N. (1973) *Strategies of biochemical adaptation*, pp. 358. Saunders, Philadelphia.

8 Laverack, M.S. (1968) On the receptors of marine invertebrates. *Oceanogr. Mar. Biol. Ann Rev.* **6,** 249–324.

9 Macdonald, A.G. (1975) *Physiological aspects of deep sea biology*. Monograph of the Physiological Society, **31,** pp. 450. Cambridge University Press, London.

10 Mara T.J. (1971) *Chemoreception in Fish Physiology* V (eds W. S. Hoar & D. J. Randall). Academic Press, New York & London.

11 Pickard G.L. (1975) *Descriptive physical oceanography*, pp. 214. Pergamon Press, Oxford.

12 Precht H., Christophersen J., Hensel H. & Larcher W. (1973) *Temperature and Life*, pp. 779. Springer Verlag, Berlin & New York.

13 Pressman A.S. (1970) *Electromagnetic fields and life*, pp. 336. Plenum Press, New York & London.

14 Ridgway S.H. (1972) *Mammals of the sea*, pp. 812. Charles C. Thomas, Illinois.

15 Riley J.P. & Skirrow G. (eds) (1975) *Chemical oceanography*. See volumes I, II & III. Academic Press, New York & London.

16 Schevill W.E., Backus R.M. & Hersey, J.B. (1962) Sound production by marine animals. In *The Sea*, Vol. I (ed. M. N. Hill) pp. 540–66. Wiley Interscience, New York & London.

17 Sleigh M.A. & Macdonald A.G. (1972) Symposium of the Society for Experimental Biology **26**. pp. 516. The effects of pressure on organisms. Cambridge University Press, London.

18 Solon A.G. & Cohen M.J. (1971) *Gravity and the organism*, pp. 474. University of Chicago Press.

19 Vigoureux P. & Hersey J.B. (1962) Sound in the sea. In *The Sea*, Vol. I (ed. M. N. Hill) pp. 476–97. Wiley Interscience, New York & London.

20 Zimmerman A.M. (ed.) (1970) *High pressure effects on cellular processes*, pp. 324. Academic Press, New York & London.

Prelude to Chapter 5

Osmotic and ionic regulation comprises a very large body of knowledge to which the student has access through numerous books and review articles. The subject is sometimes viewed as beginning with natural history and ending with biophysics. This is understandable on historical grounds but it would be more accurate to see the subject as one which links ecology and physics, comprising a most important central area of physiology.

In the treatment which follows the discussion begins with physical chemistry. It then involves a number of physiological strategies which have evolved in response to well-defined physical problems, discussing some remarkable adaptations which appear to be emerging in recently separated populations, and then returns to a discussion of the energetics of regulatory processes. The reader may find it entertaining to try to decide if the chapter is intended to teach would-be biophysicists some of the environmental implications of their subject or would-be aquatic ecologists some physical and physiological concepts. Of course, the true purpose of the chapter includes both of these aims.

Chapter 5
Ionic and osmotic regulation of aquatic animals

P.C.CROGHAN

5.1 INTRODUCTION

The osmotic and ionic regulation of the body fluid of animals has been studied extensively and well reviewed. The early book by Krogh [9] is still useful; for more recent accounts see [10, 16] and relevant chapters in [17]. Baldwin [1] gives an account at a more elementary level. The purpose of this present chapter is not to compile extensive lists of comparative data but to attempt a physical-chemical approach to a prime problem: the evolution of fresh-water organisms from a marine origin.

5.2 SOME DEFINITIONS

A number of terms are used, the meaning of which should be clearly understood. The concentration of *sea water* and *brackish water* can be defined by the *salinity* (g solute/kg solution, written S‰) or be given directly in terms of the concentration of sodium of chloride ions. The concentration of open-sea sea water varies from about 40‰ to 30‰. Water more dilute than this would be regarded as brackish water. A series of names have been given to the various dilution ranges but the value of such definitions appears limited. The definition of *fresh water* is purely arbitrary. Usually a salinity $<0{\cdot}5$‰ (7·3 mM chloride) is regarded as fresh water. It should be remembered that fresh water is, relatively speaking, enormously variable in composition and that these variations can have physiological and ecological significance.

An animal that is limited to a narrow range of external medium concentration is termed *stenohaline*. Both marine and fresh-water animals may be stenohaline. An animal that can tolerate a wide range of external concentrations is termed *euryhaline*. These are ecological terms and are relative. There is no such thing as an absolutely stenohaline animal.

The terms *isoosmotic*, *hyperosmotic* and *hypoosmotic* are frequently used. They define the relation between the osmotic pressure of a stated solution and another stated solution.

An animal that cannot regulate the osmotic pressure of its body fluid (i.e. the body fluid is isoosmotic with the external medium) is termed *poikilosmotic*. An animal that can regulate the osmotic pressure of its body fluid (e.g. the body fluid is hyperosmotic to the external medium over a range of external osmotic pressure) is termed *homoiosmotic*. These are physiological terms and are also to some extent relative.

The *osmotic pressure* of a *dilute solution* is given by the *Van't Hoff Equation*

$$\Pi = RTC \tag{1}$$

where π is the osmotic pressure and C the total concentration of non-electrolytes and ions present. Dimensionally, it is correct to express this total concentration as moles and g-ions per litre of solvent. However, it is more usual to express concentration as moles and g-ions per kg of solvent (*molal scale*). This is numerically correct in eqn. (1) for an *aqueous* solution. This total concentration is sometimes, incorrectly, termed *osmolality*. It should be stressed that eqn. (1) is only approximate in the upper range of concentration found in many biological situations. However, if the osmotic pressure of any solution is known, the ratio Π/RT defines a value C that is the *osmolality*. Osmotic pressure is frequently expressed using this *osmolal scale*. It is difficult to measure the osmotic pressure of a solution directly but other properties related to osmotic pressure can be more easily determined. These properties, called the *colligative properties*, are all determined by *water activity* in the system. The *freezing point depression* is easily determined and the relation between osmotic pressure and freezing point depression (ΔT_f) is given by

$$\Pi = K\,\Delta T_f \tag{2}$$

where K is a constant. Then

$$C = (K/RT)\,\Delta T_f \tag{3}$$

where C is the osmolality corresponding to the freezing point depression ΔT_f and RT/K is termed the *cryoscopic constant* or *molal depression constant* (1·86°C mole^{-1}kg for aqueous solutions). Although there are advantages in using the molal scale for body fluids, particularly when the protein concentration is high, it is in practice much easier to measure the concentration per litre of solution (*molar scale*). The symbol mM will be used to mean m-mole l^{-1}. The molar and molal scales converge in dilute solutions. Further information on colligative properties can be found in any physical chemistry text, e.g. [13]. Such a text may also provide a useful clarification of a number of other physical chemical phenomena discussed later in this chapter.

5.3 SOME BASIC CONCEPTS

The animals that will be discussed are the *Metazoa*. In contrast to the *Protozoa*, these animals contain two basically different cell types. Firstly, *epithelial cells*: these cells form sheets of tightly linked cells separating a *body fluid* on one side from an *external medium* on the other or in some cases separating two different body fluids. Although in this latter case these cells may be given a different name, they are essentially epithelial in form and function. These *epithelia* frequently have very different solutions on their two faces and in fact the difference between these solutions is maintained by a combination of the passive and active transport properties of these cells. These cells are *bipolar*, the inner and outer cell membranes having different properties. Secondly, all the other types of cell: these cells are immersed in the *extracellular fluid*, the composition of which is ultimately under epithelial control. These cells are *homopolar*, the membrane properties being essentially uniform over the whole area of the cell. The cell population has been described as occupying a *private pond*, isolated and different from the external medium.

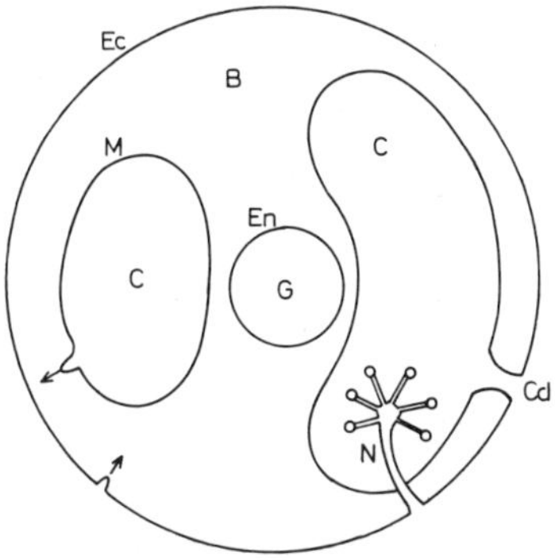

Fig. 5.1. Body-fluid spaces and duct systems in a 'typical' invertebrate (idealized *annelid*). On the left-hand side the embryological origin of the duct systems are indicated. On the right-hand side the functional systems are shown. Ec, ectoderm; M, mesoderm; En, endoderm; G, gut lumen; B, blastocoel, reducing to haemocoel or blood vascular system; C, coelom; Cd, coelomoduct; N, nephridium, which in this case is a closed nephridium (solenocytes).

In the more advanced *Metazoa*, parts of the extracellular fluid system are specialized as relatively cell-free systems. A diagrammatic representation of this is given in Fig. 5.1. The spaces are the *haemocoel*, which in some types is restricted to the *blood vascular system*, and the *coelom*. The presence of these open fluid spaces has led to the development of *convective transport systems* (*haemolymph*, *blood*, and to a lesser extent, *coelomic fluid*). This overcomes the limitation on size and activity set by diffusion in a solid mass of cells.

These spaces may be connected to the exterior by epithelial duct systems. There are two types: the *nephridial system*, of *ectodermal* origin, grows in towards the haemocoel or coelom. The internal ends of the ducts may be *closed* (*flame cells*, *solenocytes*) or, if they terminate in the coelom, may be *open*. The *coelomoduct system*, of *mesodermal* origin, grows out towards the exterior. It is an open funnel system. Many of the excretory and regulatory organs, including the *vertebrate kidney*, are derived from these duct systems.

The basic problem of adaptation to environment is that the range of environmental conditions, including chemical composition of the extracellular fluid, under which cell life can occur is limited. This is particularly so in the case of more advanced organisms with complex associations of cells in a central nervous system.

Adaptation to external media of differing chemical composition is at two levels. Firstly, the internal cells themselves can adapt to differing composition of their extracellular fluid environment. Secondly, the epithelial cells can adapt their transport functions to maintain the composition of the extracellular fluid surrounding the internal cells at a level they can tolerate. These epithelial cells may have one surface in contact with a medium very different from that of the internal extracellular fluid. Control mechanisms clearly exist within individuals and have developed in different ways during evolution.

5.4 GENERAL NATURE OF THE EVOLUTIONARY PROBLEM

It is generally considered that life originated in the sea (Chapter 3). Part of the evidence for this is the extreme variety and richness of the present-day marine fauna. The number of different phyla, families, genera and species is highest in sea water and there is a marked impoverishment as one proceeds into *brackish water* and even more into *fresh water*. This phenomenon is well seen in the stable *salinity gradient* of the *Baltic*. Many marine organisms are stenohaline, highly intolerant to dilution of the external medium, and some whole groups (e.g. *Cephalopoda*, *Echinodermata*) are virtually absent from brackish water and certainly from fresh water. The picture is essentially that of a stenohaline marine fauna from which a few persistent types have managed to adapt to and colonize brackish and ultimately fresh water. This is not to say that certain special groups cannot thrive and speciate in dilute media. The abundance of fresh water *insects* and *branchiopod crustacea* and their rarity in the sea should be noted. There is also evidence that some groups have secondarily returned from fresh water to the sea, particularly fish groups (*elasmobranchs, teleosts, coelacanths*).

Another line of evidence is from the chemical composition of the extracellular fluids of marine invertebrates. Some examples are given in Table 5.1. The composition of the body fluids is rather similar to that of sea water. In both. sodium and chloride ions predominate. The body fluids are also virtually iso-osmotic with sea water. If the *Metazoa* had evolved in sea water, this would be expected as sea water would be the medium to which unicellular organisms, from which the *Metazoa* were derived, were adapted. On this view, the hyperosmotic body fluids of brackish and fresh-water animals would be considered as a relic of a marine ancestry. Although the internal cells of these animals have been able to evolve a tolerance to a lowered body-fluid concentration, this adaptation is limited and thus adaptation to dilute media entails evolution of epithelial mechanisms, e.g. reduced permeability and active uptake of NaCl from dilute solution, that can maintain a body-fluid composition fairly similar to that of marine organisms and within the range of tolerance of the internal cells. The earlier ideas of Macallum [12] that the present-day composition of the body fluid represented the composition of sea water at the time that particular group isolated its body fluid from the external medium is now discredited. It is unlikely that different metazoan groups developed extracellular fluids at various times and phenomena such as the *hypoosmotic* behaviour of *marine teleosts* can be explained by an earlier fresh-water stage in their evolution. However, the criticism by Baldwin [1] and Potts and Parry [16] that implies that Macallum envisaged the body fluids as isolated from the external medium by impermeability is not justified. Macallum realized that, if the body fluid differed from the external medium, regulatory mechanisms (e.g. kidney) would be required to maintain the composition of the body fluid.

The development of a significant number of new types of organism in brackish and fresh water implies that there should be large areas of stable composition over significant geological time. The brackish waters of estuaries, which are small in volume, show rapid changes in composition and are transitory geological phenomena are not in this category. The *Baltic Basin*, however, seems to have the required properties. It constitutes a large and stable salinity gradient from full-strength sea water to fresh water in its northern and eastern extremities. However, this entire area was covered by the *Scandinavian ice cap* during the last ice age up to about 12,000 yrs B.C. and the subsequent history of this area has been somewhat complex. Thus, although the Baltic must now constitute an ideal region for the evolution of new brackish- and fresh-water types, the time that has elapsed is, in geological terms, insignificant. Although a number of species that occur in the Baltic show morphological differences from species in the arctic oceans and estuaries or in the fresh-water rivers and lakes from which they were derived, the extent to which these differences justify specific rank is debatable. There are further differences in the forms that occur in lakes that have been isolated from the Baltic Basin at various times since the retreat of the ice cap by *isostatic land elevation*. The isopod *Mesidotea entomon* (Fig. 5.2) is a case in

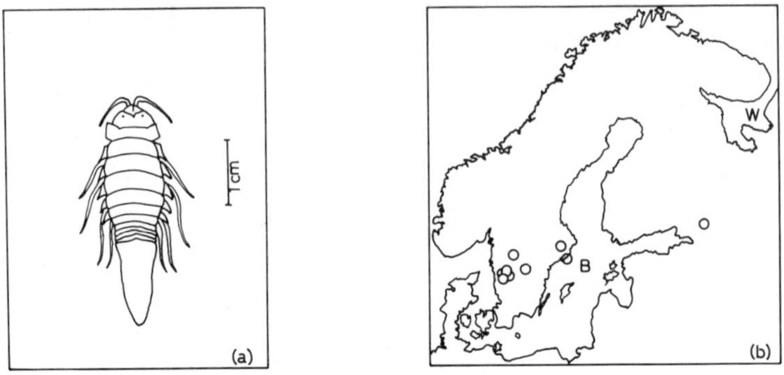

Fig. 5.2. The isopod *Mesidotea entomon*. (a) A specimen of the Lake Vättern race. Compared with the other races, the telson of the Lake Vättern race is elongated and this race has been described as a separate sub-species, *Mesidotea entomon vetterensis*. (b) Distribution of *Mesidotea entomon* in the Scandinavian region. This occurs in the White Sea, W (probably in brackish water), widely in the Baltic, B, and as isolated populations in a number of fresh-water lakes, ○. *Mesidotea entomon* also occurs in the brackish-water *Caspian Sea*.

point. The genetic basis for such differences is unknown and whether these forms are to be regarded as separate species, sub-species, varieties or races is a matter of conjecture.

It could be argued that Baltic-like situations, particularly in areas less subject to glacial catastrophes, may have played a role in the large-scale evolution of brackish and fresh-water faunas. *Continental drift* may have played a key role in the genesis of such regions. Two types of process could be involved. Firstly, the approach of continental land masses could produce a large brackish area either by simple entrapment or as a consequence of folding. The *Sarmatic Sea*, which covered an area from the Danube Basin across the Black Sea and Caspian Sea to the Aral Sea could be a case of this type. A considerable number of brackish and fresh-water species are believed to have evolved in this area. The second process could be the separation of continental land masses. During the formation of the South Atlantic, for example, there must have been a long period of brackish conditions before the widening gap led to complete mixing with oceanic sea water. Situations of the types considered could also have played a role in the reverse process of secondary colonization of the sea by groups that had previous evolutionary history in fresh water. The separate colonizations of the sea by *elasmobranch* and *teleost* fishes may possibly be related to such geological processes.

5.5 MARINE INVERTEBRATES

A very considerable number of chemical analyses have been made on the body fluids of marine invertebrates. A small selection of these data is given in Table 5.1. A close chemical similarity to sea water is apparent. However, there are certain significant differences. Almost always potassium concentration is higher and magnesium and sulphate concentration is lower in the body fluid than in the sea-water medium. It should be remembered that it is ion concentrations that are important. In the body fluid, a significant proportion of calcium may be bound to protein in a non-ionized form. Thus the actual B/M ratio for ionic calcium may be significantly less than the values given in Table 5.1. It is important to ascertain if the individual ion species are in equilibrium between body fluid and medium and, if certain ions are not in equilibrium, how the disequilibrium is maintained. The question of why there should be such differences is more difficult.

Table 5.1. Composition of sea water and of the body fluids of some marine invertebrates. Blood, or, in the case of *Arenicola*, coelomic fluid, concentration is expressed as proportion of the concentration of the sea water medium from which the animals were taken (B/M ratio). These media were not necessarily precisely identical to the specific sea-water sample given (Plymouth sea water, salinity = 35·2‰). All concentrations determined as m-moles kg water^{-1}.

	Na	K	Ca	Mg	Cl	SO_4
Sea water, m-moles kg water^{-1}	490	10·4	10·8	55·9	573	29·5
Arenicola (*Polychaeta*)	1·00	1·04	1·00	1·00	1·00	0·92
Maia (*Crustacea*)	1·02	1·22	1·29	0·81	0·99	0·50
Nephrops (*Crustacea*)	1·14	0·78	1·39	0·17	0·98	0·68
Carcinus (*Crustacea*)	1·11	1·21	1·27	0·36	1·00	0·57
Mytilus (*Lamellibranchiata*)	0·99	1·18	1·13	0·97	0·99	1·00
Sepia (*Cephalopoda*)	0·95	2·09	1·07	1·03	1·03	0·21
Equilibrium ratios for $V_m = -2$mV	1·08	1·08	1·17	1·17	0·92	0·85

The thermodynamic criterion of equilibrium of an ion between two phases is that the *electrochemical potential difference* of this ion between the two phases is zero. The electrochemical potential difference between two *similar* phases is determined by the *electrical potential difference* and by the *ratio of the concentration* (strictly *activity*) of the ion in the two phases. The relation between these terms at equilibrium is given by the *Nernst Equation*

$$E_i = -\frac{RT}{z_i F} \ln \frac{C_{iB}}{C_{iM}} \tag{4}$$

where E_i is the electrical potential difference (electrical potential of phase B (body fluid)—electrical potential of phase M (external medium) and C_{iB}/C_{iM} is the ratio of the concentration of ion i in the phase B to phase M. Note that z_i, the *valency* of ion i has both number and sign. Care is needed with the sign convention in this equation. E_i is sometimes referred to as the *Nernst potential* of ion i. E_i is the electrical potential difference that exists between the two phases if ion i is in equilibrium between the two phases. A simple qualitative kinetic appreciation of the meaning of this equation is to consider a membrane permeable to only one ion species and separating two solutions containing different concentrations of that ion. The ion will tend to diffuse down the concentration gradient across the membrane until the transfer of charge, resulting from the net movement of small amounts of this ion, builds up an electrical potential difference that opposes further net movement. The system is then in equilibrium and the quantitative relationships between the concentrations and the electrical potential difference is defined by eqn. (4).

If the Nernst potential predicted by eqn. (4) differs from the measured electrical potential difference between the body fluid and medium (*membrane potential*) there is a force acting on that ion tending to drive it in or out of the body fluid. The resultant net passive ion flux can be treated in electrical terms (*Ohm's Law*)

$$J_i = -\frac{G_i}{z_i F}(V_m - E_i) \qquad (5)$$

where J_i is the flux of the ion i, G_i is the *conductance* of the membrane to ion i, and V_m the membrane potential and the bracketed term represents the displacement of the system from the equilibrium position. With the sign convention used here, an influx is a positive quantity. If these passive fluxes are occurring, *active transport processes*, i.e. involving use of metabolic energy, in the epithelia must occur if a *steady state* is maintained.

An approach that has been frequently used, particularly by Robertson [21, 22] is *dialysis equilibrium*. A sample of body fluid is dialysed against sea water. After dialysis against sea water, any difference between the ion concentration in the body fluid and sea water would be due to the presence of proteins in the body fluid. Proteins usually carry a net negative charge at physiological pH and behave as non-diffusable anions. Thus, after dialysis equilibrium, there will be a slightly higher concentration of mobile cations and a slightly lower concentration of mobile anions in the body fluid than in the external medium. There will be a potential difference across the dialysis membrane defined by the Nernst equation. Such a situation is termed a *Gibbs–Donnan equilibrium*. If the concentration of an ion in the body fluid falls during dialysis it has been claimed that this means that this ion is above its equilibrium value in the body fluid. The fundamental fallacy in this approach is that electrical potential difference between body fluid and external medium across the epithelium is not measured and without this information the question cannot be answered. The technique would only be correct if the electrical potential difference across this epithelium was the same as that across the dialysis membrane and this could only be fortuitous. The electrical potential difference across the dialysis membrane will be small and it is also probable that the electrical potential difference across the external epithelia of marine invertebrates is also small. In which case, the conclusions drawn, e.g. that potassium ion is above its equilibrium value and magnesium ion is below its equilibrium value in the body fluid of most marine invertebrates, are probably correct, though not for the reasons claimed.

In order to decide the significance of data such as those of Table 5.1, it is *essential* to have information on the electrical potential difference between the body fluid and the medium. Unfortunately, information of this type is infrequent. Perhaps the importance of this information has not been sufficiently widely realized. The few published measurements for marine invertebrates suggest that, in sea-water medium, V_m is small and within the range 0 to -2mV (potential body fluid–potential of medium). If a value of potential difference is substituted into eqn. (4), equilibrium B/M ratios can be calculated. As an example, this has been done for $V_m = -2$mV (Table 5.1). With this potential difference, the equilibrium B/M ratio for potassium, for example, is exceeded by most of the actual ratios of the examples in Table 5.1. As the differences of concentration and of electrical potential are usually small, these measurements should be made on the same individuals. However, even if specific electrical potential differences are unknown, something can be done with the existing analytical data. An electrical potential difference, whatever its magnitude, will affect different ions in a predictable manner. Thus at equilibrium

$$\frac{(\mathrm{Na})_B}{(\mathrm{Na})_M} = \frac{(\mathrm{K})_B}{(\mathrm{K})_M} = \sqrt{\frac{(\mathrm{Ca})_B}{(\mathrm{Ca})_M}} = \sqrt{\frac{(\mathrm{Mg})_B}{(\mathrm{Mg})_M}} = \frac{(\mathrm{Cl})_M}{(\mathrm{Cl})_B} = \sqrt{\frac{(\mathrm{SO}_4)_M}{(\mathrm{SO}_4)_B}} \qquad (6)$$

Consider for example the case of the potassium ion. In some animals, the ratio $(\mathrm{K})_B/(\mathrm{Na})_B$ is about twice the value of the ratio $(\mathrm{K})_M/(\mathrm{Na})_M$. There is an enrichment of the body fluid with potassium ion relative to sodium ion. This could mean that the potassium ion is above the equilibrium value in the blood or, conversely, that the sodium ion is below its equilibrium value in the blood. It is clear, however, that both ions cannot be in equilibrium.

The principle places where passive and active transport processes between the body fluid and external medium can occur are the external epithelium and the epithelium of the excretory organ. In some animals the gut epithelium may also play a role.

In soft bodied marine invertebrates, transport may occur over the whole external surface but in some types, especially the *Crustacea*, the external surface of the animal is covered by an impermeable cuticle and significant permeability is confined to specialized structures, *gills* (*branchiae*), where the cuticle covering the epithelium is both thin and permeable. As a result of the lamellar or filamentous structure of these gills, the total permeable area may be surprisingly large. These structures are important in the exchange of respiratory gases, but, as a consequence of the large area and permeable cuticle, they are places where passive movements of water and ions occur. Unpublished observation on *Carcinus* gills indicate a very high ion permeability. These gills are also places where active transport mechanisms would be expected.

The excretory organs are of a variety of types (see Fig. 5.1). The physiology of these organs has been reviewed by Riegel [19]. One that has been studied fairly extensively is the coelomoduct excretory organ of Crustacea. A more detailed

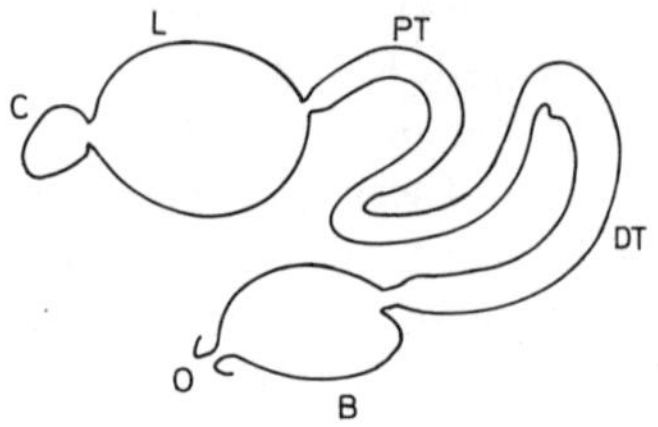

Fig. 5.3. Structure of the Antennal Gland of *Astacus*. In this diagram the components have been unravelled. C, coelomic end sac. Tubule system: L, labyrinth; PT, proximal tubule; DT, distal tubule; B, bladder; O, opening on basal segment of antenna. The epithelia of the labyrinth and tubule are extensively infolded, greatly increasing the surface area.

diagram of such an organ is given in Figs. 5.3. A *coelomic end sac*, the space of which is the coelom of the particular head segment in which the excretory organ occurs (usually either *antennal* or *maxillary* segments) is connected to the exterior by a *coelomoduct*, which may have a number of morphologically specialized regions, the details of which vary considerably in different types.

In marine animals the length of the tubule is relatively short, whereas in some fresh-water forms the tubule is relatively long. This is related to the production of a urine hypo-osmotic to the body fluid in these types.

This system is closely similar to the vertebrate *nephron* which is also a coelomic sac (*Bowman's capsule*)—coelomoduct system. There is clear evidence that this vertebrate nephron operates by *ultrafiltration*, i.e. a hydrostatic pressure difference between the blood and the fluid in the capsule drives a bulk flow of fluid, which is essentially protein-free plasma, into the capsule. Then this fluid is modified in the tubule by passive and active transport processes in either direction across the tubule epithelium to produce the final urine.

There is evidence that the crustacean excretory organ operates in the same manner. The cells of the end sac are not laterally attached to each other and have a series of interlocking 'foot' processes sitting on a basement membrane. The structure is extremely similar to that found in the vertebrate capsule. As in the vertebrates, crustacea excrete inert substance of reasonably high molecular weight and low diffusability in the urine. Substances such as inulin, ^{51}Cr-EDTA, dextrans and low-molecular weight proteins are excreted in the urine following injection into the haemolymph. The only way these substances could be excreted is by some type of bulk flow of fluid from the haemolymph into the lumen of the excretory system and the rate of excretion of these substances can be used to measure the rate of this bulk flow (ultrafiltration).

Direct chemical analysis of fluid taken from this coelomic end sac have been made in the crayfish by Riegel and the osmotic pressure and concentrations of sodium, chloride and inulin are very similar to the haemolymph, as would be expected from ultrafiltration. However, the potassium concentration in this end-sac lumen was substantially greater than that in the haemolymph and this could mean that there is additionally some active transport function of the end-sac epithelial cells. The ultrafiltrate is then modified by the tubule epithelium during its passage through the tubule system. This animal is in fact a freshwater form that produces a urine very hypoosmotic to the haemolymph, the modifications to the ultrafiltrate occurring during passage through the tubule system.

In marine invertebrates, the urine is closely isoosmotic with the body fluid. Some data are given for the crab *Carcinus* (Table 5.2). Although the urine is isoosmotic with the haemolymph, the ionic composition differs considerably from the haemolymph and this must represent active transport processes by the tubule epithelium. In particular, the concentration of magnesium and sulphate are higher and the concentration of potassium lower than in the haemolymph and this has been interpreted by Webb [29] as indicating a significant role of the

Table 5.2. Composition of haemolymph and urine of *Carcinus maenas*. Haemolymph concentration expressed as proportion of medium concentration (*B*/*M* ratio) and urine concentration expressed as proportion of haemolymph concentration (*U*/*B* ratio). All concentrations determined as m-moles kg water^{-1}.

Medium		Na	K	Ca	Mg	Cl	SO_4
Ordinary	Haemolymph	1·11	1·21	1·27	0·36	1·00	0·57
Sea water	Urine	0·95	0·78	0·94	3·90	0·98	2·24
Sea water							
enriched with	Haemolymph	1·13	—	—	0·24	0·99	0·29
$MgSO_4$	Urine	0·92	—	—	5·00	0·98	4·65

excretory organ in controlling haemolymph composition. The ratio of the concentration of inulin in the urine to the concentration in the haemolymph (*U*/*B ratio*) indicates the function of the tubule systems in reabsorbing water from the ultrafiltrate. In *Carcinus*, kept immersed in sea water, and some other marine forms, the inulin *U*/*B* ratio is about unity, indicating negligible water uptake in the tubule system. This means that the high concentration of magnesium and sulphate in the urine cannot be explained by reabsorption of the other components of the ultrafiltrate. The high concentration in the urine of both magnesium and sulphate must thus indicate that one or both of these ions is actively transported by the tubule system epithelium into the lumen. Electrical potential difference measurements across this epithelium would help to clarify the situation.

Pantin [14] considered that the maintenance of body-fluid ion concentration both above and below the presumed equilibrium values could be explained in terms of the function of the excretory organ. However, an important point to bear in mind, when considering the effects of gill epithelial and tubule epithelial transport on body-fluid composition, is that as far as outwardly directed transport is concerned the effect is identical, but for inwardly directed transport there is an important difference in the possible effects of the two epithelia. This is because the tubule epithelium can only transport inwards those substances presented to it by the ultrafiltration of body fluids and thus it can merely reduce the loss via the excretory organ. Whereas tubular transport activity alone could explain a concentration in the body fluid lower than the equilibrium value, it cannot explain a concentration in the body fluid above the equilibrium value, as this would then involve diffusion of that ion from the external medium into the body fluid against its electrochemical potential difference. Thus, if an ion is above equilibrium concentration in the body fluid it is necessary to invoke active transport from the external medium by the external epithelium.

The excretory organs are also of course excreting water from the animal. This is a simple ultrafiltration process involving a small hydrostatic pressure difference across a highly permeable body fluid-coelom barrier, the coelomic end sac wall in the case of the Crustacea or the walls of the general coelom in the case of those types with a large coelom drained by open nephridial or coelomoduct systems (e.g. annelids).

The rate of urine production can be determined by various methods. Methods that have been used include direct cannulation and collection, blocking the excretory pores and measuring initial rate of weight increase. Other methods involve measuring the concentration in the urine of a substance such as inulin that is only lost by this route. Then the rate of appearance of this substance in the external medium can be used to define urine volume flow rate or, if the U/B ratio is known, the rate of fall of concentration of this substance in the body fluid can be used to define the urine volume flow rate. Care is needed with such indirect methods, as can be seen by a critical perusal of a paper by Shaw [26] on urine volume flow rates in *Carcinus*.

The urine volume flow rates in marine invertebrates are not inconsiderable. For example, in *Carcinus* in sea water the rate is about 0·2% body weight/h although this urine flow rate estimate may not be very reliable. If the animal is maintaining a steady state, the animal must be taking up water from the external medium at the same rate. If the body fluid is hyperosmotic to the medium, there will be an osmotic influx of water. But these marine invertebrates are closely isoosmotic with the sea-water medium. The mechanism of this uptake presents a difficulty. It is possible that some active uptake process for water is occurring across the gill epithelium. However, there are various mechanisms by which water can be moved passively as an indirect result of ion transport. Various mechanisms of this type have been recently reviewed in a magnificent compendium by House [6]. Although there is no reason why water molecules should not be transported, as any other type of non-electrolyte, House cannily takes the view that the existence of active water transport is 'not proven'.

On the basis of the information discussed, it is possible to construct a model of the steady state water and ion balance of a 'typical' marine invertebrate. Much of the information discussed is derived from Crustacea but there is little

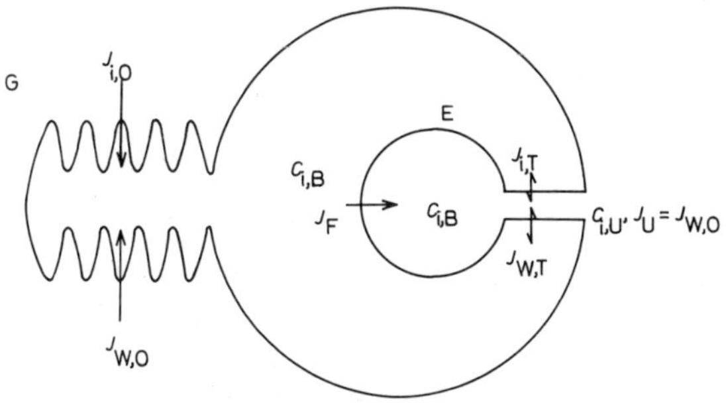

Fig. 5.4. Model of a 'typical' marine invertebrate (*Carcinus*). G, gill; E, excretory organ. $C_{i,B}$, concentration of solute species i in body fluid and coelomic end sac; $C_{i,U}$, concentration of solute species i in urine. Net fluxes, which contain passive and/or active components, indicated by arrows. $J_{i,O}$, flux of solute species i into gill; $J_{W,O}$, flux water into gill; J_F, rate of ultrafiltration; $J_{i,T}$, flux of solute species i across epithelium of tubule system; $J_{W,T}$, flux of water across epithelium of tubule system; J_U, rate of urine production.

doubt that other groups show similar phenomena. The model is summarized in Fig. 5.4. The model is based to a considerable extent on data from the shore crab *Carcinus maenas*. Although this animal is perfectly at home in sea water and is thus treated as a marine animal, it is also capable of adaptation to brackish waters.

5.6 ADAPTATION TO BRACKISH AND FRESH WATER

The question that will now be considered is how a marine organism of the type considered could undergo adaptation to brackish and fresh water. A very considerable number of brackish-water forms have been investigated. These tolerate full strength sea water and show various degrees of euryhalinity. For example *Carcinus maenas* will adapt down to about 20% of sea water, whereas the Baltic isopod *Mesidotea entomon* will survive down to much more dilute conditions (about salinity 0·8‰).

After exposure to media of various dilutions, the osmotic pressure or concentration of the body fluid can be determined. Some examples of the adaptation curves are given in Fig. 5.5. Each point on these curves represents a steady-state body-fluid composition and thus these curves can be described as *adaptation isotherms*. Some marine organisms are entirely poikilosmotic and the osmotic pressure of the body fluid would closely follow the *isoosmotic line* until death occurs. The spider-crab *Maia* and the lamellibranch *Mytilus* are examples here. It should be remembered that, although the animal may be isoosmotic with the media, the concentration of individual ions will differ from that of the external medium. Brackish-water animals are all homoiosmotic to some extent and their body fluids at the more dilute end of the adaptation range are markedly hyperosmotic to the medium. Even so, in these dilute media the concentration of the body fluid is usually considerably below that of a marine organism. Some degree

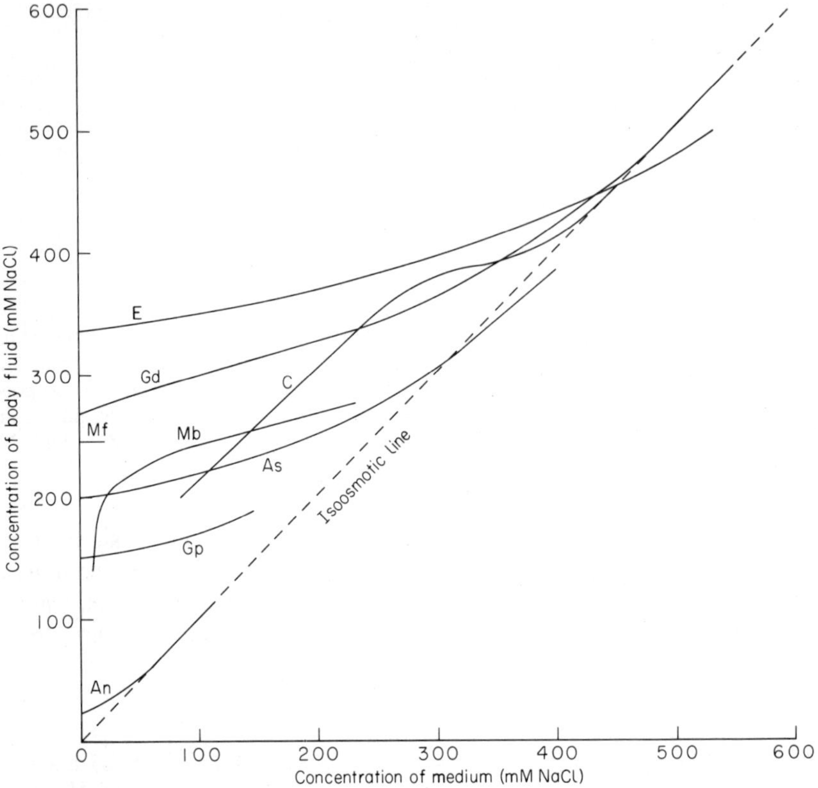

Fig. 5.5. Adaptation isotherms for some homoiosmotic organisms, particularly Crustacea. Steady-state body-fluid concentration as a function of medium concentration. In some cases osmotic pressure is plotted as equivalent isoosmotic NaCl concentration: E, *Eriocheir sinensis*; Gd, *Gammarus duebeni*; Gp, *Gammarus pulex*; An, *Anodonta cygnaea* (*Lamellibranchiata*). In other cases the sodium concentration is plotted: As, *Astacus pallipes*; C, *Carcinus maenas*; Mb, *Mesidotea entomon* (brackish-water race); Mf, *Mesidotea entomon* (fresh-water races). The upper termination of the adaptation isotherms may represent absence of data suitable for inclusion. The lower termination of the adaptation isotherms, however, represents the physiological limit to adaptation to dilute media.

of cellular adaptation to a reduced body-fluid concentration must therefore be involved and it is undoubtedly the limit of this adaptation that defines the extent of euryhalinity.

An important point is that although such adaptation isotherms define a physiological range, the actual ecological range may be more restricted. Other *physical factors*, e.g. temperature, may limit the range. Also in some cases the larval stages may have a more restricted physiological range than the adults. *Biotic factors* may have an important limiting effect. A good example of an ecologically restricted range is the virtual absence of *Gammarus duebeni* from the open water of the Baltic. Physiologically, it is perfectly capable of living in this medium and in fact occurs frequently in the very variable and sometimes extreme conditions of rockpools along the edge of the Baltic. Its absence from the open water of the Baltic must be due to biotic factors, possibly competition with *Gammarus zaddachi oceanicus*, which is abundant in the open water of the Baltic.

The problem of hyperosmotic regulation is two-fold, involving both water and ion transport. The problem can be seen by considering the predicament of a purely marine organism unkindly transferred to a dilute medium. There is a rapid initial increase in volume due to osmotic influx of water. However, water influx does not present a great problem to an excretory organ operating by ultrafiltration and the volume will tend to fall back towards the original value. However, there will be a rapid fall in body-fluid concentration towards iso-osmoticity with the external medium. This will be due to two factors: loss of ions (principally NaCl) by diffusion across the external surface of the animal and loss of ions (again principally NaCl) in the increased volume flow rate of urine iso-osmotic with the body fluid. Osmotic swelling and changes in the ion composition of the cells will occur and ultimately death occurs.

This process can be looked at quantitatively. The flux of water across a membrane can be written

$$J_V = -L_p A (\Delta P - \sigma \Delta \Pi) \quad (7)$$

where J_V is the *volume flow rate*, L_p the *hydraulic conductivity coefficient* of the membrane, A the surface area, ΔP the *hydrostatic pressure difference*, $\Delta \Pi$ the *osmotic pressure difference* and σ the *reflection coefficient*. If preferred, L_p can be expressed in terms of an *osmotic permeability coefficient* (P_{os}) where

$$P_{os} = L_p R T / \bar{V}_W \quad (8)$$

where $\bar{V}_W$ is the *partial molar volume* of water. The dimensionless reflection coefficient is a property of the membrane (not the solution). If the membrane is completely impermeable to the solutes that give rise to $\Delta \Pi$, the value of σ is unity. However, if the membrane is permeable to some or all of the solutes, the value of σ will be less, perhaps approaching zero or may even be negative (*anomalous osmosis*). It will be assumed that σ can be taken as unity. Also the ΔP term will usually be trivial compared to $\Delta \Pi$. Eqn. (7) can then be considerably simplified. In the case of ultrafiltration into the excretory organ, the situation is different. Here the barrier is very permeable and σ for ions and small molecular weight non-electrolytes tends to zero, the residual $\sigma \Delta \Pi$ being termed the *colloid osmotic pressure difference*. The hydrostatic pressure difference becomes dominant. It is because an increased influx of water into an animal would tend to increase the ΔP term, that volume regulation does not present great difficulty when the body fluid is hyperosmotic to the external medium. The ultrafiltration mechanism might thus be regarded as fortuitous pre-adaptation to dilute media.

The situation regarding ions is more complex. There are a considerable number of ion species involved and their fluxes are controlled by their concentrations, electrical potential difference, membrane permeabilities to specific ions and specific active transport mechanisms. However, the situation can be simplified if we treat the body fluid and external medium as simply NaCl solutions and treat diffusion and active transport in the simple terms of a non-electrolyte. The *net passive flux* of NaCl across the external epithelia can then be defined using the *Fick Equation*

$$J_E = P_{NaCl}\, A\, (C_B - C_M) \tag{9}$$

where J_E is the net passive flux of NaCl, P_{NaCl} is the *permeability coefficient* of the membrane for NaCl, A the surface area and C_B and C_M the NaCl concentration is in the body fluid and medium respectively. Effects of any linkage between NaCl and water flux are ignored. There will be a net passive efflux of NaCl across the external epithelium for an animal hyperosmotic to the external medium.

There will also be a loss of NaCl from the body fluid via the excretory organ. The rate at which NaCl is ultrafiltrated into the excretory organ (J_F) can be written

$$J_F = J_V\, C_B \tag{10}$$

where J_V is defined by eqn. (7). It must be admitted that this is the simplest possible model and assumes that there is no tubular reabsorption of water. The rate of which NaCl is actually lost from the animal in the urine (J_U) is then

$$J_U = J_V\, C_U \tag{11}$$

where C_U is the concentration of the urine. The rate of tubular reabsorption of NaCl (J_T) is

$$J_T = J_V\, (C_B - C_U) \tag{12}$$

In a number of forms J_T is zero and the urine is isoosmotic with the body fluid. This is the case in *Carcinus* and even in a number of fresh-water forms, e.g. the fresh-water crabs *Eriocheir* and *Potamon*. In some brackish and fresh-water types, e.g. gammarids and crayfish, however, tubular reabsorption of NaCl occurs and a urine hypoosmotic to the body fluid is produced.

The important point about the curves in Fig. 5.5 is that they represent the *steady-state situation*. The influx and efflux of water and ions balance. The excretion of the osmotic influx of water presents little problem. In the case of NaCl, in the steady state, the total rate of active uptake like the body fluid must balance the total rate of loss from the body fluid.

$$J_A + J_T = J_E + J_F \tag{13}$$

where J_A is the rate of active uptake from the external medium across the external epithelium. Combining the foregoing equations, produces a *model system* that defines a steady-state C_B as a function of C_M, the precise value of C_B being defined by the permeabilities to water and NaCl and by the active-uptake parameters.

The various factors involved in adaptation can now be considered in more detail.

5.6.1 Concentration of the body fluid

Examination of data such as that in Fig. 5.5 indicates that different animals show very varying degrees of hyperosmoticity to the external medium. Some forms, particularly fresh-water crabs such as *Eriocheir*, maintain a very high haemolymph osmotic concentration (636 m-osmolar) even in fresh water. At the other extreme are the fresh-water lamellibranchs with a very low body-fluid concentration typified by the swan mussel *Anodonta cygnaea* (haemolymph osmotic concentration 42 m-osmolar). It can be argued that the retention of a very high body-fluid concentration in brackish and fresh-water media is a primitive feature. The higher the body-fluid concentration is maintained in a dilute medium, the greater is the rate of NaCl loss from the body fluid, as defined by eqns. (9) and (10). It can be seen that in very dilute media the rate of NaCl ion by diffusion is proportional to C_B but the rate of loss by ultrafiltration is proportioned to C_B^2. Thus, with a higher body-fluid concentration there must be increased active uptake to maintain the steady state. The thermodynamic consequence of this will be considered in a later section.

Those organisms with lower body-fluid concentration have undergone further evolutionary adaptation at the cellular level. This reduces the kinetic and energetic problems of maintaining a high body-fluid concentration in very dilute media. The basic problem of cellular existence is an osmotic problem. The cell membrane is very permeable to water and the cells contain many metabolically important organic anions and neutral molecules that are osmotically active. Such a cell would tend to swell osmotically. The method of volume regulation that has developed involves active transport of sodium ions out of the cell. Then, even if all the other inorganic ions can move freely across the cell membrane, the total concentration of these ions will be less than in the extracellular medium and thus there will be an osmotic and volume steady state. However, the total intracellular concentration of organic anions and neutral molecules that can be maintained in this steady state is limited and problems consequently arise when the body fluid is diluted. Adaptation to these dilute body fluids must then entail a reduction in the concentration of the organic anions and neutral molecules. The concentration of amino acids in the cell fluid is under cellular control and there is evidence in several types that changes in body-fluid concentration are accompanied by adaptive changes in free amino acid concentration in the cell fluid [24]. Cell adaptation to very dilute body fluids could only occur with such a considerable reduction in the cell organic solute concentrations that, in the case of *Anodonta* and similar types, it is difficult to envisage how normal cell metabolism and activities can continue. A further problem relates to the excitation and propagation of the *action potential.* Although the Nernst potentials and resting potential and theoretical peak of an action potential are not themselves necessarily affected by adaptation to a dilute body fluid, there will be other significant effects. The inrush of sodium ions during the rising phase of an action potential is controlled by the sodium conductance of the membrane and this conductance would be proportional to sodium concentration. Thus, in a dilute body fluid, a slower rate of rise of the action potential would be expected. Further, the increased specific resistance of both the extracellular and intracellular fluids would, by affecting the cable properties of the system, reduce the propagation velocity. It is thus not surprising that *Anodonta* nerves have been found to have an extraordinarily long chronaxie and slow propagation velocity.

5.6.2 Permeability of the external surface

The effects of the permeability of the external surface to water and NaCl are defined in eqn. (7), eqn. (8) and eqn. (9).

The flux will normally be expressed per unit mass of animal (J_i/W) and then the other side of the equation contains the term P_iA/W. This will be termed the *overall permeability coefficient* (K_i). The reason for this is the difficulty in determining surface areas, particularly as any real animal is obviously a mosaic of areas each with different permeability properties. The most obvious case of such differences is seen in the larger crustacea, where the general cuticle is virtually impermeable and the gill area itself is not necessarily uniform. There seems to be some evidence of difference in permeability between different gills in the crayfish *Austropotamobius* (*Astacus*). A technique that has been frequently used on arthropods is *silver staining*. The animal is exposed to a low concentration of $AgNO_3$ and, after rinsing off the excess, the silver that is taken up is visualized by reduction to black metallic silver grains. The interpretations that have been put on this phenomenon are various. The simplest explanation is that it merely demonstrates those parts of the cuticle, usually in the gills, which are ion permeable and through which silver ions can enter the cuticle and tissues. A rather interesting picture emerges in *Austropotamobius* (*Astacus*). Branchial filaments constitute the main part of the considerable surface area of the gills. However, only the filaments at the basal end of the gill are silver stained. In view of problems of this type, the advantage of working with a lumped coefficient K_i, as an operational concept, are obvious.

In the case of water permeability there are problems resulting from the ways in which the permeability is determined. The physiologically significant process is the *net osmotic flow of water* into the animal. This is the volume that is excreted in the steady state and is conveniently determined by measuring the urine flow rate. Another method of determining this flow is to measure the initial rate of weight or volume change following transfer to a medium of different osmotic pressure. The coefficient that defines this osmotic flow is P_{os}. However, it is technically simpler to measure isotopic water flux (usually using THO). This flux can be treated using the simple Fick equation for a non-electrolyte solute

$$J_W^* = P_d\, A\, \Delta C^* \qquad (14)$$

where J_W^* is the flux of labelled water, ΔC^* the concentration difference of labelled water on the two sides of the barrier and P_d the *diffusional permeability coefficient* of water. If $P_{os} = P_d$, these simple experiments could be used to determine the net osmotic flow rate. However, frequently $P_{os} > P_d$. The reason for this difference is that different physical processes are being studied by the two methods. The osmotic method is measuring a bulk volume flow, whereas the isotopic method is measuring a diffusion process. The diffusion process may be limited by diffusion in the *unstirred layers* on both sides of the permeability barrier, whereas bulk flow is not limited in the unstirred layers. The possible presence of bulk flow through pores in the permeability barrier may also affect differently the values of the two coefficients. The general conclusion from all this is that water permeability data based on isotopic fluxes should be interpreted with great caution, particularly if any attempt is being made to determine the net osmotic flow.

As an example of the problems involved consider the case of *Carcinus*. Shaw [26] devised an interesting method for estimating urine flow rates which involved equating the influx of sulphate with the sulphate loss via the urine (= rate urine volume flow × urine sulphate concentration) and then calculating the volume flow rate. However, an examination of the procedure reveals a serious mathematical error and Shaw's urine flow data must be corrected by multiplying by the ratio blood sulphate concentration/medium sulphate concentration. This greatly reduces the apparent volume flow rates, particularly in dilute media. In sea water the corrected values are 1·14% body weight/day and in 40% sea water the value rises to 3·91% body weight/day. These values are substantially less than those found by occluding the excretory pores and following weight changes [29]. But these data may also be subjected to errors due to the effects of operating and handling on the animals. If the corrected Shaw data are accepted and if it is assumed that the difference between the sea water and 40% sea water urine flow rates represents the osmotic flow of water across the gills, a permeability coefficient (P_{os}) can be calculated using eqns (7) and (8). Taking $\Delta\Pi$ as 200 m-osmolar and the permeable area as 0·63 $cm^2\ g^{-1}$, then $P_{os} \simeq 1{\cdot}4 \times 10^{-6}\ ms^{-1}$, a value well towards the lower end of the range of data on animal cells reviewed by House [6]. However, in the case of crustacea, it should be remembered that there is a cuticle as well as cell membranes present. Also, although *Carcinus* can live in the sea, it is also a brackish-water animal and might be expected to have a lower osmotic permeability than a stenohaline marine type. The *Carcinus* permeability can be compared with that of some fresh-water crustacea. For example, there are data on the fresh-water *Eriocheir*, *Potamon* and *Astacus* (data reviewed in [16]). Assuming in the case of *Eriocheir* and *Potamon* that the permeable area/weight is the same as in *Carcinus*, then for *Eriocheir* $P_{os} \simeq 0{\cdot}57 \times 10^{-6}\ ms^{-1}$. In the case of *Potamon*, the urine flow rates are so insignificant that, if they are correct, P_{os} must be about an order lower than in *Eriocheir*. In the case of *Austropotamobius* (*Astacus*), the gill structure is filamentous and the filament surface area is 4·3 $cm^2\ g^{-1}$ (Croghan and Curra, unpublished). Then $P_{os} \simeq 0{\cdot}28 \times 10^{-6}\ ms^{-1}$. These values for fresh-water forms seem significantly lower than the value for the brackish-water *Carcinus*. The nature of these adaptations at the cellular level is unknown.

A real problem in determining these permeability coefficients is the evaluation of permeable surface areas. It is relatively straightforward to determine overall permeability coefficient K_{os} but adaptation could operate at the level of both the properties of the membranes and of the areas. An example illustrating this problem, considered by Potts and Parry, is the fresh-water mussel *Anodonta cygnaea*. The value of K_{os} in this form is enormous. This is undoubtedly a consequence of the modification of the gill (*ctenidium*) structure in the lamellibranchs as a complex filter-feeding system with enormous surface area. A high overall permeability is inevitable. This is undoubtedly the reason why the few fresh-water lamellibranchs have such a low body-fluid concentration. In a fresh-water medium, it would be an impossibility for them to have anything else.

The interpretation of water isotope flux data are usually more difficult. However, information of a relative or comparative nature is available. The case of *Gammarus duebeni* is of particular interest. This species lives in a wide range of brackish media and fresh-water populations occur on the western fringes of the British Isles [11]. As *Gammarus duebeni* is adapted to a decreasing external concentration, there is a decrease in P_d for water. In sea water $P_d = 15{\cdot}3 \times 10^{-7}$ ms^{-1} and in 2% sea water $P_d = 6{\cdot}64 \times 10^{-7}$ ms^{-1}. Most of this reduction occurs in the range 75–50% sea water when the body-fluid concentration begins to be maintained noticeably hyperosmotic to the medium. The change in permeability following a change in external concentration is very rapid (<5 min). The mechanism of the reduction in permeability is not known. A number of other cases of a reduction of diffusional permeability for water during adaptation of marine and brackish-water animals, particularly in crustacea but also in the polychaete *Nereis diversicola*, to reduced external concentration have also been described [25].

In the case of ion permeability, different problems arise due to the effect of any electrical potential difference between the body fluid and medium. As has been described earlier, the problem can be avoided if the situation can be treated as diffusion of NaCl as this can be treated as a non-electrolyte and a NaCl permeability coefficient P_{NaCl} or the corresponding overall permeability coefficient K_{NaCl} determined. For a single-membrane system, these coefficients can be measured directly from efflux data into distilled water.

The greatest body of flux data is derived from unidirection flux experiments, mainly using ^{22}Na. Passive fluxes of an ion across a membrane can be related to electrical potential and concentration differences by a number of models. Using the *Goldman Flux Equation*, the net passive efflux of an ion (J_i^{net}) can be written

$$J_i^{net} = P_i A \frac{z_i F\ V/2\ R\ T}{\sinh\ (z_i F\ V/2\ R\ T)} (C_{i,in} \exp\ (z_i F\ V/2\ R\ T) - C_{i,out} \exp\ (-z_i F\ V/2\ R\ T) \quad (15)$$

where V is the electrical potential difference (in – out) and $C_{i,in}$ and $C_{i,out}$ are the concentrations of the ion on the two sides. The format of the equation written in this way may be unfamiliar but has a pleasing symmetry. In fact, what is measured is a *unidirection efflux* (J_i^{efflux}) where

$$J_i^{\text{efflux}} = P_i A \frac{z_i F\ V/2\ R\ T}{\sinh\ (z_i F\ V/2\ R\ T)} (C_{i,\text{in}} \exp\ (z_i F\ V/2\ R\ T)) \tag{16}$$

If J_i^{efflux}, V and $C_{i,\text{in}}$ are known, the permeability coefficient P_i can be defined. This value substituted in eqn. (15) gives the net efflux. For some purposes it is convenient to define an operational permeability P_i' itself a function of $z_i V$. Then

$$J_i^{\text{net}} = P_i' A(C_{i,\text{in}} - C_{i,\text{out}}) \tag{17}$$

Problems may arise because all the passive efflux may not be simple diffusion. Another passive process called *exchange diffusion* may occur. This is a passive 1:1 exchange of a given ion across a membrane. A possible mechanism is a shuttling or rotating carrier that always crosses the membrane with a complexed ion. Such an exchange is unaffected by electrical potential differences and contributes nothing to membrane electrical conductance. There is no net movement of ion and, unless metabolic energy is involved at any stage, the animal is physiologically speaking unaware that anything is happening. It is a phenomenon, however, that affects isotope flux experiments. Identification and correction of measured fluxes for this phenomenon is by no means easy. However, exchange diffusion involves the reversible formation of a complex involving the ion and exchange diffusion flux would thus be a function of the concentration of the exchanged ion on both sides of the membrane. Thus, in low external concentrations, exchange diffusion flux is unlikely to be very significant.

It has usually been the case that the epithelial barrier is considered to be a single membrane across which both passive and active fluxes of ions occur. In this single membrane model, there is no necessity for an equality of the sodium and chloride unidirectional fluxes, except in the special case where the external medium is deionized water, although, unless other ions are involved, the net fluxes of sodium and chloride must always be equal. An example of the application of the single membrane model can be found in the study by Croghan and Lockwood [5] in *Mesidotea*.

However, an epithelium is essentially two membrane barriers, undoubtedly with different properties, in series. To interpret the experimental data for such a system in terms of a single membrane model might give rise to serious errors. Consider a model of the epithelial cell (Fig. 5.6). The *inner membrane* is postulated to have active ion pumps as envisaged by Koefoed-Johnsen and Ussing [8]. The *outer membrane* is postulated to have significant permeability to only sodium and chloride ions. Fluxes are indicated inwards. This is a consequence of sign convention. In fact an actual net passive flux could be outwards across either membrane. In this system the net passive fluxes of sodium and chloride *must* be equal across the outer membrane and *must* be equal to the net fluxes of sodium and chloride across the inner membrane. The relationships can be written

$$J_{i,O}^{\text{net influx (passive)}} = J_{i,I}^{\text{net influx}} = J_{i,I}^{\text{net passive influx}} + J_{i,I}^{\text{active influx}} \tag{18}$$

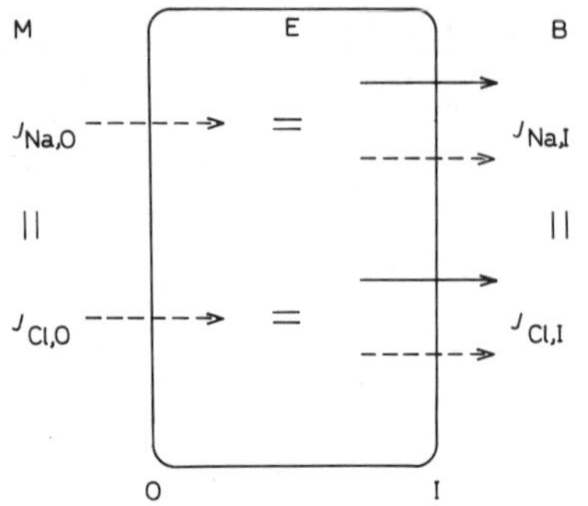

Fig. 5.6. A model of the epithelial cell. M, medium; E, epithelial cell fluid; B, body fluid; O, outer cell membrane; I, inner cell membrane. Net passive influxes indicated by broken arrows; active influxes indicated by continuous arrows.

where the subscripts O and I refer to the outer and inner cell membranes respectively and influx is used for the direction medium towards body fluid. The inner membrane is likely to have a relatively low permeability to sodium and chloride, as this would be essential for an effective pumping system. For the situation where $P'_{i,O} >> P'_{i,I}$ eqn. (18) can be expanded

$$J_{i,O}^{\text{net influx}} = J_{i,I}^{\text{active influx}} - P'_{i,I}\, C_{i,B} \qquad (19)$$

An important point is that the right-hand side must have the same value for both sodium and chloride, although the active fluxes and the permeabilities need not have the same values for each ion. In the simplest situation, the final term of eqn. (19) might be rather small. Then the active fluxes of sodium and chloride across the inner membrane would also be equal and equal to the net passive flux across the outer membrane. It would thus be possible to speak correctly about the diffusion of NaCl and the active transport of NaCl rather than of the individual ions. When the system operates in a steady-state situation with the body fluid hyperosmotic to the external medium there is actually no net diffusion of NaCl *outwards* into the external medium. Net diffusion is actually *inwards* across the outer membrane. The net diffusion and active transport across the inner membrane balance NaCl losses elsewhere in the animal, e.g. excretory organ losses.

Transport across epithelia is frequently studied by isotope flux experiments. Interpretation of these data are straightforward when a single membrane barrier is involved. However, the real situation is more complex. From the model developed above, it is possible to derive equations defining isotope efflux and influx. However, these equations are complex and not immediately useful. It can be seen qualitatively that, in an experiment measuring, for example, efflux of a labelled ion from the body fluid, efflux will be limited by the permeability of the inner membrane to that ion and also that, if this ion is actively transported across the inner membrane, some of this labelled ion will be promptly pumped back again into the body fluid and not appear in the external medium. The isotope fluxes of sodium and chloride are determined by the various permeability and active transport terms and need not be the same.

It should be apparent that there are difficulties in interpreting ion isotope flux data across epithelia. These difficulties are largely unresolved. Consequently caution is required in the interpretation of derivations of permeabilities and active transport rates that have been made from isotope flux data assuming a single membrane model. Such derivations should be treated as purely operational concepts.

As an example of ion permeability, the efflux of NaCl from the body fluid of the brackish and fresh-water races of *Mesidotea entomon* can be considered. The efflux of sodium from the body fluid was measured after transfer of animals from their medium to deionized water or a medium with very low NaCl concentration.

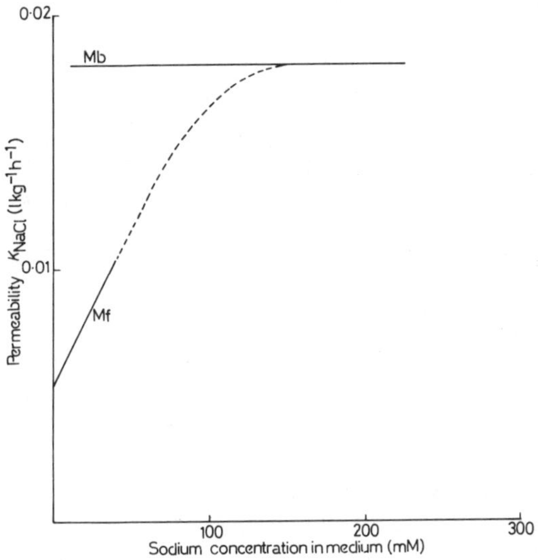

Fig. 5.7. Overall permeability, K_{NaCl}, of *Mesidotea entomon* related to the sodium concentration of the medium to which they had been adapted. Mb, brackish-water race; Mf, fresh-water races. Broken line is assumed behaviour of fresh-water races.

centration. It should be stressed that it is assumed that losses in the urine (maxillary gland) are negligible and thus that these efflux experiments define a value for overall permeability K_{NaCl}. In Fig. 5.7 data from [5, 11] and Lockwood and Croghan (in preparation) are summarized. The permeability of the fresh-water races isolated in Lake Mälaren and in Lake Vättern is, on average, considerably below that of the brackish-water Baltic race. In the case of the Lake Vättern animals, permeability was also investigated for animals adapted to a higher sodium concentration in the medium. The interpretation is that the brackish-water race is unable to reduce its permeability to NaCl on transfer to more dilute media whereas the established fresh-water races have acquired the ability to reduce NaCl permeability. There is a high degree of variability in the permeability of the brackish-water animals and it must be selection at the lower end of this range of permeability that has resulted in the lower permeability of the fresh-water races. The reduced permeability of the fresh-water races is undoubtedly an important factor in the adaptation and survival of *Mesidotea* in fresh water. Assuming that all sodium loss is via the gills, the permeability of the Lake Vättern race can be estimated as $P_{NaCl} = 0{\cdot}11 \times 10^{-7}$ ms^{-1}. This low value can be compared to the value for *Carcinus maenas*, a marine to concentrated brackish-water type where, measured by isotope efflux into sea water, $P'_{Na} = 2{\cdot}43 \times 10^{-7}$ ms^{-1} (data of Shaw, 1961). In the case of *Gammarus duebeni*, there is also evidence that adaptation to very dilute media is associated with a reduction in NaCl permeability. Euryhaline fish are interesting in this respect (Chapter 12).

5.6.3 Active uptake of ions

Active uptake of ions has been implicit in the preceding section. Direct evidence of net active uptake of NaCl exists for both the external epithelium and for the tubule epithelium of animals producing a urine hypoosmotic to the body fluid. The type of experiment carried out by Krogh [9] on a large number of homoiosmotic species provides clear-cut information. The body-fluid concentration is first reduced by placing the animals in a diluted medium or distilled water. Then the animals are returned to their normal medium, which is less concentrated than the body fluid. The concentration of the body fluid could be shown to rise towards the normal value in this medium. The experiment indicates a net transfer of NaCl from the medium to the body fluid against a NaCl concentration difference. This can only be active transport. These simple experiments do not answer whether one or other or both ions are transported actively.

Experiments have also been carried out on isolated preparations of the external epithelia. Koch [7] worked with the isolated gills of the fresh-water crab *Eriocheir sinensis*. The gills are removed from the animal and ligatured at the base. These isolated epithelial sacs can be placed in various media and the ion-uptake behaviour studied. Analysis of the medium indicates a brisk net uptake of NaCl from dilute media (43 m-moles NaCl kg gill^{-1} h^{-1}). Unidirectional isotope fluxes (^{22}Na) were also studied in this preparation. Metabolic inhibitors, as would be expected, blocked this net uptake of NaCl. Thc elegant studies initiated by Ussing on ion uptake across isolated amphibian epithelia have produced a detailed picture of transport in this group. Sodium ions are actively transported inwards. The inside medium has a positive electrical potential compared to the outside and chloride ions move inwards passively [27, 28]. It is, however, dangerous to extrapolate this well-investigated system to other transporting epithelia. For example in the isolated gills of the crayfish *Austropotamobius* (*Astacus*) the body fluid is negative with respect to a dilute external medium (−60 mV) and both sodium and particularly chloride concentration in the haemolymph are above their equilibrium concentrations as defined by the Nernst equation. Both these ions must be actively transported inwards by the gill epithelium [4].

The active uptake of NaCl follows *Michaelis–Menten* type kinetics (see [5, 11]). The rate of active uptake (J_A) can be defined

$$J_A = J_{max} C_M / K_m + C_M \tag{20}$$

where J_{max} is the maximum rate of active transport and K_m the *Michaelis Constant*. This suggests that the transport is occurring via enzyme-like carrier sites in the epithelial cell membranes.

The Michaelis constant K_m, which here is the external concentration at which the available active sites are transporting at half the maximum rate or in a simple system are half in the form of a solute-site complex, must be a feature of the particular chemical system present in the animal considered. A different value of this constant implies that a different system is present. In brackish-water animals quite high values are found, e.g. *Carcinus* $K_m \simeq 20$ mM, but, in well-adapted fresh-water animals, the values may be <1 mM and in the case of the fresh-water species *Gammarus pulex* a value as low as 0·1–0·15 mM has been found. In the case of *Mesidotea*, in the brackish-water Baltic race $K_m = 12$ mM but in the fresh-water races the value is considerably reduced and in the Lake Vättern race $K_m = 1{\cdot}23$ mM, although this value is well above a number of other fresh-water species. As the sodium concentration in Lake Vättern is only 0·26 mM, this means that the transport system is operating well below maximum capacity and thus this species cannot be regarded as well adapted to this medium. Comparison of brackish- and fresh-water races of *Gammarus duebeni* also shows a reduction of K_m in fresh water. In this species another interesting phenomenon was found. A population of *Gammarus duebeni* with a fairly high K_m was kept in Lake Windermere water which, like Lake Vättern, has a very low sodium concentration and after a period of two years the K_m of this population was found to be considerably reduced.

These differences in K_m suggest biochemical adaptation of the transport system, increasing the affinity of the carrier sites for the transported ions and adapting these animals for existence in very dilute media. However, a caution should be inserted about the application of simple Michaelis–Menten kinetics to active uptake processes. If the active transport is across the inner cell membrane of the epithelial cell as envisaged in the model in Fig. 5.6, K_m will only have a simple physical meaning if the concentration of transported ion in eqn. (20) is the concentration of the transported ion in the epithelial cell fluid. A consideration of the model indicates that the concentration of the cell fluid may not necessarily be the same as the concentration in the medium. As active uptake can, however, be described by eqn. (20), it is possible to treat K_m as an operational concept.

J_{max} would be defined by the total number of carrier sites that were in an operational state. This may be less than the total number of sites present. In the short-term adaptation of an individual, the switching of sites between the inactive and active state must be an important component of the feedback control process. The total number of sites present will vary between different types and even in an individual might be subject to long-term adaptive change. There is evidence that the activation of carrier sites is controlled by body-fluid concentration, a fall in body-fluid concentration increasing the rate of active uptake in most cases studied. For this reason, experiments to determine K_m and J_{max} should be carried out on animals with a previously somewhat depleted body-fluid concentration so that all the sites are in an active state. In the case of *Mesidotea entomon*, the value of J_{max} in the Lake Vättern race considerably exceeds the value in the brackish-water race (Table 5.3). The combination of a greater number of carrier sites together with a higher affinity of these sites for the transported ion must be an important component in the adaptation of this organism to fresh water.

Table 5.3. Transport parameters in *Mesidotea entomon.*

Parameter	Baltic Population (Askö)	Lake Mälaren Population	Lake Vättern Population
C_M, m-moles Na l^{-1}	86·0	0·67	0·26
C_B, m-moles Na l^{-1}	243	246	243
K_{NaCl}, 1 kg animal^{-1} h^{-1}	0·018	0·0054	0·0056
J_{max}, m-moles Na kg animal^{-1} h^{-1}	8·5	7·85	20·8
K_M, m-moles Na l^{-1}	12·0	3·25	1·23

5.6.4 Hypoosmotic urine

A number of brackish and even fresh-water forms have successfully colonized these media without having developed the ability to produce a urine hypoosmotic to the body fluid. The brackish-water crab *Carcinus* is a well-investigated example but this feature seems to be a general rule amongst the fresh-water crabs, e.g. *Eriocheir*, *Potamon*. The antennal glands of these types have relatively short tubule systems compared to related types such as the fresh-water crayfish *Astacus*, which produces a urine markedly hypoosmotic to the body fluid. A relationship between tubule length and ability to produce a urine hypoosmotic to the body fluid is also seen in the gammarids.

The evidence for active uptake of NaCl by the excretory tubule epithelium is simply the existence of a urine hypoosmotic to the body fluid in a number of brackish and fresh-water types. Direct evidence of the localization of function in the excretory organ is more difficult to obtain. The situation is, of course, well known in the amphibian nephron but there are much less data from the invertebrates. Ramsay [18] has shown a fall in the osmotic pressure along the length of the nephridial tubule in the earthworm (*Lumbricus*). This is an open nephridium draining the general coelom. The most detailed studies are those of Riegel on the antennal gland of the crayfish [19] that have already been mentioned. Analysis of samples from various parts of this tubule system shows that the concentration falls from isoosmoticity with the haemolymph in the coelomic end sac along the tubule system. However, the greatest relative decrease in concentration is found in the bladder, the terminal part of the tubule system. This confirms the early classic study by Peters. This might suggest that the greater part of the NaCl is reabsorbed by the bladder epithelium. However, measurements of the ratio of inulin concentration in the tubule fluid and haemolymph indicate that there is significant reabsorption of water by the epithelium in this type and thus there must also be considerable reabsorption of NaCl in the earlier parts of the tubule system. Possibly the reabsorption of water is a purely passive consequence of an active reabsorption of NaCl, a relatively small fall in the osmotic pressure of the lumen contents allowing an osmotic flow of water to occur across a possibly rather water permeable epithelium. Similar isoosmotic reabsorption is important in the vertebrate nephron. In the bladder, however, NaCl reabsorption without water reabsorption occurs and the final very dilute urine is produced. The final sodium concentration of *Astacus* urine can be as low as 1 mM compared to a haemolymph sodium concentration of 200 mM. An impressive performance by any standard.

When *Gammarus duebeni* and *Astacus* are living in media approaching the concentration of sea water, the urine is isoosmotic with the haemolymph. It is only when the animals are adapted to more dilute media that the mechanisms of tubular reabsorption operate to produce a urine hypoosmotic to the body fluid. The mechanism controlling production of a hypoosmotic urine is complex and, although it is undoubtedly related to body-fluid concentration, it also appears to involve other sensory inputs.

There is an obvious tendency to regard the continued production of a urine isoosmotic with the medium as a primitive feature. Thus the question of the advantage in producing a urine hypoosmotic to the body fluid should be considered. Eqn. (13) could still define a steady state if all the NaCl uptake was across the external epithelium. The advantages of developing a mechanism for taking up NaCl from the tubule fluid are undoubtedly due to the higher concentration of NaCl in the tubule fluid compared to the lower concentration in the external medium. There is a possible thermodynamic advantage in taking up NaCl from a medium with a high NaCl concentration and this will be discussed in detail in a later section. Another advantage is simple kinetic efficiency. With probably a limited number of carrier sites and possible a fairly high K_m, there would be a more rapid uptake from a more concentrated NaCl solution.

Where data are available for both urine concentration and urine volume flow rate, the net loss of NaCl in the urine can be determined and compared with the total net passive NaCl efflux. The losses via the urine usually turn out to be a relatively small proportion of the total loss. This is even so in the case of types such as *Eriocheir* and *Potamon* which produce a urine isoosmotic with the body fluid and this is a result of low overall water permeability. In *Potamon* the extremely low overall water permeability means that loss of NaCl in the urine is entirely negligible. In *Astacus* also the loss via the excretory organ in dilute external media is negligible, although this would not be the case if the urine was isoosmotic with the haemolymph. An exception is the fresh-water prawn *Palaemonetes antennarius*. The overall water permeability of this animal is rather high and the urine is isoosmotic with the haemolymph. This animal should clearly consider the advantages of producing a urine hypoosmotic to the haemolymph. Due to difficulties in obtaining uncontaminated samples from a maxillary gland, it has not been possible to determine the urine concentration and volume flow rate in *Mesidotea entomon* or in any other *isopod.*

5.7 CONTROL MECHANISMS AND MODEL SYSTEMS

The rates at which substances enter and leave the body fluid by various routes and mechanisms determine the way in which the composition of the body fluid varies with time and more importantly the final *steady state*. In principle it should be possible to predict the way the osmotic regulation system should behave. In practice insufficient information is known about the components of the systems to make an exact prediction. However, making a number of simplifying assumptions, *model systems* can be considered that predict a number of observed phenomena and may perhaps emphasize those aspects of osmotic regulation that require further investigation. Some biochemical events associated with osmoregulation are mentioned in Chapter 12.

The concept of *negative feedback control* (as in other areas of regulatory physiology, Chapter 20) is of great importance. This is an engineering concept that has increasing application to physiology. Such a system has two parts: a *controlled system* and a *controller*. The property of the controlled system that is being controlled, the *controlled variable*, is monitored continuously by a *sensor*. The value of the controlled variable is fed back to a *comparator* and compared with a previously determined *set point*. The difference between the value of the set point and the controlled variable is the *output error*. When suitably amplified this can be used to actuate an *effector* that acts on the controlled system in such a way as to minimize the output error. *Physiological control systems* operate in a similar way and subjects such as control of position, temperature, ventilation rate, cardiac output and mammalian kidney function have been investigated. Perusal of the literature (e.g. [20]) shows that this is a difficult field.

An attempt will be made here to apply the concepts of feedback control in a very simple manner to osmotic regulation. The various components in a *feedback system* can be related by a *block diagram*. This has been done for an osmotic regulation system (Fig. 5.8). If, for each component of such a system, the equation describing its behaviour can be derived, the simultaneous solution of these equations describes the way the controlled variable varies with time, e.g. after changing the concentration of the outer medium. In the case considered, such a solution presents little difficulty. In more complex models, computed solutions may be necessary.

The behaviour of the controlled system has been simplified. All contributions of the excretory organ to NaCl balance have been ignored. This may not be such

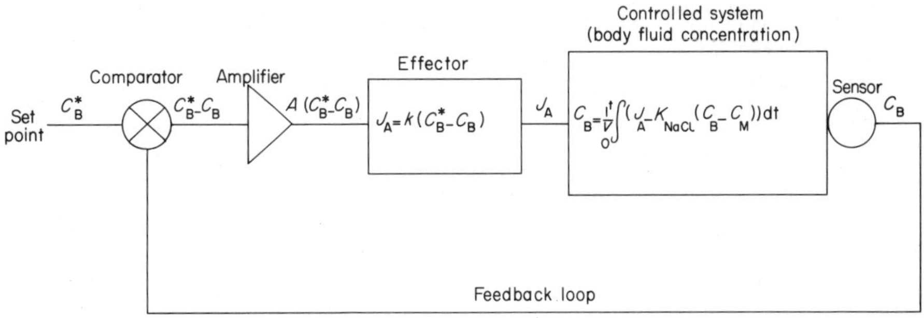

Fig. 5.8. Block diagram of a simple osmotic regulation feedback system. C_B, concentration of body fluid; C_M concentration of medium; C^*_B, set point; A, gain of amplifier; k, overall gain of controller; V, volume of body fluid; K_{NaCl}, overall permeability; J_A, rate of active uptake.

an extreme simplification, as, in the majority of fresh-water types, the greater part of NaCl loss from the body fluid is across the external surface rather than in the urine. The identity of the sense organs is unknown. They could be specific ion chemoreceptors, osmoreceptors or operate indirectly as body-fluid volume (stretch) receptors or possibly a combination of such receptors. The connections between the various components could be nervous and/or endocrine.

A possible point of oversimplification is that in the block diagram the output error is *linear*. In fact the output from many animal sense organs is *logarithmic.* This is the *Weber–Fechner Law* of sensory physiology. The mechanism and significance of this type of output is not altogether clear, although any sense organ, the response of which involves a sodium ion inrush, would have the response ultimately limited by the Nernst potential of sodium and could be expected to show non-linear response characteristics, which would approximate to a logarithmic response over part of the stimulus intensity range. If the sense organ is an ion-specific electrode, i.e. with a membrane selectively permeable to sodium or chloride ion, the membrane potential would be defined by the Nernst potential for that ion, which is logarithmically related to the concentration of that ion outside the membrane.

Assuming that the Weber–Fechner Law applies to the overall behaviour of the controller

$$J_A = k \log_e (C^*_B/C_B) \tag{21}$$

where the symbols are the same as in Fig. 5.8 except that k the *overall gain* of the controller is dimensionally different. This equation has been applied in a simple model of the steady state [3]. Ignoring NaCl loss in the urine, eqn. (13) simplifies

$$J_A = J_E \tag{22}$$

substituting from eqn. (21) and eqn. (9)

$$k \log_e (C^*_B/C_B) = K_{NaCl}\,(C_B - C_M) \tag{23}$$

This equation was solved to predict body-fluid concentration as a function of medium concentration for various arbitrary values of $k/(K_{NaCl}\,C^*_B)$. The results

(Fig. 5.9) are not altogether unlike the adaptation isotherms of a number of brackish-water animals.

More realistic models can also be developed. A finite number of transport sites can be in either the inactive or active state and it will be assumed that the number of active sites is controlled by a Weber–Fechner type relation. The sites, when active, transport at a rate determined by the Michaelis–Menten equation. Then it should be possible to approximate the behaviour of the controller by a relation of the following type

$$J_A = \left(J_{max} \frac{1}{1+1/k \log_e (C_B^*/C_B)} \right) \left(\frac{C_M}{K_m + C_M} \right) \tag{24}$$

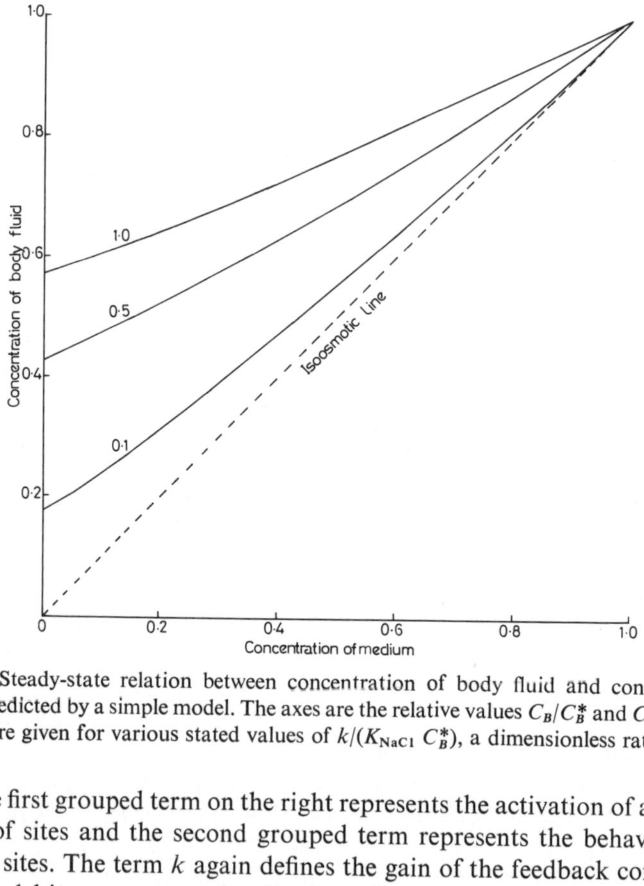

Fig. 5.9. Steady-state relation between concentration of body fluid and concentration of medium predicted by a simple model. The axes are the relative values C_B/C_B^* and C_M/C_B^* and the solutions are given for various stated values of $k/(K_{NaCl}\ C_B^*)$, a dimensionless ratio.

where the first grouped term on the right represents the activation of a finite total number of sites and the second grouped term represents the behaviour of the activated sites. The term k again defines the gain of the feedback controller but in this model is a more complex dimensionless term.

If the uptake component defined by eqn. (24) is now equated with the rate of loss of substrate from the body fluid, eqn. (9), as was done for the simpler model, a more realistic model is obtained. The steady-state relation between body-fluid concentration and medium concentration can be computed if the experimental values of J_{max}, K_m and K_{NaCl} are available. This can be attempted for the isopod *Mesidotea entomon* using data in [5, 11] and Lockwood and Croghan (in preparation). A comparison will be made between the population living in the brackish water of the Baltic and the populations isolated in fresh water in Lake Mälaren and in Lake Vättern. The experimental data used are given in Table 5.3. Adaptive differences between the populations are apparent, particularly in the case of the Lake Vättern population. In Fig. 5.10, the computed body-fluid concentration of the brackish-water population is compared with the experimental values. The set point has been assumed to be 300 mM and solutions are given for various stated values of k. The permeability

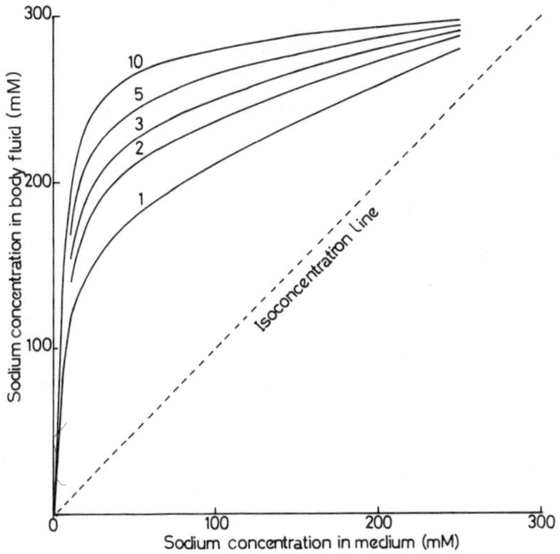

Fig. 5.10. Steady-state relation between the sodium concentration in the body fluid and medium computed using experimental parameters for *Mesidotea entomon* (brackish-water race) and various stated values of k, a dimensionless term.

is assumed to be constant at the stated value. Agreement between theory and experiment seems to be quite close, suggesting that the assumptions made in developing the model bear some relation to reality. These brackish-water animals are incapable of surviving in very dilute media and the dramatic and ultimately lethal fall in body-fluid concentration found in the more dilute media is also shown by the model.

The case of the fresh-water populations can now be considered. In the case of the Lake Mälaren animals, using the stated experimental values (Table 5.3) and assuming the set point to be 300 mM, it is just possible to predict the body-fluid concentration found in fresh water but only by taking large values of k (>1000). This means that *all* the carrier sites must be active. There is in fact experimental evidence for this, as fresh-water *Mesidotea* are incapable of increasing the influx of sodium when the body-fluid concentration is lowered below the normal value. This phenomenon is unusual in fresh-water animals and this lack of safety margin indicates that *Mesidotea* is surviving on the extreme edge of its physiological range. The value of k required to predict survival in fresh water, however, predicts a steeper rise in body-fluid concentration as the external concentration is increased than is in fact observed. However, the model assumes that permeability and k are constant but there is evidence that the low permeability of the fresh-water population is an adaptation to a high degree of dilution and that in more concentrated media the permeability rises to values more similar to that of the brackish-water population (Fig. 5.7). It is also possible that the very high values of k required can be considered as an adaptation to the extreme dilutions and that this value may fall in more concentrated media.

In the case of the Lake Vättern animals, again assuming the set point to be about 300 mM, it is possible to predict the body-fluid concentration found in fresh water using a much lower value of k (= 3), even although the sodium concentration in Lake Vättern is considerably less than in Lake Mälaren. This is a consequence of the higher value of J_{max} and lower value of K_m in the Lake Vättern animals. Again with the Lake Vättern animals, there is a steeper predicted rise in body-fluid concentration as the external concentration is increased than is in fact observed. However, the increase in permeability in the higher external concentrations and a possible decrease in k could correct this. A problem that should be mentioned is that the Lake Vättern *Mesidotea* also does not seem to be able to increase the rate of active uptake if the body fluid concentration is further reduced. Yet from the data in Table 5.3 and assuming that all the transport sites are active, eqn. (24) predicts that higher rates of active uptake should be possible. This point requires further investigation. It seems clear that with *Mesidotea entomon* there are distinct physiological races in the brackish and fresh-water habitats. The principal adaptations to fresh water being reduction of solute permeability, a larger number of carrier sites, carrier sites with a higher affinity for solute and changes in the gain of the feedback system. There are differences between the two fresh-water populations investigated. The Lake Mälaren population seems to be less well-adapted to fresh water and survival is only possible with, in terms of the model, an enormous gain in the feedback control system. The Lake Vättern population seems, with its large number of transport sites and their high affinity for solute, to be better adapted to very dilute fresh water. These two populations must have originated independently. The fresh-water habitats of *Mesidotea* in Scandinavia are a series of fresh-water lakes that became separated from the Baltic basin at various times since the end of the last ice age. Adaptations of the type considered must have evolved several times in this species over a relatively short time period.

5.8 ENERGETICS OF ADAPTATION

Transport processes are of two types: passive and active. When there is a net movement of a substance down a gradient of its electrochemical potential, the movement may be passive but when there is a net movement up a gradient of its electrochemical potential the movement must be active, which means that there must be an input of metabolic energy in some form to drive the transport process. The amount of energy required is related to the difference of electrochemical potential, which has both concentration and electrical potential terms, and to the efficiency of the transport process.

The energy input required to transport a mole (ΔG_T) of NaCl from solution A to solution B is given by

$$\Delta G_T = RT \log_e (Na_B Cl_B / Na_A Cl_A) \tag{25}$$

where the bracketed terms are the concentrations of the ions in the two media. As in most situations $Na_A \simeq Cl_A$ and $Na_B \simeq Cl_B$, the equation can usually be approximated

$$\Delta G_T = 2\, RT \log_e (\mathrm{NaCl}_B / \mathrm{NaCl}_A) \tag{26}$$

The term ΔG_T is the *free energy change* of the transport process. It is the minimum energy input required and would only be approached if the transport process was completely efficient and operating infinitely slowly, i.e. in thermodynamic terms a *reversible process*.

Direct measurements of the efficiency of transport system present problems. Perhaps the most satisfactory approach is that of Zerahn [30] using frog skin. In this convenient preparation, it was possible to measure simultaneously oxygen consumption (and thus energy production) and rate of active transport of sodium. By varying the conditions, the sodium transport could be changed and related to the change in oxygen consumption that occurred. Efficiencies of less than 50% were obtained in most cases. As ΔNa active flux/ΔO_2 consumption was essentially constant, it is clear that the efficiency varies with the conditions under which transport is occurring.

The problems in applying these equations have been considered by Croghan [3]. It is envisaged that the energy input is obtained from another reaction coupled in some specific way to the actual transport reaction. Under reversible conditions, ΔG_E of the energy supply reaction would be equal and opposite to ΔG_T of the actual transport reaction. However, any real process occurring at a significant rate will not be reversible. Then $-\Delta G_E > \Delta G_T$ and the difference is wasted as heat. Consider the situation when a given transport system is operating against a varying concentration ratio of NaCl. Under isoosmotic conditions, when the concentration is the same in both solutions, no thermodynamic transport work is in fact done and the system is thus completely inefficient. As the concentration ratio increases, the work done by the system and thus its efficiency increases until $\Delta G_T = -\Delta G_E$ when the system is operating completely efficiently but infinitely slowly.

The energy requirements for transporting NaCl from the external medium into the body fluid can be considered. The value of ΔG_T for animals showing marked hyperosmoticity in dilute external media is increased considerably. It is possible that the energy available from the energy supply reaction coupled to the transport process might be a limiting factor in adaptation to dilute media, as $-\Delta G_E$ must $>\Delta G_T$, and thus adaptation at the level of the energy supply mechanism may be required. Adaptation reducing the energy required for hyperosmotic regulation can be considered at two levels. Decrease of external permeability and/or a lowering of body fluid concentration reduces the passive efflux from the animal and thus reduces the active flux and thus energy input required to maintain the steady state. Further, a lowering of the body fluid concentration reduces the solute concentration ratio across which active uptake must occur. If advantage is to be obtained from this reduced solute concentration ratio, the energy supply process must adapt and $-\Delta G_E$ must be reduced towards the value of ΔG_T. Changes in ΔG_E may well occur in long-term evolutionary processes but are less likely in the short-term adaptation of individuals.

Attempts have been made to consider the energetics of the excretory system. Some remarkably early attempts were made by Dreser and others to consider the very complex case of the vertebrate kidney (see [23]) but the most relevant to the problems considered here is that of Potts [15]. The basis of this is that even when a urine hypoosmotic to the body fluid is produced, the fluid entering the proximal end of the excretory tubule is isoosmotic with the body fluid. This means that much of the reabsorbed solute is being transported from the tubule lumen to the body fluid across much smaller concentration ratios than that from the external medium to body fluid. The value for ΔG_T for this tubule transport can be calculated from the solution of the equation

$$\Delta G_T = \frac{2\,RT}{\mathrm{n}} \int_{C_T = C_B}^{C_T = C_U} \left(\log_e \frac{C_B}{C_T}\right) \mathrm{dn} \qquad (27)$$

where C_B is the body-fluid concentration and C_T is the tubule concentration which decreases from C_B to C_U (the final urine concentration) and n the number of moles of NaCl transported.

The value of ΔG_B calculated from this equation must always be considerably less than for a similar uptake from the external medium, as the concentration of the external medium is considerably less than the concentration at any point in the tubule lumen. Potts claimed therefore that for animals hyperosmotic to the external medium there were significant energetic advantages in producing a hypoosmotic urine.

A number of fresh-water types do in fact produce a hypoosmotic urine and, in the case of *Gammarus duebeni* and the crayfish *Astacus*, the urine, which is isoosmotic with the body fluids in media approaching sea water, becomes hypoosmotic to the body fluid in dilute brackish-water media. There must clearly be some advantage in producing a hypoosmotic urine. Although, as has been discussed here, ΔG_T is not directly relevant, it is possible that, if there are a series of different transport processes zoned along the length of the excretory tubule, the value of $-\Delta G_E$ of the reaction in each zone could be adapted so that it was not excessively greater than ΔG_T in that zone. Then there would be an energetic advantage in producing a hypoosmotic urine. The advantage would of course be more significant in more permeable forms producing larger urine flow rates. There could also be a kinetic advantage in producing a hypoosmotic urine. In maintaining a steady state, it would be easier for a limited number of carrier sites to transport solute from the relatively high concentration in the tubule lumen than to excrete an isoosmotic urine and then to reabsorb solute from the lower external concentration.

Numerous measurements have been made of the total respiratory metabolism of animals adapted to various media concentrations. The minimum energy required for regulation of the body-fluid composition is only a very low proportion of total body metabolic energy, although this must be partly a result of the adaptations discussed. However, estimates for total minimum energy requirements for regulation should also include components for regulation of intracellular composition. In conclusion, any adaptations that might tend to decrease the energy requirements of the organism must be regarded as advantageous.

5.9 REFERENCES

1 Baldwin E. (1964) *An Introduction to Comparative Biochemistry*, 4th edition. Cambridge University Press, London.

2 Conway E.J. (1943) The chemical evolution of the ocean. *Proc. Roy. Irish Acad. B.* **48,** 161.

3 Croghan P.C. (1961) Competition and mechanisms of osmotic adaptation. *Symp. Soc. Exp. Biol.* **15,** 156.

4 Croghan P.C., Curra R.A. & Lockwood A.P.M. (1965) The electrical potential difference across the epithelium of isolated gills of the crayfish *Austropotamobius pallipes* (Lereboullet). *J. Exp. Biol.* **42,** 463.

5 Croghan P.C. & Lockwood A.P.M. (1968) Ionic regulation of the Baltic and fresh-water races of the isopod *Mesidotea* (*Saduria*) *entomon* (L.). *J. Exp. Biol.* **48,** 141.

6 House C.R. (1974) *Water Transport in Cells and Tissues.* Monograph of the Physiological Society **24.** Arnold, London.

7 Koch H.J. (1954) Cholinesterase and active transport of sodium chloride through the isolated gills of the crab *Eriocheir sinensis* (M. Edw.). *Recent Developments in Cell Physiology* (ed. J. A. Kitching). Butterworth, London.

8 Koefoed-Johnsen V. & Ussing H.H. (1958) The nature of the frog skin potential. *Acta Physiol. Scand.* **42,** 298.

9 Krogh A. (1939) *Osmotic Regulation in Aquatic Animals.* Cambridge University Press, London.

10 Lockwood A.P.M. (1967) *Animal Body Fluids and their Regulation.* Heinemann, London.

11 Lockwood A.P.M., Croghan P.C. & Sutcliffe D.W. (1976) Sodium regulation and adaptation to dilute media in crustacea as exemplified by the isopod *Mesidotea entomon* and the amphipod *Gammarus duebeni*. *Perspectives in Experimental Biology*, Vol. 1 (ed. P. Spencer Davies). Pergamon Press, Oxford.

12 Macallum A.B. (1926) The palaeochemistry of body fluids and tissues. *Physiol. Rev.* **6,** 316.

13 Morris J.G. (1974) *A Biologist's Physical Chemistry*, 2nd edition. Arnold, London.

14 Pantin C.F.A. (1931) The origin of the composition of the body fluids of animals. *Biol. Rev.* **6,** 459.

15 Potts W.T.W. (1954) The energetics of osmotic regulation in brackish- and fresh-water animals. *J. Exp. Biol.* **31,** 618.

16 Potts W.T.W. & Parry G. (1964) *Osmotic and Ionic Regulation in Animals.* Pergamon Press, Oxford.
17 Prosser C.L. (1973) *Comparative Animal Physiology*, 3rd edition. Saunders, Philadelphia.
18 Ramsay J.A. (1949) The site of formation of hypotonic urine in the nephridium of the earthworm, *Lumbricus. J. Exp. Biol.* **26,** 65.
19 Riegel J.A. (1972) *Comparative Physiology of Renal Excretion.* Oliver & Boyd, Edinburgh.
20 Riggs D.S. (1970). *Control Theory and Physiological Feedback Mechanisms.* Williams & Wilkins, Baltimore.
21 Robertson J.D. (1957) Osmotic and ionic regulation in aquatic invertebrates. *Recent Advances in Invertebrate Physiology* (ed. B. T. Scheer). Oregon.
22 Robertson J.D. (1960) Osmotic and ionic regulation. *The Physiology of Crustacea* 1 (ed. T. H. Waterman). Academic Press, New York & London.
23 Robinson J.R. (1954) *Reflections on Renal Function.* Blackwell Scientific Publications, Oxford.
24 Schoffeniels E. (1976) Biochemical approaches to osmoregulatory processes in crustacea. *Perspectives in Experimental Biology* Vol. 1 (ed. P. Spencer Davies). Pergamon Press, Oxford.
25 Smith R.I. (1976) Apparent water-permeability variation and water exchange in crustaceans and annelids. *Perspectives in Experimental Biology*, Vol. 1 (ed. P. Spencer Davies). Pergamon Press, Oxford.
26 Shaw J. (1961) Studies on ionic regulation in *Carcinus maenas* (L.). 1. Sodium balance. *J. Exp. Biol.* **38,** 135.
27 Ussing H.H. (1954) Active transport of inorganic ions. *Symp. Soc. Exp. Biol.* **8,** 407.
28 Ussing H.H. (1960) The alkali metal ions in isolated systems and tissues. *Handb. Exp. Pharm.* **13,** 1.
29 Webb D.A. (1940) Ionic regulation in *Carcinus maenas. Proc. Roy. Soc. B.* **129,** 107.
30 Zerahn K. (1956) Oxygen consumption and active sodium transport in the isolated short-circuited frog skin. *Acta Physiol. Scand.* **36,** 300.

Prelude to Chapter 6

Table 4·1 (p. 50) listed the physical and chemical characteristics of aquatic environments. Some of the factors mentioned are even more significant on land, others less so. In general, aquatic environments are more stable than terrestrial ones and, consequently, land animals are exposed to far greater environmental fluctuations than are aquatic organisms. This applies particularly to temperature, humidity and radiation. At night, or when it enters a cave, for example, a desert animal experiences a very marked alteration in these factors. On the other hand, a terrestrial animal lives at a hydrostatic pressure of about 1 atm ($100\ kNm^{-2}$), which is both low and effectively constant in comparison with the pressure range in the sea. The significance of the familiar decrease in atmospheric pressure with increase in altitude lies in the reduced partial pressures of atmospheric gases, particularly oxygen.

Although poisonous, ammonia is very soluble and consequently is an efficient excretory compound for aquatic organisms. Terrestrial animals, on the other hand, with few exceptions excrete either insoluble substances such as uric acid and guanine, or else some non-toxic soluble substance like urea. The possession of insoluble nitrogenous end products is correlated with the possession of a '*cleidoic*', or enclosed egg, whose embryo would be poisoned if it were to excrete ammonia and would also be destroyed by the osmotic pressure of concentrated urea. Cleidoic eggs are characteristic of insects, reptiles and birds. The waste products of the mammalian embryo are removed through the placenta and excreted by the kidney of the mother. Thus there is no harmful build up of urea to upset the osmotic balance of the fetus. In shifting attention from aquatic to terrestrial environments, therefore, emphasis must needs be redirected to different environmental factors than those of primary importance to aquatic animals and to the new physiological adjustments that become necessary for the maintenance of homeostasis.

Chapter 6
Terrestrial environments

J.L.CLOUDSLEY-THOMPSON

6.1 INTRODUCTION

Whether or not life actually began in the sea is still unsolved (Chapter 3), but certainly animal evolution has occurred mostly in the sea. The earliest known fossils are those of marine animals and, although many large taxa of animals have no terrestrial or fresh-water representatives, there is no major group without any marine relatives [4]. Another indication of the marine origins of contemporary animals is afforded by the comparative physiology of their intra-cellular and extra-cellular body fluids (see Chapter 5).

On account of their high reproductive potential (a quality which first impressed Charles Darwin with the inevitability of evolution by natural selection [8]) living organisms rapidly populate all available ecological niches and there is continual pressure on them to exploit new ones. The conquest of the land, which has occurred independently within at least three separate phyla *viz.*, Mollusca, Arthropoda and Chordata, may well have been the result of both inter-specific and intra-specific competition. Adaptation to life on land presents animals with a number of physiological problems of homeostasis. These are associated mainly with water conservation, nitrogenous excretion, osmoregulation, respiration and locomotion, and are discussed in the following Chapters.

The atmosphere provides a high and constant concentration of oxygen which permits a fast rate of metabolism and a considerable degree of structural and physiological development. Its low thermal conductivity and heat capacity, as compared with water, enables terrestial animals to maintain a considerable differential between their bodies and the temperature of the environment. This is almost impossible for aquatic animals unless they are of sufficient size to carry substantial amounts of subcutaneous, or water-impermeable supra-cutaneous thermal insulation. Certain fishes such as the tuna and some sharks are able, by means of circulatory counter-current heat exchange structures, to maintain the temperatures of active muscles as much as 14°C above the water in which they are swimming. Muscle action, like all other chemical and biochemical processes is temperature-dependent (see Chapter 20) and the high operating temperature enables these species successfully to pursue speedy prey, such as mackerel and pelagic squids, which can swim so fast that they could not otherwise be caught. Although the force exerted by a contracting muscle is relatively independent of temperature, muscle contracts faster at higher ambient temperatures and, since the number of contractions per unit time increases, so does the power output [18]. In general, however, true tachymetabolism and homeothermy has evolved only in terrestrial birds and mammals, although some of them, including penguins, seals and whales, have subsequently returned to the sea.

6.2 SIZE AND ENVIRONMENT

The greatest physiological problem associated with a transfer to an atmospheric terrestrial environment lies in the maintenance of an aquatic internal environment despite the high rate of evaporation that inevitably occurs, especially during pulmonary respiration. Small animals, such as arthropods, have a very large surface area in proportion to their mass. Consequently, the conservation of water for the maintenance of a fairly constant aqueous internal medium is especially important to terrestrial members of that phylum. Desiccation is avoided, to some extent, by the evolution of a water-proof, epicuticular wax-layer; but gas exchange must still occur across the permeable surfaces inside spiracles, lung-books and so on. The physiology of respiration, as well as of excretion, in small terrestrial animals is thus intimately concerned with water conservation. In contrast, in larger animals with a very much lower surface to volume ratio, water conservation and respiration are less acute problems. On the other hand, the higher ratio of body mass to linear dimensions affects locomotory mechanisms (see Chapter 8), for gravity becomes an increasingly important factor in the environment of larger terrestrial animals.

The size of an animal is related to the kind of skeleton it possesses. Two main types of skeleton occur; the exoskeletons of Arthropoda and the endoskeletons of vertebrates. An exoskeleton is basically a tubular structure which is extremely resistant to twisting and bending but which, above a certain size, becomes disproportionately heavy. Tubular structures are light, but much more prone to collapse when stressed than solid girders are—as bridge builders have recently re-discovered.

The size of arthropods is also limited by the fact that animals encased in armoured skeletons can grow only by moulting. After a certain size has been reached, linear dimensions increase only slightly at each ecdysis, although the arthropod may nearly double its weight.

The skeletons of vertebrate animals are structurally and functionally related to both the size and the locomotion of the species [1, 11]. The capacity of a column to support weight per unit of transverse area varies inversely as the square of its length. It is not surprising therefore, that the leg bones of heavy vertebrates tend to be proportionately shorter than those of lighter species.

Tracheal respiration could, theoretically, be efficient, even in quite large animals, if there were sufficient air-sacs to circulate tidal air throughout the main tracheal branches so that the distances to be covered by diffusion were not great. It is, nevertheless, a deterrent to large size and it is probably significant that the biggest insects either have long, slender bodies, like dragonflies and mantids, or else they tend to be very sluggish, like Goliath and Hercules beetles. It seems probable, too, that very large terrestrial arthropods may also be limited by their vulnerability, since their exoskeletons cannot be strengthened by the deposition of calcium carbonate, as in marine Crustacea, for reasons of weight. The significance of the nocturnal habits of scorpions and Solifugae may be related to attack by predators: even dangerous stings and powerful jaws are no protection against the huge beaks of marabou storks or the hooves of antelopes [2, 5]. Thus morphology, physiology and behaviour are affected not only by the physical and chemical attributes of the environment, but also by its biotic factors. Plants and other animals are an integral part of the environment and, consequently, they affect environmental physiology as physical factors do.

The extent of the influence of different components of the environment depends to a large extent upon the size of the animal. This is particularly true of terrestrial animals whose habitats are far less homogeneous than those of marine animals. Very small animals are able to escape the rigours of life on land by seeking less stressful microhabitats such as soil crevices, leaf litter, cracks in rocks, the spaces beneath the bark of trees and so on, where the evaporating power of the air is negligible or non-existant, temperature fluctuations are almost eliminated and the light is excluded [6, 16]. The cryptozoic animals that enjoy a hidden life in such secluded surroundings have been discussed in detail [14], and some aspects of their physiology are considered in Chapter 7. In general, they avoid desiccation on land by behavioral means: they spend most, if not all of the time, in a moist environment [3, 10].

Even within orders, mean environmental temperatures may influence size and dimensions. Fishes that live in cold waters tend to be larger and to have more vertebrae than closely related species that live in warmer seas. This observation was first made by David Starr Jordan, the 19th-century American zoologist. The proportions of the body are an important factor in thermoregulation, especially among terrestrial animals. The effect of climate on the evolution of the proportions of the extremities and appendages of animals was noted by J. A. Allen of the American Museum of Natural History, also in the last century. The radiation potential of a cylinder increases in proportion to the square of its diameter. This physical fact probably lies behind the natural selection of the lean and lanky build of many of the larger vertebrates, such as goats, camels and gazelles, that inhabit hot desert and semi-arid regions of the world. Conversely, the mammals from the Arctic tend to have short legs and stocky bodies. For example, the musk ox (*Ovibos moschatus*) has legs so short that it stands only one metre high, although it is two and a half metres long. Its neck is thick, its tail very short and its ears are hidden in its furry coat.

Carl Bergmann's rule, published in 1847, states that warm-blooded mammals and birds from colder climates are larger, and therefore have proportionately less surface area from which to lose heat, than corresponding homeotherms of warmer regions. The African elephant (*Loxodonta africana*), is an apparent exception, but its surface area is increased approximately one third by its enormous ears. These have a rich blood supply and almost certainly serve as radiators for cooling the body during the heat of the day. The significance of this becomes even more obvious when we remember that an elephant may weigh as much as a million mice, but its linear dimensions are only about 100 times greater and its heat production per unit of tissue is much smaller.

The ecological significance of Bergmann's rule has recently been challenged on the ground that a position correlation of weight with latitude in homeotherms cannot normally depend upon the physics of heat exchange, and that an animal does not live on a per-gram basis, but as an intact individual [15]. Only the smallest species of a group of similar predators normally conforms to Bergmann's rule, and the most widespread mammals in North America do not do so. Instead, it has been suggested that a correlation of body size with latitude in carnivores may reflect the size of the available prey. This, in turn, is influenced by the distribution both of the prey and of other predators with which it must be shared.

The physiological implications of size are considerable. They affect all aspects of an animal's life, from its embryological development and growth to the amount and nature of the food that it requires. The relative dimensions of the different organs of the body of an animal also depend upon its size. Indeed, size is perhaps the most important single factor influencing variations in the physiological processes, as well as in the morphological relations of terrestrial animals.

A major problem of comparative physiology is therefore one of scaling—that is, of making valid comparisons between animals of different sizes. In most mammals, the size of the heart is directly related to that of the body, about 5 g and 6 g/kg body wt. The weight of the skeleton, however, increases more than proportionately. The slope of the regression line when one is plotted against the other, is 1·13. When body surface (M^2) is plotted against body weight (kg), however, the regression line has a slope of 6·7 and, when metabolic rate is plotted (kJh^{-1}) it is about 3·1. There is a tremendous increase in the metabolic rate of very small mammals compared with large species. Lung volume of mammals is scaled in simple proportion to body size, as indicated by a slope of the regression line of nearly 1·0. The same is true of the ratio of alveolar surface area to oxygen consumption. The question therefore arises, should drug doses be related to weight, metabolic rate or brain size? Scaling is not a simple problem but it is an important one, especially in environmental and comparative physiology [17].

6.3 WORLD CLIMATES

The major climatic regions of the world and the principle types of vegetation they support can be summarized as follows (Table 6.1) [7]. From this it can be seen that the type of vegetation found depends primarily on temperature and rainfall.

Table 6.1. Classification of world climates and vegetation.

A. *Hot climates:* Mean annual temperatures above 21°C.	
1. Equatorial	(Rain-forest)
2. Tropical marine	(Rain-forest)
3. Tropical continental	(Savanna)
B. *Warm temperate (or sub-tropical)*: No month below 6°C.	
1. Western margin	(Temperate forest)
2. Eastern margin	(Temperate forest)
3. Continental	(Steppe)
C. *Cool temperate*: One to five months below 6°C.	
1. Marine	(Temperate forest)
2. Continental	(Taiga or steppe)
D. *Cold climates*: Six or more months below 6°C.	
1. Marine	(Taiga)
2. Continental or boreal	(Taiga or steppe)
E. *Arctic climates*: No month above 10°C.	
	(Tundra)
F. *Desert climates*: Low rainfall.	
1. Hot: No month below 6°C.	
2. Cold: One or more months below 6°C.	
G. *Mountain climates*: Depend on latitude and altitude.	

6.4 TERRESTRIAL BIOMES

Large animals are far less able to evade the vagaries of meteorology than are cyptozoic forms: consequently, the climatic and biotic conditions of the biomes in which they live are far more significant to them. The principal terrestrial biomes of the world are described below.

(a) *Tropical forest*

A vast girdle of rain-forest encircling the earth between the tropics enjoys a humid tropical climate in which the average daily range of temperature exceeds by several times the difference between the warmest and coolest months of the year. The sun's rays are never far from vertical, and day lengths vary little throughout the year. The abundance of cloud and dense forest prevents excessive temperatures and the climate is characterized by its uniformity and monotony. There is little seasonal change and the differences between day and night are less marked than in open country.

(b) *Savanna*

Park-like savanna-woodlands are found where the dry season is longer and the rainfall less than in regions of tropical forest. Precipitation is variable, the rainy season is usually ushered in and out by violent thunderstorms and wind squalls alternating with extremely hot sunshine. Flora and fauna are dominated by the seasons: in the absence of marked changes in day length and temperature, the pronounced division of savanna climate into wet and dry seasons is the main meteorological factor affecting the environmental physiology of savanna animals.

(c) *Hot desert*

Beyond the limits of the annual swing of the equatorial rainfall belt, at the latitudes in which the trade winds blow throughout the year, lie the world's greatest deserts, where the annual precipitation is below 0·25 M. Hot deserts, such as the Sahara and Kalahari, have no cold season but, in 'cold deserts', like the Gobi and Great Basin, one or more of the winter months has a mean temperature below 6°C. Aridity, rather than high mean temperatures, is the most characteristic feature of the desert. Desert climates are subject to extremes. High temperatures and low humidity during the day are followed by comparatively cold nights. Long periods of drought are broken by torrential rainfall and flooding and, although desert rainfall tends to be seasonal, it is most erratic and unreliable.

(d) *Steppe*

Temperate grasslands occupy the interiors of continents in temperate regions where the summers are hot, the winters are cold, and the annual rainfall is low. Only on the shores of lakes and along the banks of rivers is there usually sufficient moisture for trees to grow.

(e) *Temperate forest*

This may take many forms depending on the climatic regions. In cooler latitudes the trees are mainly deciduous, but evergreens predominate in warmer regions. The three main types are: temperate deciduous, moist temperate coniferous and broad-leaved deciduous forest.

(f) *Taiga*

This is a form of coniferous forest which exists in regions where the growing season is too short to support deciduous woodlands. Because they are evergreen, coniferous trees are ready to begin photosynthesis without delay as soon as temperatures become favourable. Moreover, the coniferous type of fructification has the advantage that it is pollinated one year and dispersed the next, whereas deciduous trees have to complete the process in a single season. Length of growing season with temperatures above the threshold for growth, is clearly the most significant factor controlling forest types.

(g) *Tundra and snowlands*

Arctic climates can be divided into two types: (i) Tundra climates with a summer, however short, above freezing and (ii) Polar or perpetual frost climates in which the growth of vegetation is impossible. The inequality of the length of day and night reaches its maximum: insolation is absent in winter and continuous in summer. Tundra vegetation is exposed to extremely adverse circumstances which eliminate all but a few hardy species. A long period of frost is followed by an extremely short growing season and most of the tundra overlies deep deposits of sphagnum, resulting from the failure of dead plants to decompose at low temperature.

(h) *Mountains*

On account of the low temperatures strong winds and short summers, trees do not grow at high altitudes. The Alpine zone, above the timberline is in many ways similar to tundra and snowlands. There are certain differences, however. At high altitudes atmospheric pressure is reduced. Photoperiod is related to latitude rather than to altitude and, at high elevations, the atmosphere is thin. Consequently, insolation is powerful on mountain tops, in contrast to Arctic snowlands where the rays of the sun are strongly filtered as they pass obliquely through the atmosphere. Winds reach high speeds because frictional drag with the earth's surface is reduced.

6.5 SELECTIVE INFLUENCES

The various macro-environments described above can be classified according to their climates or by topographical features. The topography of the land and the variations of its climate represent the same part in the make up of the environment, figuratively speaking, as morphology and physiology do in the life of an animal [12]. Thus, irrespective of climate, the mammalian fauna of desert, savanna, steppe, tundra and high plateaux have certain features in common. In each, the dominant forms tend to be either large, cursorial herbivores, or subterranean rodents with social habits. The structural adaptations of limbs for running, leaping or digging, are usually similar in unrelated forms from different parts of the world. Again, the animals of tropical rain-forest, temperate deciduous forest, or of taiga, tend to show similar adaptations to arboreal life. Similarly aereal animals show parallel adaptations to flight, whether they be insects, molluscs, fishes, amphibia, reptiles, birds or mammals [13].

Seasons when conditions are unfavourable may be avoided by migration, which occurs in various phyla of the animal kingdom and, among terrestrial forms is especially conspicuous in Arthropoda, birds and mammals.

An alternative, found in less mobile animals, consists of hibernation [9] or aestivation, as the case may be, in a state of diapause (see Chapter 15).

This discussion of the adaptations of animals to terrestrial environments emphasizes, once again, the close, interdependence between morphology, physiology and ecology, all of which are, in turn, greatly influenced by size. In the following chapters various aspects of these complex relations are considered in greater detail.

6.6 REFERENCES

1 Alexander R.McN. (1968) *Animal Mechanics*. Sidgwick & Jackson, London.

2 Cloudsley-Thompson J.L. (1961) *Rhythmic Activity in Animal Physiology and Behaviour*. Academic Press, New York & London.

3 Cloudsley-Thompson J.L. (1964) Terrestrial animals in dry heat: Arthropods. In *Handbook of Physiology* (ed. D. B. Dill), Sect. 4, pp. 451–65. Amer. Physiol. Soc., Washington D.C.

4 Cloudsley-Thompson J.L. (1965) *Animal Conflict and Adaptation*. Foulis, London.

5 Cloudsley-Thompson J.L. (1968) *Spiders, Scorpions, Centipedes and Mites*, 2nd edition. Pergamon Press, Oxford.

6 Cloudsley-Thompson J.L. (1969) *The Zoology of Tropical Africa*. Weidenfeld & Nicolson, London.

7 Cloudsley-Thompson J.L. (1975) *Terrestrial Environments*. Croom Helm, London.

8 Darwin C. (1859) *On the Origin of Species by means of Natural Selection*. Murray, London.

9 Folk G.E. (1966) *Introduction to Environmental Physiology*. Lea & Febiger, Philadelphia.

10 Fraenkel G.S. & Gunn D.L. (1961) *The Orientation of Animals*, 2nd edition. Dover Publications, New York.

11 Gray J. (1968) *Animal Locomotion*. Weidenfeld & Nicolson, London.

12 Haviland M.D. (1926) *Forest Steppe and Tundra*. Cambridge University Press, London.

13 Hesse R., Allee W.C. & Schmidt K.P. (1951) *Ecological Animal Geography*, 2nd edition. Wiley, New York.

14 Lawrence R.F. (1953) *The Biology of the Cryptic Fauna of Forests*. Balkema, Cape Town.

15 McNab B.K. (1971) On the ecological significance of Bergmann's rule. *Ecology* **52,** 845–54.

16 Savory T.H. (1971) *Biology of the Cryptozoa*. Merrow, Watford, Herts.

17 Schmidt-Nielsen K. (1970) *How Animals Work*. Cambridge University Press, London.

18 Schmidt-Nielsen K. (1975) *Animal Physiology. Adaptation and Environment*. Cambridge University Press, London.

Prelude to Chapter 7

Osmotic homeostasis is a greater problem on land than it is in water. The terrestrial environment may provide easy access to oxygen, but the concomitant threat of desiccation presents physiological problems that have been satisfactorily solved by only two animal phyla, the Arthropoda and vertebrates, some of which can thrive even in the hottest and driest of desert habitats. Moist-skinned animals, such as earthworms, slugs, snails, frogs and toads, lose water by evaporation almost as rapidly as it can be transferred to the surrounding air by conduction and convection. Throughout most of their lives, therefore, they are virtually confined to damp surroundings. Desert snails are really no exception. Except at the time of rain, they remain dormant, sealed in their shells with an impermeable *epiphragm* consisting of dry mucus, sometimes associated with crystalline calcium carbonate.

Especially among smaller invertebrates, physiological mechanisms of water balance are assisted by behavioural responses to physical parameters of the environment—especially humidity, temperature and light. The terrestrial arthropods can be roughly divided on a physiological and ecological basis into two groups. The first of these consists of most woodlice, centipedes, millipedes, Collembola, and other forms that lack a discrete epicuticular layer of impervious wax. These lose water rapidly in dry air at normal ambient temperatures and, consequently, are restricted to moist, cryptozoic micro-habitats in the soil, under stones, fallen leaves and in crevices under the bark of trees. When taken into the open, they are negatively stimulated by the light and drought so that they run actively until, by chance, they reach some dark, damp spot where they come to rest. On the other hand, if their shady retreat should dry up, woodlice are not restrained by negative phototaxis until they die from desiccation for they become photopositive in dry air. This response is again reversed when they are rehydrated.

The second group contains most insects and arachnids which possess an epicuticular layer of wax which is relatively impervious to water vapour. Such animals are not usually so restricted to cryptozoic micro-habitats by their behavioural responses. Nor are they necessarily strictly nocturnal in their habits. Although most scorpions and Solifugae, for example, are strictly nocturnal in habit, they can withstand high temperatures and are extremely resistant to desiccation. It appears, therefore, that in these comparatively large and vulnerable arthropods, nocturnal behaviour is associated with the avoidance of predators rather than with the avoidance of adverse physical environmental conditions.

Behaviour plays an important part in the water balance of invertebrates and of small vertebrate animals. Indeed, it will be argued in a later chapter that behaviour and physiology are in no way separate disciplines, but that behaviour merely represents a particular type of physiological response to environmental stimulation. This type of interaction is seen in the functioning of 'biological clocks'. In their natural habitats, most organisms are entrained to a 24-hour rhythm through the daily cycles of light and dark generated by the earth's rotation. Under constant conditions, however, the period of the rhythm usually becomes slightly longer or shorter than 24 hours and hence is known as *circadian* (Latin *circa*, about, and *diem*, a day). The biological clock plays a vital role not only in regulating diurnal rhythms of activity, but also in time-compensated solar and astral navigation, as well as in the photoperiodic control of diapause and seasonal rhythms of reproduction (Chapter 15).

Chapter 7
Water balance and excretion

E.B. EDNEY AND K.A. NAGY

7.1 INTRODUCTION

Terrestrial animals first appeared in Devonian times about $0{\cdot}35 \times 10^9$ years ago (see Appendix 2, p. 444). Today there are far more species on land than in water, and the attributes usually associated with advanced evolution are found predominantly in land animals. In this chapter we consider an aspect of terrestrial life that has played an important role in determining the various evolutionary lines that have been followed; namely, the need to maintain water balance in a generally dehydrating environment.

Because nearly everything an animal does is powered by energy from its food, it should be possible to assign an energetic cost or saving to any physiological, morphological or behavioural attribute, and thus to examine by comparison with other animals the associated energetic advantage. This approach requires the assumption that chemical potential energy is always limiting, and any attribute of an animal that allows it to live on less energy, or to gather and accumulate more, will be selectively advantageous. This simple approach is often unsatisfactory when dealing with water balance adaptations, because water rather than energy may be in short supply. Attributes that favour an animal's energy balance are unimportant if the animal cannot remain in water balance. Thus terrestrial animals are exposed to selection pressures resulting from limited energy supply, limited water availability, or both as well as to other selection pressures.

There are important physical and chemical differences between aquatic and terrestrial environments, and it is the responses to these, in an evolutionary sense, which concern us. On the whole, the terrestrial environment is strongly dehydrating, and two important physical factors, temperature and water activity, vary over much wider ranges and much shorter periods on land than in water. We shall identify the main sources of water loss or gain, and consider the extent to which each is controllable. In treating each process we shall compare vertebrates and arthropods in order to show how differences in morphology and physiology dictate different means of solving similar problems.

7.2 WATER LOSS

Water is continually being lost from the bodies of animals, and must be replaced if the animal is to remain in balance.

7.2.1 Water in the environment

When air is in contact with a pure water surface in a closed system, water molecules move out of and into the water surface at equal rates and the air is said to be saturated with water vapour. The concentration of water vapour in saturated air increases exponentially with temperature—a relationship shown graphically in Fig. 7.1.

Relative humidity (*r.h.*) is the ratio between the partial pressure of water vapour in a sample of air (P_v) and the partial pressure at saturation (P^*_v), and is usually expressed as a percentage. The activity of water vapour in air (a_v) is simply related to *r.h.* by the equation

$$a_v = \frac{r.h.}{100} = \frac{P_v}{P^*_v}.$$

The difference between P^*_v and P_v (ΔP_v), the saturation deficit, or the vapour pressure deficit, at any a_v is clearly greater at higher than at lower temperatures, and since water tends to move from higher to lower vapour pressures, it does not necessarily move from higher to lower *r.h.* or a_v. For example, if air at the bottom of a scorpion's burrow is at 15°C and 90% *r.h.* ($a_v = 0{\cdot}9$), then $P_v = 11{\cdot}5$ mm Hg (or $15{\cdot}3 \times 10^2$ Pa). If at the same time air outside the burrow is at 28°C and only 50% *r.h.* ($0{\cdot}5\ a_v$), $P_v = 14{\cdot}2$ mm Hg (or $18{\cdot}7 \times 10^2$ Pa), and water vapour will move into the burrow, against the *r.h.* gradient.

The inclusion of a solute in water increases its osmotic pressure and lowers its water activity and that of air in equilibrium with the solution. The extent of the

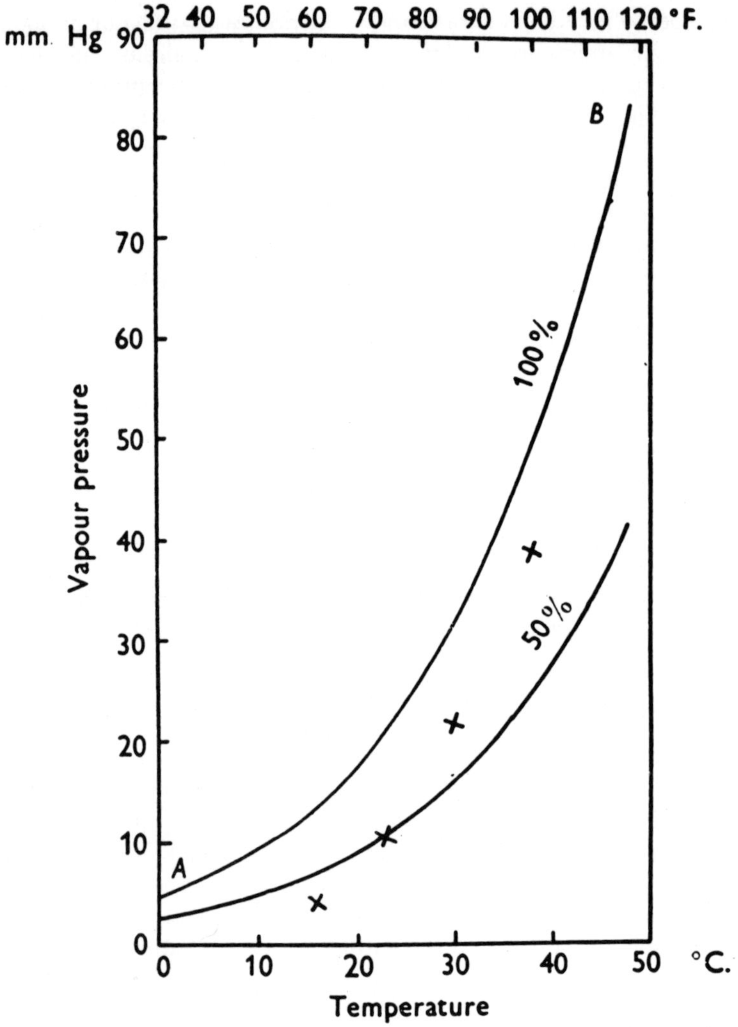

Fig. 7.1. The curve *A–B* shows the saturation vapour pressure (P^*_v) in air at various temperatures. The curve for 50% *r.h.* ($a_v = 0{\cdot}5$) is also drawn. The crosses represent vapour pressure deficits (ΔP_v) of 10 mm Hg at different temperatures. After [7].

depression of a_w by a solute is determined by the mole fraction of water in the solution (N_w), i.e. the ratio of the number of moles of water to the number of moles of all substances in the system. For example, the activity of an osmolar solution of NaCl (approximately 35 g l^{-1}) is

$$a_w = \frac{55{\cdot}55}{55{\cdot}55+1} = 0{\cdot}982.$$

This is approximately the a_w of sea water. The osmolar concentration of human blood and of insect haemolymph is about 300 mosm l^{-1}.

Osmotic concentrations are sometimes expressed in terms of freezing point depressions (Δ°C), and Δ_i and Δ_o refer to the internal and external media respectively. A 1·0 osmolar solution has Δ = 1·86°C, and this also is the Δ for sea water.

Several interesting conclusions follow. Firstly, unless the air surrounding an organism is nearly saturated with water vapour, a steep gradient between the animal's body fluids and the outside air will tend to cause loss of water by evaporation. Secondly, doubling (for example) the osmotic concentration of an animal's body fluid (Δ_i) will have only a minimal effect on water loss because the gradient will scarcely be affected. Thirdly, if there is a net movement of water inwards from anything but almost saturated air, this takes place against a very steep gradient of water activity, and once again, any biologically feasible decrease in internal a_w will not help the process significantly.

7.2.2 Evaporation

The two major avenues of water vapour loss are the integument and the respiratory system. Because the surface: volume ratio in small animals is much greater than in large animals, integumentary water loss, as percentage of body weight,

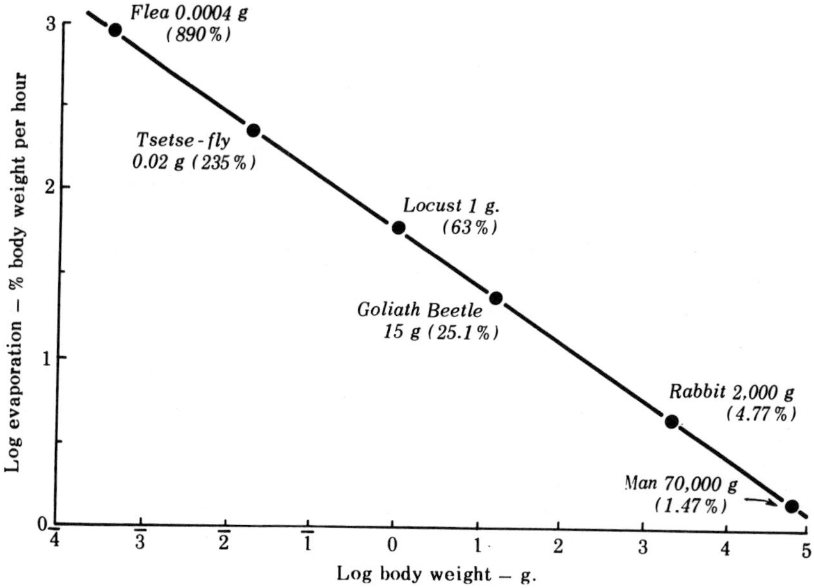

Fig. 7.2a. To maintain a given body temperature depression below ambient, water must evaporate from an animal at a particular rate per unit surface area. In desert conditions, such a rate is tolerable for some hours by a large animal because it represents only a small percentage of total weight, but a small animal would have to lose several times its own weight of water per hour. Figures in parenthesis show the amount of water, expressed as a percentage of total weight, to be evaporated each hour by animals whose weights are also shown. From [13]; data in part from [27].

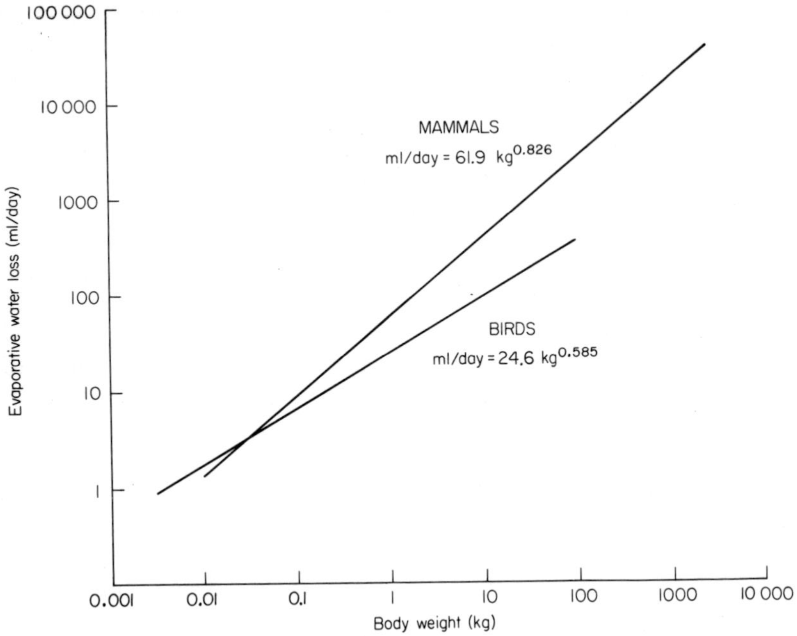

Fig. 7.2b. Relation between rate of evaporation and body size in birds and mammals resting in relatively dry air at temperatures within or below zones of thermal neutrality. Modified from [8] and [11].

can be expected to increase with decreasing body size, all other things being equal. Similarly, because weight-specific metabolic rate increases with decreasing body size, ventilation, and hence respiratory water loss, should be much greater in small than in large animals of similar taxa under identical environmental conditions. In addition to body size effects, rates of evaporation are also related to humidity and temperature, to the degree of air movement as it affects the thickness of the boundary layer surrounding the animal, and to the extent of movement of the animal itself.

The importance of this size effect is well illustrated by the following. In order to reduce body temperature by a given amount below ambient by evaporative cooling, it is necessary for an animal to lose water at a rate roughly proportional to its surface area. Figure 7.2.a shows that if the necessary rate for a man in a particular hot environment amounts to 1·47% of his total body weight each hour, the same rate per unit surface area for a locust weighing 1 g would represent 63% of its total body weight per hour, and for a flea of 0·0004 g, 890% of its body weight h^{-1} would have to be expended.

7.2.3 Integumentary water loss

This generally occurs as a result of body water diffusing through the integument and evaporating from the animal's surface. The permeability of the integument to water is therefore an important variable. Many animals possess skin glands, the ducts of which traverse the outer layers and increase water permeability. Some mammals possess sweat glands which secrete fluid onto the skin surface to cool the animal by evaporation in hot environments. Thus, the minimization of cutaneous water loss is not just a matter of forming a relatively waterproof, uniform layer over the animal; the integument has other functions, unrelated to water balance, that complicate the matter.

Arthropods

Because most land invertebrates are smaller than vertebrates the need to reduce transpiration from the integument is enhanced.

The structure and properties of the insect cuticle have been recently reviewed by Locke [17] and Neville [24]. Its varied forms are all based on the same plan, and this is shown in Fig. 7.3.

The main part of the cuticle (procuticle) which is laid down by the single layer of epidermal cells, is composed of protein and chitin (a nitrogenous polysaccharide). Part of the procuticle (the exocuticle) may be hardened and darkened by tanning and melanin deposition to give rigidity and strength. Outside this

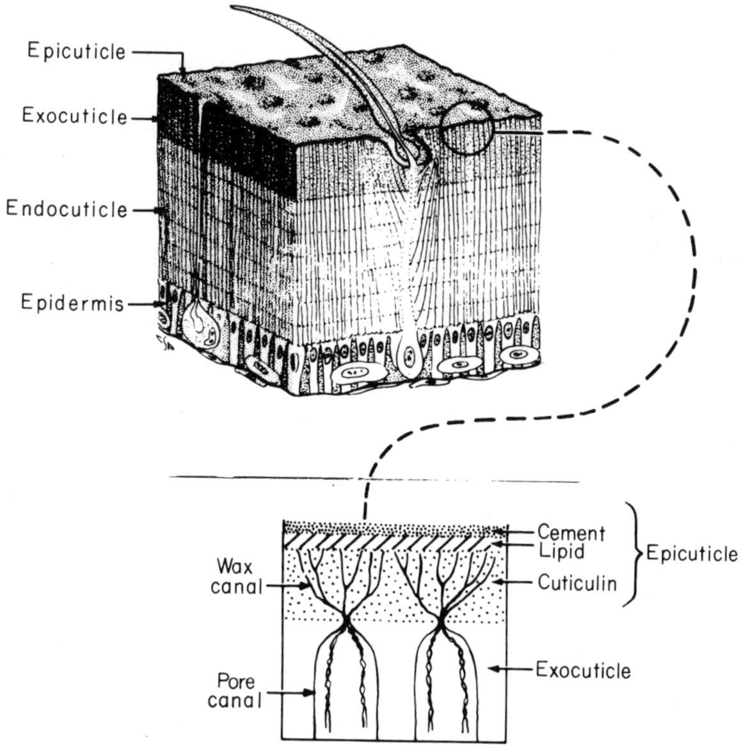

Fig. 7.3. Diagram of a generalized insect integument. From [13].

is a thin epicuticle of lipoprotein (no chitin) and finally a layer of a mixture of wax-like lipids, sometimes protected by a 'cement'. Impermeability to water is conferred partly by the hard, dark, tanned protein of the exocuticle, partly by the external lipid layer [2]. But the epicuticle need not be the only barrier, and there is evidence that the apical (outer) membranes of the living epidermal cells may contribute to the control of outward movement of water [4].

In many arthropods, including wireworms and isopods, the rate of cuticular transpiration decreases with time during exposure; and in *Locusta* at least, permeability is affected by ambient a_v [19]. Perhaps changes in cuticular permeability regulate water balance, but there is not enough evidence yet for a definite answer.

Whatever the precise nature of the water barrier or barriers, permeability of arthropod cuticles varies greatly between species, and in general is lower in species from hotter and drier habitats. Examples of this are shown in Table 7.1.

Table 7.1. Arthropod transpiration rates vs. habitat.

Species	Habitat	Rate of transpiration* $\mu g \cdot cm^{-2} \cdot h^{-1} \cdot mmHg^{-1}$
Isopod crustaceans		
Porcellio scaber	hygric	1·10
Hemilepistus reaumuri	xeric	0·32
Insects		
Calliphora erythrocephala	mesic	0·51
Blatta orientalis	mesic	0·48
Arenivaga investigata	xeric	0·12
Glossina morsitans adults	mesic-xeric	0·08
Glossina morsitans pupae	xeric	0·003
Tenebrio molitor pupae	xeric	0·01
Thermobia domestica adults	xeric	0·15
Locusta adults	xeric	0·22
Myriapods		
Lithobius sp.	hygric	2·70
Glomeris marginata	hygric	2·00
Arachnids		
Pandinus imperator (scorpion)	mesic	0·82
Androctonus australis (scorpion)	xeric	0·008
Galeodes arabs (solfugid)	xeric	0·066
Ixodes ricinus (tick)	mesic	0·60
Ornithodorus moubata (tick)	xeric	0·04

* Measured in dry air at temperatures between 20° and 30°C. For further data and authorities see [13].

Vertebrates

There are large differences in the rates of transpiration found in the four classes of terrestrial vertebrates. Depending on body size and shape, amphibians generally lose between 35–80% of their body weight per day by cutaneous evaporation in dry air [30]. Despite the remarkable ability of amphibians to survive after large body water losses (up to 50% of body weight in some desert forms [3]), and the capacity to store and later utilize large volumes of water in the urinary bladder, most amphibians would not survive long in many terrestrial habitats away from a source of free water. They would quickly dehydrate as a result of their large cutaneous water losses. Amphibians apparently cannot reduce cutaneous evaporation by physiological means, although the bullfrog (*Rana catesbeiana*) can increase skin evaporation to keep cool during hot periods by increasing skin gland secretions. Two interesting exceptions to the general pattern are the arid-land anurans *Chiromantis xerampelina* and *Phyllomedusa sauvagii* [30]: both have cutaneous water losses of about 2% of body weight per day, similar to desert lizards. The mechanisms involved in this phenomenon are not known.

In reptiles, overall evaporation rates are exceedingly variable, ranging from less than 1% of body weight per day in some desert lizards up to 150% day^{-1} in small fossorial snakes [10]. Although cutaneous and respiratory evaporation have been measured separately in but a few reptiles, indications are that cutaneous water loss accounts for about half of the total evaporation in reptiles with low rates of loss, and nearly all evaporation is cutaneous in reptiles with high loss rates. This confusing variation in reptilian evaporation rates is quickly clarified when the animals' natural habitats are taken into account: reptiles with high evaporation rates are aquatic, marine, fossorial or live in the humid tropics, while those that transpire slowly are invariably desert-dwellers [9, 10]. This habitat correlation is so great that body size effects are completely masked: young crocodiles lose up to 15% of body weight per day, while the much smaller (4 g) xeric lizard *Uta stansburiana* loses only 4% day^{-1} under similar conditions. There is some evidence that reptiles can reduce cutaneous evaporation after prolonged exposure to dry air and that skin permeability to water may decrease with decreasing *r.h.*

In birds and mammals, rates of total evaporation (cutaneous plus pulmonary) are similar in similar sized animals, and evaporation is correlated with body weight (Fig. 7.2.b). Cutaneous and pulmonary evaporation have been measured separately in only a few mammals [8], and even fewer birds [1]. These results indicate that cutaneous water loss accounts for roughly half of total evaporation, except in some desert species where cutaneous evaporation is very low. There is evidence indicating that birds [1] and mammals [8] can reduce total evaporation when water is restricted, but again, as in lizards, the means used to accomplish this are unknown.

It is apparent that a pattern exists regarding evaporative water loss and habitat among terrestrial vertebrates. Rates of evaporation are high in mesic vertebrates such as amphibians and aquatic and marine reptiles, but transpiration is low in xeric reptiles. Birds and mammals are intermediate.

7.2.4 Respiratory water loss

Because a dry membrane is much less permeable to O_2 than a moist one, respiratory surfaces in land animals are always moist, and consequently a source of water loss. In this section we consider the extent to which such loss may be minimized, and yet allow for rapid uptake of O_2 when this is needed.

Arthropods

In insects and some other land arthropods, O_2 is carried directly to the tissues by a system of ramifying tubules, the tracheae, without the intervention of a blood circulatory system.

In insects, the tracheal system opens by segmentally arranged pairs of occlusible spiracles. The lining of the tracheal branches is continuous with the cuticle and resembles it in general structure, including a waxy epicuticle. Internally, however, the tracheal branches become small, and terminate in long narrow intracellular tracheoles, the luminal surfaces of which form the membranes through which O_2 uptake occurs.

Most of the O_2 transport within tracheae results from diffusion; but in larger insects, particularly during flight or other high activity, air is either circulated through, or pumped tidally in and out of, the large tracheal trunks or air sacs, thus reducing the lengths of the diffusion paths and increasing the gradient along them. Theory suggests that there is no advantage, in terms of the ratio of O_2 uptake to water loss, in having the respiratory membranes at the internal ends of long tubes, but there is evidence that spiracular closing reduces water loss. If the spiracles of tsetse flies are kept open by CO_2, water loss is high and inversely related to ambient a_v, but if the spiracles are free to act, the rate of loss is strongly reduced at low humidities [5].

The spiracular valves of insects are operated by muscles whose responses provide a good example of adaptations associated with water balance. In dragon flies, contraction of the spiracular muscle closes the valve, and the direct action of CO_2 on the valve is to open it (thus admitting more O_2 and allowing CO_2 to escape). But the CO_2 concentration necessary for this effect is higher if the insect is short of water, or if the ambient temperature is high, and this of course has the effect of limiting spiracular water loss when such control is appropriate.

In several insects, particularly in their pupal or other inactive periods, CO_2 is eliminated discontinuously and this too may reduce water loss. In these cases the spiracles remain closed for long periods during which O_2 in the tracheal air is used up, and the resulting CO_2 goes into solution, probably as bicarbonate ions [5]. After a time the spiracles begin to flutter, providing only very small apertures through which air flows in, supposedly as a result of reduced intratracheal pressure, and this inward flow of air is sufficient to prevent outward diffusion of CO_2 and water vapour. Ultimately in each cycle the P_{CO_2} reaches a threshold which causes the spiracles to open wide allowing an efflux of CO_2. Water is lost only during the brief periods of full spiracular opening and consequently there may be an overall reduction of water loss when this mechanism is in action.

It is difficult to compare rates of cuticular and spiracular water loss because the latter depends on activity. In flying locusts between 65% and 80% of water loss is spiracular, but the fraction is very much less in resting insects [19]. In desert beetles as well as scorpions [13], tracheal loss is a very small proportion of the whole except at high temperatures. In tsetse flies, about 75% of the loss is cuticular, except in flying insects when the proportion is much lower [5].

Most spiders and all scorpions have book lungs (stacks of plate-like lamellae) instead of tracheae but again there are occlusible spiracles. Land Isopoda on the other hand do not have true tracheae nor occlusible spiracles, and O_2 uptake in these animals occurs mostly through plate-like pleopods (*Ligia*, *Oniscus*). In some species, the pleopods bear tuft-like 'pseudotracheae' (*Porcellio*, *Armadillidium*) but the rate of water loss is rather high compared with most insects (see Table 7.1). To this extent Isopoda are adapted to moist surroundings, although some, such as *Hemilepistus* and *Venezillo* live in crevices in deserts; and in spite of their apparent vulnerability to dehydration Isopoda are among the most common of all land arthropods in many mesic areas.

Finally, the possibility exists that, as in some vertebrates, water loss from the respiratory membranes could be reduced if air leaves the body at a temperature lower than that of the respiratory surface. In large insects such as the desert locust, thoracic temperature (T_{th}) during flight may be 7°C above ambient as a result of metabolic heat from the flight muscles. If some of the air saturated in the thorax is pumped to the cooler abdomen before being discharged through the abdominal spiracles, water would condense in the abdominal tracheae, and if this were re-absorbed there could be a significant saving of water. If 110 ml air g^{-1} hr^{-1} were so cycled, 4·8 mg water g^{-1} hr^{-1} would be saved; but further measurements are necessary to find whether this intriguing possibility does in fact occur [13].

Vertebrates

It is generally believed that, upon inhalation, air rapidly becomes saturated with water vapour at body temperature. Because birds and mammals are usually warmer than the air around them, and because warm air holds more vapour than cold air (Fig. 7.1), these animals supply a considerable amount of water in order to humidify inhaled air. As many reptiles and amphibians are known to achieve and maintain mammalian-like body temperatures by their behaviour (Chapter 20), these animals are also subjected to potentially large pulmonary water losses.

To discuss actual pulmonary water losses, two factors should be considered.

First, the amount of water vapour the animal must supply to inspired air depends on the absolute humidity of the ambient air. Secondly, all of the water vapour in lung air will be lost from the animal only if the air is exhaled at body temperature. In many small vertebrates, the exhaled air can be much cooler than the body, resulting in condensation and thus conservation of some of the pulmonary water vapour. This remarkable phenomenon is due to a temporal counter-current heat exchanger operating in the nasal passages of many vertebrates (Fig. 7.4). As cool air is inhaled, the nasal lining is cooled by conduction and evaporation. When the now warm and humid air in the lungs is exhaled over these cool membranes, the air is cooled and can no longer hold all its water as vapour. Some condenses on the membrane ('rain in the nose'), and is thus

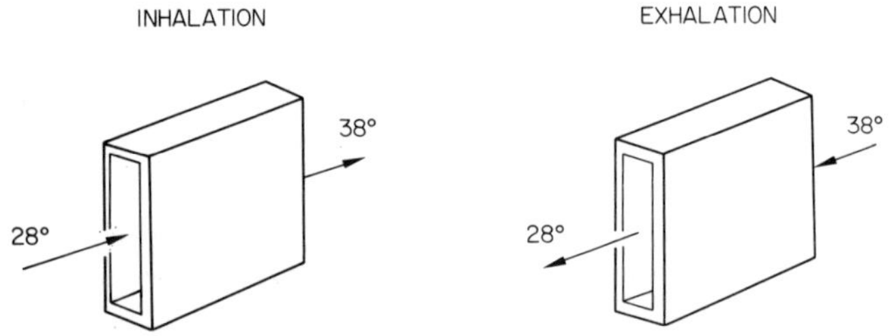

Fig. 7.4. Diagram of counter-current heat exchanger in nasal passages. Ambient air saturated with vapour at 28°C, is warmed and humidified upon inhalation. When this air is exhaled over the cool nasal membranes, it loses heat and some of its water condenses in the nose. From [28].

saved [27]. The effectiveness of this mechanism depends on the temperature and humidity of the inhaled air, and the narrowness and length of the nasal passages. Desert kangaroo rats have long, narrow, highly convoluted nasal passages, and can conserve up to 80% of the pulmonary water vapour that might otherwise be lost [28]. Small birds and mammals have potentially large pulmonary water losses, because their metabolism, and hence ventilation, is much greater on a weight-specific basis than larger endotherms. It is not surprising that many small rodents and birds have 'cold noses'. Nasal heat exchange also occurs in desert lizards [22]. Several lizards possess nasal salt glands, which secrete concentrated salt solutions and function importantly in osmoregulation [23]. These glands drain into the nasal passages, where evaporation further concentrates the salt solution and recycles even this water [22].

7.2.5 Loss by excretion and ionic regulation

General

In most animals the so-called 'excretory' system is not only concerned with the elimination of excess nitrogen but also with elimination or retention of water and other materials as may be required to maintain osmotic and ionic balance.

In most active animals at most times N is in excess as a result of the deamination of amino-acids and other metabolic processes, but water and inorganic ions may be in excess or in short supply according to several factors including diet, so that the 'excretory' system has to be able to eliminate or retain these materials according to need. Regarding diet, consider the differences in composition of the various types of foods in Table 7.2. It is obvious that an herbivore must excrete nitrogen and salts at a much higher rate than carnivores or granivores, but the high water content of vegetation provides the means for doing this without producing a highly concentrated urine.

Table 7.2. Nitrogen, salt and water content of food representative of carnivores (beef steak), granivores (millet) and herbivores (cabbage). Values are given in terms of kilojoules (energy) available from each food type in order to permit comparison between diets in a physiologically meaningful way. Values were calculated from data given in [34].

Food	Nitrogen µmol/kJ	Sodium µmol/kJ	Potassium µmol/kJ	Calcium µmol/kJ	Water ml/kJ
Beef steak (raw)	1771	29·3	96	2·1	0·50
Millet seed	1449	1·3	142	6·3	0·17
Cabbage (raw)	2592	150·7	1043	213·5	16·12

The form in which N is eliminated is usually either uric acid, urea or ammonia, and each compound has certain adaptive pros and cons depending on the animal's general way of life. Of the three compounds, ammonia is most costly in water because 3 H atoms (potential water) are lost for every N. NH_3 is also highly soluble in water and very toxic, again requiring a lot of water for its elimination. Urea, $H_2N \cdot CO \cdot NH_2$, (H/N ratio = 2) is very soluble and thus may exert a high osmotic pressure, but is relatively non-toxic. Uric acid has the lowest H/N ratio, 1·0, is non-toxic, and is relatively insoluble. On the other hand the chemical energy lost per N atom excreted is highest for uric acid, lowest in ammonia. It seems that water conservation plays a large role in determining which N end product is used: aquatic invertebrates (where water is no problem for $\Delta_i \geqq \Delta_e$) use ammonia; amphibians and mammals use urea (but see below for interesting exceptions), and reptiles, birds and most land arthropods use uric acid or guanine. Land Isopoda are exceptional in using NH_3 (as their aquatic relatives do), but they eliminate it as a gas [36].

Arthropods

In arthropods urine is elaborated by Malpighian tubules, passes from them into the hind gut where it is modified by adjustment of water or ionic concentrations, and is eliminated via the anus together with waste material from the rest of the gut. The Malpighian tubules, the ileum and the glands of the rectal walls, together form a controlling system for osmotic and ionic balance similar in

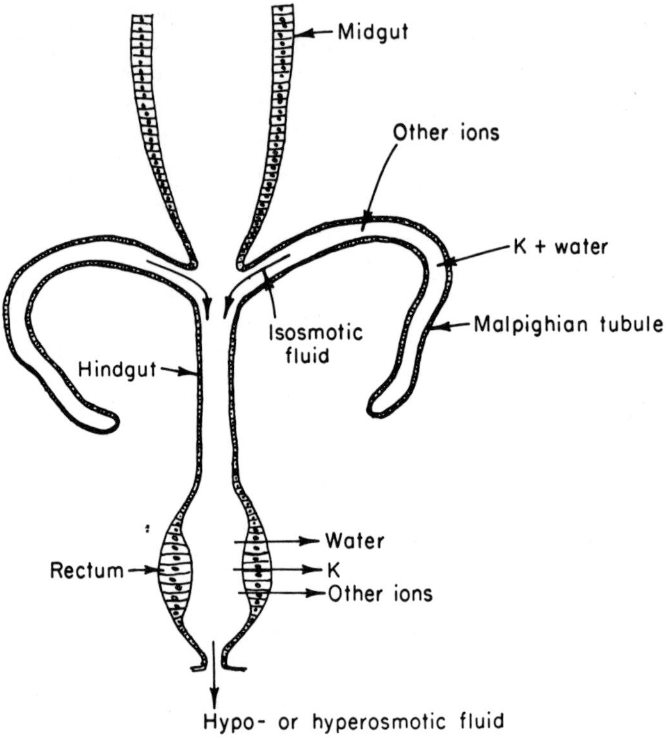

Fig. 7.5a. Diagram of water and salt circulation in the excretory system of an insect. From [32].

many ways to the nephrons of vertebrates, although the production of urine in arthropods takes place without a pressure gradient. The organs and major substances involved are shown diagrammatically in Fig. 7.5a.

In general, the water content of faecal material varies according to the state of the animal's water reserves and this may change dramatically over short time periods. For example, parasites such as ticks and tsetse flies which feed on their host's blood, may take enormous meals at long intervals. After feeding on blood a tsetse fly has a water content many times higher than normal, and this is rapidly eliminated by the production of watery faecal material, the amount of which is determined by the insect's water status before feeding. In flies whose water content is low before they feed (about 66% of body weight), only 30% of the blood meal is excreted as water, but this increases to 50% in animals whose initial water content is 73% or so [6].

In the tick *Amblyomma americanum* excess water in the blood meal is excreted back into the host by the tick's salivary glands, and the same is true of *Boophilus* and *Dermacentor* [13].

Urine produced by the Malpighian tubules is nearly always isoosmotic with the blood, and hyper- or hypo-osmoticity is brought about at a later stage in the hind gut. Uric acid in the form of its soluble potassium salt passes into the tubule lumen together with water (see p. 118). Then either in the proximal part of the tubule (*Rhodnius*) or in the hind gut (most insects) K^+ is withdrawn, the pH is reduced, and uric acid is precipitated. In the hind gut and rectum, other ions and water are withdrawn to the extent necessary, as shown in Table 7.3 [26].

Usually uptake of water from the rectum is linked to the uptake of solutes, but the process may occur against a large osmotic gradient without solute uptake in locusts [26], blow flies, cockroaches, and other insects [13]. In locusts, water is removed from the rectal lumen to the blood against osmotic gradients up to about 1 osmole l^{-1} ($\Delta = 1{\cdot}86°$), but the limiting gradient is itself determined by the water status of the insect, being greater in locusts kept in rather dry air and given saline to drink (Fig. 7.6a) [21].

Table 7.3. Ionic concentrations of locust fluids*.

Fluid	Ionic concentration (mean values in mEq/litre)		
	Na	K	Cl
Saline for drinking	300	150	450
Haemolymph			
With water to drink	108	11	115
With saline to drink	158	19	163
Rectal fluid			
With water to drink	1	22	5
With saline to drink	405	241	569

* If desert locusts are given strong saline to drink, ionic concentrations in their haemolymph rise, but not to the level of the saline. Ionic concentrations in their rectal fluid become higher than those in the saline. Data from [26].

The mechanism whereby water moves apparently against an osmotic gradient poses an intriguing problem. Of several solutions proposed, that most generally accepted was originated by Gupta and Berridge [16] for the blow fly, and since then it has been applied to several other insects. The essential feature of the model is the creation of locally high osmotic concentrations in a system of narrow intercellular spaces, channels or lamellae. This causes the movement of water from the cells into the spaces, along the narrow channels, and finally out through openings into the haemocoele, while the solutes are either recycled by re-absorption from the basal region of the intercellular spaces or recruited from the blood itself.

A further remarkable example of an adaptation that reduces water loss during excretion almost to the vanishing point is that of the cryptonephridial system found in meal worms (*Tenebrio molitor*) [15] and several other insects. Here the distal ends of the Malpighian tubules are enclosed within a membrane which surrounds the rectum. Ions, particularly K^+, are actively taken from the surrounding blood by special cells through 'windows' and secreted into the tubule lumen. In this way the gradient against which water must be absorbed from the rectal lumen is decreased, and the two steps (rectum to perinephric space to tubule lumen) in series serve to move water from the rectal material, leaving the latter virtually dry ($a_w \cong 0{\cdot}9$). It seems that water is present in the rectum as vapour and absorbed from that phase—an interesting fact that we shall refer to again (p. 128).

In general, terrestrial arthropods regulate their ionic and osmotic concentrations by a combination of means, of which the Malpighian tubule-rectal system is a very important component. In conditions leading to desiccation, the blood volume may be greatly reduced, although its osmotic concentration is regulated to a certain extent [13]. In fact the haemolymph of these animals appears to function as a buffer against the effects of water loss on living cells. Water may be withdrawn from the blood without leading to a serious shortage in the tissues.

Water storage in an even more direct form has recently been found in a desert termite and in the cockroach *Leucophaea*. The cotton stainer *Dysdercus* stores water in the form of hypotonic urine in the rectum, and regulates its blood osmotic pressure by drawing on this store [4].

There has been increasing evidence in recent years that, as in vertebrates, water balance is under hormonal control in land arthropods [21]. The hormones involved are liberated by glands in the head, the mesothoracic ganglia or the last abdominal ganglion. Both diuretic and anti-diuretic factors have been found and the target organs are the Malpighian tubules and the rectum, where rates of urine formation and water re-absorption respectively are affected.

In some cases the hormonal control mechanism is clearly adapted to the insect's mode of life: thus the stick insect *Carausius* feeds continuously on moist plant material while *Rhodnius* feeds only at long intervals (but then enormously) on vertebrate blood. Reflecting these differences, the diuretic hormone of *Carausius* is produced continuously in the head (at some distance from the target organs, which respond comparatively feebly), while in *Rhodnius*, the hormone is liberated after a meal by peripheral abdominal nerves close to the Malpighian tubules, and these respond vigorously to even small doses.

Vertebrates

Vertebrates have kidneys that are composed of thousands of closely-packed tubules called nephrons, which receive a protein-free, pressure filtrate of blood plasma at the glomerulus, and modify this fluid into urine along the length of the nephron, by means of selective secretion and absorption of substances (Fig. 7.5b). In the proximal convoluted tubule, most of the organic substances (glucose, amino acids, vitamins, hormones, etc.) are re-absorbed, and most of the NaCl and water are removed from the filtrate here. In birds and most reptiles, uric acid is actively transported into the nephron in the proximal tubule. In the distal convoluted tubule, more NaCl and water can be re-absorbed, and H^+,

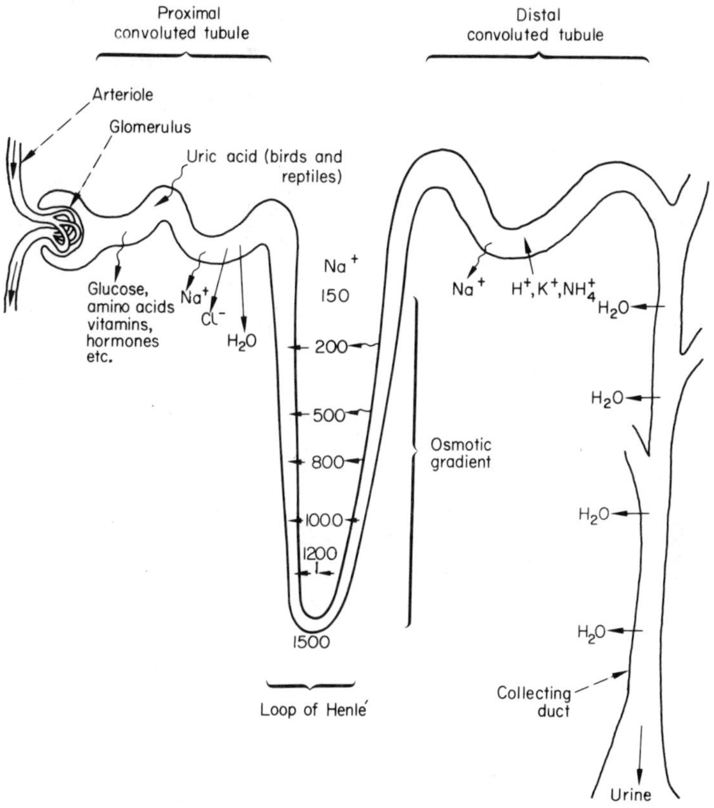

Fig. 7.5b. Diagrammatic representation of mammalian nephron. Fluid enters the proximal convoluted tubule after being filtered through the glomerulus by hydrostatic pressure in the blood vessels. The filtrate is modified in the convoluted tubules by active transport (wavy arrows) and passive diffusion or osmosis (straight arrows). The loop of Henle maintains an osmotic gradient by active sodium transport, and the filtrate is dehydrated osmotically while passing through this gradient via the collecting duct. The water permeability of the collecting duct is regulated by antidiuretic hormone.

K^+ and NH_4^+ ions are transported here to regulate body pH. The middle segment of the nephron in mammals and many birds contains a hairpin turn, called the loop of Henle, which functions to establish and maintain a concentration gradient that increases toward the turn in the loop. This is accomplished by active transport of Na^+ and by water impermeability in the ascending portion of the loop. The advantage of this is that as fluid flows down the collecting duct, through this concentration gradient, water can be removed from the urine by osmosis through the collecting duct walls, thus making the urine nearly as concentrated as the fluid at the tip of Henle's loop. The longer the relative length of the loop of Henle, the more concentrated the urine can be. Several desert rodents have extremely long loops, and can produce urine up to 9000 mosm l^{-1} [20]. Among mammals, there is a fair correlation between kidney concentrating ability and the aridity of the habitat. In many birds, a large fraction of their nephrons contain loops of Henle, and most birds can produce somewhat hyperosmotic urine [29]. The salt marsh-dwelling savannah sparrow can produce urine of 2000 mosm l^{-1}, the highest concentration yet measured in birds [49]. Reptiles and amphibians do not have loops of Henle, and their kidneys do not produce hyperosmotic urine.

Despite the fact that reptiles and most birds do not form highly concentrated urine, their excrement can be fairly dry. This occurs because these animals excrete nitrogenous wastes primarily as precipitated uric acid or urates. When the urine and faeces reach the cloaca, water can be reabsorbed osmotically, following active transport of ions, in much the same manner as in arthropods, although the details of the mechanism in vertebrates are not known. Thus, in birds and most reptiles, the combination of kidney, uric acid and cloaca can reduce net excretory water losses to levels comparable with those in desert rodents. Amphibians can completely stop urine production during periods of water deprivation, but in nature, these animals often must eliminate excess water, and urine output rates as high as 160% of body weight per day have been measured [3]. The anurans *Chiromantis xerampelina* and *Phyllomedusa sauvagii*, mentioned above as having very low rates of evaporation, are exceptional in another regard: whereas other amphibians excrete ammonia or urea these animals produce uric acid as their primary nitrogen excretory product, and are thus similar to reptiles in two ways.

Many birds and reptiles possess other organs that excrete excess electrolytes with little water loss: the salt glands. These glands produce concentrated (1000–2000 mosm l^{-1}) solutions of NaCl, in the case of carnivores and marine animals, or KCl in terrestrial herbivores. Birds and reptiles that have salt glands often live in osmotically stressful habitats, such as deserts (many lizards, roadrunners, desert partridge) and marine environments (sea turtle, sea snake, marine iguana, many sea birds). However, several freshwater birds (ducks, flamingos) and tropical reptiles (green iguana) also have salt glands [3, 29].

Regulation of the rate of urine production can occur in two ways: by varying the rate at which filtrate enters the nephrons, and by altering the amount of filtrate re-absorbed in the collecting ducts. Amphibians, reptiles and birds can vary filtration rate, but mammals apparently do not. The permeability to water of the collecting ducts, and hence the amount of filtrate re-absorbed, is under the control of two antidiuretic hormones: argenine vasopressin in most mammals, and argenine vasotocin in birds, amphibians and reptiles. These hormones are secreted by the posterior pituitary gland in response to changes in plasma osmotic pressure. Regulation of salt gland secretion is apparently under gross control of the autonomic nervous system, with more subtle regulation by hormones, particularly the steroids [29, 31], as occurs in the kidneys [3].

7.3 WATER GAIN

Water must be gained to offset loss, although temporary imbalances or long-term trends do occur. During active growth or egg production, more water must be gained than lost. At other times water may be stored in the salivary reservoir, blood or other compartments (p. 120). But even land animals not uncommonly have more than enough water and then there is no question of storage or conservation—the problem is how to get rid of it. This may happen, for example, when meal worms and other stored products insects are kept at very high a_v.

7.3.1 Uptake with food and by drinking

Arthropods

Most invertebrates drink water if the need and opportunity arise, and they do so to an extent that keeps them in water balance. This has been shown in bees, flies, *Arenivaga* and many other insects. Spiders drink from moist surfaces, sometimes against high suction forces, as do millipedes and isopods [13]. It would be interesting to know more about the extent of this process, which would seem to be particularly valuable in areas where no free water is available.

But all food contains water, and although the content may be very low (about 10–15% in 'dry' grain), flour moths and meal worms live with no other source. Meal worms eat more in dry than in moist conditions and so do isopods, but these animals are more active in dry than in moist air and consequently their need for energy is greater, so that this, rather than the water content, may be the reason for eating more food. In *Tenebrio*, however, the excess food is passed through the gut undigested, suggesting that it had been eaten for the sake of its water content.

Vertebrates

The diet of carnivores generally contains 60–70% water, and green vegetation typically is 80–95% water. For vertebrates living in mesic habitats where evaporative water losses are likely to be low, the diet could well provide more than enough water to meet requirements. However, in arid lands, growing seasons are often short, and carnivores may suffer from seasonal scarcity of prey, while herbivores are often faced with very dry vegetation. Various behavioural strategies are used by many of these animals, such as migration, either to water holes or to another climate altogether, or avoidance such as aestivation and hibernation. But some animals continue to carry on normally in these habitats, even without drinking. For example, two African antelopes can obtain sufficient dietary water to remain in balance by eating dry shrubs at night. During the day, these shrubs contain only 1% water, but as the temperature drops at night and the *r.h.* increases as a result (Fig. 7.1) the shrubs take up water from the air hygroscopically, and their water content can increase to above 40% [33]. Desert kangaroo rats can obtain enough water in their dry seed diet, along with oxidation water (see below), to maintain water balance without drinking, so long as the *r.h.* is higher than about 10% [27]. There is evidence that some seed-eating desert birds also survive without drinking [1].

Although most vertebrates will drink given the opportunity, amphibians generally do not. This is probably related to their high rates of cutaneous water uptake (see below). Vertebrates that live in or near sea water are of considerable interest from a water balance viewpoint, because sea water can be quite dehydrating.

7.3.2 Oxidation water

General

When food is oxidized water is formed. As Table 7.4 shows, the amount of oxidation water produced depends upon the amount and nature of the fuel used, and the water so produced then becomes a part of the general water pool of the animal concerned. The significance of oxidation water in the water balance of all animals depends upon the size of all other components: thus in most desert animals the total water flux is low and oxidation water forms a large part of water gain, while for animals living in more hygric environments the reverse is true.

Two questions are often asked: can and do animals in water stress increase their metabolic rate and thus derive more oxidation water, and does a switch from other substrates to fat result in overall water gain?

Firstly, although doubling the metabolic rate results in doubling the rate of water production, it also requires twice the rate of O_2 uptake, and this may result

Table 7.4. The relationship between oxygen consumed and energy and water produced when various classes of food materials are oxidized to CO_2, and that proteins go as far as urea. Values are representative approximations, since different foods within the same class behave differently. From [13] and [27].

Food	g water per g food	litres O_2 per g food	litres O_2 per g water	kJ per g food	g water per kJ	R.Q.
Carbohydrates	0·56	0·83	1·49	17·58	0·032	1·0
Fats	1·07	2·02	1·89	39·94	0·027	0·71
Proteins	0·40	0·97	2·44	17·54	0·023	0·79

in a greater loss of water by ventilation. However, the extent to which extra O_2 uptake necessitates extra water loss is uncertain. In tsetse flies, while the metabolic rate increases twenty-twofold during flight, water loss increases only sixfold [5]. Secondly, Table 7.4 shows 1 g fat yields about 1·07 g water, while 1 g carbohydrate yields only 0·56 g water. But more O_2 per g water is required if fats are used, so that the question of additional water loss as a result of additional O_2 uptake is again raised. More important, however, is the fact that fat yields more than twice as much energy as an equal weight of carbohydrate, so that in terms of equal energy yields, fat produces less water than carbohydrate. Thus switching from carbohydrate to fat metabolism is counter-productive for water conservation.

Arthropods

The interplay between environmental conditions, gain of water by oxidation and loss by transpiration is well illustrated by the desert locust.

In flying locusts, ventilation through the thorax rises to about 320 ml air g^{-1} hr^{-1}, a tenfold increase over the resting state. This results in both a rapid loss of water and an increase in oxidation water, and the question arises as to how these balance out. Water loss depends on ambient a_v since dry air passing through the tracheal system will carry away more water than moist air. In addition, the higher the temperature of an insect the greater the water loss, since saturated air has a higher water content at higher temperatures, and both ambient temperature and the intensity of solar radiation affect this parameter.

In Fig. 7.6b the relationship of these variables is shown. Each curve represents, for one radiation level, those combinations of air temperature (T_a) and a_v that will just permit the insect to remain in water balance. The rate of metabolism during flight is fixed at about 270 J g^{-1} hr^{-1}, and it has been estimated that oxidation water amounts to 8·1 mg g^{-1} hr^{-1} [35]. At T_a = 30° and a_v = 0·60, T_{th} is 36°C in the absence of radiation, and in these conditions an insect

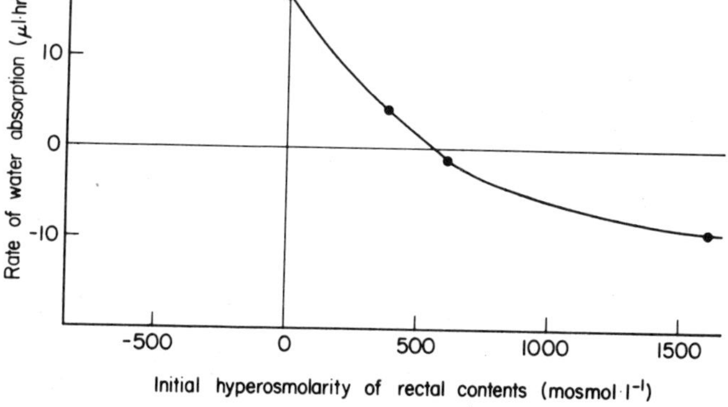

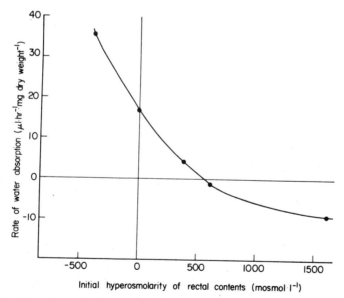

Fig. 7.6a. The relationship between the initial osmotic pressure gradient and net rate of water movement across the rectal wall in the desert locust, *Schistocerca*. A positive sign indicates movement from the lumen outwards (ordinate), or that the rectal fluid is more concentrated than the haemolymph (abscissa). From [26].

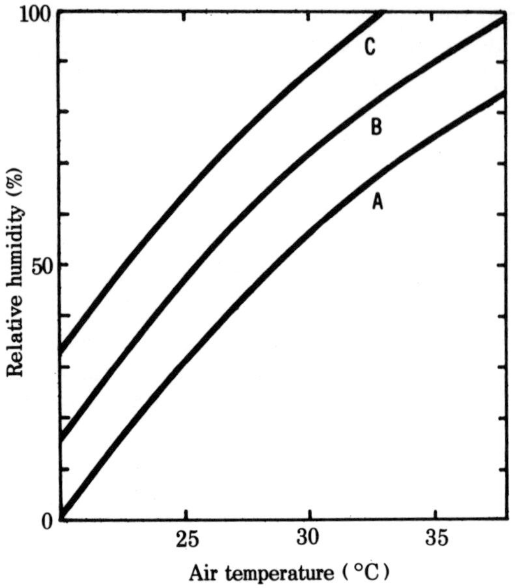

Fig. 7.6b. The relationship between the relative humidity and air temperature at which flying desert locusts lose water by evaporation and through the spiracles at the same rate as water is produced by the oxidation of fat. (A) no net radiative heating; (B) thoracic temperature increased by 2°C relative to A by net absorption of radiation; (C) increased by 4°C. For points above the curves locusts gain water, while they lose water at points below the curves. From [35].

loses about 8·0 mg g^{-1} hr^{-1}, and so remains in water balance. If solar radiation were to raise T_{th} by 2° or 4° (curves B or C), then either T_a must be lower or a_v higher if the insect is to avoid dehydration.

In fact by flying very high and using thermals to get there, locusts are in much cooler air, where they can fly all day without net water loss. The advantage of using fat is clear: it provides many more kJ g^{-1} than other foods do.

Vertebrates

No reptiles or amphibians are known to be able to maintain water balance on dry food and oxidation water alone. However, several small desert rodents and birds can survive on the performed water contained in seeds and the oxidation water produced from them. This feat is possible only because water losses are exceedingly low in these animals. Of primary consideration here is the reduction of pulmonary evaporation by nasal counter-current heat exchange. Even though large endotherms have smaller surface to volume ratios and lower weight-specific metabolic rates, which result in lower weight-relative water losses by evaporation in large animals, the effectiveness of the nasal exchanger is determined by the narrowness of the nasal passages. Clearly, the ratio of pulmonary loss to oxidative production is the critical value, and the small animal can reduce this ratio further because its nasal exchanger would probably be more effective. This prediction may account for the observation that no large animals are known to be able to survive on dry food and oxidation water as can kangaroo rats. This raises the question of how bears sleeping through the winter months, and large migratory birds on long-distance, non-stop flights are able to avoid lethal dehydration. Unfortunately, little is understood about these interesting questions.

7.3.3 Other avenues

Cutaneous, etc.

The major avenue of water gain in amphibians is through the skin by osmosis. Many anurans have specialized areas of skin on their abdomens and thighs ('seat patch'). The animal simply sits in hypo-osmotic water, and takes up water at rates as high as 360% of body weight per day. The permeability of the skin to water is apparently regulated by argenine vasotocin [3]. If the animal is not completely submerged, it will also be losing water by evaporation rapidly. Microscopic channels have been found on the surface of toad skin, which draw water up from the substrate by capillarity and over the skin. This water substitutes for internal water and thus reduces the dehydrating effects of cutaneous evaporation. A similar mechanism occurs in the Australian desert lizard *Moloch*. This animal also has cutaneous capillary grooves, which lead to the mouth. When the animal sits in water, the grooves conduct water to the mouth where it is swallowed.

Although no vertebrate is known to take up water vapour from moist air as some arthropods can (see below), some ectothermic vertebrates may be able to gain water from vapour by condensing it from the air first. If an animal's surface temperature is below the dew point of the air immediately next to it, water will condense on the animal and may then be taken in by drinking, or perhaps directly through the skin or cuticle. Laboratory measurements have shown that desert lizards, toads and tarantulas gained weight when placed in warm moist air, because water condensed on their surfaces. Desert sand dune beetles, *Lepidochora*, and snakes, *Bitis*, are known to allow water to condense on their integuments in advective fog, and than to take in the water by drinking [18].

Uptake from the vapour phase by arthropods

A physiologically more puzzling process has been found so far only in arthropods, a few of which (Table 7.5) are able to absorb water vapour directly from the air, even from an a_v as low as 0·5 in some cases. Certain regularities exist in the distribution of this ability. Species in which it has been observed are all either insects, ticks or mites. No winged insect is included, which means that the ability is restricted to larval forms except for the wingless adults of thysanurans, psocids and lice. The neotenic wingless adult female *Arenivaga* is able to absorb, but the winged male is not. The restriction to wingless forms is probably no

Table 7.5. Some arthropods that are known to take up water vapour from unsaturated air and their critical equilibrium humidities. For further data and authorities see [14].

	r.h.% (= a_v . 100)
Arachnida	
Ixodes ricinus	92·0
Rhipicephalus sanguineus	84·0–90·0
Acarus siro	75·0
Laelaps echidnina	90·0
Insecta	
Thermobia domestica	45·0
Liposcellis bostrychophilus	60·0
Xenopsylla brasilinensis	50·0
Tenebrio molitor larvae	88·0
Arenivaga investigata	82·5

coincidence, but reflects the adaptive significance of a process which enables its possessor to live in niches where free water is not available or is in short supply. Caterpillars, for example, which feed on moist plants, do not possess the ability and winged forms can usually fly to a source of water.

The lowest a_v that permits absorption varies greatly between species, but in all cases the limit is independent of temperature or vapour pressure deficit.

As we saw earlier in this chapter, the a_w of arthropod haemolymph is usually 0·99, and is thus in equilibrium with air at 99% *r.h.* But absorption by firebrats, for example, occurs in air down to $a_v = 0{\cdot}5$, so that there is an osmotic gradient of 55·5 osmoles l^{-1}, or 126 J.cm^{-3} against which the water has to move. Several proposals have been made to account for the process [13] including absorption through the tracheal system and the cuticle. But the rectum is the site for which there is currently most evidence, at least in the firebrat *Thermobia* [25]. In ticks this may not be so and the mouth has been implicated. We recall that meal worms can reduce the a_w of their fecal material to 0·9 and that the rectum contains air with this a_v.

Although the site has been identified in some arthropods (and there is no reason why it should be the same in all), the mechanism is still incompletely understood. So far as energetics are concerned there is no difficulty, for although the gradient is impressively steep, the energy involved is but a small fraction of the animal's standard metabolic rate. *Arenivaga* nymphs, for example, absorbed 60 mg g^{-1} day^{-1} from $a_v = 0{\cdot}9$ [12]. The amount of energy required to concentrate this amount of water through the gradient involved may be derived from the equation $\bar{G} = -nRT \ln (a_2/a_1)$, where $\bar{G}$ is the Gibbs free energy, n the number of moles of water, R the gas constant, T the absolute temperature and a_1 and a_2 the water activities in the initial and final states, respectively. The result shows that a 100 mg insect would use 0·0778 J day^{-1} in absorbing 6 mg water.

The standard metabolic rate for such an insect is about 10·6 J day^{-1}, so that even allowing for thermodynamic inefficiency the energy involved is proportionately small.

7.4 CONCLUSIONS

In arthropods water loss from the respiratory surfaces is much lower than that from the cuticle (except when the animal is very active) as a result of efficient spiracular closing devices. Loss with nitrogenous excretion is insignificant as compared with that from other sources as a result of uricotely. The cuticle is relatively impermeable where necessary (desert beetles, ticks and tsetse flies for example) and this is very appropriate for animals of small size. Cuticular water loss may be controllable; loss from the respiratory system, and from the elimination of waste nitrogen and salts certainly is.

On the uptake side, the main source of water gain depends very much on an arthropod's mode of life. In caterpillars or aphids, most water goes in with the food, as it does in ectoparasites that feed on blood, and water in these animals may be temporarily in excess. Direct uptake by drinking is known to be a balance mechanism, but whether or not food is ingested for the sake of its water content is open to investigation.

Insects that live in the absence of free water, such as stored products pests, may use nearly dry food, and then oxidation water is the most important source of gain. But there is no evidence that the production of oxidation water is adjusted as a means of water balance control. Finally, direct absorption of water vapour, in those arthropods where it occurs, is certainly a major component of water gain (it may be the only source, as in pre-pupal fleas), and is clearly regulatory in its effects since it can be switched on or off according to need.

Respiratory water loss in vertebrates is determined primarily by the breathing rate required to support energy metabolism, which in turn depends on the animal's body size, and whether it is endothermic or ectothermic. Respiratory evaporation is reduced by the nasal counter-current exchanger operating in many smaller vertebrates. Cutaneous water loss varies greatly, between species, and vertebrates living in arid habitats have the lowest rates of evaporation from the skin. Urinary water losses vary about as much as do evaporative losses. Again, xeric vertebrates tend to have the lowest urinary losses. In small desert vertebrates, low cutaneous water permeability, effective nasal water condensation and low urinary losses (resulting from either highly concentrated urine as in rodents, or uric acid or urate excretion in birds and lizards) combine to yield total water requirements as low as 3% of body weight per day. In amphibians and hygric reptiles, total water losses can be more than 200% of body weight per day.

As in arthropods, vertebrates gain water in a variety of ways depending on their life style, habitat and morphology. In humid habitats, evaporation may be so low and the diet so moist that water excretion rather than water conservation may be the rule. Even in deserts, birds and larger mammals are sufficiently mobile to travel to water holes to drink. Of particular interest are the small desert vertebrates, which may never drink water. Most of these are carnivorous or herbivorous, and can maintain water balance with the water in their food when this is available; when it is not, these animals generally aestivate or hibernate. Most striking are the few desert rodents and birds that can live on dry seeds: these animals show the greatest reduction in all avenues of water loss.

Terrestrial environments include a well-nigh unlimited variety of niches, from an open desert surface to the litter on a forest floor, and there is a correspondingly vast array of animals variously adapted to this range of places to live. Are there any general considerations, based on water balance, that help to make this heterogenous assemblage more comprehensible? Certain regularities are worth considering. Chief of these are the basic attributes of the taxonomic group to which an animal belongs. Thus mammals are endothermic homeotherms, with particular respiratory, excretory and integumental systems, and they usually weigh 10 g or more, while land arthropods are exothermic poikilotherms, usually weighing less than 1 g. These differences in size mean differences in restraints and opportunities. Small animals such as arthropods are more vulnerable to dehydration than larger ones, and they cannot afford evaporative cooling. On the other hand, being small, they take advantage of crevices to avoid extremes of drought and temperature; and water vapour absorption through the surface, where it occurs, is significant.

Evolution is opportunistic, and representatives of many diverse phylogenetic groups may be adapted to any one habitat. Thus beetles, spiders, millipedes, lizards and mammals all occur in desert sand dune country, and certain arthropods, mammals and birds, can all thrive on dry seeds with no other exogenous source of water. But, again, quite closely related animals may be adapted to very different environments. *Arenivaga* and *Periplaneta* are both cockroaches, yet the first has an impermeable cuticle, absorbs water vapour and 'swims' in loose sand, while the latter loses water ten times faster, does not absorb water vapour, has long, thin appendages adapted to fast running, and is largely domestic.

In general the minimum water requirements of both arthropods and vertebrates decrease with increasing aridity of their habitats, and the extent to which such requirements have been reduced by natural selection is testimony to the remarkable plasticity of living material. Certain interesting questions remain. For example, what prevents desert rodents or desert isopods, well adapted as they are to water conservation in a 'difficult' environment from colonizing adjacent less arid areas? The answers will become clear only when we have a better understanding of animal biology and the mechanisms of evolution than we have at present.

7.5 REFERENCES

1 Bartholomew G.A. (1972) The water economy of seed-eating birds that survive without drinking. *Proc. XVth Intern. Ornithol. Congr.*, 237–54.

2 Beament J.W.L. (1961) The water relations of the insect cuticle. *Biol. Rev. Cambridge Phil. Soc.* **36,** 281–320.

3 Bentley P.J. (1971) *Endocrines and Osmoregulation.* Springer Verlag, Berlin, Heidelberg & New York.

4 Berridge M.J. (1970) Osmoregulation in terrestrial arthropods. In *Chemical Zoology*, Vol. 5, Arthropoda, Part A (eds M. Florkin & B. T. Scheer) pp. 287–320. Academic Press, New York & London.

5 Bursell E. (1970) *An Introduction to Insect Physiology.* Academic Press, New York & London.

6 Bursell E. (1974) Environmental aspects—humidity. In *The Physiology of Insecta*, Vol. II (ed. M. Rockstein) pp. 44–84. Academic Press, New York & London.

7 Buxton P.A. (1931) The law governing the loss of water from an insect. *Proc. Entomol. Soc. Lond.* **6,** 27–31.

8 Chew R.M. (1965) Water metabolism of mammals. In *Physiological Mammalogy*, Vol. II (eds W. V. Mayer & R. G. Van Gelder) pp. 43–178. Academic Press, New York & London.

9 Claussen D.L. (1967) Studies of water loss in two species of lizards. *Comp. Biochem. Physiol.* **20,** 115–30.

10 Cloudsley-Thompson J.L. (1971) *The Temperature and Water Relations of Reptiles.* Merrow, Watford, Herts.

11 Crawford E.C. Jr. & Lasiewski R.C. (1968) Oxygen consumption and respiratory evaporation of the Emu and Rhea. *Condor* **70,** 333–9.

12 Edney E.B. (1966) Absorption of water vapour from unsaturated air by *Arenivaga* sp. (Polyphagidae, Dictyoptera). *Comp. Biochem. Physiol.* **19,** 387–408.

13 Edney E.B. (1974) Desert arthropods. In *Desert Biology*, Vol. 2 (ed. G. W. Brown) pp. 311–84. Academic Press, New York & London.

14 Edney E.B. (1975) Absorption of water vapour from unsaturated air. In *Physiological Adaptation to the Environment* (ed. J. Vernberg). Intext Education Publishers, New York.

15 Grimstone A.V., Mullinger A.M. & Ramsay J.A. (1968) Further studies on the rectal complex of the mealworm, *Tenebrio molitor* L. (Coleoptera, Tenebrionidae). *Phil. Trans. Roy. Soc. Lond.* **253,** 343–82.

16 Gupta B.L. & Berridge M.J. (1966) Fine structural organization of the rectum in the blowfly *Calliphora erythrocephala* (Meig.) with special reference to connective tissue, tracheae and neurosecretory innervation in the rectal papillae. *J. Morph.* **120,** 23–82.

17 Locke M. (1974) The structure and formation of the integument of insects. In *The Physiology of Insecta*, Vol. VI (ed. M. Rockstein) pp. 124–213. Academic Press, New York & London.

18 Louw G.N. (1972) The role of advective fog in the water economy of certain Namib Desert animals. In *Comparative Physiology of Desert Animals* (ed. G. M. O. Maloiy) *Symp. Zool. Soc. Lond.* **31,** 297–314. Academic Press, New York & London.

19 Loveridge J.P. (1968) The control of water loss in *Locusta migratoria migratorioides* R. and F. *J. Exp. Biol.* **49,** 1–29.

20 MacMillen R.E. & Lee A.K. (1969) Water metabolism of Australian hopping mice. *Comp. Biochem. Physiol.* **28,** 493–514.

21 Maddrell S.H.P. (1971) The mechanisms of insect excretory systems. *Advances in Insect Physiol.* **8,** 199–331.

22 Murrish D.E. & Schmidt-Nielsen K. (1970) Exhaled air temperature and water conservation in lizards. *Respir. Physiol.* **10,** 151–8.

23 Nagy K.A. (1972) Water and electrolyte budgets of a free-living desert lizard, *Sauromalus obesus*. *J. Comp. Physiol.* **79,** 39–62.

24 Neville A.C. (1975) *The Biology of Arthropod Cuticle.* Springer-Verlag, Berlin, Heidelberg & New York.

25 Nobel-Nesbitt J. (1970) Water balance in the firebrat, *Thermobia domestica* (Packard). The site of uptake of water from the atmosphere. *J. Exp. Biol.* **52,** 193–200.

26 Phillips J.E. (1964) Rectal absorption in the desert locust, *Schistocerca gregaria* Forskal. *J. Exp. Biol.* **41,** 15–80.
27 Schmidt-Nielsen K. (1964) *Desert Animals: Physiological Problems of Heat and Water.* Clarendon Press, Oxford.
28 Schmidt-Nielsen K. (1972) *How Animals Work.* Cambridge University Press, London.
29 Shoemaker V.H. (1972) Osmoregulation and excretion. In *Avian Biology*, Vol. II (eds. D. S. Farner & J. R. King) pp. 527–74. Academic Press, New York & London.
30 Shoemaker V.H., Balding D., Ruibal R. & McClanahan L.L. Jr. (1972) Uricotelism and low evaporative water loss in a South American frog. *Science* **175,** 1018–20.
31 Shoemaker V.H., Nagy K.A. & Bradshaw S.D. (1972) Studies on the control of electrolyte excretion by the nasal gland of the lizard *Dipsosaurus dorsalis. Comp. Biochem. Physiol.* **42A,** 749–57.
32 Stobbart R.H. & Shaw J. (1974) Salt and water balance: excretion. In *The Physiology of Insecta*, Vol. V (ed. M. Rockstein) pp. 361–446. Academic Press, New York & London.
33 Taylor C.R. (1968) Hygroscopic food: a source of water for desert antelopes? *Nature, Lond.* **219,** 181–2.
34 Watt B.K. & Merrill A.L. (eds) (1963) *Composition of Foods.* U.S. Dept. of Agriculture Handbook No. 8, U.S. Govt. Printing Off., Wash., D.C.
35 Weis-Fogh T. (1967) Respiration and tracheal ventilation in locusts and other flying insects. *J. Exp. Biol.* **47,** 561–87.
36 Wieser W. & Schweizer G. (1970) A re-examination of the excretion of nitrogen by terrestrial isopods. *J. Exp. Biol.* **52,** 267–74.

Prelude to Chapter 8

The diversity of form and structure found in the animal kingdom is matched by a comparable diversity of locomotory mechanisms, each posing its own mechanical and physiological problems. These differ according to the environment in which an animal lives and the way in which it exploits that environment. There may appear to be little in common between the flight of a bird and the movement of a snail but, whatever the form of an animal, or the environment in which it lives, its locomotion will depend upon certain basic principles that are incorporated in Newton's three Laws of Motion. According to the first of these, a body that is at rest can be set in motion only by the application of an external force. This is often obvious, as when a locust jumps, but it is less so in the cases of buoyancy and gliding. In order to elicit such a force from the environment, an animal must actively move part or all of its body. According to the second law, the velocity imparted to the body is directly proportional to the magnitude of the force and the duration of time in which it acts, and inversely proportional to the mass of the body. Newton's third law states that for every action there must be an equal and opposite reaction. In other words, to subject its body to a propulsion force an animal must exert an equal force against the environment, but in the opposite direction.

These physical principles are not the only things in common between the locomotion of a bird and a snail. Both animals may move for similar reasons—to reach a new source of food, to escape from an unfavourable environment, or to find a mate. In the following chapter the reader will be introduced to the physiology and mechanics of movement in different environments—water, air, soil and on firm surfaces—to energy sources, structural materials, co-ordinating mechanisms, and the functions of locomotion in relation to the environments in which animals live.

Chapter 8
Locomotion

R. D. HARKNESS

8.1 INTRODUCTION

Locomotion is a central feature in the life of most animals. A simple consideration of body composition illustrates its importance; a terrestrial mammal contains about 40% by weight skeletal muscle and 5–20% skeleton [22, 90, 91, 221, 264]. There is a large literature on many aspects of the subject including evolution [44, 94, 153, 216, 260] summarized in this chapter with particular attention to some of its more neglected aspects.

8.2 ENVIRONMENTAL FACTORS AFFECTING LOCOMOTION

8.2.1 Water

The nature of the aquatic environment largely determines the mechanism of propulsion, the shape of the body and, possibly, the nature of its surface [59]. The direct action of gravity is relatively unimportant. Many animals have buoyancy mechanisms (Chapter 18) that reduce it, as for example, the swim-bladders of fishes [53, 54, 55]. Pangolins are terrestrial animals with a high average density on account of their heavily armoured skin; but even they can float by taking air into the alimentary canal (up to 18% of body volume) [177]. Indeed, many animals that do not live in water, including bats [240], are able to swim.

An important characteristic of the aquatic environment is the variation in pressure with depth, which creates problems for diving animals [66, 137, 138]. The principal characteristic is that it is continuous, over great distances. Many parasites are adapted to finding moving hosts in such a large space. A problem of keeping fish confined in a small space is that parasites may find them too easily, and multiply excessively.

8.2.2 Air

The need to move in an aerial environment also determines to a large extent the design of the body. The highest speeds are achieved in it and the greatest distances of movement for it also is continuous.

8.2.3. Surfaces

Gravity is the predominating influence on land, and most animals show specializations for surface contact. Special problems of locomotion arise on vertical or tilted surfaces. Running up a vertical surface requires more energy than on a horizontal one. It is easier for small animals than large as, for them, the relative increase in energy required to run vertically at the same speed as horizontally is less [229]. A special category of surface is that occurring between air and water [9, 172].

8.3 EFFECT OF BODY SIZE ON LOCOMOTION

The absolute size of an animal's body affects its functions [2, 89, 115, 207, 210].

8.3.1 Body size and movement in a fluid medium

With objects of the same shape, surface area varies as the square of the linear dimensions, volume as the cube. Thus, *Paramecium aurelia* has a length of about 130 μm, a diameter of 40 μm, a volume about 100,000 μm^3 and a surface area of about 10,000 μm^2[256]: its surface to mass ratio is about 1000 $cm^2\ g^{-1}$ compared with about 0·5 $cm^2\ g^{-1}$ for man. The energy available for movement is related to an animal's bulk, resistance to movement to its surface area. *Paramecium* at an interface, half in air half in water, would be subject to a force of surface tension about ten thousand times its body weight. So most small organisms live in a single fluid medium. For reasons connected with this scale effect, smaller animals tend to move more slowly than larger ones, but speeds differ little when expressed in terms of the animal's linear dimensions. The maximum speed of *Paramecium* is 1–3 mm sec^{-1} (3–10 m h^{-1}), or up to 15 lengths sec^{-1}. Because of their low speeds the movement of small creatures over distances depends largely upon translocation of the medium, water or air, as is produced by convection currents. Even 'still' air indoors moves about 10 cm sec^{-1} (0·5 k h^{-1}) [242]. There is an up current over the skin of the human body of up to 25 cm sec^{-1} [144] which carries shed epithelial cells that may have pathogenic bacteria on them [174]. Like many plant seeds [193] the smallest airborne animals are equally dependent on air movement as for example newly hatched spiders, that use a silk thread for airborne dispersal [70] or small insects like *Drosophila* (about 1 mg weight) [254].

Gravity becomes increasingly important for larger animals. In the mg to kg range, an addition to the area of surface in the form of wings makes it relatively easy for animals to fly. There is an upper limit to the size of flying animals, imposed by the nature of the materials from which the wings are made, and the source of power, skeletal muscle. The largest existing bird, which seems to be near the limit for self-propelled flight, is the Kori bustard (*c.* 12 kg [181]). In even larger flying animals external air movement again becomes important, as it must have been to the extinct flying reptiles such as *Pteranodon* [31], which had a wing span up to 10 m or more [142].

Buoyancy permits large size in an aqueous medium. Most fish swim at speeds of up to 10 body lengths sec^{-1}, but some, like tunny, are specialized for fast movement and can achieve 20 lengths sec^{-1} (up to 75 k.p.h.) for short distances. Difficulty in locomotion is probably not an important factor limiting the sizes of animals. Intrinsic physiological factors, like blood supply, are more important. Thus, in a vertebrate, if per unit of body weight the output of power were constant, as one might expect, the output of the heart per unit of body weight would also have to be constant. But the cross sectional area of the aorta varies as the square of the linear dimensions in related animals. So an increase in cardiac output in larger forms must be achieved by raising the length of the column of blood pumped out at each beat—that is, by raising the velocity. But the work necessary to accelerate the blood increases as the square of the velocity, and the largest animals seem to have reached a size at which such work is impossible [115]. Consequently they have had to reduce their output of power per unit of bulk.

8.3.2 Body size and terrestrial locomotion

In terrestrial locomotion the importance of air resistance has not been carefully examined but is probably small. For man it becomes important only when speeds of 35 k.p.h. or so are achieved as in skating [10]. But the effects of gravity are more severe. As size increases, the cross-sectional area of weight-bearing bones becomes smaller per unit of body weight, unless there is a change in skeletal configuration. There is no evidence that larger animals have developed stronger bones, but clear evidence of a change in the configuration of the skeleton [16]. Stresses at joint surfaces increase less than one would expect in larger mammals [215] and can be reduced by behaviour: elephants do not jump like horses. Effects of gravity limit the weight of arboreal animals; for example, much of the available food in trees is at the ends of finer branches [84]. It is difficult for an animal weighing more than a kilogram or two to reach it directly. Trees undoubtedly provide a refuge for lighter animals from heavier predators.

8.4 THE FUNCTIONAL BASIS OF LOCOMOTION

8.4.1 Sources of energy

There are two main sources of mechanical energy for locomotion in animals; cilia and related structures of small aquatic animals, and muscle in larger animals. Occasionally other sources are used, for example, in the limbs of spiders where hydrostatic force is used for extension, muscle only for flexion [263]. Cilia provide a rather special source of power as they are small and their action depends on the combined effect of large numbers [12, 29, 33, 41, 136, 219,

247]. Their diameter is commonly only 0·1–0·5 μm and their length about 20 μm. The *Paramecium* discussed above bears about 20,000 cilia on its surface.

Muscle

Much general information about the properties of muscle is available [11, 83, 148, 165, 187, 214, 250]. Invertebrate muscle varies more in properties than vertebrate, e.g. from very slow as in movement of skeletal structures by fluid under pressure (hydrostatic skeletons [42, 64], to very fast, as in insect wing muscles [187]). Among vertebrates in general, and mammals in particular, there is less variation, mainly in maximum rate of contraction. The individual contractile units (sarcomeres) are constant in length (2–3μ) and can produce tension within 20% of maximal (about 0·3 MNm^{-2} or 3 kgm/cm^2) over a range of variation in length of about 50%. The maximum energy production for a single contraction seems to be about 0·05 Jg^{-1} [see 181]; the quantity of muscle used in locomotion varies e.g. bird's in flight–a fifth of body weight [181]; bush baby in jumping—a tenth [96]. In vertebrates there appear to be at least two kinds of skeletal muscle, 'white' and 'red', whose properties are respectively adapted to short rapid actions, and to prolonged [97, 256].

Muscular activity raises physiological problems in supply of energy, and dissipation of heat, since at most 30% of the energy of fuel is available for mechanical work, the rest being lost as heat [115]. This may be used to raise the temperature and consequently the work output of the tissues, as in the flight muscles of many insects [20, 109, 110, 111, 112]. Specialized mechanisms for the dissipation of heat are found only in some animals, mammals, birds (e.g. [229]) and insects [37, 108]. A relatively unexplored subject is the cooling effect of forced air flow resulting from an animal's own movement [164].

Over short periods (secs–mins) energy may be obtained without the consumption of oxygen by the conversion of glycogen to lactic acid. Over longer periods, oxygen is necessary, supplied by the cardiovascular and respiratory systems. Muscle has a capacity for work of up to 1/3 watt (1/3 J/sec) per g [see 176] over periods of seconds, but less over longer. The cardiovascular system is also involved in the dissipation of heat, but the amount of blood required is small, probably less than 5% of maximal cardiac output in man.

8.5 STRUCTURAL MATERIALS

Three types of structural material, *simple* (providing mechanical stability and transmitting force) *energy storing* and *surface contact material* can be distinguished.

8.5.1 Simple structural materials

Chitin is the most important structural material of invertebrates [123, 202] used mainly for form exoskeletons. It is a polymer of N-acetylglucosamine, primarily of carbohydrate origin and so may be regarded as biologically cheap. It is strong —insect cuticle has a tensile strength about 10^8 Nm^{-2} [122]. Chitin is a fibrous material associated with cross-linked scleroprotein [173] and sometimes also with calcium salts. These may form structures almost alone with little other material in mollusc shells [87, 130, 261]. Collagen is found, but not extensively, for example, in soft internal structures in Arthropods. In vertebrates collagen is the principal structural material making probably an important contribution to their success [13, 100]. Its molecule has a unique structure [76, 185, 190]; three polypeptide chains of about 100 turns, like the strands in a rope. The molecules, about 3000 Å long and 15 Å in diameter, are assembled in an orderly fashion [58, 163, 185] to form cylindrical fibrils, later crosslinked [14, 15, 162, 228]. Collagen is used to resist tension along the length of the fibrils. These are, in general, between 50 and 150 mm in diameter and can be a centimetre long in the cornea [see 99]. They may well be much longer in, for example, tendons, but there is no direct evidence. The strength of collagen under slowly applied tensile stress along the direction of the fibrils (as in tendons) is of the order of 10^8 Nm^{-2} [23, 65, 101, 159, 243] about the same as mild steel on a weight for weight basis (excluding water). Though relatively inextensible (Young's modulus, about 10^9 Nm^{-2}) tendons can store functionally useful amounts of energy, up to about 5 Jg^{-1} [4, 25]. Collagen forms about 90% of the dry weight of such structures [100] which, in life, contain about 75% water. Little work has been done on the properties of tendons under rapidly applied stresses, although these may be of critical importance in locomotion, as when a horse lands from a jump [197, 226].

Though collagen is primarily a tensile material, it can also be used to create structures that resist compression as in cartilage, found predominantly in vertebrates [19, 74, 157, 211] but also in invertebrates [184]. Cartilage consists of a three-dimensional meshwork of collagen fibres, distended by water, attracted by anionic charges fixed to polysaccharide material, and their counter ions, mostly Na^+ [157]. This material (proteoglycan) of a high molecular weight (up to 10^6), is trapped in the mesh of the collagenous framework [106, 198]. It is made of polysaccharide chains of about 50 disaccharide repeating units attached to serine in a protein core (about 300 nm long, serines every 3 nm). These cores are attached in turn to a molecule of hyaluronic acid [141] to make an even larger structure [167, 168]. Cartilage contains about 20% collagen and 6% wet weight of such material with up to 150 meq charged groups per kg. Its mechanical properties depend on the density of the fixed charge groups which is limited by the amount of serine in the core protein. The degree of sulphation can be altered to a limited extent. Elasmobranchs that have no bone possess highly sulphated cartilage.

In bone which is more rigid than cartilage, collagen (30%, fresh weight) is still the basis, but the polysaccharide material is replaced by calcium phosphate crystals (hydroxyapatite, 60% of fresh weight) [61]. Its mechanical importance lies in its high compressive strength, up to about 2×10^8 Nm^{-2} under slowly increasing stress, its tensile strength in tendon being much like that of collagen. There is little information on the behaviour of bone under rapidly changing stress, as occurs in locomotion but what there is shows it, if anything, to be stronger than under slowly changing stress [38]. Bone is also mechanically stronger than mollusc shell [48].

Forces in movement may also be transmitted through fluid [spiders, 263].

8.5.2 Energy storing materials

Both collagenous and chitinous structures can be used to store energy. Two proteins that have this as their main function are *resilin* in arthropods and *elastin* in vertebrates [6, 73, 178, 255]: nearly all of the energy put into these can be retrieved. Both can be extended to a greater extent than collagen (up to about double their unstressed length) but, in general, they operate with smaller changes than this. Their moduli of elasticity in tension are lower than that of collagen (of the order of 5×10^5 Nm^{-2} approximately). Their capacity to store energy is also lower (about 2 Jg^{-1}). How they work is still not clear. The most important function of elastin as an energy store is in blood vessels such as the aorta. In vertebrate locomotion collagen is more important as an energy store, elastin being used in special places as in the ligamentum nuchae in ungulates holding up the head. Resilin, on the other hand, is used as an energy store in rapid, reciprocating movement. Insect wing muscles pull one way, resilin the other. Resilin is used where material is needed in a small space in connection with a muscle of wide cross sectional area. Collagen and chitin are used to provide energy storage in a smaller volume and with smaller extension. For example, in the jump of the locust, movement of the end of the limb is about 30 times greater than that of the chitinous energy store [25].

8.5.3 Surface contact materials

It does not seem that any special materials are involved in invertebrates, other than those used for the exoskeleton in general. In vertebrates, on the other hand, *keratins* [201] are involved. These are inert insoluble materials stabilized by disulphide cross links. Their importance is in the special structures formed of them—feathers, hooves and claws, and in softer pads covered with less rigid epidermal keratin. They also form hair which is associated with locomotion on the soles of the feet of mammals adapted to cold [93, 225]. Keratin can form an energy store and was used in China for making bows.

8.6 STRUCTURES

8.6.1 Joints

The majority of the structures involved in animal locomotion are composed of rigid or semi-rigid members united by joints (for a general account see [149]). The simplest joint consists of flexible material as is found between the segments of arthropods. The structure of the material may be sophisticated. Reversible extensions of up to ten times have been described in the membranes between the segments of the locust ovipositor, and also an interesting reversible process of work softening [244, 245, 246]. Flexible joints may be formed of cartilage in the mammalian ribcage. A more elaborate form is the intravertebral disc [75, 227], consisting of a central core of soft material enclosed by a flexible collagenous sheath.

In more complex joints two surfaces slide over one another. In arthropods they form hinges that allow movement in one plane. Universal movement in limbs is achieved by several joints in different planes. In vertebrates [18, 132] universal joints consist of a spherical head moving in a cup, as the human hip joint. Such a joint allows freedom of movement, but has the disadvantage that muscular power, which might otherwise be used for propulsion, is needed to stabilize it. The commonest form of joint is a modified hinge, as in the human knee. This is stabilized in one plane, mainly by collagenous ligaments. It is not a simple hinge, however, since movement does not take place about a fixed axis [223]. Two features are critical in the design of such joints. First, the nature of the surfaces and, secondly, their shape. The important feature of the surface is a low coefficient of friction—about 0·05 or less [43]. How this is achieved is not clear [266]. The joints have in them synovial fluid, containing hyaluronic acid. The cartilage at the surface differs from that beneath in having less fixed charge material, so that it is probably softer, spreading the load, on to more rigid cartilage beneath. Cartilage is thicker in larger animals; for example, in the knee of a mouse it is about 0·03 mm thick and in a cow 3 mm [215]. The reason is not exactly clear but presumably connected with getting the surface to fit together. They are not circular and are only fit (are 'congruent') at a certain angle of the joint, usually that in which the animal is standing with its weight on the limb [197]. Irregularity of the surface, as produced by a fracture in the underlying bone, may, in time, cause a failure in the joint owing to wearing away of the cartilage [5].

8.6.2 Lever systems

The lever systems that make up limbs are varied and show great mechanical sophistication (see [230]). Only a few general points are considered here. The work required to move a limb depends on the viscosity of the system and on the necessity to decelerate and accelerate parts that move back and forth in reciprocating motion. An ideal system would be a wheel moving on a flat surface. The centre of gravity does not move up and down and there is no reciprocating motion. A terrestrial animal's limbs in action seem to approximate to the efficiency of a wheel as far as movement of the centre of gravity is concerned. It is impossible, however, to avoid reciprocating movement but the work needed can be minimized by good design. The limb of a horse, say, behaves like a pendulum and can only be moved economically at its natural frequency. For high frequency the centre of gravity of the limb must be kept as near the axis of rotation as possible. So the ends of the limbs are made light and the weight of muscle concentrated near the axis of rotation. Economy of energy can be achieved on the return swing by curling up the limb to raise the centre of gravity. A similar trick is used by arboreal monkeys in brachiation. There the whole body is used as a pendulum [72].

8.6.3 Wings

The principles of wing construction are admirably described by Pennycuick [182]. For reasons like those just discussed the weight of a wing must be reduced as far as possible, and concentrated near the axis of rotation [182]. The design of wings varies with the requirement. For manoeuverability a high angle of attack, high camber, low aspect ratio and wing loading are required as in most bats. (*Angle of attack* is the angle between the plane of motion and that through the front and rear edge of the wing; *camber* is the curvature of the wing from front to back; *aspect ratio* is the length of the wing divided by the width or, if the shape of the wing is irregular, wingspan^2 wing area^{-1}). For fast flight the opposite is needed. This is seen in the longer, narrower wings of bats that fly fast and far, and of swallows. Aspect ratios in bats are usually in the range 5–10, wing loading in the range of 1–3 kg M^{-2} [241]. Some wings can be altered in shape during flight (birds, bats); others not (insects). The only animals that can alter the camber are the bats. They can also alter area by muscle in the wing but less than birds that can change the overlap of feathers. Feathers also have the advantage that they can be thin enough to reduce air turbulence at the tips and trailing edges of wings; and they are a non-living tissue, less easily damaged by, for example, sunlight. This can injure bats' wings which may partly explain why these animals are largely nocturnal.

8.7 SURFACE CONTACT STRUCTURES

8.7.1 Surface contact in smaller animals

Adhesion is important for small animals on flat surfaces and makes possible movement on smooth surfaces, even against gravity. Claws are commonly employed with a counter force, such as may be provided with the help of a frictional pad; as, for example, in the foot of a cat and in the adhesive organs of some parasites (e.g. *Entobdella* [133]). Claws have had little study though they seem to show sophisticated features of design. The keratin beneath the surface of the outer side of some mammalian claws is harder than elsewhere and is slightly calcified to form, it seems, a self-sharpening device [179]. Adhesion may be achieved by wet adhesive organs associated with mucus secretion. Many molluscs move by lifting an area of foot, sliding forward and repeating the process [166, 204]. Caterpillars move similarly [118] but use a different mode of adhesion.

Special modes of adhesion consisting of areas covered with fine hair-like processes are found in insects (e.g. [62]) and some reptiles (e.g. [203]). How such adhesive pads operate is not clear, but it seems likely that they employ the surface tension of a small quantity of liquid between the hair tips and the surface. The main problem is perhaps not so much how to make a pad adhere, but how to detach it.

8.7.2 Ground contact in larger animals

Contact structures may have a more sophisticated design than appears at first sight. Snow builds up under a rigid wooden clog but not under a rubber boot with a flexible sole [222]. In my experience an unshod foal does not accumulate snow under its hooves as its shod mother does. No detailed study of contact structures such as these appears to have been made or of the relation to the surfaces on which they are used. Information on specialization in birds' feet is given in [225]. Functionally important factors appear to be the avoidance of

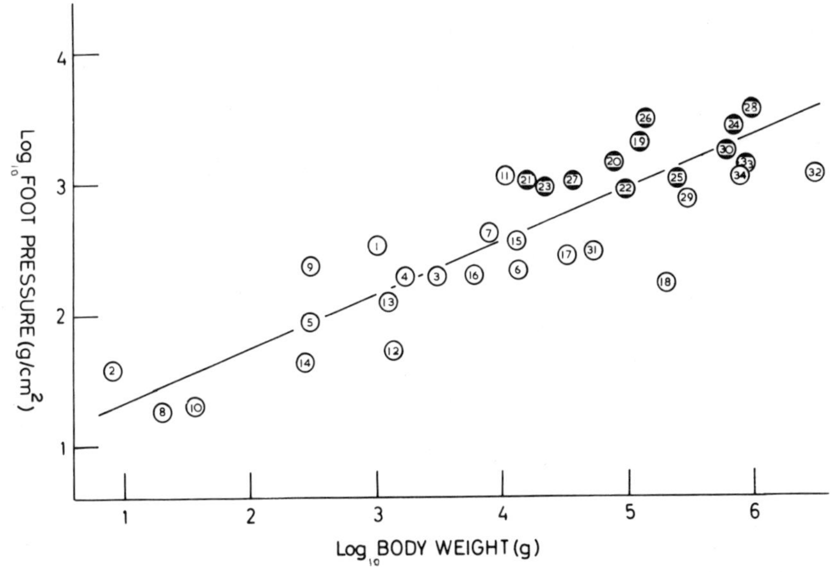

Fig. 8.1. Pressure on surface of feet. Pressure is calculated from body weight and area of hooves (●) or pads (○) in foot prints except for elephant, giraffe and bactrian camel which are based on measurements made on feet, and kindly provided by Dr Brambell and Miss Sue Matthews from the Zoological Gardens, London. The line is drawn by eye and has a slope of 0·41. The information for other animals was obtained from [17]. 1 Hedgehog; 2 Shrew; 3 Hare; 4 Rabbit; 5 Red squirrel; 6 Beaver; 7 Coypu rat; 8 Field vole; 9 Rat; 10 Wood mouse; 11 European lynx; 12 Pine marten; 13 Polecat; 14 Stoat; 15 Badger; 16 Fox; 17 Wolf; 18 Brown bear; 19 Wild boar; 20 Fallow deer; 21 Muntjac deer; 22 White-tailed deer; 23 Roe deer; 24 Elk (moose); 25 Reindeer; 26 Mouflon sheep; 27 Chamois; 28 Cattle; 29 Camel (one humped); 30 Horse; 31 Man (author); 32 Elephant; 33 Giraffe; 34 Camel (bactrian).

mechanical damage to the contact surfaces, or to the animal (not slipping), protection from thermal damage by a layer of inert material, e.g. nails in the desert lizard *Acanthodactylus*, or the feathers on the feet of ptarmigan [225], and resistance to wear during prolonged use. Weight on unit of area of surface of feet increases with body weight in the animals as one would expect (Fig. 8.1). A good example of an elaborate design is seen in the foot of a camel. This resembles a tyre filled with fat instead of air and is formed from the pads of the terminal phalangeal bones of two digits [8]. It consists (Fig. 8.2) of a bag con-

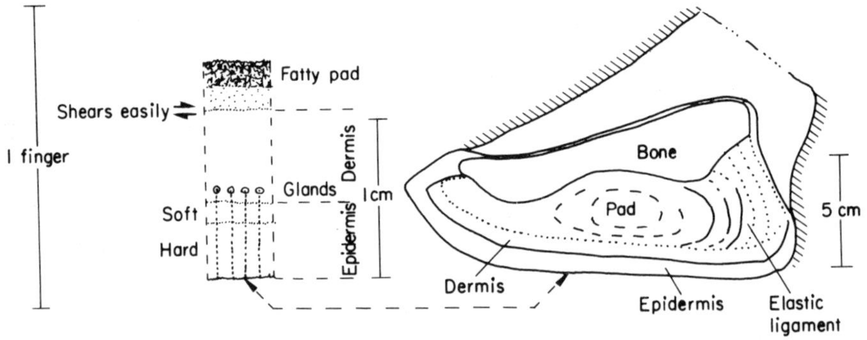

Fig. 8.2. Longitudinal section through foot of camel (*Camelus dromedarius*) with (on the left) the sole shown in greater detail.

taining long fatty pads separated by collagenous septa and surrounded by a strong collagenous wall, except at the rear end which contains a good deal of elastin. Above the fatty pads is bone and below, closely attached to the collagenous wall, a layer 1 cm or so thick of rubbery epidermis, kept flexible by moisture from sweat glands whose ducts run through it. This epidermal layer has a fibrous structure organized in a manner reminiscent of the interlacing prisms in tooth enamel [30]. When wetted it swells in a direction at right angles to its surface. The fat in the pad is mostly neutral triglyceride containing 75% of unsaturated fatty acids. Such fat is liquid at relatively low temperatures, a feature that could enable an animal to walk on cold surfaces without its pads solidifying.

8.7.3 Structures used in boring and burrowing

Some animals bore through rock by chemical means, using mechanical structures to scrape out the weakened material [39, 40]. Burrowing involves making a hole either by displacement and compression of the substrate or by its removal by digging, and is dependent on the texture of the substrate. Thus for displacement it must be soft, e.g. wet sand, and contain water or air-filled spaces [234]. A common method is to insert a thin wedge of material (muscle, hydrostatic skeleton) and expand it [233, 235]. In vertebrate reptiles (e.g. Amphibisbaeniaens) a hard, wedge-shaped head is thrust forward [78]. Burrowing by displacement is found only in animals with anatomical specializations for the purpose. Digging is more common and may also involve specialization of limbs or claws, as in the mole [82]. The mouth parts are often used by digging insects, such as ants, and by some fossorial mammals, e.g. the mole rat *Spalax*. Digging involves the separation of pieces of medium and the work involved is proportional to the area of the surface created in separating them; the larger the pieces and the ratio surface to volume, the more economical the work. The forces required to separate particles of substrate depend on the shape and structure of what is inserted and

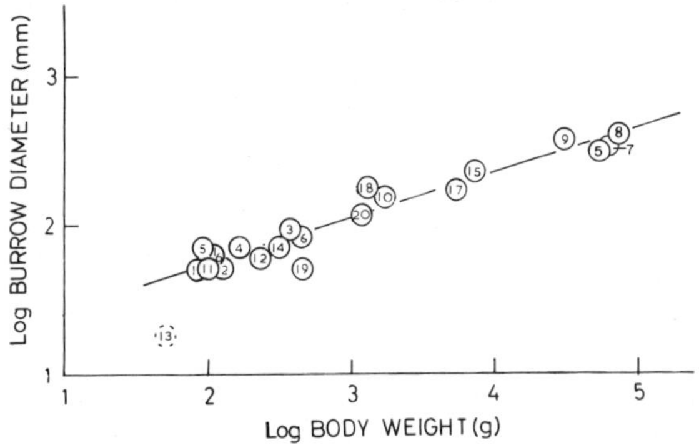

Fig. 8.3. Relation between body weight and diameter of burrow. The diameter of the burrow is taken as the average of the height and breadth where these are different. The species and sources of information are as follows: 1 Mole, *Scalopus aquaticus* [34]; 2 Pika, *Ochotona* princeps [155]; 3 Pocket gopher, *Pappogeomys* castanops [191]; 4 Pocket gopher, *Thomomys* bettae [191]; 5 Wolf *Canis lupis* [161]; 6 Ground squirrel, *Citellus columbianus* [154, 262]; 7 Badger, Meles meles [174a]; 8 Aardvark, *Orycteropus afer* [177]; 9 Pangolin, *Manis gigantea* [177]; 10 Rabbit, *Oryctolagus cuniculus* [231]; 11 Mole, *Talpa europea* [82]; 12 Tenrec, *Setifer setosus* [63]; 13 Tenrec, *Microgale talazaci* [63, uncertain burrow identification]; 14 Water vole, *Arvicola terrestris* [17]; 15 Fox, *Vulpes vulpes* [17]; 16 Cururo, *Spalacopus cyaneus* [192]; 17 Marmot, *Marmota monax* [71]; 18 Musk rat, *Ondatra zebithicus* [17]; 19 Tucotuco, *Ctenomys talarum* [253]; 20 Prairie dog, *Cyanomys ludovicianus* [212].

how. These same factors have to be considered in the design of equipment for mining coal [68]. The mechanism of digging by moles has been examined [217, 267] but not from this point of view. The diameters of burrows made by mammals appear to be proportional to the cube root of the body weight, or approximately to the linear dimensions of the animal (Fig. 8.3). Parasites that bore and burrow in animal tissues use both chemical and mechanical means [79, 143, 224].

8.7.4 Water/air interfaces

Only a few animals move at water/air interfaces: for example, molluscs of the genus *Ianthina*, some adult and larval insects, and many birds. The problem is that of controlling movement of water and the wetting of surfaces [194].

8.8 MECHANISMS OF LOCOMOTION

Locomotor mechanisms have been studied in detail (see [85]). Similar mechanisms may involve different structures [e.g. 195].

8.8.1 Aquatic locomotion

A few animals, such as frogs, use their limbs with a rowing motion. Others, such as cephalopods [127, 176], and some insects propel themselves with a jet of water. The majority perhaps of those specially adapted for swimming use a sinuous motion of the body in which waves are propagated backwards from the front. The principles of this method of propulsion are discussed by Lighthill [146; see also 3, 80, 85, 104, 113]. Mechanisms of aquatic locomotion seem to be designed to provide maximum effect, e.g. speed, for minimum expenditure of energy.

8.8.2 Flying

A number of animals jump, glide or fall considerable distances [92], and many are able to fly under their own power. Mechanisms of flight have received much attention (insects, [188]; birds [182, 28]; bats [241]). Special adaptations that use natural air movements to provide lift (soaring), combined with gliding can provide a means of travelling with less expenditure of energy than in simple powered flight [152]. Limitation on design may be imposed by the need to be able to take off from a surface.

8.8.3 Terrestrial locomotion

Limbless locomotion

The locomotion of snakes [21] and limbless lizards involves sinuous motion in all but exceptional cases, such as 'side winding' [24]. The functional significance of the loss of limbs is obscure.

Limbed locomotion

Locomotion involves 2, 4, 6 or, more rarely, 8 or more limbs (hexapedal, tetrapedal, bipedal or octopedal [36]). Bipedal differs from the others in being always unstable in the sense that there is no time in the cycle of movement when it can be arrested without the animal falling over.

Hexapedal locomotion is typical of Arthropoda [118] and involves at its simplest the simultaneous movement of the middle leg on one side and the fore and hind limbs on the other, while the remaining three limbs provide support. There is much detailed information from which it is difficult to generalize. The mechanism seems intrinsically simple with difficulty only in detail, as in arranging that the limbs do not hit one another.

Tetrapedal locomotion is typical of terrestrial vertebrates, and is most highly developed in mammals. It also occurs in hexapods whose front limbs have been modified for predation (e.g. preying mantids). In vertebrates, limb movement varies with different speeds of travel [77, 117]. In the slowest, the *walk*, legs are moved one at a time so that the animal is always on a stable base of three. The usual sequence is left front, right hind, right front, left hind. The forward phase of the limb's movement is called *protraction*; the backward, *retraction*. In the *trot* two legs come off the ground simultaneously on opposite sides of the body; in the *pace*, on the same side. In the *gallop* all four feet are off the ground at the same time in at least one phase of the stride. The design of the mechanism is, it seems, to minimize energy expenditure, for example to bring the footfalls as nearly as possible on a line beneath the centre of the animal, so that the legs exert no couple that could rotate the animal's body about its vertical axis. The fore and hind limbs do not normally touch the ground together and level with one another. The first is termed the leading limb. In the *transverse gallop* (horses) the leading fore and hind limb are on the same side of the body, in the *rotatory gallop* (dogs) they are on opposite sides. Individual species use one or other gallop consistently. If the movement is such that the two limbs (fore or hind) in any phase are moving together in the same direction, the lead can be changed easily, as in the cheetah [114]. This makes high speed possible over rough ground. The gallop is used only for short periods (mins), the walk, trot or pace for long periods (hours). Animals vary in choice of trot or pace. Thus dogs trot but the pace is characteristic of camels [50]. Many aspects of biological importance in limbed locomotion are not understood. Thus, compared with wolves, caribou go faster up hill than down [161]; hares similarly compared to dogs [67].

Bipedal locomotion has no obvious advantage except to free the fore limbs for flight or other activity, or for jumping. This last characteristic bipedal activity requires application of force by each limb simultaneously, a problem that is presumably too difficult to solve with more than two limbs. It usually involves energy storage, high acceleration (flea [199], click beetle [69], up to 300 g), and features of design that allow the application of force over a long time through long limbs [4, 25]. Bipedal locomotion may involve the two legs moving together in a series of jumps ('hopping') or alternatively. Energy loss in hopping, by up and down movement of the animal's weight is minimized by the use of tendons as energy reservoirs (kangaroos [52]).

8.8.4 Climbing and arboreal locomotion

This type of locomotion may involve only modifications of movements used on flat surfaces, or specialized ones (e.g. [72, 121]. Adhesion is a particular problem.

8.9 CO-ORDINATION OF LOCOMOTOR MECHANISMS WITH OTHER FUNCTIONS

An animal must be able to use its senses, particularly vision, while moving. This is possible, partly because the image that moves across the retina can be understood, and partly because there are complex mechanisms for stabilizing the head and eyes so that they remain fixed on a given object (man [56]). The human eyes can be well stabilized to movements with a frequency of up to 5 sec^{-1} [27] by means of the vestibular system and the semi-circular canals of the ear [129]. The locomotor mechanisms themselves when rapid seem to involve no feedback and are pre-set. The vertebrate cerebellum particularly is involved possibly as a timing device [119]. Other animals can perform complex processes with less nervous tissue [140], but their behaviour is less versatile.

8.10 PRESERVATION OF THE LOCOMOTOR SYSTEM

Locomotion involving unstable movement at speed carries a risk of accidental injury. Protection from injury by collision is achieved to some extent by the skin [102], which is so organized that it provides little resistance to movement [124]. The main factor in preventing accidental injury, however, is probably skill and the ability to avoid dangerous activities. An important factor in preserving skill is the avoidance of fatigue, as this increases proneness to accidents.

Many animals in locomotion use the structural materials of their body nearly to the limit of their mechanical capacity. Thus, for example, athletes and race-horses often damage themselves [197, 226]. Wild animals also become lame [161]. Young mammals are particularly prone to damage at the weak junction between the bone shaft and the epiphysis. This may be stabilized against shear by its shape, for example, at the lower end of the femur. No-one seems to have examined these junctions in detail from a mechanical point of view. An especially weak junction is at the head of the femur, which can be displaced in a dog by its pulling on a lead, and in man by playing rugby football [171].

Overloading of structural tissue may be avoided in a number of ways. Tendons may be large enough to withstand loads several times greater than the maximum their muscles can put on them, e.g. five times, pigeon flight muscle [183]. There are mechanoreceptors in the tendons (Golgi tendon organs [160, 218]) closely associated with collagen bundles [32]. They measure tension and can cause reflex relaxation of the muscle in whose tendons they lie [200]. Some mammalian muscle has a property that can be regarded as a safety device to protect the tendon from excessive stress. It gives way under severe stress [131], acting then as a viscous damper. Pain may provide warning of stress or strain, threatening rupture. It arises primarily from connective tissues [145]. Damage can be produced insidiously by repeated rapidly-applied stresses. So running on a hard surface can lame a horse. Damage by such rapid shocks cannot be avoided reflexly but only by avoiding the circumstances that give rise to them. The connective tissues of limbs are provided with shock detectors in the form of Pacinian corpuscles [149], for which no-one has found a convincing function [86].

Stresses arising indirectly from locomotion may involve mechanisms to protect particular parts of the body, as for example the central nervous system, whose function can be disorganized by mechanical shocks (though just how is not clear [249]).

Small animals may also use structural material to the limit of its mechanical capacity, for example, fleas [26] jumping and locusts ([25] safety factor about 50%).

8.11 FUNCTIONS OF LOCOMOTION IN RELATION TO THE LIFE AND ENVIRONMENT OF THE ANIMAL

8.11.1 Dispersal and aggregation

Dispersal may be important in finding sites for feeding or reproduction [170] but the extent to which it is limited by the locomotor system is not clear. Lepidoptera and other insects may be attracted over distances of kilometres by olfactory stimuli. For such purposes the animal must have a good enough locomotor system to allow it choice of direction and sufficient distance, for example, against a wind [181]. Many animals have reproductive forms with enhanced mobility (e.g. ants [125]).

8.11.2 Food gathering

Carriage of loads

Carnivorous mammals like the wolf take at one meal about 30% of their body weight [161]. Bats can take in even more, vampires [46, 265] up to 50%, others up to 70% of their body weight [51, 128]. Snakes occasionally ingest even larger loads of food [186]. Herbivorous mammals with fermenting material in the rumen or colon may carry 10% of their body weight [22, 91, 264]. Many carnivorous mammals can carry heavy loads in their mouths. Lions may carry a quarter to a third of their body weight [206]. Wolves may carry food 15 km or more to their young [169]. Domesticated transport animals can carry up to about 40% of their body weight (asses 50–60 kg, camels 150 kg, elephants 500 kg) [116]; men can carry up to 25 kg or more for 10 km per day [116]. Pregnant female mammals, including bats, may carry fetuses that weigh up to nearly half their own weight (Fig. 8.4). The weight of a single bat fetus at term is more than that of an egg in a bird of the same weight. Male mammals may bear antlers that weigh up to 10% of their total body weight [7, 81].

Very little is known of the effect of a load on locomotor ability. One pound added to the weight carried slows down a racehorse by about half a length (1·3 m) over a distance of 1·5 km [258]. This added weight is less than one thousandth that of the horse. Carriage of a fetus could clearly have a much larger effect, but it is not known.

8.11.3 Locomotion and predator–prey relationships

Locomotion is of critical importance in relation to predation. Predators may be divided roughly into two types, *pouncers* and *coursers*. Pouncers wait for the prey and attack it suddenly. A bush baby projects its whole body more than 2 m with an average acceleration of about 4 g and a take-off velocity of about 15 k.p.h. [95]. Squid can accelerate at up to 3 g to about 10 k.p.h. [236]. A num-

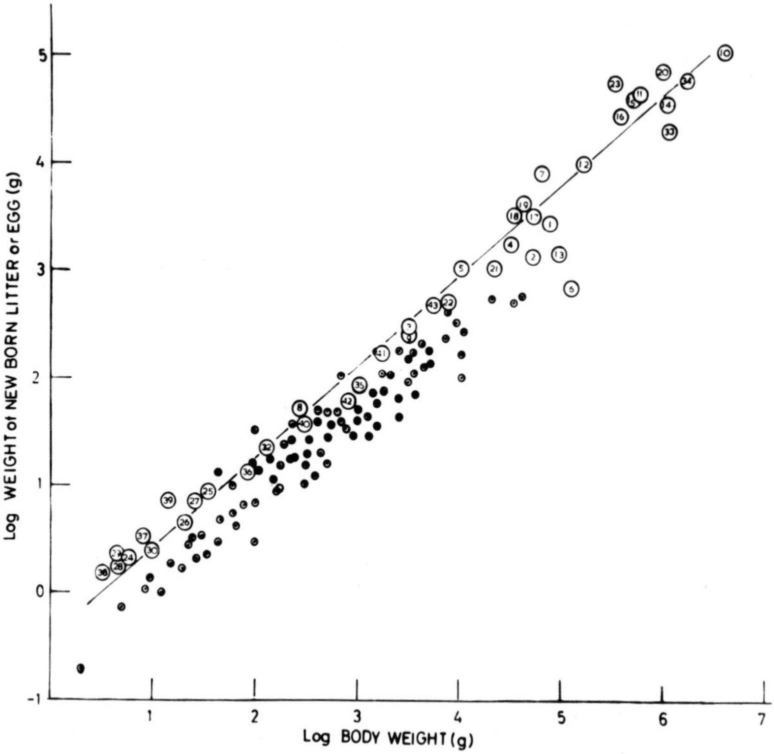

Fig. 8.4. Relation between weight of litter of newborn mammals and mother's weight (○) and between weight of an egg and bird (⊙). Information from [90, 107, 175, 206, 220]. 1 Jaguar; 2 Leopard; 3 Domestic cat; 4 Wolf; 5 Jackal; 6 Brown bear; 7 Common seal; 8 Rat; 9 Rabbit; 10 Elephant; 11 Domestic horse; 12 Domestic pig; 13 Barbirussa; 14 Pygmy hippopotamus; 15 Cattle; 16 Eland; 17 Rocky mountain goat; 18 Indian antelope; 19 Domestic sheep; 20 Giraffe; 21 Red brocket deer; 22 Pudu-deer; 23 One-humped camel; 24 Bat (*Balantiopteryx plicata*); 25 Bat (*Artibeus lituratus*); 26 Bat (*Choeronycteris mexicana*); 27 Bat (*Sternoderma rufus*); 28 Bat (*Myotis lucifugus*); 29 Bat (*Myotis austroriparius*); 30 Bat (*Plecotus townsendii*); 31 Bat (*Antrozaus pallidus*); 32 Bat (*Rousettus aegypticus*); 33 Black rhinoceros; 34 Indian rhinoceros; 35 Hedgehog; 36 Mole; 37 Shrew; 38 Pygmy shrew; 39 Water shrew (*Neomys fodicus*); 40 Red squirrel; 41 Rabbit; 42 Ferret; 43 Red fox.
The very light young of the one species of bear shown (6) is not unrepresentative; other bears have very small young.

ber of animals can accelerate a part of their body very fast—for example, chameleons, frogs and salamanders project their tongues to catch smaller animals. *Chamaeleo jacksoni* with a body length of about 12 cm can project its tongue up to 20 cm (maximum acceleration about 50 g, to about 20 k.p.h. [98]). The forelimbs of preying mantids can attain speeds up to 0·4 k.p.h. [45] in 30 m.sec. The head of a striking rattlesnake can attain a speed of 18 k.p.h. [186]. Coursers select their prey, particularly weak or lame individuals, and run it down over distances of up to several kilometres in mammals. The important locomotor characteristics in predators and prey are acceleration, speed and stamina. Predators must balance the energetic cost of movement against the quantity of food obtained by it [e,g. 150].

Acceleration

The ability to accelerate diminishes with increased size of body because the force exerted by muscle contraction is proportional to the square of the linear dimension of an animal, its weight to the cube. This may limit the size of the prey that a predator can catch without using more energy than it gets by eating it. In mammals the weight of the prey is usually about one-third that of the predator, though it can be larger [206]. Little information is available about acceleration in relation to predation. Friction may limit horizontal acceleration (as at the start of a sprint race). Small differences in the ability to accelerate may be important. Hares can avoid greyhounds by dodging [67] and are said to find greater difficulty in avoiding whippets that are slightly smaller. Small antelope (and other animals [e.g. 196]) may avoid predators by dodging [206].

Speed

Speed is important to predator and prey alike. Many predators will only go fast over a short distance. If they are outpaced for more than a minute, cheetahs and wolves will break off the chase

Stamina

Some predators catch their prey by exhausting it. Beagles may chase a hare for half-an-hour [67] while a greyhound catches it within a minute or not at all. The African hunting dog runs down its prey, as does the hyaena [139]. What physiological mechanisms limit ability to go on running is not clear, but several factors may be involved; *metabolic acidosis* from the production of lactic acid [105]; *overheating* may occur in heavily furred animals and has been recorded on marathon runners [189], associated with cessation of sweating; *partial failure of energy* supply is indicated by a fall in the blood glucose level. Other less obvious factors may also be concerned. Moose may collapse during a short run after a hard winter [169], but the reason is not known. A fit man can run for long periods at not more than 80% of his maximum rate of work. By chasing them in relays, predators may force an animal to run at speeds they cannot keep up.

8.11.4 Ranges and migration

Ranges

In general animals move in a limited area related to a 'home', a place for shelter, food storage, or reproduction. The distances over which animals move can be determined by simply following them [e.g. 103] or in various more complex ways [205, 213]. The area of the range is approximately proportional to the 2/3 power of body weight in land mammals [151], and in non-predatory birds, but to 4/3 power in predatory birds [209]. Many animals spend a large proportion of their time in movement. Wolves are on the move for up to 12 hours a day and travel distances up to 80 km or more during this time.

Migration

Migrating animals may travel long distances (e.g. [57, 158]) many hundreds of miles, particularly flying animals (e.g. [88]). The limiting factor is in general probably the amount of food reserves that the animal can carry. Fuel consumption per unit body weight for a given distance travelled decreases with the size of the animal [208, 238]. It is generally lower in flying animals [e.g. 239]. Fort he same energy expenditure, a bird weighing 100 g can go roughly ten times as far as a terrestrial animal of the same weight. The lightest fuel is fat. Glycogen is about eight times heavier because it has a lower caloric value, and can only be stored with about three times its weight of water. Before migration birds can lay down fat to the extent of 50% of their body weight [126, 135] on which a 100 g bird could go about 2000 km.

Navigation and pathways

Problems of navigation arise in travelling to and fro. No special mechanisms seem to be involved near a home base and many clues are used including ones laid down by the animal itself. Many animals make paths through vegetation that they follow repeatedly. Different species may follow the same paths. The frequency of use may be low [180]. Trails may be marked (insects [120, 147]; snails [257]). More elaborate mechanisms are used over long distances, e.g. solar navigation [156] which may be time compensated [248]. Animals tend to use almost every kind of available information, including the recognition of landmarks and the direction of the wind, e.g. ants [35, 60, 252], and birds [134, 158].

8.11.5 Communication

The problem of direction-finding brings us naturally to that of communicating direction from one animal to another, as bees do with a special form of movement [147]. Locomotion patterns are used by other animals for transmitting information, e.g. by birds [47], fish [232], and mammals, as for example probably in the curious behaviour of some ungulates, called 'stotting' [251].

8.12 REFERENCES

1 Alexander R.McN. (1968) *Animal Mechanics*. Sidgwick & Jackson, London.
2 Alexander R.McN. (1971) *Size and shape*. Institute of Biology Studies in Biology No. 29. Arnold, London.

3 Alexander R.McN. (1974) *Functional Design in Fishes.* Hutchinson, London.

4 Alexander R.McN. (1974) The mechanics of jumping by a dog (*Canis familiaris*). *J. Zool., Lond.* **173,** 549–73.

5 Ali S.Y., Elves M.W. & Leaback D.H. (eds) (1974) *Normal and Osteo-arthrotic Articular Cartilage.* Institute of Orthopaedics, London.

6 Andersen S.O. (1971) Resilin. In *Comprehensive Biochemistry* (eds M. Florkin & E. H. Stotz) Vol. 26C, pp. 633–58. Elsevier, Amsterdam, London & New York.

7 Anon (1954) *Jagd und Hege in aller Welt.* pp. 356–84. Heinzwolf Kölzig, Düsseldorf.

8 Arnautovic I. & Abdalla O. (1969) Elastic structures of the foot of the camel. *Acta anat.* **72,** 411–28.

9 Ashole N.P. (1971) Sea bird ecology and the marine environment. In *Avian Biology* (eds D. S. Farner, J. R. King & K. C. Parkes) Vol. 1, pp. 223–86. Academic Press, New York & London.

10 Åstrand P-O. & Rodahl K. (1970) *Textbook of Work Physiology.* McGraw Hill, New York.

11 Atwood H.L. (1972) Crustacean muscle. In *The Structure and Function of Muscle* (ed. G. H. Bourne) Vol. 1, pp. 422–90. Academic Press, New York & London.

12 Baba S.A. (1972) Flexural rigidity and elastic constant of cilia. *J. exp. Biol.* **56,** 459–67.

13 Bailey A.J. (1968) The nature of collagen. In *Comprehensive Biochemistry.* (eds M. Florkin & C. H. Stotz) Vol. 26B, pp. 297–424. Elsevier, Amsterdam, London & New York.

14 Bailey A.J. & Robbins A.P. (1973) Development and maturation of cross links in collagen fibres of skin. In *Ageing of Connective Tissues—Skin* (eds L. Robert & B. Robert) pp. 130–56. Karger, Basel.

15 Bailey A.J., Robins S.P. & Balian G. (1974) Biological significance of the inter-molecular cross links of collagen. *Nature, Lond.* **251,** 105–9.

16 Bakker R.T. (1971) Ecology of brontosaurs. *Nature, Lond.* **229,** 172–4.

17 Bang P. & Dahlstrom D. (1972) *Animal Tracks and Signs* (translated by G. Vevers). Collins, London.

18 Barnett C.H., Davies D.V. & MacConaill M.A. (1971) *Synovial Joints.* Longman, London.

19 Barrett A.J. (1971) Cartilage. In *Comprehensive Biochemistry* (eds M. Florkin & C. H. Stotz) Vol. 26B, pp. 425–74. Elsevier, Amsterdam, London & New York.

20 Bartholomew G.A. & Heinrich B. (1973) A field study of night temperatures in moths in relation to body weight and wing loading. *J. exp. Biol.* **58,** 123–5.

21 Bellairs A.deA. (1969) *The Life of Reptiles.* Weidenfeld & Nicolson, London.

22 Benedict F.G. (1936) *The Physiology of the Elephant.* Carnegie Institute, Washington.

23 Benedict J.V., Walker L.B. & Harris E.H. (1968) Stress strain characteristics and tensile strength of unembalmed human tendon. *J. Biomechan.* **3,** 181–9.

24 Bennet S., McConnell T. & Trubatch S.L. (1974) Quantitative analysis of the speed of snakes as a function of peg spacing. *J. exp. Biol.* **60,** 161–5.

25 Bennet-Clark H.C. (1974) Energy storage in jumping animals. *Proc. 50th Anniversary Meeting, Soc. Exp. Biol.* (eds P. Spencer-Davies & L. Sunderland). Pergamon Press, Oxford.

26 Bennet-Clark H.C. & Lucy E.C.A. (1967) The jump of the flea; a study of the energetics and a model of the mechanism. *J. exp. Biol.* **47,** 59–76.

27 Benson A.J. (1970) Interactions between semicircular canals and graviceptors. *Recent Ads. Aerospace Med.* (ed. D. E. Busby) pp. 249–61. Reidel, Dordrecht.

28 Berger M. & Hart J.S. (1974) Physiology and energetics of flight. In *Avian Biology* (eds D. S. Farner & J. R. King) Vol. 4, pp. 415–77. Academic Press, New York & London.

29 Blake J.R. & Sleigh M.A. (1974) Mechanics of ciliary motion. *Biol. Rev.* **49,** 85–125.

30 Boyd A. (1969) Electronmicroscopic observations relating to the nature and development of prism decussation in mammalian dental enamel. *Bull. Group. Int. Rech. Sc. Stomat.* **12,** 151–207.

31 Bramwell C.D. & Whitfield G.R. (1974) Biomechanics of pteranodon. *Phil. Trans. R. Soc., Lond.* B. **267,** 503–81.
32 Bridgman C.F. (1968) The structure of tendon organs in the cat. *Anat. Rec.* **162,** 209–20.
33 Brokaw, C.J. (1966) Mechanics and energetics of cilia. *Amer. Rev. Resp. Dis.* **93,** 32–40.
34 Brown L.N. (1972) Unique features of tunnel systems of the eastern mole in Florida. *J. Mammal.* **53,** 394–5.
35 Burkhalter A. (1972) Distance measuring as influenced by terrestrial clues in Cataglyphis bicolor (Formicidae, Hymenoptera). In *Information Processing in the Visual Systems of Arthropods* (ed. R. Wehner) pp. 281–6. Springer Verlag, Berlin, Heidelberg & New York.
36 Burrows M. & Hoyle G. (1973) The mechanism of rapid running in the ghost crab, *Ocypoda ceratophthalma. J. exp. Biol.* **58,** 327–49.
37 Bursell F. (1974) Environmental Aspects—Temperature. In *The Physiology of Insects.* (ed. M. Rockstein) Vol. II, pp. 2–43. Academic Press, London.
38 Burstein A.H., Currey J.D., Frankel P.V.H. & Reilly D.T. (1972) The ultimate properties of bone tissue: The effects of yielding. *J. Biomechan.* **5,** 35–44.
39 Carriker M.R., Scott D.B. & Martin N.M. (1963) Demineralisation mechanism of boring gastropods. In *Mechanisms of Hard Tissue Destruction* (ed. R. G. Sognnaes) pp. 55–89. American Association for Advancement of Science, Washington.
40 Carriker M.R. & Van Zandt D. (1970) Predatory behaviour of a shell-boring muricid gastropod. In *Behaviour of Marine Animals.* (ed. H. E. Winn & B. L. Olla) pp. 157–244. Plenum Press, New York.
41 Carson S., Goldhamer R. & Carpenter R. (1966) Mucus transport in the respiratory tract. *Amer. Rev. Resp. Dis.* **93,** 86–92.
42 Chapman G. (1958) The hydrostatic skeleton in the invertebrates. *Biol. Rev.* **33,** 338–71.
43 Charnley J. (1959) The lubrication of animal joints. *Symposium on Biomechanics,* pp. 12–19. Inst. of Mech. Engineers, London.
44 Clark R.B. (1964) *Dynamics of Metazoan Evolution.* Clarendon Press, Oxford.
45 Cloarec A. (1969) Étude descriptive et expérimentale du comportement de capture de *Ranata linearis* au course de son ontogènese. *Behaviour* **35,** 84–113.
46 Crespo R.F., Burns R.J. & Linhart S.B. (1970) Load lifting capacity of the vampire bat. *J. Mammal.* **51,** 627–8.
47 Cullen J.M. (1972) Some principles of animal communication. In *Nonverbal Communication* (ed. R. A. Hinde). Cambridge University Press, London.
48 Currey J.D. & Taylor J.D. (1974) The mechanical behaviour of molluscan hard tissues. *J. Zool. Lond.* **173,** 395–406.
49 Curry J.D. (1970) *Animal Skeletons.* Institute of Biology Studies in Biology No. 22. Arnold, London.
50 Dagg A.I. (1974) The locomotion of the camel (*Camelus dromedarius*). *J. Zool., Lond.* **174,** 67–78.
51 Davis R. & Cockrum E.L. (1964) Experimentally determined weight lifting capacity of five species of Western bats. *J. Mammal.* **45,** 643–4.
52 Dawson T.J. & Taylor C.R. (1973) Energetic cost of locomotion in kangaroos. *Nature, Lond.* **246,** 313–14.
53 Denton E.J. (1961) The buoyancy of fish and cephalopods. *Prog. Biophys.* **11,** 177–234.
54 Denton E.J. (1974) On buoyancy and the lives of modern and fossil cephalopods. *Proc. R. Soc. Lond. B.* **185,** 273–99.
55 Denton E.J. (1974) Buoyancy in marine animals. *Oxford Biology Readers No.* 54 (ed. J. J. Head). Oxford University Press, Oxford.
56 Ditchburn R.W. (1973) *Eye Movements and Visual Perception.* Clarendon Press, Oxford.
57 Dorst J. (1962) *The Migrations of Birds.* Translated by C. D. Sherman. Heinemann, London.
58 Doyle B.B., Holmes D.J.S., Miller A., Parry D.A.D., Piez K.A. & Woodhead-Galloway J. (1974) A D-periodic narrow filament in collagen. *Proc. R. Soc.* B. **186,** 67–74.

59 Dubois A.B., Cavagna G.A. & Fox, R.S. (1974) Pressure distribution on the body surface of swimming fish. *J. exp. Biol.* **60,** 581–91.
60 Duelli P. (1972) The relation of astromenotactic and anemomenotactic orientation mechanisms in desert ants, *Cataglyphis bicolor* (*Formicidae, Hymenoptera*). In *Information Processing in the Visual Systems of Arthropods* (ed. R. Wehner) pp. 281–6. Springer-Verlag, Berlin, Heidelberg & New York.
61 Eastoe J.E. (1975) The composition and chemical dynamics of bone. In *Scientific Fundamentals of Dentistry* (eds I. R. H. Kramer & B. Cohen) Ch. 48. Heinemann, London.
62 Edwards J. S. & Tarkanian, M. (1970) The adhesive pads of Heteroptra: a re-examination. *Proc. R. ent. Soc. Lond.* **45,** 1–5.
63 Eisenberg J.F. & Gould E. (1970) The tenrecs: A study in mammalian behaviour and evolution. *Smithsonean Contrib. Zool.* No. 27, 1–126.
64 Elder H.Y. (1973) Direct peristaltic progression and the functional significance of the dermal connective tissues during burrowing in the Polychaete *Polyphysia Crassa* (Oersted) *J. exp. Biol.* **58,** 637–55.
65 Elliott D.H. (1965) Structure and function of mammalian tendon. *Biol. Rev.* **40,** 392–421.
66 Elsner R. (1969) Cardiovascular adjustments to diving. In *The Biology of Marine Mammals.* (ed. H. T. Andersen) pp. 117–46. Academic Press, New York & London.
67 Evans G.E. & Thomson D.R.A. (1972) *The Leaping Hare.* Faber & Faber, London.
68 Evans I. & Pomeroy, C.D. (1966) *The Strength, Fracture and Workability of Coal.* Pergamon Press, Oxford.
69 Evans M.E.G. (1972) The jump of the click beetle (*Coleoptera, Elateridae*)—a preliminary study. *J. Zool. Lond.* **167,** 319–36.
70 Fabre J.H. (1912) *The Life of the Spider.* Translated by A. Teixelira de Mattos. Hodder & & Stoughton, London.
71 Fisher W.H. (1893) Investigations of the burrows of the American marmot. *J. Cincinnati Soc. Natural Hist.* **16,** 105–23.
72 Fleagle J. (1974) Dynamics of brachiating simiang (*Hylobates* (*symphalangus*) *syndactylus*) *Nature*, **248,** 259–60.
73 Franzblau C. (1971) Elastin. In *Comprehensive Biochemistry* (eds M. Florkin & E. H. Stotz) Vol. 26C, pp. 659–712. Elsevier, Amsterdam.
74 Freeman M.A.R. (ed.) (1973) *Adult Articular Cartilage.* Pitman Medical, London.
75 Galante J.O. (1967) Tensile properties of the human lumbar annulus fibrosus. *Acta Orthop. Scand.* Supp. 100.
76 Gallop P.M., Blumenfeld O. & Seifter S. (1972) Structure and metabolism of connective tissue proteins. *Ann. Rev. Biochem.* **41,** 617–72.
77 Gambaryan P.P. (1974) *How Mammals Run.* Translated by H. Hardin Wiley, New York.
78 Gans C. (1974) *Biomechanics.* Lippincott, Philadelphia.
79 Garnham P.C.C. (1966) Locomotion in the parasitic protozoa. *Biol. Rev.*, **41,** 561–86.
80 Gaskin D.E. (1972) *Whales, Dolphins and Seals.* Heineman, London.
81 Geist V. (1966) The evolution of horn-like organs. *Behaviour* **27,** 175–214.
82 Godfrey G. & Crowcroft P. (1960) *The Life of the Mole.* Museum Press, London.
83 Gould R.P. (1972) The microanatomy of muscle. In *The Structure and Function of Muscle* (ed. G. H. Bourne), Vol. 2 pp. 185–241. Academic Press, New York & London.
84 Grand T.I. (1972) A mechanical interpretation of terminal branch feeding. *J. Mammal.* **53,** 198–201.
85 Gray J. (1968) *Animal Locomotion.* Weidenfeld & Nicolson, London.
86 Gray J.A.B. (1960) Pacini and his corpuscle. *Sperimentale*, **110,** 372–92.
87 Grégoire Ch. (1967) Sur la structure des matrices organiques des coquilles de mollusques. *Biol. Rev.* **42,** 653–88.
88 Griffin D.R. (1970) Migrations and homing of bats. In *Biology of Bats* (ed. W. A. Winsatt) Vol. 1, pp. 233–64. Academic Press, New York & London.
89 Günther B. (1975) On theories of biological similarity. *Fortschritte. exp. u. Theoret. Biophys.* **19,** 1–111.

90 Guggisberg C.A.W. (1966) *S.O.S. Rhino*. Deutsch, London.

91 Hakonson T.E. & Whicker F.W. (1971) The contribution of various tissues and organs to total body mass in the mule deer. *J. Mammal.* **52,** 628–30.

92 Haldane J.B.S. (1928) On being the right size. In *Possible Worlds*, pp. 18–26. Chatto & Windus, London.

93 Hall E.R. (1951) *American Weasels*. University of Kansas Publications, No. 4, 1–466 (p. 64).

94 Hall T.S. (1969) *Ideas of Life and Matter. Studies in the history of general physiology* 600 *BC*–1900 *AD*. University of Chicago Press, Chicago.

95 Hall-Craggs E.C.B. (1965) An analysis of the jump of the Lesser Galago (*Galago senegalensis*). *J. Zool.* **147,** 20–4.

96 Hall-Craggs E.C.B. (1974) Physiological and histochemical parameters in comparative locomotor studies. In *Prosimian Biology* (eds R. D. Martin, G. A. Doyle & A. C. Walker) pp. 829–45. Duckworth, London.

97 Hall-Craggs E.C.B. (1974) Mammalian skeletal muscle and its innervation. In *Essays on the Nervous System* (eds R. Bellairs & E. G. Gray) pp. 106–30. Clarendon Press, Oxford.

98 Harkness L.I.K. (1975) Personal communication.

99 Harkness M.L.R. & Harkness R.D. (1973) The use of mechanical tests in determining the structure of connective tissues. *Biorheology* **10,** 157–63.

100 Harkness R.D. (1961) Biological functions of collagen. *Biol. Rev.* **36,** 399–463.

101 Harkness R.D. (1968) Mechanical properties of collagenous tissues. In *Treatise on Collagen* (ed. B. S. Gould) Vol. 2A, pp. 248–310. Academic Press, New York & London.

102 Harkness R.D. (1971) Mechanical properties of skin in relation to its biological function and its chemical components. In *Biophysical Properties of the Skin* (ed. H. R. Elden) pp. 393–436. Wiley, New York.

103 Harkness R.D. (1976) Duration and lengths of foraging paths of *Cataglyphis bicolor* (*Hymenoptera, Formicidae*) *Ent. mon. Mag.* in press.

104 Harrison R.J. (1972) *Functional Anatomy of Marine Mammals*. Academic Press, New York & London.

105 Harthoorn A.M., van der Walt K. & Young E. (1974) Possible therapy for capture myopathy in captured wild animals. *Nature, Lond.* **247,** 577.

106 Hascall V.C. & Heinegård D. (1975) The structure of cartilage proteoglycan. In *Extracellular Matrix Influences on Gene Expression* (eds H. C. Slavkin & R. C. Greulich) pp. 423–44. Academic Press, New York & London.

107 Heimroth O. (1930) In *Tabulae Biologicae* (eds C. Oppenheimer & L. Pincussen) Band VI, pp. 716–41. Junk, Berlin.

108 Heindrich B. (1970) Thoracic temperature stabilization by blood circulation in a free-flying moth. *Science, N.Y.* **168,** 580–2.

109 Heindrich B. (1971) Temperature regulation of the sphinx moth *Manduca sexta* I. Flight energetics and body temperature during free and tethered flight. *J. exp. Biol.* **54,** 141–52.

110 Heindrich B. (1971) Temperature regulation of the sphinx moth *Manduca sexta* II. Regulation of heat loss by control of blood circulation. *J. exp. Biol.* **54,** 153–66.

111 Heindrich B. & Bartholomew G.M. (1971) An analysis of pre-flight warm-up in the sphinx moth *Manduca sexta*. *J. exp. Biol.* **55,** 223–34.

112 Heindrich B. & Kammer A.E. (1973) Activation of the fibrillar muscles in the bumble bee during warm-up. Stabilization of thoracic temperature and flight. *J. exp. Biol.* **58,** 677–88.

113 Hertel H. (1969) Hydrodynamics of swimming and wave-riding dolphins. In *The Biology of Marine Mammals* (ed. H. T. Anderson) pp. 31–64. Academic Press, New York & London.

114 Hildebrand M. (1959) Motions of the running cheetah and horse. *J. Mammal.* **50,** 481–95.

115 Hill A.V. (1949) The dimensions of animals and their muscular dynamics. *Proc. Roy. Inst.* **34,** 450.

116 Hobley C.W. (1914) Transport Animals. In *The Frontiersman's Pocket Book*, pp. 182–98. Murray, London.

117 Howell A.B. (1944) *Speed in Animals.* University of Chicago Press, Chicago.
118 Hughes G.M. & Mill P.J. (1974) Locomotion: Terrestrial. In *The Physiology of Insecta* (ed M. Rockstein) Vol. 3, pp. 335–81. Academic Press, New York & London.
119 Ito M. (1974) The control mechanisms of cerebellar motor systems. In *The Neurosciences* (eds F. O. Schmitt & F. G. Worden) pp. 293–303. M.I.T. Press, Cambridge, Mass.
120 Jacobson M. (1974) Insect Pheromones. In *Physiology of Insecta* (ed. M. Rockstein) Vol. 3, pp. 229–79. Academic Press, New York & London.
121 Jenkins F.A. (ed.) (1974) *Primate Locomotion.* Academic Press, New York & London.
122 Jensen M. & Weis-Fogh T. (1962) Biology and biophysics of locust flight. V. Strength and elasticity of insect cuticle. *Phil. Trans. R. Soc. B.* **245,** 137–69.
123 Jeuniaux C. (1971) Chitinous structures. In *Comprehensive Biochemistry* (eds M. Florkin & E. H. Stotz) Vol. 26, pp. 595–632. Elsevier, Amsterdam.
124 Johns R.J. & Wright V. (1962) Relative importance of various tissues in joint stiffness. *J. appl. Physiol.* **17,** 824–8.
125 Johnson C.G. (1974) Insect migration: Aspects of its Physiology. In *The Physiology of Insecta* (ed. M. Rockstein) Vol. 3, pp. 280–334. Academic Press, New York & London.
126 Johnston D.W. (1970) Caloric density of avian adipose tissue. *Comp. Biochem. Physiol.* **34,** 827–32.
127 Johnson W., Soden P.D. & Trueman E.R. (1972) A study in jet propulsion: an analysis of the motion of the squid, *Loligo vulgaris. J. exp. Biol.* **56,** 155–65.
128 Jones C. & Suttkus R.D. (1971) Wing loading in *Plecotus rafinesquii. J. Mammal.* **52,** 458–60.
129 Jones G.M. & Spells K.E. (1963) A theoretical and comparative study of the functional dependence of the semicircular canal upon its physical dimensions. *Proc. Roy. Soc.* **B. 157,** 403–19.
130 Jope M. (1971) Constituents of Brachiopod Shells. In *Comprehensive Biochemistry* (ed. M. Florkin & C. H. Stotz) Vol. 26C, pp. 749–84. Elsevier, Amsterdam.
131 Joyce G.C., Rack P.M.H. & Westbury D.R. (1969) The mechanical properties of cat soleus muscle during controlled lengthening and shortening movements. *J. Physiol.* **204,** 461–74.
132 Kapandji I.A. (1970) *The Physiology of Joints.* Translated by L. H. Honore. Churchill Livingstone, Edinburgh & London.
133 Kearn G.C. (1964) The attachment of the monogenean *Entobdella soleae* to the skin of the common sole. *Parasitology,* **57,** 327–35.
134 Keeton W.T. (1974) The orientation and navigational basis of homing in birds. *Advanc. Study Behaviour* **5,** 47–132.
135 King S.R. (1972) Adaptive periodic fat storage by birds. *Proc. XV Ornithol. Congress,* (ed. K. H. Voons). pp. 200–17. Brill, Leiden.
136 Kinosita H. & Murakami A. (1967) Control of ciliary motion. *Physiol. Rev.* **47,** 53–82.
137 Kooyman G.L. (1975) Behaviour and physiology of diving. In *The Biology of Penguins* (ed. B. Stonehouse) pp. 115–38. Macmillan, London.
138 Kooyman G.L. & Andersen H.T. (1969) Deep diving. In *The Biology of Marine Mammals* (ed. H. T. Andersen) pp. 65–94. Academic Press, New York & London.
139 Kruuk H. (1972) *The Spotted Hyaena.* Chicago University Press, Chicago.
140 Land M.F. (1974) A comparison of the visual behaviour of a predatory arthropod with that of a mammal. In *The Neurosciences* (ed. F. O. Schmitt & F. G. Worden) pp. 411–18. M.I.T. Press, Cambridge, Mass.
141 Laurent T.C. (1972) The ultrastructure and physical chemical properties of the interstitial connective tissue. *Pflugers Arch* **336,** Suppl. 21–42.
142 Lawson D.A. (1975) Pterosaur from the latest cretaceous of West Texas: discovery of the largest flying creature. *Science* **187,** 947–8.
143 Lewert R.M. (1958) Invasiveness of helminth larvae. *Rice Institute Pamphlet* **45,** 97–113.
144 Lewis H.E., Foster A.R., Mullan B.J. Cox R.N. & Clark R.P. (1969) Aerodynamics of the human microenvironment. *Lancet* **1,** 1272–7.

145 Lewis T. (1942) *Pain*. Macmillan, New York.
146 Lighthill M.J. (1969) Hydromechanics of aquatic animal propulsion. *A. Rev. Fluid Mech.* **1,** 413–46.
147 Lindauer M. (1974) Social behaviour and mutual communication. In *The Physiology of Insecta* (ed. M. Rockstein) Vol. 3, pp. 150–228. Academic Press, New York & London.
148 Lockhart R.D. (1972) Anatomy of muscles and their relation to movement and posture. In *The Structure and Function of Muscle* (ed. G. H. Bourne) Vol. 1, pp. 1–23. Academic Press, New York & London.
149 Loewenstein W.R. (1971) *Mechano-Electric Transduction in the Pacinian Corpuscle* (ed. W. R. Loewenstein) Vol. 1, pp. 269–90. Springer-Verlag, Berlin, Heidelberg & New York.
150 MacArthur R.H. & Pianka E.R. (1966) On optimal use of a patchy environment. *Amer. Nat.* **100,** 603–9.
151 McNab B.K. (1963) Bio-energetics and the determination of home range size. *Amer. Nat.* **97,** 133–40.
152 McGahan J. (1973) Gliding flight of the Andean Condor in nature. *J. exp. Biol.* **58,** 225–37.
153 Manton S.M. (1972) The evolution of arthropodan locomotry mechanisms. Part 10. Locomotory habits morphology and evolution of the hexapod classes. *Zool. J. Linn. Soc.* **51,** 203–400.
154 Manville R.H. (1959) The Columbian ground squirrel in North Western Montana. *J. Mammal.* **40,** 26–45.
155 Markham O.D. & Whicker F.W. (1972) Burrowing in the Pika (*Ochotona princeps*) *J. Mammal.* **53,** 387–8.
156 Markl H. (1974) Insect behaviour: functions and mechanisms. In *The Physiology of Insecta* (ed. M. Rockstein) Vol. 3, pp. 3–149. Academic Press, New York & London.
157 Maroudas A. (1973) Physico-chemical properties of articular cartilage. In *Adult Articular Cartilage* (ed. M. A. R. Freeman) pp. 156–70. Pitman Medical, London.
158 Matthews G.V.T. (1968) *Bird Navigation*. Cambridge University Press, London.
159 Matthews L.S. & Ellis D. (1968) Viscoelastic properties of cat tendon; effects of time after death and preservation by freezing. *J. Biomechan.* **1,** 65–71.
160 Matthews P.B.C. (1972) *Mammalian Muscle Receptors and Their Central Actions*. Arnold, London.
161 Mech L.D. (1966) The wolves of Isle Royale. *Fauna of the National Parks of United States.* Series 7, p. 78.
162 Mechanic G.L., Kuboki Y., Shimokawa H., Nakamoto K., Sasaki S. & Kawanishi Y. (1974). Collagen cross links; direct quantitative determination of stable structural cross links in bone and dentin collagens. *Biochem. biophys. Res. Commun.* **60,** 756–763.
163 Miller A. & Wray J.S. (1971) Molecular packing in collagen. *Nature, Lond.* **230,** 437–9.
164 Mitchell D. (1974) Convective heat transfer from man and other animals. In *Heat Loss From Animals and Man.* (ed. J. L. Monteith & L. E. Mount) pp. 59–76. Butterworth, London.
165 Monod H. (1972) How muscles are used in the body. In *The Structure and Function of Muscle* (ed. G. H. Bourne) Vol. 1, pp. 24–74. Academic Press, New York & London.
166 Morton J.E. (1964) Locomotion. In *Physiology of Mollusca* (ed. K. M. Wilbur & C. M. Yonge) Vol. 1, pp. 383–423.
167 Muir H.M. & Hardingham T.E. (1974) The functions of hyaluronic acid in proteoglycan aggregation. In *Normal and Osteoarthritic Cartilage* (eds S. Y. Ali, M. W. Elves & D. H. Leaback) pp. 51–8. Institute of Orthopaedics, London.
168 Muir H.M. & Hardingham T.E. (1974) Hyaluronic acid in cartilage and proteoglycan aggregation. *Biochem. J.* **139,** 565–81.
169 Murie A. (1944) The wolves of Mount McKinley. *Fauna of the National Parks of the United States*, Series 5.
170 Murray B.G. (1967) Dispersal in vertebrates. *Ecology* **48,** 975–7.
171 Murray R.O. (1974) Aetiology of degenerative joint disease—a radiological re-assessment.

In *Normal and Osteoarthritic Articular Cartilage* (eds S. Y. Ali, M. W. Elves & D. H. Leaback) pp. 125–7. Institute of Orthopaedics London.
172 Nachtigall W. (1974) Locomotion: mechanics and hydrodynamics of swimming in aquatic insects. In *The Physiology of Insecta* (ed. M. Rockstein) Vol. 3, pp. 381–432. Academic Press, New York & London.
173 Neville A.C. (1975) Biology of the Arthropod cuticle. *Zoophysiology and Ecology*, Vol. 415. Springer-Verlag, Berlin, Heidelberg & New York.
174 Noble W.C. (1968) Ward infections. *Trans. St John's Hosp., Dermatol. Soc.* **54,** 83–8.
174a Ognev S.I. (1962) *Mammals of Eastern Europe and Northern Asia*, Vol. 2. S. Monson: Jerusalem.
175 Orr R.T. (1900) Development prenatal and postnatal. In *Biology of Bats* (ed. W. A. Wimsatt) Vol. 1, pp. 217–31. Academic Press, New York & London.
176 Packard A. (1969) Jet propulsion and the giant fibre response of Loligo. *Nature, Lond.* **221,** 875–7.
177 Pages E. (1970) Sur l'écologie et les adaptations de l'orycterope et des pangolins sympatriques du Gabon. *Biologia gabonica* **6,** 28–92.
178 Partridge S.M. (1970) Isolation and characterization of elastin. In *Chemistry and Molecular Biology of the Intercellular Matrix* (ed. E. A. Balazs) Vol. 1, pp. 593–616. Academic Press, New York & London.
179 Pautard F.G. (1963) Mineralization of keratin and its comparison with the enamel matrix. *Nature, Lond.* **199,** 531–5.
180 Pearson O.P. (1959) A traffic survey of *Microtus reithrodontomys* runways. *J. Mammal.* **40,** 169–80.
181 Pennycuick C.J. (1969) The mechanics of bird migration. *Ibis* **111,** 525–56.
182 Pennycuick C.J. (1972) *Animal Flight.* Institute of Biology Studies No. 33. Arnold, London.
183 Pennycuick C.J. & Parker G.A. (1966) Structural limitation on the power output of the pigeon's flight muscles. *J. exp. Biol.* **45,** 489–98.
184 Person P. & Philpott D.E. (1969) The nature and significance of invertebrate cartilages. *Biol. Rev.* **44,** 1–16.
185 Piez K. & Miller A. (1974) The structure of collagen fibrils. *J. Supramolec. Struct.* **2,** 121–37.
186 Pope C.H. (1962) *The Giant Snakes.* Routledge, London.
187 Pringle J.W.S. (1972) Arthropod muscle. In *The Structure and Function of Muscle* (ed. G. H. Bourne) Vol. 1, pp. 491–541. Academic Press, New York & London.
188 Pringle J.W.S. (1974) Locomotion: Flight. In *The Physiology of Insecta* (ed. M. Rockstein) Vol. 3, pp. 433–76. Academic Press, New York & London.
189 Pugh G. (1972) The gooseflesh syndrome (acute anhidrotic heat exhaustion) in long-distance runners. *Brit. J. Physical. Educ.* 9–12.
190 Ramachandran G.N. (ed.) (1968) *Treatise on Collagen.* Vol. 1, Chemistry of Collagen. Academic Press, New York & London.
191 Reichman O.J. & Baker R.J (1972) Distribution and movements of two species of Pocket Gopher (Geomyidae) in an area of sympatry in the Davis Mountains, Texas. *J. Mammal* **53,** 21–33.
192 Reig O.A. (1970) Ecological notes on the fossorial octodont rodent, *Spalacopus cyanus* (Molina). *J. Mammal.* **51,** 592–601.
193 Ridley H.N. (1930) *The Dispersal of Plants Throughout the World.* Reeve, Ashford.
194 Rijke A.M. (1970) Wettability and phylogenetic development of feather structure in water birds. *J. exp. Biol.* **52,** 469–79.
195 Robinson P.L. (1975) The functions of the hooked fifth metatarsal in Lepidosaurian reptiles. *Problèmes actuels de Paléontologie.* (Evolution des Vertébrés). Editions du CNRS, Paris.
196 Roeder K.D. (1965) Moths and ultrasound. *Sci. Amer.* 216–24.
197 Rooney J.R. (1969) *Biomechanics of Lameness in Horses.* Williams & Wilkins, Baltimore.

198 Rosenberg L., Margolis R., Wolfenstein-Todel C., Pal J. & Strider W. (1975) The organization of extracellular matrix in bovine articular cartilage. In *Extracellular Matrix Influences on Gene Expression* (eds H. C. Slavkin & R. C. Greulich) pp. 415–21. Academic Press, New York & London.
199 Rothschild M., Schlein Y., Parker, K. & Sternberg S. (1972) Jump of the oriental rat flea, *Xenopsylla cheopis* (Roths). *Nature, Lond.* **239,** 45–8.
200 Ruch T.C. & Patton H.D. (1965) *Physiology and Biophysics* 19th ed., p. 195. Saunders, Philadelphia.
201 Rudall K.M. (1968) Intracellular fibrous proteins and the keratins. In *Comprehensive Biochemistry* (ed. M. Florkin and C. H. Stotz) Vol. 26B, pp. 559–91. Elsevier, Amsterdam.
202 Ruddall K.M. & Kenchington W. (1973) The chitin system. *Biol. Rev.* **49,** 597–636.
203 Ruibal R. & Ernst V. (1965) The structure of digital setae of lizards. *J. Morph.* **117,** 271–94.
204 Runham N.W. & Hunter P.I. (1970) *Terrestrial Slugs.* Hutchinson, London.
205 Sanderson G.C. (1966) The study of mammal movements—a review. *J. Wild Life Mgr.* **30,** 215–35.
206 Schaller G.B. (1972) *The Serengeti Lion.* University of Chicago Press, Chicago.
207 Schmidt-Nielsen K. (1970) *Animal Physiology.* Prentice Hall, New Jersey.
208 Schmidt-Nielsen K. (1972) Locomotion energy cost of swimming, flying and running. *Science, N.Y.* **177,** 222–8.
209 Schoener T.W. (1968) Sizes of feeding territories among birds. *Ecology* **49,** 123–41.
210 Schoener T.W. (1969) Models of optimal size of solitary predators. *Amer. Nat.* **103,** 277–313.
211 Serafini-Fracassini A. & Smith J.W. (1974) *The Structure and Biochemistry of Cartilage.* Churchill-Livingstone, Edinburgh & London.
212 Sheets R.G., Linder R.L. & Dahlgren B.B. (1971) Burrow systems of prairie dogs in South Dakota. *J. Mammal.* **52,** 451–2.
213 Shirer H.E.W. & Fitch H.S. (1970) Comparison from radio tracking of movements and denning habits of the raccoon, striped skunk and opossum in North Eastern Kansas. *J. Mammal.* **51,** 491–507.
214 Simmons R.M. & Jewell B.R. (1974) Mechanics and models of muscular contraction. In *Recent Advances in Physiology* (ed. R. J. Linden) pp. 87–147. Churchill Livingstone, Edinburgh & London.
215 Simon W.H. (1970) Scale effects in animal joints. 1. Articular cartilage thickness and compressive stress. *Arthritis and Rheumatism* **13,** 244–56.
216 Simpson G.G. (1950) *Horses.* Oxford Univ. Press, New York.
217 Skoczen S. & Rozmus S. (1973) A device for testing the strength of moles. *Acta Theriol.* **18,** 490–2.
218 Skoglund S. (1973) Joint receptors and kinaesthesis. In *Handbook of Sensory Physiology* (ed. A. Iggo) Vol. 2, pp. 111–36. Springer-Verlag, Berlin, Heidelberg & New York.
219 Sleigh M.A. (1969) Co-ordination of the rhythm of beat in some ciliary systems. *Int. Rev. Cytol.* **25,** 31–54.
220 Southern H.N. (1964) *Handbook of British Mammals.* Blackwell Scientific Publications, Oxford.
221 Stara J.F. (1965) Tissue distribution and excretion of Cesium-137 in the guinea pig. *Health Phys.* **11,** 1195–202.
222 Steele S.F. (1972) Footgear—Its history, uses and abuses. *Clin. Orthop.* **88,** 119–30.
223 Steindler A. (1955) *Kinesiology of the Human Body.* Thomas, Springfield.
224 Stirewalt M.A. (1966) Skin penetration mechanisms of helminths. In *Biology of Parasites* (ed. E. J. L. Soulsby). Academic Press, New York & London.
225 Storer R.W. (1971) Adaptive radiation of birds. In *Avian Biology* (eds D. S. Farner, J. R. King & K. C. Parkes) Vol. 1, pp. 149–88. Academic Press, New York & London.
226 Strömberg B. (1971) The normal and diseased superficial flexor tendon in race horses. *Acta Radiol.* Supp. 305.
227 Szirmai J.A. (1970) Structure of the inter-vertebral disc. In *Chemistry and Molecular*

Biology of the Intercellular Matrix (ed. E. A. Balazs) Vol. 3, pp. 1279–1308. Academic Press, New York & London.
228 Tanzer M.L. (1973) Cross-linking of collagen. *Science* **180,** 561–6.
229 Taylor C.R. (1974) Exercise and Thermoregulation. In *Environmental Physiology* (ed. D. Robertshaw) pp. 163–84. *MTP International Review of Science* (ed. A. C. Guyton & D. Horrobin) Vol. 7. Butterworth, London.
230 Thompson D'A.W. (1942) *On Growth and Form.* Cambridge Univ. Press, London.
231 Thompson H.V. & Worden A.N. (1956) *The Rabbit.* Collins, London.
232 Tinbergen N. (1951) *The Study of Instinct.* Clarendon Press, Oxford.
233 Trueman E.R. (1968) The mechanism of burrowing of some naticid gastropods in comparison with that of other molluscs. *J. exp. Biol.* **48,** 663–78.
234 Trueman E.R. (1970) The mechanism of burrowing of the mole crab, *Emerita. J. exp. Biol.* **53,** 701–10.
235 Trueman E.R. & Ansell A.D. (1969) The mechanisms of burrowing into soft substrate by marine animals. *Oceanogr. Mar. Biol. Ann. Rev.* **7,** 316–66.
236 Trueman E.R. & Packard A. (1968) Motor performances of some cephalopods. *J. exp. Biol.* **49,** 495–507.
237 Tryon C.A. (1947) The biology of the pocket gopher *Thomomys talpoides* in Montana. *Montana State College of Agricult. Exp. Sta. Tech. Bull.* **448,** 1–30.
238 Tucker V.A. (1970) Energetic cost of locomotion in animals. *Comp. biochem. Physiol.* **34,** 841–6.
239 Tucker V.A. (1973) Bird metabolism during flight: evaluation of a theory. *J. exp. Biol.* **58,** 689–709.
240 Twente J.W. (1959) Swimming behaviour of bats. *J. Mammal.* **40,** 440–1.
241 Vaughan T.A. (1970) Flight patterns and aerodynamics. In *Biology of Bats* (ed. W. A. Wimsatt) pp. 195–216. Academic Press, New York.
242 Vernon H.M. & Bedford T. (1930) A study of heating and ventilation in schools. *Industrial Health Research Board Report No.* 58. *H.M. Stationery Office, London.*
243 Viidik A. (1973) Functional properties of collagenous tissues. *Int. Rev. Connect. Tissue Res.* 127–215.
244 Vincent J.F.V. (1975) Locust oviposition: stress softening of the extensible intersegmental membranes. *Proc. R. Soc. B.* **188,** 189–201.
245 Vincent J.F.V. & Prentice J.H. (1973) Rheological properties of the extensible intersegmental membrane of the adult female locust. *J. Materials Sci.* **8,** 624–30.
246 Vincent J.F.V. & Wood S.D.E. (1972) Mechanism of abdominal extension during oviposition in *Locusta. Nature, Lond.* **235,** 167–8.
247 Vivier E. (1972) Contractile structures in some protozoa (ciliate and gregarines). In *The Structure and Function of Muscle* (ed. G. H. Bourne) Vol. II. Academic Press, New York & London.
248 Walcott C. & Michener M.C. (1971) Sun navigation in homing pigeons—attempts to shift sun co-ordinates. *J. exp. Biol.* **54,** 291–316.
249 Walker A.E. (1973) Mechanisms of cerebral trauma and the impairment of consciousness. *Neurol. Surg.* **II,** 936–49.
250 Walls E.W. (1960) The microanatomy of muscle. In *The Structure and Function of Muscle* (ed. G. H. Bourne) Vol. 1, pp. 21–61. Academic Press, New York & London.
251 Walther F.R. (1969) Flight behaviour and avoidance of predators in Thomson's gazelle, (*Gazella thomsoni*, Guenther 1884). *Behaviour* **34,** 184–221.
252 Wehner R. & Flatt, I. (1972) The visual orientation of desert ants, *Cataglyphis bicolor*, by means of terrestrial clues. In *Information Processing in the Visual Systems of Arthropods* (ed. R. Wehner,) pp. 295–302. Springer-Verlag, Berlin, Heidelberg & New York.
253 Weir B. (1971) A trapping technique for Tuco-tucos (*Ctenomys talarum*) *J. Mammal.* **52,** 836–9.
254 Weis-Fogh T. (1971) Energetics of hovering flight in humming birds and in *Drosophila. J. exp. Biol.* **56,** 79–104.

255 Weis-Fogh T. & Andersen S.O. (1970) Elasticity and thermodynamics of elastin. In *Chemistry and Molecular Biology of the Intercellular Matrix* (ed. E. A. Balazs) Vol. 1, pp. 671–81. Academic Press, New York & London.
256 Wells J.B. (1965) Comparison of mechanical properties between slow and fast mammalian muscle. *J. Physiol.* **178,** 252–69.
257 Wells M.J. & Buckley S.K.L. (1972) Snails and trails. *Anim. Behav.* **20,** 345–55.
258 Whitford D. (1974) *Sporting Life Racehorse Ratings.* The Sporting Life, London.
259 Wichterman R. (1953) *The Biology of Paramecium.* Blakiston, New York.
260 Wigglesworth V.B. (1973) Evolution of insect wings and flight. *Nature, Lond.* **246,** 127–9.
261 Wilbur K.M. & Simkiss K. (1968). Calcified shells. In *Comprehensive Biochemistry* (ed. M. Florkin & C. H. Stotz) Vol. 26A, pp. 229–95. Elsevier, Amsterdam.
262 Wilson E.P. (1964) *Mammais of the World.* John Hopkins Press, Baltimore.
263 Wilson R.S. (1970) Some comments on the hydrostatic system of spiders (Chelicerata, Araneae). *Z. Morph. Tiere* **68,** 308–22.
264 Wilson V.J. & Edwards P.W. (1965) Data from a female rhinoceros and foetus (*Diceros bicornis* Linn) from the Fort Jameson district. *Puku.* **3,** 179–80.
265 Wimsatt W.A. (1969) Transient behaviour, nocturnal activity patterns and feeding efficiency of vampire bats (*Desmodus rotundus*) under natural conditions. *J. Mammal.* **50,** 233–44.
266 Wright V. (ed.) (1969) *Lubrication and Wear in Joints.* Sector, London.
267 Yalden Z.W. (1966) The anatomy of mole locomotion. *J. Zool. Lond.* **149,** 55–64.

Prelude to Chapter 9

In most animals, the energy required for locomotion and other vital functions is obtained from aerobic metabolism. A few parasites, and other animals that live in anaerobic environments can utilize chemical energy from organic material in the absence of oxygen; but the complete oxidation of such matter would provide up to twenty times more energy. Although life on land provides easy access to oxygen, it engenders problems of water conservation. The significance of respiratory water loss has been considered in Chapter 7: an account of the physiology of gas exchange is given in the following chapter. The inter-relation between the environment and various aspects of the physiology of the animals that inhabit it can be illustrated by consideration of the problems of water balance, gas exchange, reproduction and thermal biology that are associated with life in water and on land.

Chapter 9
Gas exchange

P. J. BUTLER

9.1 INTRODUCTION

The exchange of oxygen and carbon dioxide between animals with aerobic metabolism and their environment is linked to the rate of oxidative metabolism in the tissues. Oxygen is the final hydrogen ion acceptor in the respiratory chain leading to the formation of water, while carbon dioxide is produced during glycolysis and in the tricarboxylic acid cycle. The utilization of oxygen for the complete degradation of food greatly increases the efficiency of intermediary metabolism. During anaerobic metabolism, 2 mole of ATP are formed per mole of glucose, whereas complete oxidation of glucose to CO_2 and water produces 38 mole of ATP per mole of glucose. In order to maintain this level of efficiency, the metabolizing cells of aerobic animals must be continuously supplied with oxygen, while at the same time carbon dioxide must be continuously removed.

9.2 PHYSICAL PROPERTIES OF OXYGEN AND CARBON DIOXIDE IN WATER AND AIR

The percentage of the respiratory gases in air are: oxygen 20·95%, and carbon dioxide 0.03%. These values do not give any indication of the quantity of the gas, i.e. the number of molecules. Three variables affect the condition of a gas, *viz.* temperature (T) which is a measure of the kinetic energy of the gas molecules, pressure (P) and volume (V). The relationship between these three variables is given in the gas equation:

$$PV = RT \text{ where } R \text{ is the gas constant } (8{\cdot}31\ J.\ {}^{\circ}\mathrm{K}^{-1}.\ \mathrm{mole}^{-1})$$

At a constant volume, a rise in temperature will cause an increase in pressure; at constant pressure, a rise in temperature will cause an increase in volume. Thus, when describing gas volumes it is common practice to correct them to standard temperature (273°K = 0°C) and pressure (760 mmHg = 760 torr) i.e. STP. This then gives an indication of the quantity of the gas, because at STP 1 mole of any gas occupies 22·4 l and contains $6{\cdot}03 \times 10^{23}$ molecules (Avogadro's number).

It is useful to think of the pressure of a gas resulting from the bombardment of a solid object by the gas molecules. It is therefore related to the activity (kinetic energy) of the gas. If the volume of a gas within a vessel is decreased by compression, the number of collisions the molecules make with the sides of the vessel will increase, also if the temperature of the gas rises, the motion of the gas molecules will become more rapid (i.e. their kinetic energy will increase). In both cases, the pressure exerted by the gas rises, even though the total number of gas molecules remains the same.

The atmosphere consists of a mixture of gases, and the partial pressure exerted by any one of these gases is the percentage concentration of that gas × the total pressure exerted by all of the gases (Dalton's law of partial pressure). At STP, the partial pressure of oxygen (Po_2) in air is:

$$\frac{20{\cdot}95}{100} \times 760 = 159 \text{ mmHg}$$

$$P\mathrm{CO}_2 = \frac{0{\cdot}03}{100} \times 760 = 0{\cdot}2 \text{ mmHg}$$

When calculating the partial pressure of individual gases in a gas mixture it is necessary initially to deduct water-vapour pressure (P_w) from barometric pressure (P_B). Thus at 20°C (where water has a vapour pressure of 17·5 mmHg) and at a relative humidity of 50%; $P_w = 17{\cdot}5 \times 50/100 = 8{\cdot}75$ mmHg.

$$\text{If } P_B = 760 \text{ mmHg, } Po_2 = \frac{20{\cdot}95}{100} \times (760 - 8{\cdot}75) = 157 \text{ mmHg.}$$

If atmospheric pressure decreases, the partial pressure of any particular gas will decrease, even though its percentage concentration may remain the same. At a height of approximately 5500 m above sea level, atmospheric pressure is half of its sea level value. This means that in a given volume of air, and at a given temperature, there will be half as many gas molecules at 5500 m above, than at sea level. Also, the partial pressure of the individual gases will be half as much at 5500 m above sea level compared with their sea level values.

Gases also exert a pressure when they are dissolved in water. If water at 20°C is equilibrated with air at a P_B of 760 mmHg, Po_2 of the water will be:

$$\frac{20{\cdot}95}{100} \times (760 - 17{\cdot}5) = 155 \text{ mmHg, where } P_w = 17{\cdot}5 \text{ mmHg}$$

Table 9.1. Solubility coefficients (α) for CO_2 and O_2 in fresh water and sea water at three different temperatures (ml . ml^{-1}. atm^{-1}).

		O_2	
°C	CO_2	0‰ Cl (F.W.)	20‰ Cl (S.W.)
0	1·713	0·0489	0·0379
10	1·194	0·0380	0·0301
20	0·878	0·0310	0·0251

Each of the atmospheric gases dissolves in water according to its partial pressure and its solubility coefficient (α). The solubility coefficient is different for different gases and decreases for each gas as temperature and the amount of dissolved solids (salinity) increases (Table 9.1). The amount of oxygen dissolved in fresh water at 0°C equilibrated with atmospheric air with $P_B = 760$ mmHg will be:

$$\frac{159}{760} \times 0{\cdot}0489 = 0{\cdot}0103 \text{ vol/vol}$$

which is 1·03 ml O_2/100 ml fresh water or 1·03 vol %. Under the same conditions the value for O_2 dissolved in sea water will be:

$$\frac{159}{760} \times 0{\cdot}0379 = 0{\cdot}0079 \text{ vol/vol i.e. } 0{\cdot}79 \text{ vol } \%$$

Excluding the condition of supersaturation, the maximum amount of O_2 that can be dissolved in a volume of water is approximately 20 × less than is found in an equal volume of air. At any given temperature and salinity there is a linear relationship between $P\text{O}_2$ of water and the amount of oxygen in the water. The values of α for CO_2 when applied to distilled water can be used, as illustrated above for O_2, to calculate the amount of CO_2 in water at a particular $P\text{CO}_2$. When a gas mixture containing CO_2 is equilibrated with distilled water, the CO_2 combines with water to form H_2CO_3, so that 'free' carbon dioxide consists of CO_2 itself and H_2CO_3 in solution and in equilibrium with each other:

$$H_2O + CO_2 \leftrightharpoons H_2CO_3 \leftrightharpoons H^+ + HCO_3^-$$

It is this free carbon dioxide that exerts a partial pressure. The amount of carbon dioxide in natural waters at any given $P\text{CO}_2$ will be higher than that in distilled water because it will be incorporated as carbonates and bicarbonates. This extra reservoir of CO_2 is known as the carbonate alkalinity. Figure 9.1(a)

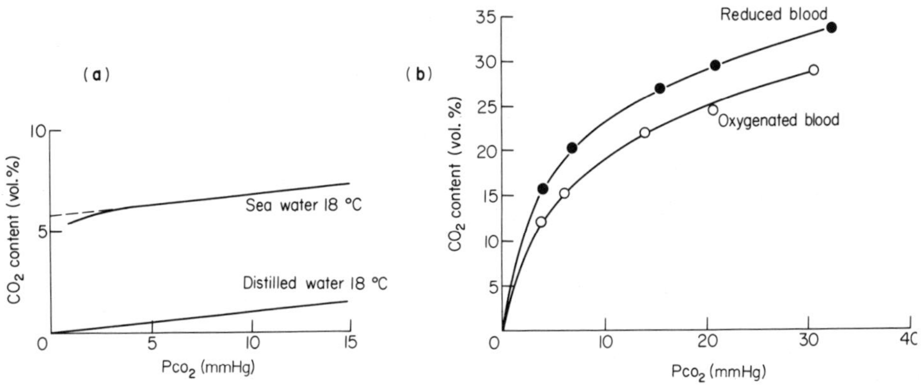

Fig. 9.1. The relationship between CO_2 content and $P\text{CO}_2$ in (**a**) sea water and distilled water at 18°C [23]; (**b**) *Neoceratodus* blood. Note that reduced blood has a higher CO_2 carrying capacity than oxygenated blood (Haldane effect) [32].

shows the relationship between $P\text{CO}_2$ and CO_2 content in distilled water and sea water. At a $P\text{CO}_2$ above 3–5 mmHg the curve for sea water is linear and the slope indicates the physical solubility of carbon dioxide in sea water, i.e. the increase in free CO_2 as $P\text{CO}_2$ increases. This physical solubility is affected by temperature and salinity. Below a $P\text{CO}_2$ of 3–5 mmHg, the sea-water line becomes curvilinear [23]. This is because at low $P\text{CO}_2$, bicarbonate forms CO_2 and H_2O with the hydrogen ions coming from the bicarbonate/carbonate buffer system resulting in a decrease in chemically bound CO_2. This curvilinear part of the CO_2 dissociation curve in sea water is in the physiological range of $P\text{CO}_2$ values (see later) and is therefore of physiological interest.

As well as the different physical properties of the respiratory gases in air and water, the two media themselves have different properties. For example, water is about 830 × denser than and 55 × more viscous than air at 20°C. Water has 3000 × greater heat capacity than air.

9.3 FACTORS AFFECTING DIFFUSION OF GASES

There is no evidence that active secretion of O_2 or CO_2 occurs across any biological membrane not even in the swimbladder were Po_2 is higher than in arterial blood. Passive diffusion is the only way in which respiratory gases pass across cell walls. The rate of diffusion of a gas is described by a form of Fick's Law of diffusion:

$$\dot{V} = \frac{K.A.}{x}(P_1 - P_2)$$

where $\dot{V}$ = volume of gas diffusing per unit time (ml STP . min^{-1})
A = area of exchange surface (m^2)
x = thickness of exchange surface (m)
P_1 & P_2 = partial pressure of gas on each side of the exchange surface (mmHg)
K = diffusion constant (ml . min^{-1} . atm^{-1})

The diffusion constant indicates the rate at which a particular gas diffuses through a particular substance of given surface area and thickness with a given pressure difference across it. This constant is proportional to the solubility of gas in the substance, but inversely proportional to the square root of the molecular weight of the gas, i.e. $K \alpha Sol/\sqrt{M.W.}$ Thus in air,

$$\frac{K_{CO_2}}{K_{O_2}} = \frac{\sqrt{32}}{\sqrt{44}} = 0{\cdot}85,$$

therefore O_2 diffuses slightly faster than CO_2 in air. In water at 20°C,

$$\frac{K_{CO_2}}{K_{O_2}} = \frac{0{\cdot}878}{0{\cdot}0310} \times \frac{\sqrt{32}}{\sqrt{44}} = 24.$$

thus CO_2 diffuses much faster than O_2 through water and tissue. Table 9.2 gives values of K for O_2 at 20°C, and it can be seen that O_2 diffuses 260,000 times faster in air, than through water.

Table 9.2. Diffusion constants (K) of oxygen in air, water and some animal tissue at 20°C (ml . min^{-1} . atm^{-1}).

Air	11·0
Water	0·000042
Muscle	0·000014
Connective tissue	0·0000115
Chitin	0·0000013

9.4 LIMITATIONS OF DIFFUSION—STRATEGIES AVAILABLE TO OVERCOME THESE LIMITATIONS

The earliest aerobic organisms relied simply on diffusion of gases between themselves and the surrounding water across their body surface. Krogh [18] calculated that diffusion alone would supply the oxygen needs of an idealized spherical cell, provided it was less than 2 mm in diameter, its oxygen uptake was no higher than 0·1 ml $O_2 \cdot g^{-1} \cdot h^{-1}$, and the surrounding water was equilibrated with air. For animals above a certain size, diffusion alone will not supply sufficient oxygen to regions further than 1 mm from the surface. Therefore diffusion must be augmented in larger animals. The possible strategies open are to a certain extent reflected in Fick's Law of diffusion.

The diffusion constant (K) for biological materials such as connective tissue and muscle are very similar. It is, therefore, unlikely that any changes in the diffusion resistance of the tissues have occurred during evolution. However, any gas-exchange surface covered with chitin, would presumably be less permeable to respiratory gases than surfaces covered with normal epithelium (Table 9.2). An increase in the surface area and a decrease in the thickness of the gas exchange area would obviously increase the rate of gas exchange, as also would a convection system. An internal circulatory system, perfusing one side of the exchanger with liquid would obviously assist the process of gas exchange by removing CO_2 from and supplying O_2 to the metabolizing cells. External ventilation of the exchanger takes this one stage further by removing the CO_2 from the exchanger and supplying it with fresh external fluid with a high P_{O_2}. Perfusion and ventilation not only have these convective functions they also greatly augment diffusion by maintaining large pressure gradients across the exchanger (high external and a low internal P_{O_2}, *vice versa* for P_{CO_2}).

Insects, diplopods, chilopods and arachnids possess a system of branching tracheae, which penetrate from the body surface down to the metabolizing cells. Air is transported along these either by diffusion alone in smaller forms, or by convection and diffusion in larger insects, so that gaseous oxygen reaches the cells. Only over the final short distance in the blind-ending tracheoles does diffusion occur through a liquid [21]. In its simplest form, an internal convection system exists in the Protozoa where protoplasmic streaming enhances gas transport above that achieved by diffusion alone. In echinoderms, annelids, molluscs, crustaceans and vertebrates there is a discrete internal circulatory system.

If the general body surface is permeable and richly supplied with circulating body fluid (blood) it will function as a gas-exchange organ. Annelids such as earthworms, *Tubifex* and most Hirudinea rely entirely upon the general body surface for gas exchange. Although the body surface may be important in a number of other animals, particularly aquatic forms, there are usually specific areas specially developed to facilitate gas exchange. These are the gills of aquatic animals and lungs of terrestrial animals. Gills and lungs comply with the requirements of the law of diffusion in order to meet necessary oxygen demands.

In aquatic animals the gills range in complexity from simple extensions of the body to elaborate structures contained in a special chamber. Simple extensions of the body are found in a number of invertebrates, e.g. *Arenicola*, *Nephthys*, *Artemia*, *Daphnia*, *Asterias*, *Echinas*. The methods of ventilation of these gills include the action of cilia on the gills themselves (in *Asterias* and *Nephthys*), irrigation of the burrow in which the animal lives by rhythmic undulations of the body (in *Arenicola*), movements of the gills in the water (in *Echinas*), and muscular ventilation of the gills associated with movement of appendages during locomotion or feeding activity (in *Artemia*). Several larval fish, e.g. Polypteridae, Dipnoi and larval Amphibia also have comparatively simple external gills. More complex internal gills which are either highly branched or consist of a series of flattened plates, lamellae, stacked upon one another, are contained within a special chamber which is ventilated by a special water-pumping apparatus, as in gastropod and cephalopod molluscs, decapod Crustacea and fish. A similar range of complexity is seen in terrestrial gas-exchange organs. Pulmonate gastropods rely simply upon the diffusion of air into the mantle cavity, when the pneumostome opens, whereas in terrestrial vertebrates and the larger insects, muscular activity is involved in ventilating the lungs or tracheae.

In larger, more active animals, one side of the gas-exchange surface is ventilated by the external medium, and the other side of the gas-exchange surface is perfused with blood (except in some arachnids and most insects). Thus, although the exchange of respiratory gases across the cell membrane at the external gas-exchange surface and at the metabolizing cells is by passive diffusion, one of the conditions for this diffusion (a pressure gradient) results from the active, i.e. energy consuming, convection of blood and water or air.

9.5 CHARACTERISTICS OF BLOOD PIGMENTS

On the face of it, a tracheal system has a higher capacity for transporting oxygen than a liquid circulatory system. The concentration of oxygen in air-equilibrated water at 0°C is at least 20 × less than in air, and increases in temperature and salinity widen the difference. The blood of some animals, e.g. echinoids (sea urchins) and the so-called 'ice fish' transport respiratory gases in physical solution only, but the blood of many other animals contains a respiratory pigment. The function of the pigment is to increase the amount of oxygen a given volume of blood can carry at a given P_{O_2}, i.e. to increase α.

There are two main pigments in animal blood, haemocyanin and haemoglobin. Less frequent are chlorocruorin and haemerythrin. Haemoglobin consists of haem, which is a porphyrin ring with Fe^{++} in the centre, attached to a polypeptide chain, globin. One molecule of oxygen combines with a single ferrous ion. In haemocyanin, the metal ion copper, is attached directly to the polypeptide chain, and one molecule of oxygen is bound by two copper atoms [16]. In all blood pigments, oxygenation is related to the P_{O_2} with which the pigment is equilibrated: ($Hb + O_2 \rightleftharpoons HbO_2$). The proportion of the total pigment molecule in the oxygenated state (percentage saturation) is related to the Po_2, but this is not a linear relationship as with water. It is often sigmoid (Fig. 9.2a) and the functional significance of this is that the increase in percentage saturation as Po_2 rises is greatest over the physiological range. The Po_2 at which the pigment is 50% saturated is known as the P_{50} (Fig. 9.2a). Clearly, the lower the P_{50} the higher is the affinity of the pigment for oxygen and pigments from different animals have different P_{50} values. In *Arenicola*, the haemoglobin has a P_{50} of approximately 2 mmHg and therefore has a very high affinity for oxygen. This is related to the fact that when the tide goes out the animal is no longer able to irrigate its burrow and the environmental Po_2 falls. In man, who does not usually experience a reduction in environmental Po_2, the P_{50} of the blood is approximately 30 mmHg and the haemoglobin has a low affinity for oxygen. The P_{50} of the pigment in any one animal may be affected by a number of factors.

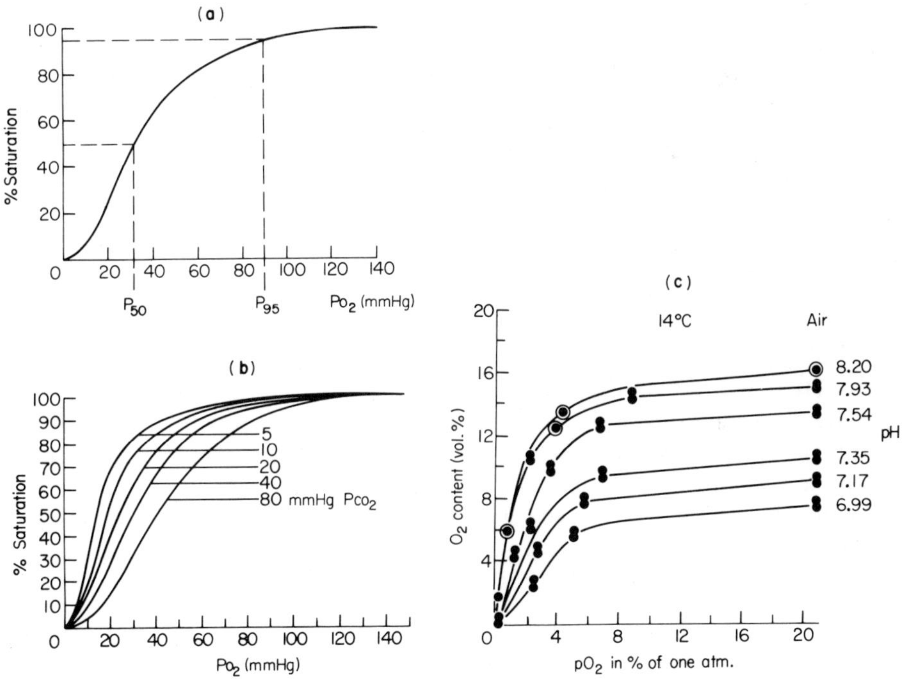

Fig. 9.2. Oxygen dissociation curves for haemoglobin.
(a) Hypothetical curve showing relationship between % saturation and Po_2. The Po_2 at which the pigment is 50% saturated is known as the P_{50}, whereas the Po_2 at which the pigment is 95% saturated is known as the P_{95}.
(b) Effect of Pco_2 on oxygen dissociation curve of human blood [32]. As Pco_2 increases (or pH falls) there is a decrease in the affinity of the blood for O_2 (Bohr effect). A similar shift in the dissociation curve is caused by a rise in temperature or an increase in organic phosphate in the red blood cells.
(c) Effect of pH on oxygen dissociation curve of eel blood [32]. As pH falls (or Pco_2 rises) there is not only a decrease in affinity of the pigment for oxygen, but also a reduction in oxygen carrying capacity of the blood (Root effect).

An increase in P_{CO_2} or reduction in pH may increase the P_{50}, i.e. decrease the affinity (Fig. 9.2b). This is the Bohr effect. An increase in temperature or in the concentration of organic phosphates in the blood may have the same effect. The maximum amount of oxygen that any blood can carry is known as the O_2 carrying capacity and will depend upon the characteristics and concentration of the pigment. This varies from animal to animal and often relates to their relative oxygen requirements. The haemocyanin-containing blood of *Carcinus* has an oxygen carrying capacity of 1 vol % and the carrying capacities of some haemoglobin-containing bloods are as follows: *Arenicola* 8 vol. %, *Scyliorhinus* (dogfish) 5 vol %, *Salmo* (trout) 9 vol %, man 20 vol %, Weddell seal 32 vol %. An increase in P_{CO_2} or reduction in pH can also reduce the oxygen carrying capacity of the blood, particularly of teleost fish, and this is known as the 'Root effect' (Fig. 9.2c).

Blood also transports CO_2 from the tissues to the gas-exchange surface. As well as the free CO_2 and bicarbonate that are present in the plasma, CO_2 is also chemically bound to the blood pigment as carbamino-haemoglobin. The relationship between CO_2 concentration and P_{CO_2} is not linear, but generally hyperbolic (Fig. 9.1b). The largest portion of the total CO_2 content of the blood is present as bicarbonates and the actual amount is determined by the ionic composition and the buffering capacity of the blood. Haemoglobin has a large buffering capacity, and can shift the following equation to the right:

$$CO_2 + H_2O \leftrightarrows H_2CO_3 \leftrightarrows H^+ + HCO_3^-,$$

thus more CO_2 is taken up. As HbO_2 becomes dissociated, this buffering capacity increases and *vice versa*. This effect of oxygenation of Hb on the CO_2 capacity of the blood is the Haldane effect. (Fig. 9.2b). The Bohr effect of the O_2 dissociation curve and the Haldane effect of the CO_2 dissociation curve are physiologically significant. In metabolizing cells, where P_{CO_2} is high, the affinity of Hb for O_2 decreases (Bohr effect) thus assisting the release of O_2. As Hb becomes deoxygenated, its buffering capacity increases, thus enhancing CO_2 uptake by the blood (Haldane effect). The opposite occurs at the external gas-exchange surface. The CO_2 carrying capacity of blood from various animals is: *Octopus* 7·5 vol %, *Scyliorhinus* 10 vol %, *Salmo* 20 vol %, *Protopterus* 45 vol %, man 51 vol %.

9.6 AQUATIC GAS EXCHANGE

9.6.1 Water and blood flow

Ventilation is usually unidirectional in animals with their gills in a special chamber. In prosobranch molluscs, cilia on the gills cause the flow of water, in decapod crustaceans, the scaphognathites perform this function whereas, in teleost fish, a buccal force pump and an opercular suction pump maintain a more or less continuous flow of water over the gills [30]. The energy expended in moving water across the gills is largely dependent upon the viscosity and density of the water, only the visco-elastic forces developed in the respiratory system are independent of the water itself [30]. A recent study has shown that in normally breathing, resting trout in aerated water, the proportion of total oxygen uptake that is used by the respiratory muscles is approximately 10%. This proportion will be greater in an animal with an elevated rate of ventilation, when actively swimming or as a result of being exposed to oxygen deficient water, or to high ambient temperatures, and there will be a point at which increased ventilation will supply no more oxygen than is required by the respiratory apparatus itself [13]. Active pelagic fish, such as tuna and mackerel, make use of their locomotory muscles to ventilate their gills. The mouth stays open during forward movement, and ventilation can be regulated by the size of the mouth and opercula. Other pelagic fish, such as sharks also cease ventilatory movements when swimming quickly and make use of 'ram-jet' ventilation.

In invertebrates, the dorsally placed heart receives oxygenated blood from the gills and then pumps this blood round the body, either via an open circulatory system (molluscs except cephalopods and arthropods) or via a closed system (cephalopods, annelids). The heart of crustaceans is confined within a rigid pericardium. As it contracts it aspirates blood from the gills and forces blood into the haemocoel. In cephalopods, there are accessory hearts at the base of the gills which assist the return of the blood to the major heart. In fish, the ventrally placed heart receives deoxygenated blood from the body via the venous system. The muscular ventricle ejects the blood along the ventral aorta and via the afferent branchial arches to the gills. Oxygenated blood reaches the dorsal aorta via the efferent blood vessels and flows round the body. It has been calculated that the oxygen demand of the cardiac pump of carp is approximately 5% of the total oxygen uptake of the resting animal. Again, as the oxygen demand of the animal increases, so the work done by the heart will increase, and both the cardiac and respiratory pumps make a significant contribution in limiting maximum oxygen uptake in fish.

9.6.2 Structure of gills

The complex gills of most aquatic animals consist of a main axis bearing filaments. In some Crustacea such as crayfish, the filaments are unbranched projections, whereas in others, e.g. *Carcinus*, and in gastropod and cephalopod molluscs and fish, the filaments are flattened and stacked one above the other. In fish there are typically four gill arches on each side of the pharynx, and each gill arch bears two alternating rows of filaments (Fig. 9.3a). Each gill filament bears a series of alternating projections (secondary lamellae) on its dorsal and ventral surfaces. Secondary lamellae are also found on the gill filaments of cephalopods. In most teleost fish the two rows of gill filaments on each gill arch are separate for most of their length (Fig. 9.3a) whereas, in elasmobranchs, they are joined together for most of their length by a vertical sheet of connective tissue, the interbranchial system. This septum extends beyond the

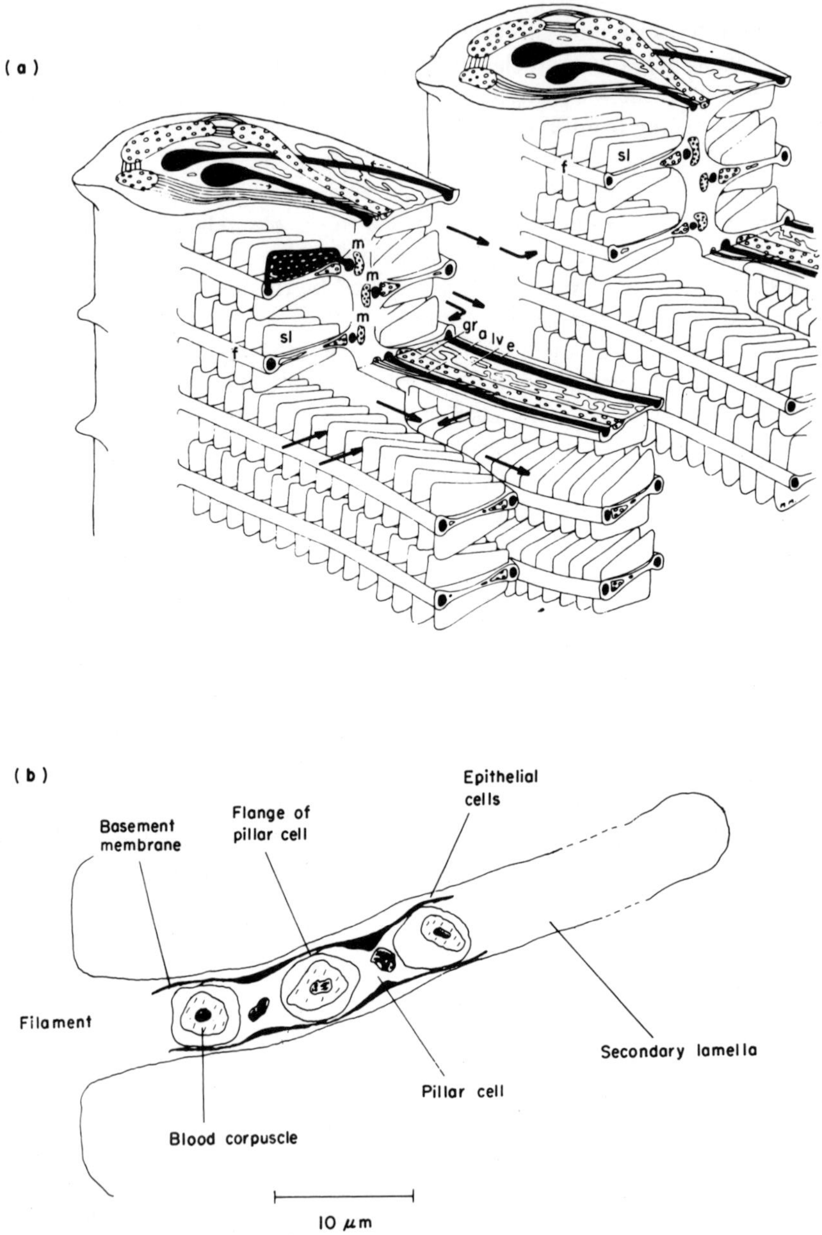

Fig. 9.3. The gills of teleost fish.
(a) Diagram of part of two adjacent gill arches of the trout, lv-filament lymph vessels, gr—gill ray, m—muscle blocks of gill filament, sl—secondary lamellae, f—filament. Solid arrows indicate direction of water flow, broken arrows show direction of blood flow [22].
(b) Diagram of section through a secondary lamella of trout.

end of the gill filaments to form a flap covering each gill slit. The separate gill filaments of each gill arch of teleosts are collectively covered by a bony articulated flap, the operculum. Each series is moved by adductor and abductor muscles [12]. The afferent and efferent blood vessels, sensory and motor nerve fibres, and skeletal elements, run longitudinally in each gill arch. Each afferent branchial blood vessel sends an afferent filament artery along the inner border of each filament which supplies each secondary lamella via the afferent lamellar arterioles. Gas exchange occurs across the secondary lamellae, and oxygenated blood leaves the lamellae via efferent lamella arterioles which join an efferent filament artery running along the outer border of each gill filament [12]. A secondary lamella consists of a network of interconnecting blood spaces, delimited by flanges of the pillar cells (Fig. 9.3b). There is evidence which indicates that the functional surface area of fish gills can change [3]. Whether this results from changes in the amount of blood passing through non-respiratory shunts [33], or from changes in the number of secondary lamellae that are perfused [3, 22] is not known. The fact that it can, and most likely does, occur under natural conditions indicates that the morphological data on the surface area of gills from various animal species, indicate the maximum surface area available for gas exchange and not necessarily the area that is functional.

The secondary lamellae of fish greatly increase the surface area available for gas exchange, and the diffusion distance between the water and blood is small. In Crustacea, the gills do not possess secondary lamellae, and yet the gill area per unit body weight is comparable with that of fish (Table 9.3). The more active fish and Crustacea have a larger gill area and the more active fish have a smaller blood–water distance. Terrestrial forms have a smaller gill area than the rest. Water and blood flow in opposite directions over the gills of gastropod molluscs, brachyuran crustaceans and fish and this is known as 'counter-current' flow.

9.6.3 Analysis of gas exchange

Gas exchange in fish has given rise to a number of important concepts and analytical techniques which can be applied to water-breathing animals in general. The following account is based upon the work of Hughes and Shelton [13] Randall [27], and Piiper and his co-workers [24, 25].

If the surface area (A) of the gas-exchange organ were sufficiently large, and the diffusion barrier (x) between the blood and water sufficiently small then, with a counter current flow, it is theoretically possible that oxygen tension in the arterial blood ($P\text{a},\text{O}_2$) would equal the oxygen tension in the inspired water ($P\text{I},\text{O}_2$) and the oxygen tension in the expired water ($P\text{E},\text{O}_2$) would equal the oxygen tension in the mixed venous blood ($P\bar{\text{v}},\text{O}_2$) (Fig. 9.4a). This situation has never been found to occur in fish [27, 24] or Crustacea [15]. However, the fact that $P\text{a},\text{O}_2$ is greater than $P\text{E},\text{O}_2$ in a number of animals, indicates that there is not a parallel flow arrangement (Fig. 9.4b). A counter current flow arrangement is thought to exist in fish and Crustacea, and there are a number of explanations for the inability of the two respiratory media to equilibrate.

Table 9.3. Morphological and physiological data from the gills of selected Crustacea and fish.

	Gill area ($mm^2 . g^{-1}$)	Mean blood-water distance (μm)	To_2, ($ml. min.^{-1} kg^{-1}. mmHg^{-1}$)	Ew,o_2, (%)	Eb,o_2, (%)
CRUSTACEA					
Callinectes (sublittoral)	1367 [10]	—	—	—	—
Cancer (sublittoral)	—	—	0·0093 [15]	17 [15]	95·6 [15]
Carcinus (intertidal)	777	—	—	—	—
Ocypode (terrestrial)	325 [10]	—	—	—	—
FISH					
Dogfish	210 [12]	11·27 [12]	0·0087 [24]	66 [24]	79·0 [24]
Rainbow trout	197 [12]	6·37 [12]	0·0056 [28]	10–30 [28]	95–100 [28]
Skipjack tuna	1350 [12]	0·598 [12]	0·115 [34]	90 [34]	—
Climbing perch	64 [12]	10·0 [12]	—	—	—

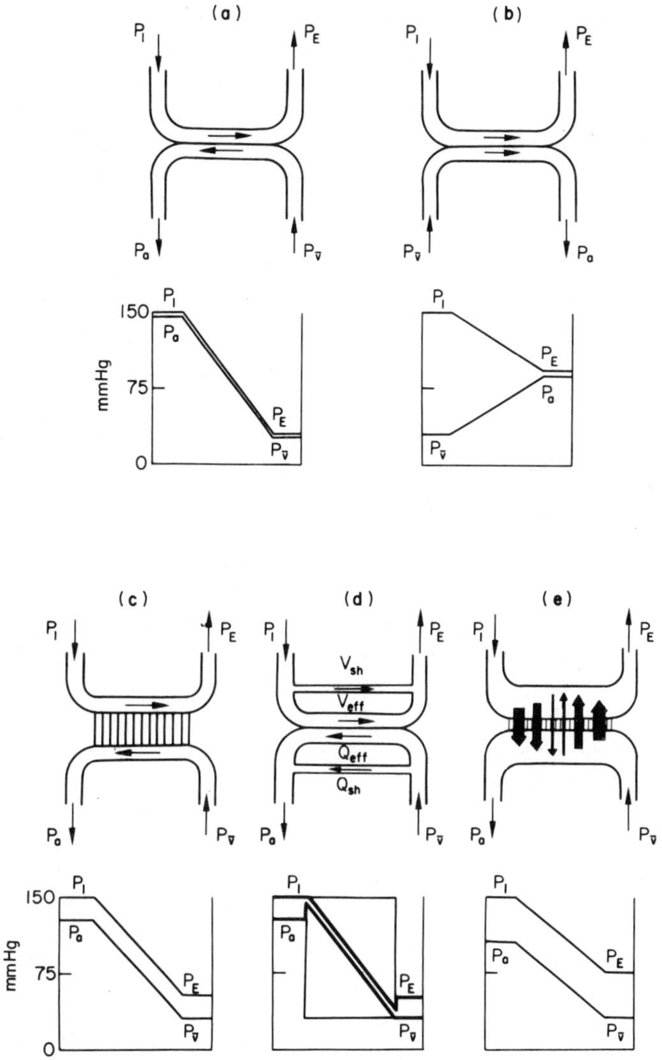

Fig. 9.4. Models for gas exchange in gills.
(a) Ideal conditions, with water and blood flowing in opposite directions (counter current).
(b) Ideal conditions, with water and blood flowing in same direction (co-current).
(c) Counter current, with diffusion resistance.
(d) Counter current, with blood and water shunts. In this case, some blood and water is thought of as completely equilibrating and therefore as being effective ($\dot{Q}_{eff}$ and $\dot{V}_{eff}$ respectively), while the rest of the blood and water, which undergo no gas exchange, can be thought of as being ineffective and constituting shunts ($\dot{Q}_{sh}$ and $\dot{V}_{sh}$).
(e) Counter current, with combination of diffusion resistance and shunts. Arrows represent gas exchange by diffusion with the thickness indicating the degree of equilibration over the distance denoted by the length. Beyond a certain distance no gas exchange occurs within the time that the liquids are in contact.
Graphs indicate changes in $P\text{O}_2$ in water and blood under each of the above conditions (based on [24]).

Diffusion resistance

This includes the reaction time of oxygen with haemoglobin, which will be slow at low temperature, plus the features incorporated in Fick's law of diffusion, i.e. surface area (A) and the thickness of the gas exchanger (x) and the diffusion constant (K) of the respiratory media (i.e. water, tissue and blood). Diffusion resistance can account for the lack of equilibration between the respiratory media (Fig. 9.4c).

The term KA/x from the diffusion law characterizes the diffusion properties of the gas exchanger and has been termed diffusing capacity for lungs (D) or transfer factor for gills (T). Thus,

$$T\mathrm{O}_2 = \frac{V\mathrm{O}_2}{\Delta P_g} \text{ ml . min}^{-1}\text{ . mmHg}^{-1}$$

where $\Delta P_g (\equiv P_{\mathrm{I}} - P_2)$ is the mean pressure difference across the gills and has been defined [28] as:

$$\frac{(P\mathrm{I,O}_2 + P\mathrm{E,O}_2)}{2} - \frac{(P\mathrm{a,O}_2 + P\bar{\mathrm{v}}\mathrm{,O}_2)}{2}$$

The lower the value of T, the greater the diffusion resistance; and T will increase with increases in effective surface area, and a reduction in effective diffusion distance of the gas exchanger. In most aquatic animals, $T\mathrm{O}_2$ is approximately 0·01 ml . kg^{-1} . min^{-1} . mmHg^{-1}. In the tuna, where it is an order of magnitude greater, the surface area of the gas exchanger is greater and the blood–water distance is smaller (Table 9.3).

Water shunt

Some water may not pass through the sieve formed by the secondary lamellae and therefore may never come into contact with the gas exchange area of the gills. A large water shunt is thought to occur in *Cancer* [15]. Whether complete equilibration occurs between the blood in the gills and the water that does flow through the lamella will depend upon the closeness of the water to the lamella and the time of contact between the two liquids. As the diffusion of O_2 through water is very slow, the water farthest from the secondary lamella participates less in gas exchange, if at all, than the water closest to the lamella. Water participating in gas exchange, but equilibrating incompletely, can be considered as consisting of a component that completely equilibrates, and of another component that takes no part in gas exchange at all (i.e. functionally similar to the water that completely by-passes the gas-exchange surface) [24]. Thus total water flow ($\dot{V}$t) can be divided into ineffective or shunted water ($\dot{V}$sh) and effective water ($\dot{V}$eff) which equilibrates with mixed venous blood. (Fig. 9.4d).

Blood shunt

Whether some of the blood leaving the ventral aorta passes through non-respiratory shunt vessels [33] or not [22], the total blood flow ($\dot{Q}$t) can still be thought of as consisting of a shunt component and an effective component [36], i.e. $\dot{Q}t = \dot{Q}sh + \dot{Q}eff$ (Fig. 9.4d). In reality, the limitations of the gas-exchange system consist of a combination of diffusion resistance and shunts (Fig. 9.4e), and there is a continuous transition from diffusion resistance to shunt.

Unequal distribution of blood and water flow

It is possible that some secondary lamellae may not be perfused or ventilated. If the same lamellae are not perfused or ventilated, this would merely reduce the effective surface area of the gas exchanger itself causing a reduction in gas exchange. If some lamellae are perfused but not ventilated, or *vice versa*, there is then a water or a blood shunt. Between these two extreme conditions and the optimum ratio between ventilation and perfusion, there are intermediate conditions where lamellae may be under-perfused or under-ventilated. Such inequalities in ventilation and perfusion will reduce the efficiency of the gas exchanger.

Efficiency of gas exchange

The combined effects of the factors affecting gas exchange can be quantified and the concepts involved are important in the physiology of gas exchange. The maximum possible rate of oxygen uptake in an aquatic animal equals the ventilation volume, ($\dot{V}_t$) multiplied by the difference in oxygen content of inspired water ($C\text{I},\text{O}_2$) and of water equilibrated with mixed venous blood ($C\bar{\text{v}},\text{eq},\text{O}_2$), i.e. if the counter current system is 100% efficient:

$$\dot{V}\text{O}_2,\ \text{max} = \dot{V}\text{t}(C\text{I},\text{O}_2 - C\bar{\text{v}},\text{eq},\text{O}_2)$$

Actual oxygen uptake can be calculated from the Fick principle:

$$\dot{V}\text{O}_2 = \dot{V}\text{t}\ (C\text{I},\text{O}_2 - C\text{E},\text{O}_2)$$

where $C\text{E},\text{O}_2$ is the oxygen content of expired water.

Therefore, the ratio of the actual to maximum possible amount of oxygen removed from the water can be expressed as:

$$\frac{\dot{V}\text{t}\ (C\text{I},\text{O}_2 - C\text{E},\text{O}_2)}{\dot{V}\text{t}\ (C\text{I},\text{O}_2 - C\bar{\text{v}},\text{eq},\text{O}_2)}$$

This is known as the effectiveness (Ew) of delivery of O_2 (or removal of CO_2) by the water pumped by the animal. It is usually multiplied by 100 and expressed as a percentage.

In general terms,

$$E\text{w} = \frac{\alpha\text{w}\ (P\text{I} - P\text{E})}{\alpha\text{w}\ (P\text{I} - P\bar{\text{v}})}$$

where αw = solubility of gas in water.

For oxygen, where only the physical solubility is concerned, αw is constant and cancels out. This is not the case for CO_2 (Fig. 9.1).

Similarly, the effectiveness of O_2 uptake or CO_2 elimination by the blood is:

$$Eb = \frac{\alpha b\,(Pa - P\bar{v})}{\alpha b\,(P_I - P\bar{v})}$$

where αb = solubility of gas in the blood at a particular partial pressure. Because of the complex relationship between blood gas content and tension, it is better if the concentration of the gas in the blood is measured directly. The tuna has a very high value of Ew_{O_2} and $Eb,_{O_2}$ is greater than $Ew,_{O_2}$ in both dogfish and trout (Table 9.3). A contributory factor to the latter phenomenon is undoubtedly the shape of the blood dissociation curve for O_2. As long as $Pa,_{O_2}$ is close to the top of the curve, raising $Pa,_{O_2}$ to the value of $P_I,_{O_2}$ does not greatly affect the ratio

$$\frac{\alpha b\,(Pa,_{O_2} - P\bar{v},_{O_2})}{\alpha b\,(P_I,_{O_2} - P\bar{v},_{O_2})}$$

Actual oxygen uptake (or CO_2 removal) of an animal cannot only be calculated from the change in gas content of the water flowing over the gills, e.g.

$$\dot{V}_{O_2} = \dot{V}t\,(C_I,_{O_2} - C_E,_{O_2}),$$

but also from the change in gas content of the blood flowing through the gills:

$$\dot{V}_{O_2} = \dot{Q}t\,(Ca,_{O_2} - C\bar{v},_{O_2}),$$

therefore

$$\frac{\dot{V}t\cdot\alpha w,_{O_2}\,(P_I,_{O_2} - P_E,_{O_2})}{\dot{Q}t\cdot\alpha b,_{O_2}\,(Pa,_{O_2} - P\bar{v},_{O_2})} = 1$$

The ratio,

$$\frac{\dot{V}t\cdot\alpha w}{\dot{Q}t\cdot\alpha b}$$

is known as the ventilation–perfusion conductance ratio [25] or the capacity-rate ratio [13]. Analyses have shown that the high efficiency of gas exchange by a counter current system is only evident when this ratio is close to unity. This is in fact the situation in dogfish [24] and teleosts [27], and as αw is much less than αb (because of the blood pigment), $\dot{V}t$ must be much greater than $\dot{Q}t$. In fact $\dot{V}t/\dot{Q}t$ or $\dot{V}g/\dot{Q}$ as it is commonly written, is around 10–20 for fish and other aquatic animals [15, 27]. In ice fish, which have no haemoglobin, $\dot{V}g/\dot{Q}$ is between 1–3. As $\alpha w,_{CO_2}$ is approximately 30× greater than $\alpha w,_{O_2}$, it follows, that with an equal exchange of CO_2 and O_2 (i.e. gas exchange ratio $R = 1$), $P_I,_{O_2}$ will fall by 30 mmHg for every 1 mmHg increase in $P_E,_{CO_2}$. In aquatic animals, therefore, $Pa,_{CO_2}$ should rarely exceed 5 mmHg.

9.6.4 The effects of hypoxia, temperature and exercise on gas exchange

All water breathing animals are poikilotherms, so an increase in environmental temperature of 10°C within the physiological range may cause at least a transient increase in oxygen demand by a factor of 2–3. Coupled with this, the amount of oxygen in the water will decrease by 18%. This problem may be partially offset as the viscosity of the water will decrease, and the rate of diffusion of gases through the water will increase. The increased demand for oxygen is met by increases in both $\dot{V}g$ and $\dot{Q}$ with $\dot{V}g/\dot{Q}$ remaining more or less constant, but To_2 decreases as temperature rises. In fish that are acclimated to high temperatures, there is an increase in the packed cell volume of the blood (haematocrit) and this appears to be related to an increase in the oxygen-carrying capacity of the blood [4].

The availability of oxygen can be reduced in the aquatic environment, particularly in stagnant water, where bacterial action can cause a reduction in Po_2 of the water (hypoxia). During a progressive reduction in oxygen tension over a period of a few hours, an animal may maintain its oxygen uptake (regulate) or allow it to fall with $P\text{I},o_2$ (conform). Different animals have been labelled as O_2 regulators or conformers, although it has been shown that the same species may be a conformer at high temperatures and a regulator at low temperature [4]. For fish at higher environmental temperatures, heart rate decreases during hypoxia although cardiac output stays reasonably constant [4]. Ventilation volume increases, so that there is a rise in $\dot{V}g/\dot{Q}$. This leads to a reduction in $E\text{w},o_2$ in fish. As $P\text{I},o_2$ falls, so does $P\text{a},o_2$, but this is partly compensated for by an accompanying reduction in $P\bar{\text{v}},o_2$, i.e. the animal extracts more oxygen from the blood, and To_2 increases. All these adjustments may serve to maintain $\dot{V}o_2$. When the respiratory and cardiovascular systems can no longer maintain $\dot{V}o_2$, there is increased anaerobiosis and the level of lactic acid in the blood rises. Long-term exposure to hypoxia in eels causes a reduction in $\dot{V}o_2$ and an increase in lactic acid production during the first few days. Eventually (after about one week) the acidosis subsides. This is related to a rise in the oxygen affinity of the blood as the concentration of GTP (guanosine triphosphate) falls in the red blood cells [35] and to an increase in the oxygen-carrying capacity of the blood [37].

During exercise, an animal's oxygen demand will increase above the resting level. Moderate exercise in trout leads to an increase in $\dot{V}g$ and $\dot{Q}$, with $\dot{V}g/\dot{Q}$ remaining the same. As $\dot{V}o_2$ rises so does To_2 with the mean pressure difference across the gills ($\Delta\, Pg$) remaining constant [27]. As To_2 increases, so do the rates of Na^+ efflux and of water influx. Aquatic animals, particularly fresh water forms, are faced with the problem of balancing their gas-exchange requirements with water and ionic stability. It is probable that at rest, only a few proximal secondary lamellae are ventilated and perfused, thus allowing sufficient gas exchange and yet restricting ionic and water fluxes. During activity more secondary lamellae could be ventilated and perfused, causing an increase in functional surface area of the gills thus maximizing gas exchange but also allowing undesirable fluxes of ions and water [3, 13]. Mackerel and tuna have many modifications associated with their active existence. Gill area is high, water–blood distance is small and To_2 is high (Table 9.3). These fish utilize the 'ram-jet' method of ventilation when swimming, and the cost of respiration lies between 1 and 3% of total metabolism at basal swimming speed in the skipjack tuna. In the tuna there is some fusion between the secondary lamellae of adjacent gill filaments to form a perforated lamina which may serve to support the thin secondary lamellae [12] and prevent the filaments being forced apart at high flow rates. Blood-oxygen capacity is high in very active fish (17 vol % in mackerel compared with 9 vol % in trout and 7 vol % in carp).

9.7 AERIAL GAS EXCHANGE

There are three typical routes for gas exchange in air: by the general body surface, by tracheae which lead air directly to the tissues, and by lungs and a circulatory system. The significance of the general body surface will be mentioned later when discussing bimodal gas exchange. The tracheal system of terrestial arthropods is a highly effective respiratory system which is different in basic design from the systems involving a circulatory system [32].

9.7.1 Air and blood flow

Of the air breathing vertebrates, birds and mammals illustrate the culmination of evolutionary changes associated with the passage from water to air, as far as respiratory and circulatory systems are concerned. In both, the heart is divided into two atria and two ventricles. Deoxygenated blood returns from the body to the right atrium, passes to the right ventricle and is pumped to the lung. From the lung, oxygenated blood enters the left atrium, passes to the left ventricle and is pumped round the body. The lungs of both birds and mammals are ventilated by an aspiration pump. Because air is less dense and less viscous than water, the amount of energy expended on ventilation is relatively small. Man at rest for example, uses between 0·6–3·2% of his total oxygen uptake on ventilation. When ventilation increases by 3–4 times, the oxygen cost of breathing rises to 2–10% of total $\dot{V}O_2$.

9.7.2 Structure of lungs and gas exchange in mammals

In both birds and mammals the trachea branches into right and left bronchi. In mammals the main bronchi divide into smaller and smaller tubes and become terminal bronchioles (Fig. 9.5a). All of these bronchi are the convecting airways and take no part in gas exchange. They constitute anatomical deadspace, the volume of which is about 150 ml in man. The terminal bronchioles divide into respiratory bronchioles which have occasional sacs (alveoli) budding from them. Finally, there are the alveolar ducts which are completely lined with alveoli and terminate in the alveolar sacs. Gas exchange occurs in the alveolar region in the lung, which has a volume of approximately 2·5 l and a surface area of 50–100 m^2 in man. The diffusion distance between the blood and the air is approximately 0·5 μm. The pulmonary blood vessels also form a series of branching tubes. The

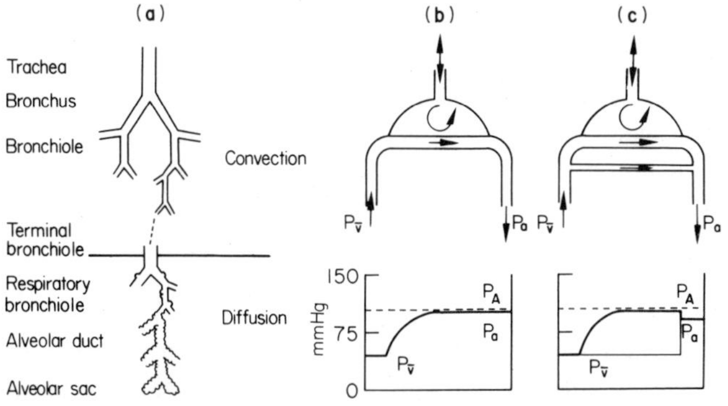

Fig. 9.5. The mammalian lung.
(a) Diagramatic representation of the human lung based on [36]. Air is transported down to the terminal bronchioles by convection and from there, gas movement is by diffusion.
(b) Ideal model for gas exchange in the mammalian lung based on the uniform pool model [25]. During its passage through the pulmonary capillaries, blood equilibrates with the alveolar gas ($Pa,O_2 = PA,O_2$).
(c) Model with blood shunt. The majority of blood equilibrates with alveolar gas but then mixes with blood which has undergone no gas exchange. Pa,O_2 is thus reduced from the ideal value.

arteries divide into smaller and smaller vessels, arterioles, which eventually form a dense network of capillaries in the walls of the alveoli. The lengths of the capillary segments are so short that this network forms an almost continuous sheet of blood in the alveolar wall.

Expired air is a mixture of gas from the anatomical deadspace, which has the same composition as inspired air, and alveolar gas which has undergone gaseous exchange. The gas in the alveoli is not exchanged by convection. Tidal volume in man is approximately 500 ml, and 150 ml of this remains in the anatomical deadspace, leaving 350 ml to supply the total alveolar volume. The final passage of gas is by diffusion through air as well as across the blood–air barrier into the blood itself. The composition of the air in the alveoli results from a balance between the rate at which fresh air is presented to the respiratory bronchioles, and the rate at which O_2 is transported away and CO_2 is released by the blood. Under normal resting conditions, alveolar gas has a PO_2 of approximately 100 mmHg and a PCO_2 of approximately 40 mmHg.

The relationship between the flow of the respiratory fluids in mammalian-type lungs is quite different from the situation in the gills of aquatic animals. The mammalian system has been called a uniform pool [25]. Capillary blood equilibrates with air in the alveoli, in which the partial pressures of gas are nearly uniform, mainly as a result of rapid diffusion (Fig. 9.5b). Under ideal conditions, the partial pressure of gases in arterial blood would equal those of mixed alveolar gas (Fig. 9.5b). This is never achieved, Pa,O_2 is lower and Pa,CO_2 is higher than mixed alveolar values, and the possible reasons for this reduced efficiency of the lung are much the same as those discussed earlier for water breathing animals, i.e. diffusion resistance, shunts and ventilation-perfusion inequalities.

Diffusion resistance

Air does not contribute to diffusion resistance as water does in aquatic breathers. The major resistances to diffusion in the lung are the tissues themselves, the small layer of liquid lining the alveolar wall and the reaction time of O_2 with haemoglobin. Because of its high rate of diffusion through tissues, CO_2 elimination is not adversely affected by diffusion resistance. The thickness of the diffusion barrier between the external medium and the blood is not vastly different in water- and air-breathing animals. Birds and mammals have a much higher oxygen demand than most poikilotherms and the diffusing capacity for oxygen ($D\text{O}_2$) in the lung of the dog and chicken is approximately 1 ml . min^{-1} kg^{-1} . mmHg^{-1}, a much higher value than $T\text{O}_2$ for any fish (Table 9.3). This is at least partly the result of the large surface area of the lungs of the dog (72 m^2). Under normal conditions, the difference in $P\text{O}_2$ between alveolar gas and end capillary blood resulting from incomplete diffusion is immeasurably small in mammalian, and bird lungs.

Shunts

The second factor that could reduce the efficiency of the lung is the passage of blood through non-ventilated areas (Fig. 9.5c). In normal animals this includes part of the bronchial venous blood which drains directly into the left ventricle. In normal animals, these contributions are equivalent to 1–2% of total cardiac output and the resulting decrease in $P\text{a,O}_2$ is less than 5 mmHg.

Unequal distribution of ventilation and perfusion

Unlike the situation in water breathers, where diffusion resistance and blood and water shunts are probably the most likely causes of reduced efficiency, in air-breathing vertebrates, particularly in the upright primates, it is ventilation-perfusion inequalities which are the most important factors. In mammals, the ratio between alveolar ventilation ($\dot{V}\text{A}$) and perfusion ($\dot{Q}$), i.e. $\dot{V}\text{A}/\dot{Q}$, is approximately 1. As the oxygen-carrying capacity of most mammalian blood is similar to that of air (between 20–22 vol %), a $\dot{V}\text{A}/\dot{Q}$ ratio of unity gives a ventilation-perfusion conductance ratio of approximately 1. This is for the lung as a whole, but different regions of the lung behave in different ways.

In the upright lung, the column of blood produces a hydrostatic pressure which increases perfusion pressure and therefore blood flow at the base of the lung. Ventilation also increases down the lung, but not to such a great extent. Thus, at the apex of the human lung there are alveoli with almost no blood flow and moderate ventilation where $\dot{V}\text{A}/\dot{Q} = 3{\cdot}3$, while at the base of the lung, blood flow is much larger, but ventilation is only slightly increased and $\dot{V}\text{A}/\dot{Q} = 0{\cdot}63$. West [36] has shown how these inequalities in $\dot{V}\text{A}/\dot{Q}$ can contribute to differences in $P\text{a,O}_2$ and $P\text{O}_2$ of mixed alveolar gas ($P\text{A,O}_2$). These $\dot{V}\text{A}/\dot{Q}$ inequalities are not so pronounced in quadruped vertebrates where the lung is horizontal.

9.7.3 Structure of the lung and gas exchange in birds

In birds, the respiratory organ is divided into a gas exchange part, the lungs, and into a ventilating system, the air sacs. The left and right primary bronchi, which divide from the trachea, continue through the lung and connect with the abdominal air sac which is in the abdominal cavity dorsal to the viscera. The primary bronchus divides into the secondary bronchi (Fig. 9.6a). As it enters the lung it gives off four ventrobronchi which ramify across the ventral surface of the lung. It passes for a short distance free of branches, and then gives off 7–10 dorsobronchi which extend and ramify at the lateral and dorsal surface of the lung. These two sets of secondary bronchi are joined together by the anastamosing tertiary bronchi, or parabronchi. These are the functional units of the lung, for it is here that gas exchange takes place. Opposite to the entrance of the dorsobronchi another group of secondary bronchi, the laterobronchi, originate ventrally from the primary bronchus. The largest of this group enters the posterior thoracic air sac. The cervical air sac arises from the anterior branch of the first ventrobronchus, while the interclavicular air sac and the anterior thoracic air sac are connected to the initial portion of the third ventrobronchus. This basic arrangement is present in all birds that have been investigated and forms the basis of all earlier descriptions of the avian lung. It has been called the 'palaeopulmo' by Duncker [5, 6]. Penguins and emus have a lung that consists entirely of this palaeopulmo, and it is also obvious in the lung of storks and cormorants. In all other birds, that have been studied, an additional network of parabronchi originates from the lateral side of the primary bronchus and of the dorsobronchi and laterally enters the funnel-shaped openings of the laterobronchus and primary bronchus into the posterior air sacs. This network of parabronchi, unlike the palaeopulmo, lies in series with air flow from the primary bronchus to the posterior air sacs, and has been named the 'neopulmo' [5, 6] (Fig. 9.6b). The neopulmo is still poorly developed in cormorants, storks and cranes, but becomes larger in pigeons, ducks and gulls. In fowl-like birds and song birds, the neopulmo extends cranially and becomes connected to the lateral branches of the anterior ventrobronchi and to the anterior air sacs. Even where best-developed, the neopulmo never exceeds 20–25% of total lung volume.

The differences in structure between avian lungs and those of other vertebrates are further exemplified when the parabronchi are studied in detail. These are completely anastamosing, none is blind-ending. Each parabronchus is surrounded by a roughly hexagonal-shaped thin layer of connective tissue (Fig. 9.6c). This delimits the gas exchange area, for the wall of each parabronchus is pierced by numerous openings which lead to atria. From these develops a complex network of fine anastamosing air capillaries which are intimately interlocked with blood capillaries to form the exchange area. The blood–gas barrier in the avian lung consists of the epithelial cell of the air capillary, a common basement membrane and the endothelial cell of the blood capillary. The thickness of this barrier is, on average, 0·35 μm in the chicken and 0·10–0·14 μm in the pigeon.

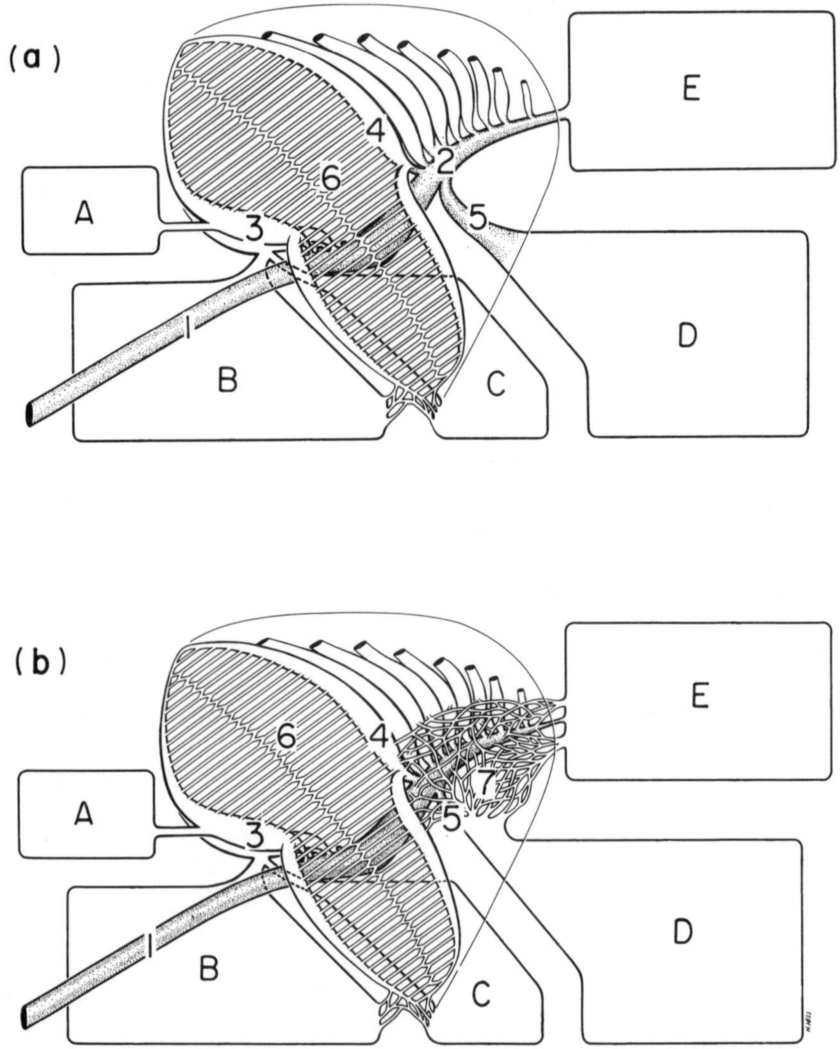
(a)
A
B
C
D
E
1
2
3
4
5
6
(b)
A
B
C
D
E
1
3
4
5
6
7

(c)

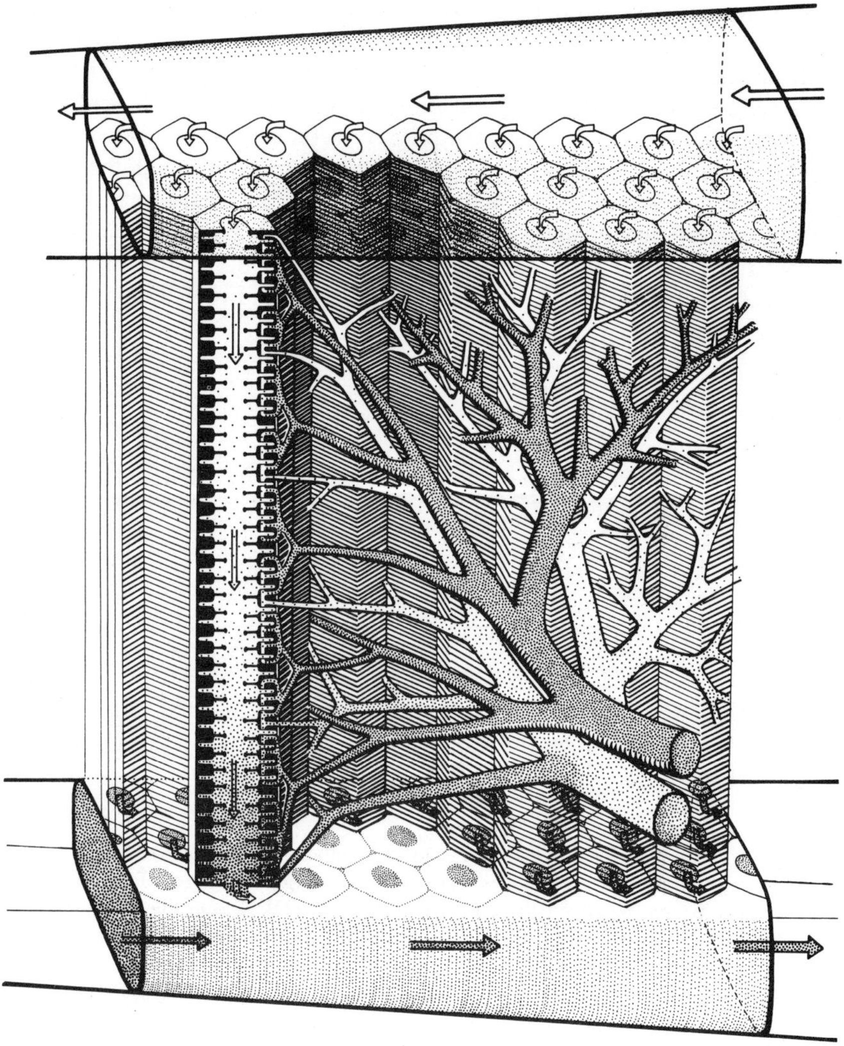

Fig. 9.6. Diagrammatic representation of the structure of the lung in birds [5].
(a) The palaeopulmo and its air sac connections 1-trachea, 2-primary bronchus, 3-ventrobronchi, 4-dorsobronchi, 5-laterobronchus, 6-parabronchi. A-cervical air sac, B-interclavicular air sac, C-anterior thoracic air sac, D-posterior thoracic air sac, E-abdominal air sac.
(b) The palaeopulmo and a small neopulmo with connections to the large posterior air sacs. Symbols, as in **(a)** with the addition of 7-parabronchial net known as neopulmo. In this diagram it connects only with the posterior air sacs, but in some birds it may extend cranially [5, 6].
(c) Representation of the arterial (dense stippling) and venous (light stippling) arrangements in the avian lung with reference to the parabronchi [6]. Inspired air (white arrows) flows through a branch of the dorsobronchus into the parabronchi which are hexagonal in cross section. On its passage through the parabronchi, air diffuses along the air capillaries which are supplied with blood capillaries. Gas exchange occurs here, and expired air (stippled arrows) flows through a branch of the ventrobronchus.

During inspiration in birds, air flows through the lungs into the air sacs and it is the air sacs, not the lung, which increase in volume. During expiration, the air sacs decrease in volume and air flows out through the lung. Air flows through the parabronchi in the same direction during both phases of ventilation [26]. During inspiration, air enters the primary bronchus, some goes directly to the posterior air sacs, and some goes via the dorsobronchi through the parabronchi and then via the ventrobronchi to the anterior air sacs. During expiration, the air from the anterior air sac passes directly to the primary bronchus, whereas that from the posterior sacs takes the following path; dorsobronchi, parabronchi, ventrobronchi, primary bronchus (Fig. 9.7a & b). From the parabronchi, the

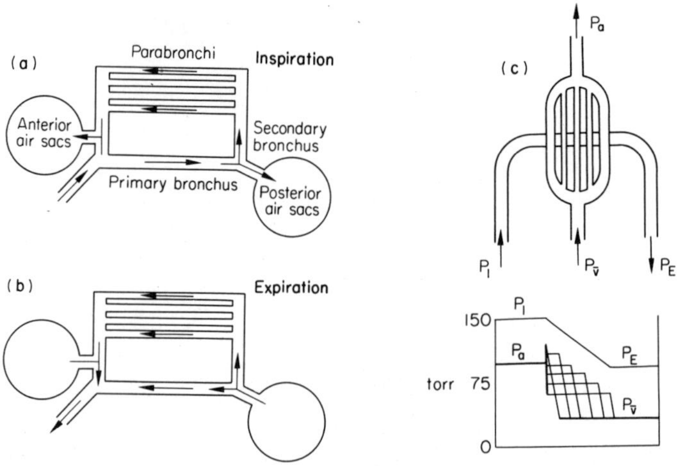

Fig. 9.7. Air flow in the bird lung.
Diagram to illustrate the direction of gas flow through the avian lung **(a)** during inspiration and **(b)** during expiration. The arrows indicate the direction of gas flow. **(c)** Model for gas exchange in the avian lung, based on the cross-current model [26]. Graph illustrates the changes in Pa,O_2 in the blood and air during their passage through the lung.

exchange of gas down to the air capillaries is thought to be by diffusion. Constriction of the parabronchi, particularly of the openings into the air capillaries, could reduce the ventilation of the exchange area and therefore reduce the diffusing capacity of the lung.

From the above description of air flow through the lung, the gas composition of the posterior air sacs should be similar to that of inspired air. This is not the case in the chicken where PO_2 is lower and PCO_2 is higher in the posterior air sac than in inspired air. The explanation is probably that during inspiration, air passes through the parabronchi of the neopulmo before entering the posterior air sacs. Gas leaving these sacs during expiration is also thought to pass through the neopulmo. Since the parabronchi of the neopulmo seem to be ventilated bidirectionally, it would appear that unidirectional air flow is not essential for gas exchange in the parabronchi. In fact it has been shown that reversing the direction of air flow through the parabronchi experimentally, does not alter the blood-gas tensions [26]. This finding leads to the proposal that in the bird lung, air and blood flow at right angles to each other in a 'cross-current' [26] (Fig. 9.7c). In such a situation it would be possible for there to be some overlap between expired and arterial gas tensions. This has been found to be the case in birds breathing air as far as CO_2 is concerned, i.e. $P_{E,CO_2} > P_{a,CO_2}$, and for both O_2 and CO_2 in birds breathing a high CO_2, low O_2 gas mixture. In this case $P_{E,O_2} < P_{a,O_2}$ and $P_{E,CO_2} > P_{a,CO_2}$. When breathing room air, $\dot{V}_A/\dot{Q}$ inequalities and/or shunts could prevent the overlapping of O_2.

9.7.4 Gas exchange at high altitude and during exercise

At high altitude, birds and mammals are exposed to environmental hypoxia as there is a reduction in P_{I,O_2}. Ventilation increases, which substantially reduces the difference between inspired P_{O_2} and P_{O_2} in the aveolar gas. Associated with this rise in ventilation there is also a reduction in P_{a,CO_2} which gives rise to alkalosis in new arrivals to a high altitude. Over a period of a few days, the kidneys remove HCO_3^- and blood pH is returned to normal. The diffusion capacity of the lung increases such that $P_{A,O_2} - P_{a,O_2}$ is less in residents at high altitude compared with sea-level residents. This is at least partly related to an increase in the ratio of alveolar volume to total lung volume, and may be also the result of a reduction in the blood–air diffusion distance. Adaptations also occur in the circulatory system. Both cardiac output and the oxygen-carrying capacity of the blood are higher in animals living at high altitude. The latter is related to a rise in haematocrit. The oxygen affinity of the blood of a number of mammals at high altitude, including man, decreases, and this is related to an increase in the level of organic phosphate (2,3-diphosphoglycerate or 2,3-DPG). This is thought to assist in the removal of O_2 from the blood at the tissues. The blood of the vicuna and llama has a higher O_2 affinity than that of mammals living at sea level, so the response of the dissociation curve to hypoxia varies from animal to animal [19]. Birds are able to tolerate lower values of P_{I,O_2} than mammals, although in birds at simulated high altitudes, there is no change in the concentration of inositol hexaphosphate (IHP), one of the major organic phosphates in avian red blood cells.

The responses to exercise are similar in aquatic and terrestrial animals. A pigeon for example flying at 10 m . sec^{-1} has a $\dot{V}_{O_2}$ which is ten times the resting value. This is achieved by increases in ventilation, cardiac output and in the difference in oxygen content of arterial and mixed venous blood ($C_{a,O_2} - C_{\bar{v},O_2}$). The latter is the result of a large reduction in $C_{\bar{v},O_2}$ indicating that the tissues extract a greater amount of O_2 from the blood than they do when the bird is at rest. Ventilation may be aided by the locomotory muscles in pigeons, as there is synchrony between wing beat and ventilation. It has been shown that in mammals the diffusing capacity of the lungs increases during exercise. Many birds contend with the dual problem of exercise and high altitude, which must place extraordinary demands on the cardiovascular and respiratory systems. It could be that high flying birds possess a considerable resistance to tissue hypoxia [26].

9.8 BIMODAL BREATHING AND THE EMERGENCE FROM WATER ONTO LAND

There are a number of ways in which early fish could have developed the ability to obtain oxygen from air and eventually give rise to completely terrestrial vertebrates. A number of living fish demonstrate some of these possibilities. Modification of the mouth or pharynx may occur, e.g. *Symbranchus*, and the eel *Anguilla* use their modified gills for air breathing, whereas the electric eel, *Electrophorus* has foldings and papillations of the buccal epithelium projecting into the buccal cavity. These form extensive vascular surfaces for aerial gas exchange. In the climbing perch, *Anabas*, opercular diverticuli extend inside the skull to form labryinthine organs and suprabranchial chambers which function as air-breathing organs. The air–blood barrier in these organs is 0·12–0·3 μm, which compares extremely well with the bird lung. Another group of fish have portions of the gastro-intestinal tract, either the stomach or small intestine, modified to function as gas-exchange organs between blood and rhythmically swallowed air, e.g. *Plecostomus* and *Hoplosternum*.

In the fish mentioned so far, the air-breathing organ is supplied with its normal arteries and the oxygenated blood drains into the general venous circuit by its normal veins. Thus, only where the gills themselves are used for air breathing, or where the air-breathing organ is in parallel with the gills, does the oxygenated blood from the air-breathing organ drain into the efferent branchial circulation [14]. The heart remains with a single atrium and a single ventricle.

In a third group of modern fish, there is a distinct air bladder which functions as an air-breathing organ. Amongst the Actinopterygii, the Chondrostei (*Polypterus*) and Holostei (*Amia* and *Lepisosteus*) use the air bladder as a respiratory organ, but in the vast majority of Teleostei that have an air bladder it serves a buoyancy function. Amongst the Sarcopterygii are the Dipnoi (lung fish), which have lungs, and these animals are related to the Rhipidistia (Crossopteryii) from which the Amphibia were derived. It is therefore the Dipnoi that may give clues as to the evolutionary changes that may have been taken by the early vertebrates. Many of the living fish which possess air-breathing organs either live in areas where dissolved oxygen may become scarce, because of drought or depletion of oxygen in the water itself, or spend part of their time on land moving from one body of water to another. It is precisely these environmental pressures which were thought to have conferred an advantage on fish which possessed air-breathing organs. During the Devonian period there seems to have been widespread conditions of seasonal drought and those fresh-water fish which could obtain oxygen from air and had limbs to move them to another water pool stood the best chance of survival.

The modern Dipnoi are probably living relatives of those early air-breathing vertebrates. There are three genera, *Neoceratodus* from Australia has one lung and is predominately an aquatic breather with efficient gills, *Protopterus* from Africa, and *Lepidosiren* from South America are predominately air breathers with an associated reduction in their gills. They all possess fairly complex lungs which resemble those of frogs and turtles. The blood–air distance is about 0·5 μm, and the ultrastructure is similar to that of the lung of birds and mammals. The significant development is a separate vascular supply to the lungs from the last branchial arch. This is the pulmonary artery. Draining the lung and sending oxygenated blood back to the heart from the lung is the pulmonary vein. Thus, in the lungfish we see the beginnings of the double circulation that reaches its zenith in the birds and mammals. Two blood streams enter the heart, deoxygenated blood from the body, and oxygenated from the lungs. There are two atria to maintain separation of these two streams, but the ventricle is not completely divided. The presence of an air-breathing organ means that it, as well as the gills, must be ventilated.

Ventilation of lungs

Both living lungfish and amphibians fill their lungs using a buccal force-pump. The lungfish ventilate their gills in a way similar to teleosts and elasmobranchs. When they surface for air, the mouth opens in air, the opercula shut, the glottis opens and as the mouth closes, air is forced into the lungs. In frogs, fresh air is taken in through the nostrils and when the buccal cavity is full of fresh air, the nostrils close, the glottis opens, the floor of the buccal cavity is raised and air is forced into the lungs. These similarities between living fish, lungfish and amphibia, led physiologists to propose that the earliest land vertebrates used a buccal force pump to ventilate their lungs thus making use of a system already present in aquatic fish [20]. However, it has been argued that early air-breathing vertebrates used a costal suction pump [8, 29] and that the method of lung ventilation as well as rib reduction seen in modern amphibians are secondary conditions [29].

Blood flow and the circulatory system

Further evidence of the modern amphibia being a specialized offshoot of the main line of vertebrate evolution can be seen in the structure of the heart [7]. In lungfish there is an interventricular system which incompletely divides the ventricle and maintains some degree, although not complete, separation of the oxygenated and deoxygenated blood. There is little contamination of the blood going to the lung, but more contamination of the blood to the system arches. Therefore shunts occur in the heart whereby some deoxygenated blood from the body mixes with the oxygenated blood from the lungs. In lungfish, blood can circulate preferentially to the particular gas-exchange organ being used at the time. When the animal is submerged in aerated water, blood flow to the gills is high and blood flow to the lungs is low. During lung ventilation the situation is reversed. Thus $\dot{V}g/\dot{Q}$ and $\dot{V}_A/\dot{Q}$ are reasonably well matched. This selective distribution is probably achieved by vasoconstriction in the non-ventilated gas-exchange organ.

Although most modern amphibia have lost their gills and rely predominately on their lungs for oxygen uptake, the ventricle of the heart has only a single chamber. Despite this, there is still a good degree of separation between oxygenated and deoxygenated blood in its passage through the heart, particularly in the Anura where the spiral valve in the conus arteriosus is important in this respect. Reptiles have an incompletely divided ventricle. In the Squamata and Chelonia the interventricular septum is incomplete whereas in the Crocodilia, this septum is complete, but there is a small hole (foramen of Panizza) between the left and right systemic arches. When amphibians and reptiles are ventilating their lungs fairly rhythmically, there is a small degree (Amphibia, Chelonia and Squamata) or no mixing (Crocodilia) of the oxygenated and deoxygenated blood. During periods of apnoea (cessation of breathing) or during submersion, there is a gradual reduction in blood flow to the lungs as $P\mathrm{a,O_2}$ falls, until blood flow along the pulmonary circuit is virtually zero. Systemic blood flow changes very little. During this time there is a large increase in pulmonary vascular resistance. When lung ventilation begins there is an almost immediate increase in flow to the lungs and pulmonary vascular resistance decreases. Thus the incomplete divisions between the left and right side of the ventricle, while they may lead to some inefficiencies in gas exchange during breathing, mean that during apnoea, unnecessary perfusion of the unventilated gas-exchange organ need not occur. This is not possible in birds and mammals where complete anatomical separation of the right and left sides of the heart occurs.

Gas exchange in bimodal breathers

The oxygen capacity of water is low, which means that water-breathing animals have high ventilation rates in order to maintain an adequate $P\mathrm{a,O_2}$ (70–90 mmHg). As $\alpha\mathrm{w,CO_2}$ is much greater than $\alpha\mathrm{w,O_2}$, $P\mathrm{a,CO_2}$ is always low in water breathers (<5 mmHg). The oxygen capacity of air is 20–30 × greater than that of water, which means that ventilation volume in an air-breathing animal need be only 1/30–1/20 that of a water breather in order to maintain a similar $P\mathrm{a,O_2}$ at a given oxygen uptake. However, the 'solubilities' of CO_2 and O_2 in air are the same so that the lower ventilation volume leads to an increase in $P\mathrm{a,CO_2}$ in terrestrial vertebrates (30–40 mmHg). To prevent such a drastic increase in $P\mathrm{a,CO_2}$ (and hence a change in acid/base balance) during the transition from aquatic to aerial breathing, there must have been an effective system of CO_2 elimination in the earliest air-breathing vertebrates. In modern amphibia the skin can be the prime area for oxygen uptake at low temperatures, or the lung can predominate at higher temperatures (>10–13°C), whereas the skin is always the major area for CO_2 elimination. For this reason, it has been assumed that the skin was the major site for CO_2 elimination during vertebrate evolution [11], although palaeontological evidence suggests that the early amphibians were completely covered in their bony scales and that there was an internal gill system capable of dealing with CO_2 discharge [29]. In modern lungfish there is a trend from *Neoceratodus*, where the gills are almost entirely responsible for exchange of both oxygen and carbon dioxide, to *Protopterus* and *Lepidosiren*, where nearly all of the oxygen uptake is via the lungs, and a greater proportion of CO_2 expulsion occurs via the lungs. Thus when *Neoceratodus* and *Protopterus* are taken from water to air, the former can neither maintain its Pa,O_2 at a high value nor its Pa,CO_2 at a low level. In *Protopterus*, both Pa,O_2 and Pa,CO_2 increase slightly (Fig. 9.8). The fact that Pa,CO_2 is high in *Protopterus* even when it is in water is an indication of the reduced efficiency of the gills as gas-exchange organs. Similarly the lung of *Neoceratodus* is not adequate to sustain a high Pa,O_2 when in air. This is the result of low blood perfusion of this organ because PO_2 of blood in the pulmon-

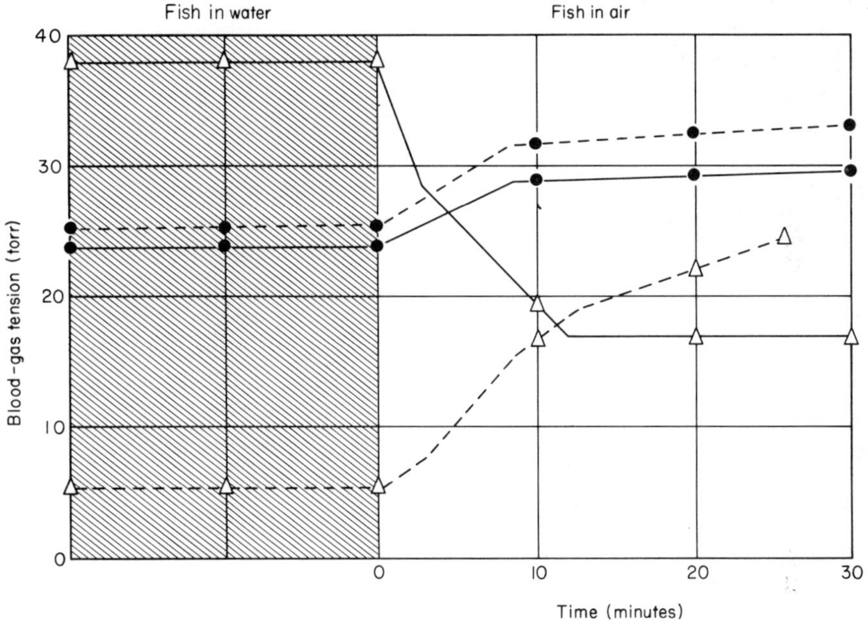

Fig. 9.8. A comparison of the changes in Pa,O_2 and Pa,CO_2 after removal from water to air of *Neoceratodus* (△) and *Protopterus* (○). Broken lines, Pa,CO_2; solid lines, Pa,O_2 [14].

ary vein actually rises from 40 mmHg to 90 mmHg upon exposure of the animal to air [14]. Accompanying the increase in Pa,CO_2 with increased air breathing in lungfish, is a rise in the CO_2 carrying capacity of the blood and a decrease in the Bohr effect.

Ventilation of the lung is often intermittent in poikilotherm vertebrates, and Pa,O_2 falls quite steadily between breaths and rises at the next breath in lungfish and Amphibia. In *Protopterus* there is quite a large difference between lung PO_2 and PO_2 in the pulmonary vein at all times, indicating a low diffusing capacity. This may result from a large diffusion resistance in the lung or $\dot{V}A/\dot{Q}$ inequalities. On the other hand, in *Amphiumia*, a urodele amphibian, there is very little difference in lung PO_2 and pulmonary vein PO_2 immediately after a breath, although the difference becomes quite marked during a period of diving apnoea, indicating a decrease in DO_2 presumably as a result of the reduced blood flow through the lung during apnoea. Oscillations in Pa,CO_2 associated with intermittent breathing and apnoea were almost non-existent with Pa,CO_2 around 10 mmHg, indicating that CO_2 removal through the skin into the surrounding water is important. In terrestrial reptiles which show intermittent breathing, it would be expected that Pa,CO_2 would oscillate in much the same way as Pa,O_2.

In both *Protopterus* and *Amphiumia*, PO_2 in the dorsal aorta is substantially less than that in the pulmonary vein, suggesting that in both animals, oxygenated blood from the lung is being contaminated with deoxygenated blood from the body. This reduces the overall efficiency of the gas-exchange organ and can be classified as a blood shunt.

Although reptiles are generally thought of as possessing a tough impermeable skin, with the lungs being the exclusive organs for gas exchange, there has been recent evidence to suggest that both aquatic and terrestrial animals from this group can obtain O_2 and get rid of CO_2 across the skin when placed in water [9, 31], and extrapulmonary gas exchange in some aquatic chelonians resulting from buccopharyngeal breathing has also been reported [2].

Birds and mammals are unable to exchange gases with the aquatic environment. This is a disadvantage for those aquatic birds and mammals that spend long periods of time under water. Such diving animals show a number of other adaptations to their aquatic habit. Blood volume and oxygen carrying capacity are higher than in their completely terrestrial relatives [1], but, more important, they are able drastically to reduce blood flow to somatic and splanchnic muscle. Consequently nearly all the oxygen contained within the blood is made available to the CNS and the heart, which cannot withstand long periods of asphyxia.

Acknowledgement

I should like to thank Dr E. W. Taylor for his useful comments and criticisms.

9.9 REFERENCES

1 Andersen H.T. (1966) Physiological adaptations in diving vertebrates. *Physiol. Rev.* **46,** 212–43.

2 Belkin D.A. (1968) Aquatic respiration and underwater survival in two freshwater turtle species. *Respir. Physiol.* **4,** 1–14.

3 Bergman H.L., Olson K.R. & Fromm P.O. (1974) The effects of vasoactive agents on the functional surface area of isolated-perfused gills of rainbow trout. *J. comp. Physiol.* **94,** 267–86.

4 Butler P.J. & Taylor E.W. (1975) The effect of progressive hypoxia on respiration in the dogfish. (*Scyliorhinus canicula*) at different seasonal temperatures. *J. exp. Biol.* **63** 117–30.

5 Duncker H-R. (1972) Structure of avian lungs. *Respir. Physiol.* **14,** 44–63.

6 Duncker H-R. (1974) Structure of the avian respiratory tract. *Respir. Physiol.* **22,** 1–19.

7 Foxon G.E.H. (1955) Problems of the double circulation in vertebrates. *Biol. Rev.* **30,** 196–228.

8 Gans C. (1970) Strategy and sequence in the evolution of the external gas exchangers of ectothermal vertebrates. *Forma et Functio* **3,** 61–104.

9 Graham J.B. (1974) Aquatic respiration in the sea snake. *Pelamis platurus. Respir. Physiol.* **21,** 1–7.

10 Gray I.E. (1957) A comparative study of the gill area of crabs. *Biol. Bull. mar. bio. Lab., Woods Hole* **112,** 34032.
11 Hughes G.M. (1967) Evolution between air and water. In *Development of the Lung* (eds A. V. S. de Reuck & R. Porter). Churchill Livingstone, Edinburgh & London.
12 Hughes G.M. & Morgan M. (1973) The structure of fish gills in relation to their respiratory function. *Biol. Rev.* **48,** 419–75.
13 Hughes G.M. & Shelton G. (1962) Respiratory mechanisms and their nervous control in fish. *Advan. Comp. Biochem. Physiol.* **1,** 275–364.
14 Johansen K. (1970) Air breathing in fishes. In *Fish Physiology* (eds W. S. Hoar & D. J. Randall) Vol. 4. Academic Press, New York & London.
15 Johansen K., Lenfant C. & Mecklenburg T.A. (1970) Respiration in the crab, *Cancer magister. Z. vergl. Physiol.* **70,** 1–19.
16 Jones J.D. (1972) *Comparative Physiology of Respiration.* Arnold, London.
17 Jones D.R. & Johansen K. (1972) The blood vascular system of birds. In *Avian Biology* (eds D. S. Farner & J. R. King) Vol. II. Academic Press, New York & London.
18 Krogh J. (1941) *Comparative Physiology of Respiratory Mechanisms.* University of Pennsylvania Press, Philadelphia.
19 Lenfant C. (1973) High altitude adaptation in mammals. *Am. Zool.* **13,** 447–56.
20 McMahon B.R. (1969) A functional analysis of the aquatic and aerial respiratory movements of an African lungfish. *Protopterus aethiopicus* with reference to the evolution of the lung-ventilation mechanism in vertebrates. *J. exp. Biol.* **51,** 407–30.
21 Miller P.L. (1974) Respiration-aerial gas transport. In *Advances in Insect Physiology*, 2nd edition (ed. M. Rockstein) Vol. VI. Academic Press, New York & London.
22 Morgan M. & Tovell P.W.A. (1973) The structure of the gill of the trout, *Salmo gairdneri* (Richardson). *Z. Zellforsch* **142,** 147–62.
23 Piiper J. & Baumgarten-Schumann D. (1968) Transport of O_2 and CO_2 by water and blood in gas exchange of the dogfish (*Scyliorhinus stellaris*). *Respir. Physiol.* **5,** 326–37.
24 Piiper J. & Baumgarten-Schumann D. (1968) Effectiveness of O_2 and CO_2 exchange in the gills of the dogfish (*Scyliorhinus stellaris*). *Respir. Physiol.* **5,** 338–49.
25 Piiper J. & Scheid P. (1972) Maximum gas transfer efficiency of models for fish gills, avian lungs and mammalian lungs. *Respir. Physiol.* **14,** 115–24.
26 Piiper J. & Scheid P. (1973) Gas exchange in avian lungs: models and experimental evidence. In *Comparative Physiology* (eds L. Bolis, K. Schmidt-Nielsen & S. H. P. Maddrell). North Holland, Amsterdam.
27 Randall D.J. (1970) Gas exchange in fish. In *Fish Physiology* (eds W. S. Hoar & D. J. Randall) Vol. 4. Academic Press, New York & London.
28 Randall D.J., Holeton G.F. & Stevens E.D. (1967) The exchange of oxygen and carbon dioxide across the gills of rainbow trout. *J. exp. Biol.* **46,** 339–48.
29 Romer A.S. (1972) Skin breathing—primary or secondary? *Respir. Physiol.* **14,** 183–92.
30 Shelton G. (1970) The regulation of breathing. In *Fish Physiology* (eds W. S. Hoar & D. J. Randall) Vol. 4. Academic Press, New York & London.
31 Standaert T. & Johansen K. (1974) Cutaneous gas exchange in snakes. *J. comp. Physiol.* **89,** 313–20.
32 Steen J.B. (1971) *Comparative Physiology of Respiratory Mechanisms.* Academic Press, New York & London.
33 Steen J.B. & Kruysse A. (1964) The respiratory function of teleostan gills. *Comp. Biochem. Physiol.* **12,** 127–42.
24 Stevens E.D. (1972) Some aspects of gas exchange in the tuna. *J. exp. Biol.* **56,** 809–23.
35 Weber R.E., Lykkeboe G. & Johansen K. (1976) Physiological properties of eel haemoglobin: Hypoxic acclimation, phosphate effects and multiplicity *J. exp. Biol.* (in the press).
36 West J.B. (1974) *Respiratory Physiology—the essentials.* Blackwell Scientific Publications, Oxford.
37 Wood S.C. & Johansen K. (1973) Organic phosphate metabolism in nucleated red cells: influence of hypoxia on eel HbO_2 affinity. *Neth. J. Sea Res.* **7,** 328–38.

Prelude to Chapter 10

A species is ‘successful’ when securely established in an ecological niche by virtue of its particular structural and functional adaptations. Whether or not a species becomes established depends on the ability of sufficient individuals to survive to maturity and to sustain the population by reproducing. Thus efficient reproduction is an essential component of the processes of adaptation by which organisms are able to exist in greatly varying environments.

Adaptation of processes involved in reproduction is imperative for survival in different environments, but reproduction also provides the means of the more general functional and structural diversifications involved in genotypic adaptation. In asexual reproduction two identical units are created from one. Mutations occur and create a gene pool, but the advent of sexual reproduction in which two gametes from different individuals combine to form the new individual, had the effect of blending the genetic material and greatly speeding up the formation of, and diversifying, the gene pool of a species. This increases the chances of there being in existence individual organisms capable of withstanding a change in the environment which might otherwise threaten the continuation of the species. Thus, although the individual organism, of finite life span, may seem nothing more than a stepping stone in the progression of life, the existence of individual organisms with ‘personal’ mixtures of genetic material, provides the means whereby species have become genotypically adapted to the varied environments in which life exists.

Most metazoic forms of life reproduce sexually and, since this involves the meeting of two ‘naked’ germ cells, the union has to be an aqueous event. Thus, wherever life has become established, there must be a means of mating by which the sperm can swim to the ovum. There must also be provision for a sustained aqueous environment in which the fertilized egg can develop into a new individual. As might be expected from the above consideration, both the broad and fine aspects of reproductive physiology vary greatly between species, and the great majority of these variations relates to the historical and contemporary environments of the species. Yet, as with most else in biology, there remains a large common denominator of fundamental cell physiology upon which these many variations in detail are superimposed.

Chapter 10
Reproduction

J. BLIGH

10.1 INTRODUCTION

The many different forms and functions of living things which have evolved in the course of approximately 3000 million years can all be related, directly or indirectly, and historically or contemporaneously, to the great variety of grossly or subtly differing ecological circumstances within which life has been sustained. The principal process by which life has diversified and established itself in these differing environmental circumstances has been by the natural selection of random genetic mutations which have somehow increased the chances of the individual organism to survive to maturity and to reproduce. The retention of the ability to reproduce in changed circumstances, and the survival of the individual organism for long enough to do so, form the keystones of every evolutionary bridge by which life has remained compatible with these changes in the environment.

Thus it is not surprising that the reproductive processes of different organisms vary greatly in detail. There is no space here to discuss the many different ways in which male and female gametes meet, and in which the fertilized ovum develops into a new individual which has to take its chance in a competitive or even hostile environment of fulfilling the role of parent before it dies. We can only take examples of how reproductive patterns and processes relate to the particular ecological circumstances in which different species occur.

A point to be kept in mind, however, is that despite the diversity of life and the complexities of multicellular structures, the unit of life remains the cell. At the cellular level life has a large common denominator which has remained virtually unchanged since the environment of life was entirely aqueous, and before the divergence of plant and animal life. An important consequence of this is that even in the most complex of multicellular organisms now living in terrestrial and atmospheric macro-climates, the environments of the constituent cells remain aqueous. Each individual life starts, of course, as a single cell, and whether reproduction is the asexual division of a diploid cell as in many protozoa and in some metazoa, or the sexual fusion of two haploid cells as in most multicellular organisms, it must occur in an aqueous phase. So must the subsequent processes of cellular multiplication by which the new individual of multicellular species is produced from the fertilized ovum.

Thus the first consideration must be that of how the processes of reproduction, which have become greatly diversified in species in different ecological circumstances that are quite alien to those which can be tolerated by individual cells, have at the same time remained wholly aqueous.

10.2 FERTILIZATION

As a general rule the cell membrane divides the largely aqueous endoplasm from a chemically different but still largely aqueous extracellular environment. In terrestrial organisms cells of the outer tegument may seem to be exceptions to this generalization, but the dermal cells are mostly dead or dying before they form the toughened outer layer which divides the aqueous internal environment from the atmospheric external environment. Some unicellular organisms, in an encapsulated form, can survive long periods of aridity in a state of suspended animation, but cannot multiply until they are restored to an aqueous or, at least a moist, environment. The ovum and the sperm, like other cells in active phases, must have an aqueous phase on either side of their cell membranes.

The fusion of male and female gametes occurs in many different ways according to the particular environmental circumstances in which fertilization has to be effected, but always the transfer of gametes, and their fusion, occurs in an aqueous macro- or micro-environment. Where the macro-environment is aquatic (e.g. fishes), or where an otherwise terrestrial species returns to an aquatic environment to spawn (e.g. amphibians), fertilization may occur inside or outside the body. The many different patterns of gamete transfer and fertilization to be found in these classes of animals, must relate to other environmental influences such as the need for protection from predators, or periods of drought, perhaps at an earlier phase in the evolutionary history of the species.

In animals confined to a terrestrial and atmospheric environment, sperm and ovum must still meet in an aqueous environment, and the subsequent development of the fertilized egg must also be in an aqueous environment. The intimate juxtaposition of the male and female genitalia during copulation ensures the release of the sperm close to the ovum, and the mixing of sperm and seminal fluid in the ejaculate provides an aqueous vehicle for the sperm on its journey to the ovum.

10.3 POST-FERTILIZATION ENVIRONMENT

There are three ways by which terrestrial animals can provide a suitable aqueous environment for the subsequent development of the fertilized egg. The first is to return to water to spawn as do most amphibians. Another method, adopted by many insects and arachnids, most reptiles and all birds, is for the fertilized egg to be enclosed within a water-impermeable casing together with the fluid and nutrients necessary for its development. This encapsulated fertilized egg can then be expelled and deposited where the physical environment is suitable, and where the egg is reasonably safe from predators as in most reptiles, or protected in a nest built by the parents as in birds. The third possibility is the retention of the fertilized egg within a parent until hatching, as in tetse flies, scorpions and some reptiles, or its retention within a uterus, in which it is bathed in amniotic fluid and 'plumbed in' to its mother for nutrients, until it has developed sufficiently to be expelled and to begin its individual life aided by varying degrees of parental care.

Despite their permanently aqueous habits, the fishes show a remarkable diversity in the micro-environments in which the fertilized egg develops. Some species leave the eggs to develop entirely by themselves. The elasmobranchs possess a genital system which allows internal fertilization, and the production of encased eggs which contain the nutrients (yolk) necessary for development, but not the water which becomes available to the egg when it is expelled. In a few species of teleost fishes the fertilized egg develops within the mother. Whatever the evolutionary significance of these quite different conditions under which fish eggs develop, the spectrum is apparently attributable to conditions other than the need to provide an aqueous environment. Since in Amphibia the sperm pass through the kidney while modern fishes have acquired separate urinary and genital ducts, Young [32] suggested that the Amphibia diverged at an early stage of the evolution of the vertebrate stock. Thus the spectrum of fish reproduction may be unrelated to the comparable spectrum in amphibians, reptiles, birds and mammals. In amphibians the pattern ranges from the shedding of eggs and sperm into the water (e.g. *Rana temporaria*) to various forms of viviparity. The eggs of *Rhinoderma darwini*, a small South American frog, are transferred by the male to his large vocal sacs which extend over the whole ventral surface, from whence they hatch. The eggs of another anuran (*Gastrotheca*) are stored in a pouch on the back of the female, the young being hatched as tadpoles in some species, and in the adult form in others [23]. Most arthropods, some reptiles and all birds discharge shell-encased eggs, while other arthropods, some reptiles and all metatherial (pouched) and eutherial (placental) mammals retain the fertilized egg within the female until various degrees of development have taken place (see section 10.6). It is apparent that the encased eggs of arthropods and birds and the viviparity of mammals, relate both to the need to provide aqueous environments for the development of the eggs of terrestrial organisms, and to the need to provide a protection from other components of the environment.

The interuterine environment of the mammalian embryo, poses a quite fundamental biological problem. Medawar [18] first pointed out that viviparity consists of a temporary parabiotic union between two organisms of dissimilar genetic constitution, but the maternal immune mechanism fails to identify and reject the fetus as non-self. Thus a unique sequence of events must obtain at the time of implantation.

In a recent consideration of this problem, Amoroso and Perry [3] point out that there is no category of function more influenced by endocrine secretions than those associated with the induction, maintenance and termination of pregnancy (see later). Chorionic gonadotrophins can inhibit an immunological system dependent on antigen recognition and act synergistically with steroids in this function. Since the implanting mammalian blastocyst has the ability to synthesize both oestrogens and gonadotrophins in sufficient quantities to be a factor in the local survival of the trophoblast, Amoroso and Perry suggest that both the placenta and the fetus are involved in the local hormonally-operated suppression of immunological reactions which permit the fetus to be retained within the uterus.

10.4 THE TIMING OF THE REPRODUCTIVE CYCLE

The most obvious physiological problem created by the emergence of life from a wholly aquatic environment into a terrestrial and atmospheric one was the preservation of the aqueous environment of every constituent cell, but for its colonization to be successful, the organism had to evolve solutions to many other problems. Of immediate pertinence to reproduction was the exposure of the organism to the direct and indirect influences of the seasons, which are much greater in terrestrial than in marine biotopes (Chapter 6). The seasonal effects of ambient temperature and precipitation, acting directly on the organism, and indirectly through food and water supplies, exert powerful influences on the success or otherwise of reproduction.

Birds, like most other wild vertebrates, show a distinct time pattern in their reproductive activity, and the evolution of periodic rather than continuous breeding is an adaptation that ensures that the young are produced when factors favouring survival tend to be optimal. In this context, food for the young and for the breeding adults appears to be the main determinant [14,19]. For any particular species, therefore, the annual reproductive pattern is precisely defined and, in the avifauna of the middle and high latitudes, natural selection has defined a pattern in which conception and egg-laying are usually confined to spring and early summer. Only in this way will the chicks be sufficiently mature to withstand the cold and famine conditions of winter, or a long migratory flight. The sandpipers (genus *Calidris*) which breed in arctic regions are an example [30]. Since these birds feed on adult insects which reach peak emergence at the time of the snow melt, the nests must be prepared and the eggs fertilized and laid sufficiently in advance of the snow melt to allow the hatching of the eggs and the emergence of the insects to coincide.

The seasonal pattern of food supply exerts a similar influence on the timing of the reproductive cycle of many mammals at high latitudes. To achieve adequate growth and fat storage to enable the young to survive the first winter, birth must occur in early spring. Since the gestation of the larger mammals takes several months it is necessary for spermatogenesis and rutting in the male, and ovulation and oestrus in the female, to occur in the autumn. The undomesticated red deer and the domesticated sheep provide examples of this need for the reproductive cycle of the organism to 'anticipate' the regular cyclic events in the environment.

The delayed implantation of the roe deer [1] is a curious elaboration of the time relations between fertilization of the ovum and the birth of the young. Mating occurs in July or August soon after the summer solstice. The slowly developing blastocyst then remains free within the uterus until the winter solstice, when it starts to grow more rapidly into an embryo. It becomes implanted into the endometrium soon after, but true gestation with the formation of the placental interface between mother and embryo does not occur until about March. True gestation is relatively short, and birth occurs during May. This unusual pregnancy pattern is, presumably, related somehow to the ecology of the roe deer, but also poses questions about the interuterine environment of the blastocyst during delayed implantation. Aitken [1] has studied the control of the growth of the blastocyst by endometrial glands during its long period of freedom within the uterus, but the environmental advantage of this particular reproductive pattern has yet to be clarified. The occurrence of a similar delayed implantation of the blastocyst in some of the pouched mammals (e.g. kangaroos) until the previous occupant (joey) has left the pouch and the nipple, clearly has logistic merit, although the biological advantage of delayed implantation over appropriately timed fertilization remains obscure. In some instances, such as that of the roe deer, delayed implantation may prolong the duration of pregnancy when the interval between the opportunity to mate and the occurrence of environmental conditions most suitable for birth exceeds the duration of gestation. Delayed implantation in pouched mammals presumably avoids the possible trauma of co-habitation of the pouch by joeys at different stages of development, yet also avoids the need for mating to be confined to shortly after the previous incumbent joey has finally left the pouch.

There are two possible ways by which anticipatory physiological changes could be geared to the annual cycle of environmental changes: (i) changes in daylength or ambient temperature, or some other environmental clue (e.g. rainfall—particularly at equatorial latitudes), could provide a stimulus to 'trigger' physiological changes, or (ii) there could be an internal 'biological clock' in perfect synchrony with the annual time course of external changes, so that sexual preparation would occur without an environmental trigger.

10.4.1 Photoperiodicity

Of all the seasonal changes in the environment, that of the length of the day is the most regular, being directly related to the fixed tilt of the earth, and the fixed rotation of the earth round the sun. There is much evidence that variations in the length of the day—either daylength *per se*, or the rate of change in the length of the day—trigger off the physiological preparations for breeding in many species of both invertebrates and vertebrates. However, the sensing of daylength or of the rate of change of daylength is a complex biological function which remains largely unexplained.

Scharrer [28] (Fig. 10.1A) suggests that in transparent organisms light can exert a direct effect on the gonads. Organisms with an opaque integument may have a transparent window which admits light to a part of the brain, in which photic stimuli are converted into chemical messages by neurosecretory cells which reach organs such as the gonads whose functions are light-dependent, but to which light can no longer penetrate (Fig. 10.1B). Scharrer [28] quotes the pupa of the Tussah silkworm, *Antherea pernyi* as an example of this. Embryologically-speaking, the retina is a specialized light-sensitive tissue of central nervous origin, and in vertebrates (except fishes) there is a pathway from the retina which is distinct from that of the visual system (Fig. 10.1C & D). This goes to the hypothalamus, reaching the median eminence, from which releasing factors flow via the hypophysial portal vessels to the adenohypophysis which releases the gonad stimulating hormones (Fig. 10.2). The neuro-endocrine relations between hypothalamus and the gonads will be considered later. The current evidence is that the influence of light on mammalian reproduction is wholly or principally via this pathway from the retina to the hypothalamus. The pineal body is often considered to play some part in light sensitivity, but there is evidence of species differences in its role in mammals. In some mammalian species pinealectomy changes the effects of light on the gonads, and it has been suggested that light and pinealectomy operate independently to reduce the availability of the same inhibitory factor [31]. In hamsters there is good evidence that the pineal gland is involved in the gonadal atrophy that occurs after blinding, or exposure to short light periods [25]; and in pinealectomized hamsters the normal decrease in spermatogenesis during December and January did not occur. On the other hand Roche *et al.* [26] found no effect on oestrus, ovulation and luteinizing hormone secretion in ewes after pinealectomy. While much remains

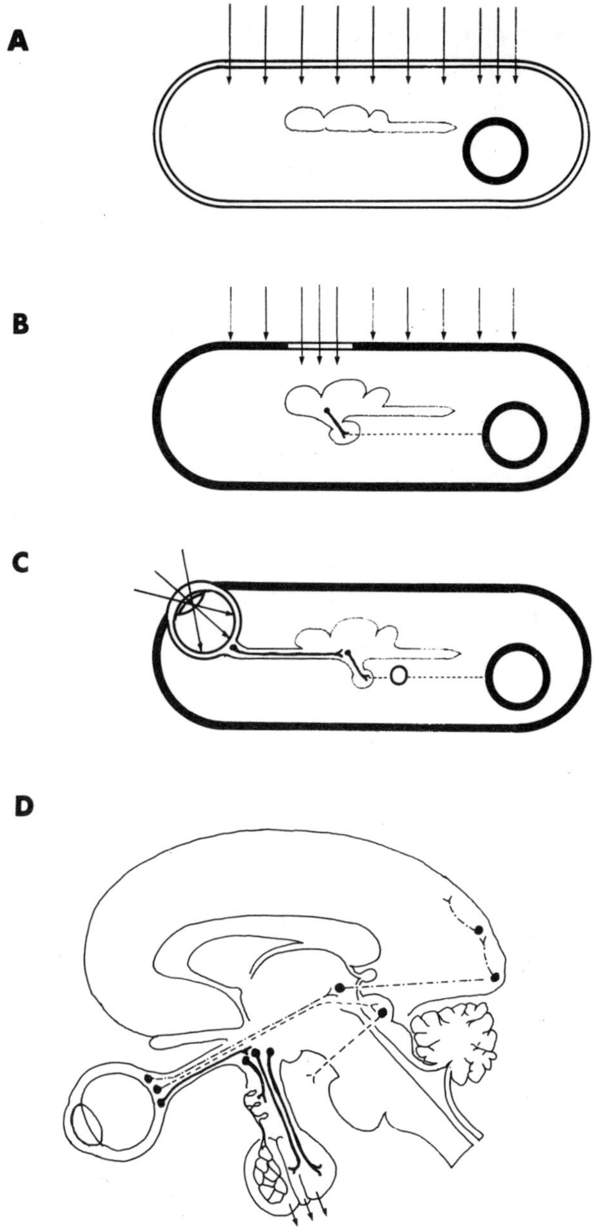

Fig. 10.1. Scharrer's representation of the influence of light on the gonads. (A) In transparent animals light can exert a direct effect on internal organs including the central nervous system and the gonads. (B) Where an opaque integument excludes light from internal structures a transparent window may admit light to photosensitive parts of the brain, where the photic stimuli are converted by neurosecretory cells into chemical messages which reach organs whose functions are light dependent but to which light can no longer penetrate. (C) A system by which light acting on the retina activates hypothalamic neurones by a nervous pathway. Neurosecretion(s) (releasing factor(s)), pass from the hypothalamus to the pituitary gland, which responds with the release of gonad stimulating hormone(s) into the blood stream. The gonad stimulating hormone thus reaches its target. (D) The system described above (C) as in vertebrates (except fishes). The broken-line pathways relate to the visual system; the solid-line pathways relate to the photo-neuro-endocrine system, and participate in the control of autonomic functions via the lobes of the pituitary.

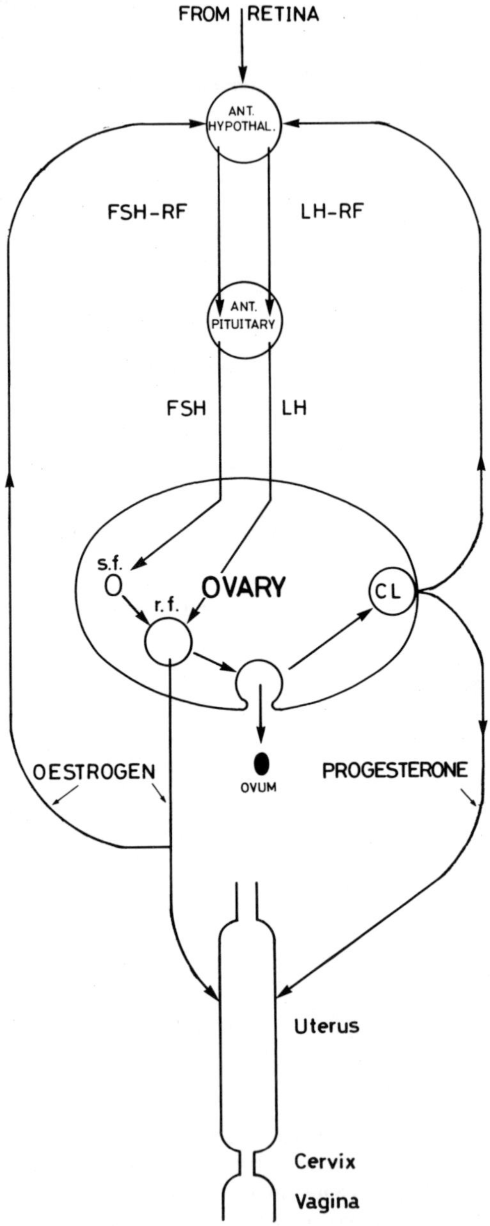

Fig. 10.2. The principal endocrine pathways involved in the control of the ovarian function in a mammal. FSH-RF, follicular stimulating hormone releasing factor; FSH, follicular stimulating hormone; LH-RF, luteinizing hormone releasing factor; LH, luteinizing hormone; s.f., small follicle; r.f., ripe follicle; CL, corpus luteum.

to be discovered about the pineal gland, there is, at least, no evidence that it functions as a primary light-sensor in mammals.

Although the seasonal gonadal stimulation of blinded ducks is less than that of ducks with undamaged eyes and optic tracts, retinal photoreceptivity is not essential for photoperiodic control of gonadal activity. Ducks blinded by enucleation or transection of the optic nerve will still respond to long days by gonadal development [4, 5]. It has also been shown [6, 7] that light applied to the hypothalamic region by means of implanted light-conducting mineral (e.g. quartz) stimulated the development of the testes of the drake. This suggests that some light may still penetrate the skull of the duck and act on intracranial sensors.

Although daylength exerts a powerful influence on the breeding patterns of perhaps the majority of both birds and mammals, and especially those at high latitudes, the effect of light varies not only between species but also between breeds. Ortovant *et al.* [22] re-examined the conclusion of Hafez [12] that the period of sexual activity in some mammals, such as the horse and donkey, is during the long daylight season, while in others, such as the sheep and goat, it is during the short daylight season, and in yet other species such as the pig and rabbit the period of sexual activity is independent of photoperiod. Ortovant *et al.* [22] found that the activity of the gonads of all domesticated species was affected by photoperiod to some extent. In sheep of the northern hemisphere the occurrence of ovulation is highest in September to November, and the occurrence of spermatogenesis is highest at a daylength of 10 hours. In some breeds of sheep, however, and in other species oestrus occurs with longer daylength. In rabbits the optimum daylength for oestrus is 11–16 hours and it is 12–16 hours in the horse. The conclusion was that there is no essential difference in the photosensitive mechanism of short-day and long-day animals. In both there is an endogenous refractory period which is longer in breeds genetically adapted to high latitudes. The implication of this finding is that the length of daylight which acts as the trigger for sexual preparation is fixed by some physiological cycle of responsiveness and refractoriness to light (see later and Fig. 10.3).

10.4.2 Endogenous rhythmicity

There is indeed evidence of an endogenous circannual clock, in some species at least, for the annual reproductive cycle may continue with a periodicity of approximately a year during the experimental denial of clues of photoperiodicity, and of all other seasonal changes in the environment. Endogenous rhymicity is discussed in general terms in Chapter 15. Its role in the reproductive cycle is still not completely clear. Sadleir [27] has concluded that in the sheep the seasonal nature of breeding is entirely dependent on responses to external environmental stimuli, and that there is no need to postulate any inherent annual rhythm in this group.

Light could be the causal factor in the timing of reproduction, or only an environmental clue (*zeitgeber*) which synchronizes an internal rhythmicity,

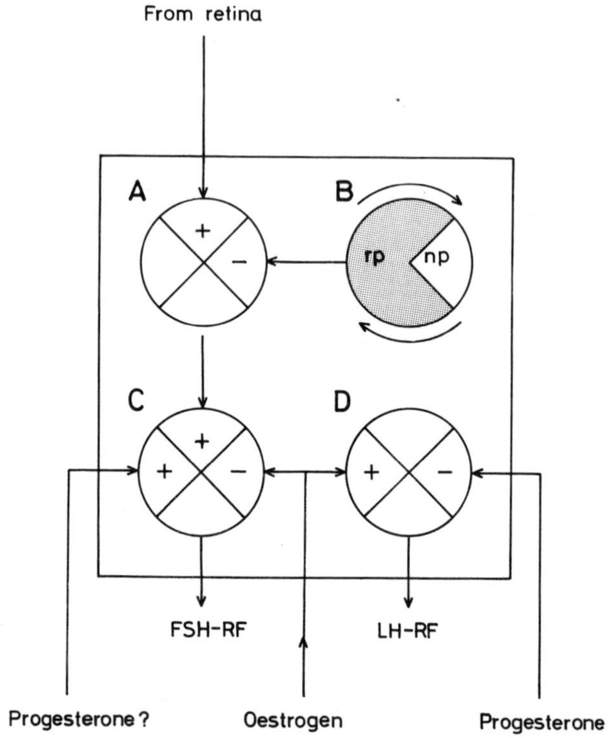

Fig. 10.3. An idealized representation of the possible relations between the 3 components of the hypothalamic involvement in the control of the reproductive cycle: (i) the neural input from photosensors; (ii) an endogenous circannual rhythmicity involving periods of refraction (light-insensitivity) and non-refraction (light-sensitivity); (iii) hormonal feedback from the reproductive organs.

Light, falling on the retina activates a neural pathway to the hypothalamus. This environmental influence is shown here as acting on a signal gate A. An endogenous signal generator B operates in a circannual cyclic manner. During the refractory period rp an inhibitory influence acts on signal gate A, blocking the passage of the signal from the retina. During the non-refractory period np there is no endogenous inhibitory influence on A, and a signal from the retina of sufficient intensity (above the threshold) then passes through gate A and reaches the second gate C. In the absence of any hormonal feedback from reproductive structures to the hypothalamus (see Fig. 10.2), the signal passes through this gate and causes the release of follicular stimulating hormone releasing factor, FSH-RF. The sequence of subsequent events is dominated by the hormonal feedback as illustrated in Fig. 10.2, and as discussed in greater detail in Perry's account of the ovarian cycle [23]. The rise in circulating oestrogen feeds back to exert an inhibitory action on gate C and an excitatory action on gate D, thus cutting off the release of FSH-RF and activating the release of luteinizing hormone releasing factor, LH-RF. This, in turn, results in the production of progesterone which feeds back again modifying the output from gates C and D. Soon after the initial exogenous (light) signal has triggered off events by passing through gate A during the non-refractory phase of the endogenous signal generator, the entry of the endogenous signal generator into a refractory phase cuts off the influence of light. Thereafter the reproductive cycle is virtually uninfluenced by the environment.

rendering it precisely annual rather than approximately (*circa*) annual. A current theory is that environmental clues and an endogenous cycle act together and provide a means of 'phase-locking'. There is clear evidence in the sheep, for example, of an endogenous seasonal refractory period: ewes cannot be kept on heat by keeping them at a daylength of 10–11 hours which is optimal for oestrus induction. Nor does spermatogenesis remain constant when daylight is held at the optimum length for its induction. It seems that the light stimulus will only influence reproduction when it coincides with the non-refractory phase of an endogenous rhythmicity.

Figure 10.3 is an attempt to summarize some of the evidence and define the area of dispute rather than to establish any kind of hypothesis. To avoid any pretence of reality, signal-mixers, borrowed from engineering convention, have been chosen rather than neuronal synapses which operate in a very similar manner. In this model the internal circannual rhythmicity is represented by a signal generator which exerts an inhibitory influence on the pathway from light sensors throughout a 'refractory period'. Obviously the ratio of the refractory period to the non-refractory period could vary between species and this variability gives expression to the view that there is no essential difference in the photosensitive mechanism of short-day and long-day animals. Species variations in the threshold of light sensitivity (photoresponsiveness), discussed by Murton and Kear [20] in relation to wildfowl, can find expression in the variable intensity of a residual inhibitory influence during the non-refractory period.

Of all possible environmental clues to the time of year, daylength is the most invariable. Thus this would seem to be an adequate and reliable trigger and that therefore the phase-locking of an endogenous clock and the change in daylength is an unnecessary precaution against the reception of erroneous or spurious environmental information in natural conditions. If, however, the environmental clue to season were not the rate of change and direction of change of length, but daylength *per se*, then confusion would be possible because at the spring and autumn equinoxes the days are of equal length: reproductive disaster could result from any confusion about the temporal context of these two equal daylengths. A different physiological responsiveness to the declining daylengths of the autumn and the increasing daylengths of the spring, based on the active and refractory periodicity of an endogenous 'clock' might be a means by which such confusion is avoided. Follett [10] provides an interesting discussion of how daylength awareness might depend on a phase-locking interaction between the incidence of light and a circadian endogenous rhythmicity which consists of photoinducible and non-photoinducible phases. (See also Chapters 13 and 15). However, the precise relations between circannual endogenous rhythmicity and environmental clues in the regulation of annual cyclic events have yet to be determined.

The species which are strongly influenced by photoperiodicity, are mostly those at high latitudes. In low (equatorial) latitudes the annual photoperiodic change is small and may be inadequate for the timing of an annual reproductive cycle. Yet the annual cycle of reproduction which is of distinct survival value for most avian species at least, persists in many if not most species in these latitudes. Here, although the circannual internal rhythmicity may be strong, the reproductive cycles may be synchronized by environmental clues other than light. In animals occupying arid desert environments the occurrence of rainfall triggers the processes of reproduction in some species [see 17].

In those well-studied mammals, man and the laboratory rat, a clear correlation between the reproductive cycle and solar-linked environmental events is apparently lacking. Whether this is because these species are of equatorial origin, or because they have been long buffered from seasonal events, or because of some other reason, is not clear. It is perhaps because of the lack of any strong influence of the environment on the reproductive activities of these particular species that discussions of the ovarian cycle tend to concentrate on the feedback of hormones produced by the sex organs onto the hypothalamus, with little or no emphasis on the influence of the environment as the primary trigger [24].

10.5 NON-PHOTOPERIODIC ENVIRONMENTAL INFLUENCES ON REPRODUCTION

By controlling the occurrence of spermatogenesis, ovulation and oestrus, photoperiodicity plays an essential and perhaps dominant role in the timing of sexual activity, but other environmental factors exert influences either on the functions of the testes and the ovaries, or on the mating behaviour. Heat, touch, vision and smell are variously involved in different species.

Heat, or temperature, has a direct effect on the rate of reproduction of most unicellular organisms and many bradymetabolic (poikilothermic) multicellular organs. This is a manifestation of the general effect of temperature on metabolism (Q_{10} effect). In the tachymetabolic (homeothermic) mammals and birds, temperature has no marked stimulatory effect on reproduction, but has a deleterious effect on spermatogenesis. Local heating of the testes can cause infertility by impairing spermatogenesis in both birds and mammals. Waites [29] has quoted social evidence that an environmental heat load which impairs the capacity of the human male to impregnate is without effect on his libido. The female reproductive processes are adversely affected by heat stress, but the harmful effect of heat on the embryonic development resulting in abortion may be due, in part at least, to precoital heat stress on spermatogenesis in the male, rather than upon the ovum before or after fertilization. In the brown rat (*Rattus norvegicus*) the cessation of breeding during the coldest time of the year is not due to a prolonged anoestrus in the female, but to the cessation of spermatogenesis in the male. The testes become withdrawn into the abdominal cavity, and the temperature of testicular tissue is thus raised to that of the body core [24].

The special senses and touch have their principal effects on mating behaviour rather than on the gonadal preparation for reproduction. Visual and olfactory signals and tactile sensations are important to the processes of meeting and mating at almost all levels of multicellular life.

Where the activities and social structure of a species is such that there is no pair-bonding and mating is, so to speak, a matter of chance encounter and sudden impulse, the induction of ovulation by mating (cervical stimulation), as in the rabbit, is evidently an adaptation to a particular circumstance. Where ovulation is a seasonal or periodic event, the need for the female to signal her physiological preparedness to the male is obvious. Pheromones are widely employed. Perry [24] points out that olfactory stimuli are of particular importance in the higher primates that have a menstrual cycle as distinct from an oestrous cycle, and in which the phenomenon of 'heat' is less obvious. Apart from the signal of the particular time of sexual receptivity, most mammals deliberately saturate their local environment with their own odour derived from special skin glands. According to Mykytowycz [21] this smell of home is important for the completion of various stages of reproduction.

10.6 EMBRYONIC DEVELOPMENT OF THE FERTILIZED EGG

The influence of the external environment on reproduction in birds and mammals is largely confined to the events leading up to fertilization. The subsequent ontogenetic events within the avian egg-shell, and the mammalian uterus, are essentially independent of climatic and other components of the environment, and are outside the scope of this discussion. However, the sequel to these events—the hatching of the chick and mammalian parturition—must not occur until the new individual has reached that stage of development necessary for it to cope with the totally different and much less buffered environment that lies outside the egg-shell and the uterus. Since genetic selection depends on survival to maturity and reproduction, there must obviously have been powerful environmental influences on the evolution of internal control processes by which the buffered environments of avian and mammalian embryos are sustained for so long as is necessary, to ensure the survival of the new lives.

The duration of embryonic development is more-or-less the same for each individual of a species, but the final events of expulsion from egg-shell or uterus seem to be activated by development-monitoring processes rather than by some precise independent 'clock' within the system which was switched on at the time of copulation or implantation. In mammals these processes, as indicated in Fig. 10.2, involved the pattern of changes in the level of production of oestrogen and progesterone by the reproductive structures and their feedback, via the circulating blood, onto the hypothalamic 'centres' which control the outflow of gonadal stimulating hormones, follicular stimulating hormone (FSH) and luteinizing hormone (LH). In some species the hypothalamus seems to be the central controller of gestation and the smooth progression of embryological development depends largely on the feedback to the hypothalamus of hormonal evidence of different stages of development.

However, the hormonal control systems concerned with the maintenance of pregnancy and the induction of parturition differ widely among mammalian species, and no general statement can be made about the roles of the maternal hypothalamus and hypophysis. Thus Fig. 10.2 and the lower part of Fig. 10.3 are neither accurate nor general. Figure 10.3 is an attempt to represent the changeover of control from an external trigger to an internal pattern of hormonal events based largely on hormonal feedback from the reproductive structures. If there are phased discharges of two or more releasing hormones, which are not solely the consequence of an internal clock mechanism, then the feedback resulting from the release of one releasing hormone, may be acting negatively on that drive, and positively on the control of another releasing hormone. However, in some species the placenta and the fetus, as well as the ovaries contribute to the symphony of hormones, and it is evident that the maintenance of pregnancy, and the timing of parturition is largely independent of feedback to and discharges from the hypothalamo-hypophysial axis in some mammalian species. In the guinea-pig maternal hypophysectomy blocks the onset of parturition, but does not cause the termination of pregnancy whereas in the pregnant sheep hypophysectomy interferes with neither the pregnancy, nor the onset of parturition [9].

In some species the fetus plays an important role in the induction of parturition. In the sheep, for example, there is evidence that the time of parturition is influenced by a system that involves the fetal pituitary and adrenal glands [15, 16]. In other species the presence of the fetus has little if any effect on the time of parturition. In the ferret, for example, the duration of pregnancy and pseudopregnancy is very similar and in rats and mice the placenta will survive the removal of the fetuses, to be delivered at normal term. This has been interpreted as evidence that the cycle of events is essentially a maternal affair.

In so far as any general statement is possible, it might be fair to say that the lower part of Fig. 10.3 is representative of a basic principle of the hormonal control of the oestrous cycle and pregnancy, but that many variations on the theme have evolved among the mammals. The extent to which the hypothalamo-hypophysial axis remains in control of the pattern of events depends on the extent to which the placenta and the fetus have become involved in the production of hormones and have facilitated the development of control processes which are independent of maternal central nervous co-ordination. One may suppose, on the basis of the underlying theme of this volume, that the diversity of environmental conditions in which reproduction must be sustained has strongly influenced this diversity of control of mammalian reproduction, but so far little attempt has been made to establish this relation systematically.

10.7 THE DEGREE OF MATURITY AT BIRTH

Since each new individual starts as a single cell, it is inevitable that the duration of embryological development is a function of the size of the new individual at hatching or birth. However, a close correlation could not be expected because newborn reptiles, birds and mammals vary greatly in the extent to which they are ready at birth to embark on an independent life.

Obviously a newborn bird and mammal must be able to breathe, to make such movements as are immediately necessary to find its mother and to take sustenance. These are minimum and invariable requirements even of a marsupial young which is expelled from the uterus in an exceptionally premature stage of development; it must still find its way to a nipple in its mothers pouch before development can proceed. The point in its development, beyond the ability to perform these essential functions, at which an embryo can emerge from its shell, or the uterus, and have a chance of survival, depends on the environment into which it emerges.

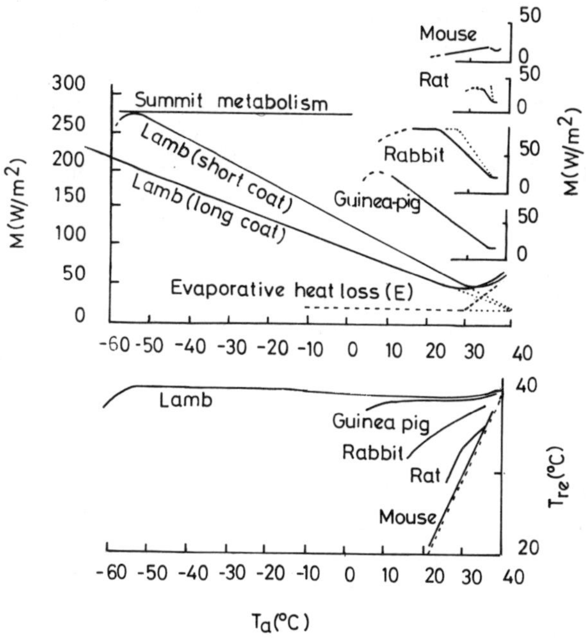

Fig. 10.4. Curves relating ambient temperature, T_a, to deep body temperature, T_{re} and to metabolic rate, M, for newborn lambs, with short or long coat, and for newborn guinea-pigs, rabbits, rats and mice. From [7].

The totally unmothered turtle must take immediate steps to reduce the hazards of predators and of dehydration as soon as it has emerged from its shell, and must then start searching for its own food. Newborn hoofed mammals of the open African plains will be nurtured by their mothers provided the newborn animals can keep with their mothers while the herd moves about in search of pastures and to avoid predators. Thus the survival of the newborn wild ungulate depends on its immediate mobility. By contrast, many newly-hatched birds and newborn mammals are quite helpless at birth and totally dependent on maternal care and protection. Newborn mice, rabbits and dogs, for example, are blind, virtually immobile except within a nest, and are unable to maintain body temperature if removed from the mother and from the thermally insulated nest prepared by her. Whether the eyes are open or shut, whether the animal is mobile, and whether the animal can thermoregulate are therefore used as indices of the degree of physiological development at birth.

The extent to which a newborn mammal can maintain its body temperature (T_{re}) when exposed to variations in ambient temperature (T_a) has been reviewed by Gelineo [11], Hull [13] and Alexander [2]. Figure 10.4 from Alexander shows that the newborn mouse has no capacity to increase heat production in response to a fall in T_a. As a result T_{re} falls rapidly. The rat, rabbit and guinea-pig show, respectively, progressively greater abilities to increase heat production in response to a fall in T_a, and progressively less pronounced falls in T_{re}. The guinea-pig can maintain a stable T_{re} while T_a varies between 10° and 30°C but the lamb demonstrates a much greater capacity to thermoregulate at birth. Largely by means of its capacity to increase metabolism progressively as T_a falls, the newborn lamb can prevent a fall in T_{re} at an ambient temperature of −50°C. This remarkable capacity for homeothermy is consistent with the environmental conditions into which the lamb may be jettisoned in birth. The ewe seeks no shelter and the lamb, still soaked in amniotic fluid, may be expelled into high winds and deep snow.

Precocial newborn mammals such as the lamb can increase metabolic rate by shivering or by non-shivering thermogenesis, and can reduce heat loss by peripheral vasoconstriction, piloerection and such behavioural activities as huddling.

All but the precocial newborn mammals depend on maternal warmth, usually in the microclimate of a nest, for the maintenance of body temperature compatible with essential vital activities.

10.8 THE ENVIRONMENTAL IMPACT OF BIRTH ON A MAMMAL

It has been explained earlier that since individual cells must be in an aqueous environment, the fertilization of the ovum and its subsequent development into a new individual must also take place in an aqueous environment. So far as the whole organism is concerned (though not, of course, for its constituent living cells), the act of birth of a land mammal involves the abandonment of the ancestral aqueous macroclimate, and the abrupt emergence into the atmospheric environment to which mammals are now genetically adapted. The newborn mammal is called on in one moment to replace the placental system of oxygen supply and carbon-dioxide disposal with a new system employing the hitherto unused lungs. It is also suddenly exposed to many new environmental factors such as a change in temperature, exposure to light and sound, the tactile sensations of contact with solid objects, and the exchange of the weightlessness of intrauterine existence with the full impact of gravity. Thus the act of birth is perhaps the most dramatic change of environment that any living thing can experience and survive. This emphasizes the importance to the baby of not being expelled from the uterus until it is capable of effecting the physiological adjustments which birth demands.

The new environmental experiences cited above cause a sudden bombardment of the central nervous system with signals from a variety of sensors. Presumably it is this influx of afferent signals that induces the reflex responses of the first gulp

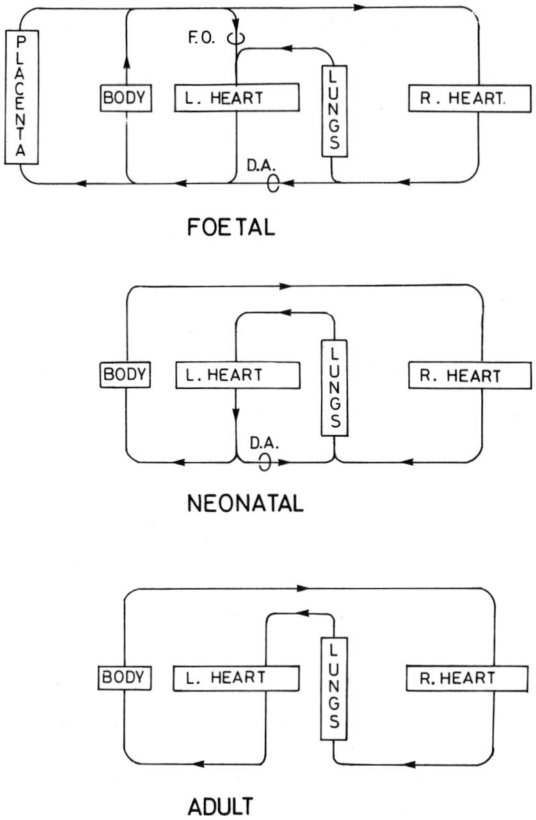

Fig. 10.5. Much simplified diagrams to illustrate the changes in mammalian circulation at birth, as briefly described in the text. In A the two ventricles are working in parallel to drive blood from the great veins to the arteries. B is the condition reached a few minutes after birth when the umbilical cord is severed and the foramen ovale, F.O., closes. When the ductus arteriosus, D.A., finally closes the adult circulation C is established with the two ventricles working in series. From [8].

of air, the opening of the lungs, and the accompanying circulatory changes. The traditional *coup de vie* of the midwife augments this sensory influx when the natural trauma of birth has not provided sufficient stimulus to induce the first breath.

The details of this abrupt physiological adaptation to an atmospheric environment are given in most standard textbooks of physiology. They are summarized in Fig. 10.5 [8]. In the circulation of the fetal lamb, the heart has to pump blood through the placenta as well as the lungs. The blood passes back from the placenta to the liver or via the ductus venosus to the inferior vena cava. During the act of birth the umbilical cord is ruptured and the umbilical artery constricts. This results in an abrupt increase in peripheral resistance and a fall in the arterial blood oxygen content. The inflation of the lungs (see previous paragraph) results in a decrease in pulmonary vascular resistance. As a result the blood flow through the lungs increases five- to ten-fold within a minute or so. Pressure in the left atrium of the heart rises and the pressure in the inferior vena cava falls, and the valve in the foramen ovale closes. Thus within a minute of breathing all venous blood entering the right atrium passes through the lungs instead of through the foramen ovale to the left side of the heart. Within about a week of birth the foramen valve has become fused to the atrial wall, and the ductus venosus has closed by collapse or contraction of its junction with the umbilical vein, probably as a result of the decrease in transmural pressure when the umbilical flow was arrested.

The primary biological task of each individual organism—to reproduce—has been fulfilled. Another air-breathing mammal has arrived in the dryland of its adoption, but the journey right up until the first gulp of air has been a wholly aqueous adventure. Indeed, the two haploid cells from which the new life had been created, and their progenitors through the eons of time, had never been exposed to anything but a wholly aqueous environment, and the germ cells of this newborn mammal are likewise still bathed in fluid within its body.

10.9 REFERENCES

1 Aitken R.J. (1974) Delayed implantation in roe deer (*Capreolus capreolus*). *J. Reprod. Fert.* **39,** 225–33.

2 Alexander G. (1975) Body temperature control in mammalian young. *Brit. Med. Bull.* **31,** 62–8.

3 Amoroso E.C. & Perry J.S. (1975) The existence during gestation of an immunological buffer zone at the interface between maternal and foetal tissues. *Phil. Trans. R. Soc. Lond. B.* **271,** 343–61.

4 Benoit J. (1935a) Stimulation par la lumiere artificielle du developpement testiculaire chez des Canards aveugles par section du nerf optique. *C.R. Soc. Biol.* **120,** 133–5.

5 Benoit J. (1935b) Stimulation par la lumière artificielle du developement par enucléation des globes oculaires. *C.R. Soc. Biol.* **120,** 136–8.

6 Benoit J. (1938) Action de divers éclairements localisés dans la région orbitaire sur la gonadostimulation chez le Canard mâle impubère. Croissance testiculaire provoquée par l'éclairement direct de la région hypophysaire. *C.R. Soc. Biol.* **127,** 909–14.

7 Benoit J. (1970) Etude de l'action des radiations visibles sur la gonado-stimulation, et de leur pénétration intra-cranienne chez les Oiseaux et les Mammifères (eds J. Benoit & I. Assenmacher). C.N.R.S. Editeur, Paris, pp. 121–46.

8 Born G.V., Dawes G.S., Mott J.C. & Widdicombe J.G. (1954) Changes in the heart and lungs at birth. *Cold spr. Harb. Symp. quant. Biol.* **19,** 102–8.

9 Denamur R. & Martinet J. (1961) Effets de l'hypophysectomie et de la section de la tige pituitaire sur la gestation de la brebis. *Annals Endocr.* **22,** 755–9.

10 Follett B.K. (1973) Circadian rhythms and photoperiodic time measurement in birds. *J. Reprod. Fert.*, Suppl. **19,** 5–18.
11 Gelineo C. (1959) The development of homeothermy in mammals. *Usp. Sovrem. biol.* **47,** 108–20 (In Russian).
12 Hafez E.S.E. (1951) Inhibitory action of artificial light on the sexual season of the ewe. *Nature, Lond.* **168,** 336–7.
13 Hull D. (1973) Thermoregulation in young mammals. In *Comparative Physiology of Thermoregulation. Vol. III—Special Aspects of Thermoregulation* (ed. G. C. Whittow) pp. 167–200. Academic Press, New York & London.
14 Lack D. (1968) *Ecological Adaptation for Breeding in Birds.* Methuen, London.
15 Liggins G.C. (1969) The foetal role in the initiation of parturition in the ewe. In *Foetal Autonomy* (eds G. E. W. Wolstenholme & M. O'Connor) pp. 218–31. Ciba Foundation Symposium. Churchill Livingstone, Edinburgh & London.
16 Liggins G.C., Grieves S.A., Kendall J.Z. & Knox B.S. (1972) The physiological roles of progesterone, oestradiol-17β and prostaglandin $F_{2\alpha}$ in the control of ovine parturition. *J. Reprod. Fert.* Suppl. **16,** 85–103.
17 Marshall A.J. (1970) Environmental factors other than light involved in the control of sexual cycles in birds and mammals. In *La Photorégulation de la Reproduction chez les Oiseaux et Les Mammifères* (eds. J. Benoit & I. Assenmacher). C.N.R.S. Editeur, Paris, pp. 53–64.
18 Medawar P.B. (1953) Some immunological and endocrinological problems raised by the evolution of viviparity in vertebrates. In *Symp. Soc. exp. Biol.* VII. *Evolution,* pp. 243–6. Cambridge University Press, London.
19 Murton R.K. & Isaacson A.J. (1962) The functional basis of some behaviour in the woodpigeon *Columba palumbus. Ibis,* **104,** 503–21.
20 Murton R.K. & Kear J. (1973) The nature and evolution of the photoperiodic control of reproduction in wildfowl of the family Anatidae. *J. Reprod. Fert.* Suppl. **19,** 67–84.
21 Mykytowycz R. (1973) Reproduction of mammals in relation to environmental odours. *J. Reprod. Fert.* Suppl. **19,** 433–46.
22 Ortovant R., Mauleon P. & Thibault C. (1964) Photoperiodic control of gonadal and hypophyseal activity in domestic mammals. *Ann. N.Y. Acad. Sci.* **117,** 157–93.
23 Parker T.J. & Haswell W.A. (1947) *A Textbook of Zoology* (6th edition, Vol. 2, revised by C. Forster-Cooper). Macmillan, London.
24 Perry J.S. (1971) *The Ovarian Cycle of Mammals.* Oliver & Boyd, Edinburgh & London.
25 Pflügfelder O. (1956) Physiologie der Epiphyse. *Verhandl. Deut. Zool. Ges.* **50,** 53–75.
26 Roche J.F., Karsch F.J., Foster D.L., Takagi S. & Dzuik P.J. (1970) Effect of pinealectomy on estrus, ovulation and luteinizing hormone in ewes. *Biol. Reprod.* **2,** 251–4.
27 Sadleir R.M.F.S. (1969) *The Ecology of Reproduction in Wild and Domestic Mammals.* Methuen, London.
28 Scharrer E. (1964) Photo-neuro-endocrine systems: general concepts. *Ann. N.Y. Acad. Sci.* **117,** 13–22.
29 Waites G.M.H. (1973) Ambient temperature: introductory remarks. *J. Reprod. Fert.* Suppl. **19,** 151–4.
30 West G.C. & Norton D.W. (1975) Metabolic adaptations of tundra birds. In *Physiological Adaptation to the Environment* (ed. F. J. Vernberg) pp. 301–29. Intext Educational Publ., New York.
31 Wurtman R.J., Axelrod J. & Kelly D.E. (1968) *The Pineal.* Academic Press, New York & London.
32 Young J.Z. (1955) *The Life of Vertebrates,* p. 322. Clarendon Press, Oxford.

PART IV
ACQUIRED ADAPTATIONS

Chapter 11
Introduction to acclimatory adaptation—including notes on terminology

J. BLIGH

11.1 GENOTYPIC AND PHENOTYPIC ADAPTATIONS TO ENVIRONMENTAL CHANGES

The evolution of the diversity of life has been achieved by the natural selection of chance mutations which gave individual organisms some inheritable quality (i.e. a variation in form or function) affording a marginally improved chance of surviving to maturity and of reproducing in the particular environmental circumstances to which it is exposed. The genetically determined forms and functions of a species are the **genotypic adaptations** of organisms to the environments in which they occur.

None of the environmental circumstances which constitute an ecological niche is fixed. All are subject to random (unpatterned) and regular (patterned) changes. If the organism can tolerate an environmental change without effecting compensatory changes in itself, it may be unresponsive to the disturbance. An organism with a fairly highly developed central nervous system (CNS) can 'learn' that an environmental event is innocuous, and may then cease to respond to it. This phenomenon is known as **habituation**, and since it requires the ability to profit from past experience, it may be a faculty limited to multicellular organisms with a well-developed CNS.

More generally it is necessary for an organism to respond to a change in its environment in a positive (reactive) way. The immediate response of multicellular organisms to environmental events involve reflexes of various degrees of complexity, all of which involve neural pathways from sensors to the CNS and from the CNS to effector organs. These immediate reflex responses are discussed in the last section of this book. Here we are concerned with more slowly developing changes which occur in unicellular and multicellular organisms alike in response to slowly developing or long maintained changes in the environment, and which serve to limit the effect of the environmental change on the organism and its viability. These changes are **phenotypic adaptations**, since they occur within the lifetime of individual organisms in response to particular environmental circumstances, and decay when these circumstances no longer exist. There are, however, genetically fixed limits to the array and magnitude of protective responses which the individual of any species can employ.

11.2 ACCLIMATIZATION AND ACCLIMATION

In nature all, or practically all, the slowly developing or long-sustained changes in the environment to which an organism responds with phenotypic adaptations, relate directly or indirectly to the position of the earth in the solar system. Seasonal changes in the meteorological components of the environment, or in the consequences of such changes including the occurrence of rainfall, the availability of food and the presence of competitors and predators, induce almost all the naturally occurring phenotypic adaptations. Thus these changes in the organism are called **processes of acclimatization.**

Seasonal changes in the natural environment are invariably multi-factorial, and it can be difficult to decide whether a change within the organism is induced by a change in ambient temperature, the length of the day, the availability of food, or several other environmental influences, all of which may occur concurrently. Thus as a matter of necessity, the experimental study of acclimatory processes usually consists of the observation of a particular adaptive response to a particular change in the environment. One might, for example, observe the effect of a raised ambient temperature on sweat rate or on the concentration of antidiuretic hormone in the blood; or the effect of a lowered ambient temperature on the thickness of subcutaneous fat, the level of metabolism or the release of hormone from the thyroid gland. The physiological responses induced by the artificial variation of a single environmental factor may, however, be quite different from those which would occur as part of several concurrent responses to the natural seasonal changes which include this particular environmental factor [8]. It is necessary, therefore, to distinguish between natural seasonal changes in the environment and experimentally induced changes in a simulated environment. Accordingly, the term **acclimatization** is now reserved for the physiological response to natural changes in the environment, and the term **acclimation** is used only for physiological changes caused by experimentally induced stressful changes in particular climatic factors [5, 7].

11.3 ADAPTATION IN SINGLE CELLS

Acclimatization is a general phenomenon of life, occurring in both unicellular and multicellular organisms. Essentially, therefore, it is based on intracellular processes, and its understanding must be sought in terms of cellular biochemical and biophysical changes (see Chapter 12). With unicellular organisms, a change in the environment may constitute a direct threat to the cell and survival may depend on an appropriate change in its physiology which is an adequate adjustment to the new condition. The response almost certainly involves qualitative or quantitative changes in the cellular protein, and changes in the structure and activity of the cell membrane. The effect of these changes in structure and function is to minimize the disruptive effect of the environmental change on the intracellular processes which constitute life. Hochachka and Somero [9] have lucidly discussed the strategies of biochemical adaptation at the cellular level, both genotypic and phenotypic.

11.4 ADAPTATION IN MULTICELLULAR ORGANISMS

In multicellular organisms the majority of the constituent cells are not affected directly by changes in the environment of the whole organism. Claude Bernard [2] was the first to appreciate that the role of many organs and systems of the body is the maintenance of the *relative* constancy of the immediate aqueous environment of the constituent living cells despite an external environment which is quite different from that in which the cell had evolved, and in which quite large fluctuations can occur. Later, Cannon [4] coined the word **homeostasis** as an 'umbrella' term for the many regulatory processes which maintain the stability of the various constituents of the extracellular fluids within multicellular organisms.

It is important to note that *homeo* means 'similar' (*homo* = same). Neither Bernard nor Cannon ever implied that there is an absolute constancy of the internal environment. Indeed, quantitative changes in the chemistry of extracellular fluids are occurring continuously as a result of changes in the relations between the organism and its environment. For example, changes in blood gases and lactic acid concentration occur during exercise, and changes in the levels of the nutrients in the blood and extracellular fluids occur during the absorption of food. There are also nychthemeral (24-hourly) changes in the levels at which the chemical and physical properties of the extracellular fluids are regulated.

The basic machinery of life became 'fixed' during its long evolutionary history in an aqueous environment. During these eons unicellular organisms, and simple multicellular organisms, were continuously bathed in what amounted to a constant, or a very slowly changing external environment, because the volume of the extracellular fluid was vast compared with that of the organism. Thus the elaborate homeostatic functions of multicellular organisms which now reside in a terrestrial and atmospheric environment are to maintain that relative stability of the immediate environment of the cells more-or-less as it had been for perhaps 2000–3000 million years. However, the chemical constituents of the cell are quite different from those of its aqueous environment, and whether free-living within the ocean or surrounded by intracellular fluid within an organism, each cell must perform work to maintain ionic and other differentials, as well as absorb nutrients and discharge waste matter. Thus every cell is doing work continuously to pump chemical substances into or out of itself. The order of the work done at the cell membrane is indicated by a recent estimate that 20%–45% of heat production of a cell occurs at the cell membrane [6]. Since virtually all the heat produced within a multicellular organism is released within the constituent cells (a small amount is frictional), this means that up to 45% of the total heat production of all organisms relates to membrane work.

11.5 THE CONTROL OF CELLULAR ADAPTATION IN MULTICELLULAR ORGANISMS

In the next chapter, on cellular adaptations to the environment, emphasis is placed on the essential cellular nature of adaptive changes and of the capacity of all cells to respond to changes in their immediate environments with changes in themselves. The environmental factors to which the constituent cells of multicellular organisms are continuously responding in an adaptive way include the proximity of other cells. Such cellular interactions play a large part in the embryological development of multicellular organisms, and the whole science of immunology is really one of cellular environmental physiology which deals with the processes by which cells recognize foreign biological material (antigens) and react with the formation of protective antibodies.

The following chapters (Chapters 13, 14 and 15) are concerned with the processes by which the internal extracellular environment is restrained within limits which are much closer together than those of the external environment. Prosser [10] identified acclimatory processes as complex interrelated regulatory events occurring in a co-ordinated fashion at various levels of organization. The essential feedback nature of the control of acclimatory processes was recognized by Adolph [1] who visualized a regulatory function of the central nervous system which responds to an environmental disturbance which he called an **adaptagent,** with an output which effected a physiological response, and which he called an **adaptate.** A negative feedback of the signal which activates the adaptate, or of some manifestation of the adaptation, onto the regulator function creates a closed-loop regulatory system (Fig. 11.1b). This serves to prevent the over-response to the stimulus which is a feature of open-loop control systems (Fig. 11.1a).

The representation of a slowly acting acclimatory function in this way is indistinguishable from that of a regulatory reflex by which an organism effects an immediate response to a disturbance. There are, however, three functional differences between reflex responses and acclimatory responses: (i) an acclimatory response takes much longer than a reflex response—hours, days or weeks; (ii) acclimatory responses usually have a hormonal link in the pathway from the central nervous controller to the effector cells, whereas reflex responses are entirely nervous; (iii) the acclimatory effect is often to change (or enhance) the ability of an effector cell or organ to respond reflexly to a disturbance.

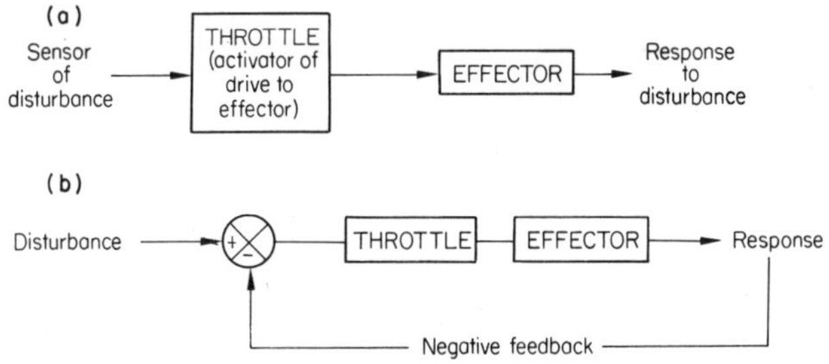

Fig. 11.1. (a) A representation of a simple open-loop control function. The magnitude of the effector activity is proportional to that of the disturbance, but the effect on the system is unregulated.
(b) A representation of a simple closed-loop regulator function. The negative feedback of effectiveness of the effector response mixes with that of a disturbance signal and so reduces the extent of over-compensation which the open-loop system could not prevent. Note that the signal mixer (⊗) could be before *or* after the throttle.

Quantitative enhancement or qualitative change in the ability of an organism to respond reflexly to a thermal stimulus resulting from processes of acclimatization, occur in many homeostatic functions such as those of thermoregulation. So far as is known there are not two sets of disturbance sensors relating to the two orders of response (reflex and acclimatory). The 'centres' which receive signals from disturbance sensors and from which the neural and humoral signals to autonomic homeostatic effectors stem are principally, but not exclusively, in the hypothalamic region of the brain. It might be supposed, then, that every time there is an input to the hypothalamus from disturbance sensors—thermosensors, for example—both reflex and acclimatory effector pathways are activated [3]. However, whereas activation of the reflex effector pathway results in the immediate activity of the effector organ, the influence of the activation of the acclimatory effector pathway is only evident if the stimulus has occurred for long enough, or often enough, for the induction of biochemical changes in the effector cells.

The activation of many acclimatory functions involves a chain of command. The first stage in the efferent pathway from the hypothalamus to the effector or 'target' cells is in many instances the generation of activity in a neurohumoral pathway from the hypothalamus to the pituitary gland. In response to this hypothalamo-hypophysial activity particular cells of the pituitary form and discharge a releasing (or first-order) hormone into the blood-stream. This releasing hormone reaches a second-order endocrine gland where it causes the release of a second-order hormone. This then circulates round the body and acts upon those cells which are specifically responsive to it. The effect of this 'second-order' hormone on the 'target cell' is to induce the acclimatory changes in the function of that cell.

In the particular case of temperature regulation, an acclimatory effect of a low ambient temperature is via the pituitary (thyroid stimulating hormone) and the thyroid gland (thyroxine). Thyroxine has the general cellular effect of elevating basal metabolism and a particular effect on some cells of increasing their capacity to produce heat reflexly in response to a cold stimulus. The negative

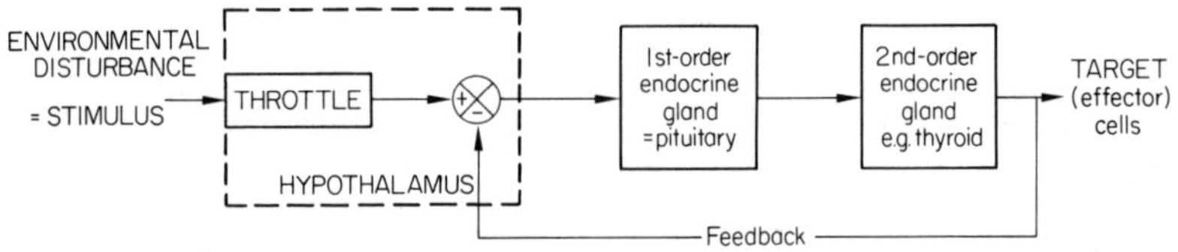

Fig. 11.2. A representation of the relation between a disturbance signal feeding into the hypothalamus and hormonally induced acclimatory influence on target (effector) cells. The feedback of the second-order hormone onto the hypothalamic control of the first-order endocrine gland (the pituitary) is represented by the action of the circulating second-order hormone on a signal mixer in the hypothalamus. The only reason for placing the signal mixer after the throttle in this figure is to facilitate the construction of Fig. 11.3 in which separate signal mixers are needed to represent the feedback of the consequences of reflex (neuronal) activation of an effector organ, and the feedback of the final hormone in the slow acclimatory pathway of command.

feedback of the circulating second-order (terminal) hormone onto as yet undefined hypothalamic 'sensors' serves to control the release of the first-order hormone from the pituitary. This, in turn, controls the rate of release of the second-order hormone and the extent of the change induced in the cells which are responsive to it.

This very generalized and simplified account of the relations between the primary stimulus and slowly developing acclimatory responses to environmental disturbances can be expressed as in Fig. 11.2. The general relation between slowly-activated hormonally-induced acclimatory changes in the effector cells, and the immediately-activated neurally-induced responses of these cells to an environmental stimulus is represented diagrammatically in Fig. 11.3.

11.6 AN EXAMPLE OF A MODIFIED RESPONSE TO AN ENVIRONMENTAL STRESS AS ACCLIMATION PROCEEDS

Figure 11.3 gives no indication of the temporal pattern of events as a reflex response to an environmental disturbance change as an animal becomes acclimated, nor does it give expression to the take-over by one effector function from another as acclimation proceeds. Figure 11.4 (from Sitaraman and Rao, personal communication) is a graphical expression of the sequential change from one response to another when the rat is exposed to a sustained cold environment. Shivering thermogenesis is rapidly activated upon exposure to cold, but after

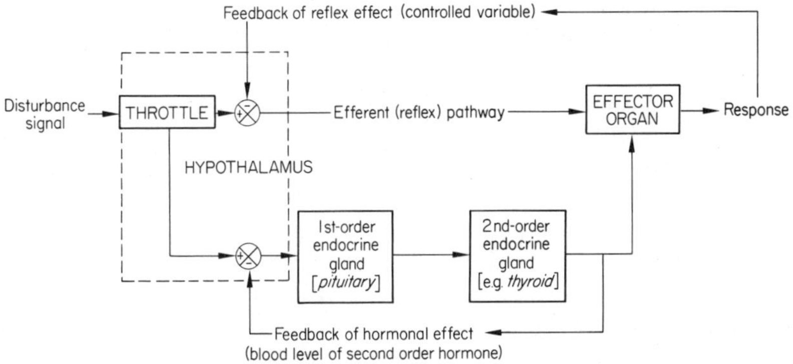

Fig. 11.3. A diagrammatic representation of the immediate neurally operated reflex activation of an effector organ, and the more slowly activated hormonal influence on the same effector organ by which its capacity to respond reflexly is modified (and generally improved). A common disturbance signal is assumed. The feedback of the consequences of reflex effects, and of the second-order hormone, are represented as acting on separate hypothalamic signal mixers on the two distinct pathways. Single lines indicate neural connexions, double lines indicate transmission via the blood stream.

a few days shivering is progressively replaced by non-shivering thermogenesis (NST), the change-over being completed within three weeks. Ultimately, however, another response to cold—an improvement in thermal insulation (an increase in subcutaneous fat and in pelage thickness and quality)—allows the progressive reduction in non-shivering thermogenesis as well as in shivering thermogenesis.

At one time it was thought that the sustained rate of oxygen consumption as the shivering disappeared was due to a change in the activity of muscle cells in response to cold. A biochemical change in the cells which allowed the uncoupling of the process of oxidation from phosphorylation, and permitted the generation of heat in the muscle cells without them doing the work of contraction, was proposed. Since the muscles of the cold acclimated rat can still be used normally for locomotion, the animal will still shiver when exposed to a temperature lower than that to which it has been acclimated, and the heat production of shivering and non-shivering thermogenesis can be additive, there can be no fundamental change in muscle biochemistry during cold acclimation.

It is now evident that the brown coloured multi-lobular deposits of fat (brown adipose tissue, abbreviated to BAT), which occur particularly in the thoracic area and beneath the scapular, but which may also be more sparsely distributed in many other tissues, play an important role in NST in the rat. In the unacclimated rat, cold-exposure has little effect on BAT metabolism, but in the cold-acclimated animal, cold exposure causes a rapid rise in the metabolism and temperature of this tissue. During this period of cold-acclimation, the cold-induced increase in the release of thyroid hormone has the effect on BAT cells of sensitizing them to the action of noradrenaline, which is released at the terminals of efferent nerves within the BAT as a reflex consequence of the stimulation of cold-sensors.

Edelman and Ismail-Beigi [6] consider it likely that at least one of the actions of thyroxine is on the cell membrane, and that it causes a modification to the membrane transport system. The immediate rise in heat production in BAT when the cold acclimatized rat is exposed to cold could be due, in part at least, to the action on the cell membrane of noradrenaline released at sympathetic nerve terminals. The action of noradrenaline could be to alter several of the properties of the cell membrane, especially the pumping action of the membrane on Na^+ and K^+. It should be noted that this brief account of the involvement of BAT in cold acclimation relates particularly to the rat. In some other species, BAT is already capable of instant thermogenesis in the newborn animal, but soon disappears and is replaced by shivering. BAT also plays an important role in the periodic re-warming of hibernating animals [see 3].

11.7 HIERARCHICAL CONTROL OF ACCLIMATION

It must now be evident why there is such difference between the response of an organism to a single artificially-induced environmental change (*acclimation*), and the responses of an organism to the natural concurrent overlapping or sequential changes in many environment factors that occur with the progression of the seasons (*acclimatization*). A single environmental disturbance can set off a chain of events of different temporal dimensions, which may then interact with, or feedback onto, each other. Where several environmental changes are influencing the organism at the same time, where each disturbance is activating a sequence of events (Fig. 11.4) and where the stimuli, the responses and the intervening processes may be interacting with each other, the physiological events are too complex for analysis and description. This, of course, is equally true of all physiology, and the artificial division of the teaching of the subject into special senses, nerve-muscle, water balance, circulation and so on, is largely a matter of scholastic convenience. However, since acclimatization involves the whole organism it is less amenable to artificial sub-division.

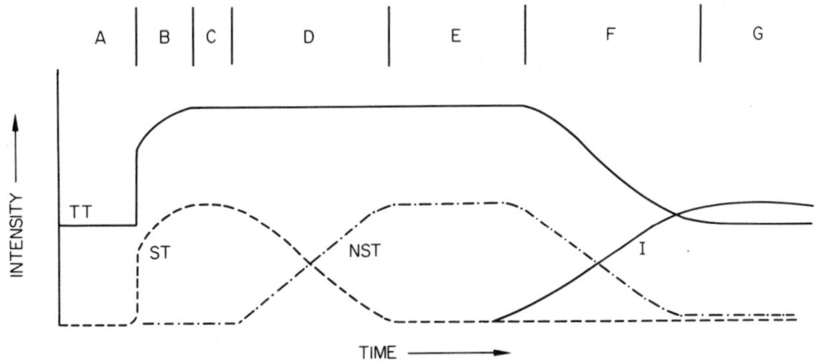

Fig. 11.4. A diagrammatic expression of the sequence of the responses of a small mammal such as the laboratory rat to a sustained low ambient temperature. TT = total thermogenesis; ST = shivering thermogenesis; NST = nonshivering thermogenesis; I = insulation (pelage and/or subcutaneous fat). Period A = period at thermoneutrality; A/B interface = point at which ambient temperature is lowered; period B = period of acclimatory improvement in ST; period C = period of maximum ST; period D = period of increase in NST and decrease in ST; period E = period of maximum and sustained NST; period F = period of increase in I and decrease in NST; period G = period of adequate I and near-basal TT. (Adapted from Sitaraman and Rao, personal communication).

Sitaraman and Rao (personal communication) have proposed that hierarchical control principles can afford a means of visualizing, and perhaps of analysing, acclimatory processes. At the lowest level of organization—perhaps at the cellular level, or at a simple reflex level, a stimulus/response relation can be regarded as a single control function. This is referred to as the *infimal* level of control, which apart from activating an effector, also exerts an upward influence on one or more *supremal* controllers, and receives *interventive* influences from them. These influences modify the primary response to the disturbance (Fig. 11.5).

Each 'supremal' interface is also receiving information from and passing information to other interfaces 'above' and/or 'below' itself. The diagrammatic representation of such a stack of interfaces indicates that the response to any stimulus at any level of the central nervous system, or at the level of the single cell, will depend on the patterns of other influences (interventions) acting on the interface, while at the same time the primary environmental influences acting at that particular interface will be contributing to many other environment/organism interactions.

11.8 A COMMENT ON THE GENERALITY OF CELLULAR ADAPTATION

From the above discussion it might be inferred that acclimation or acclimatization consists essentially of changes in the responsiveness of effector cells in reflex pathways. This is a gross over-simplification. As was noted above, cells in

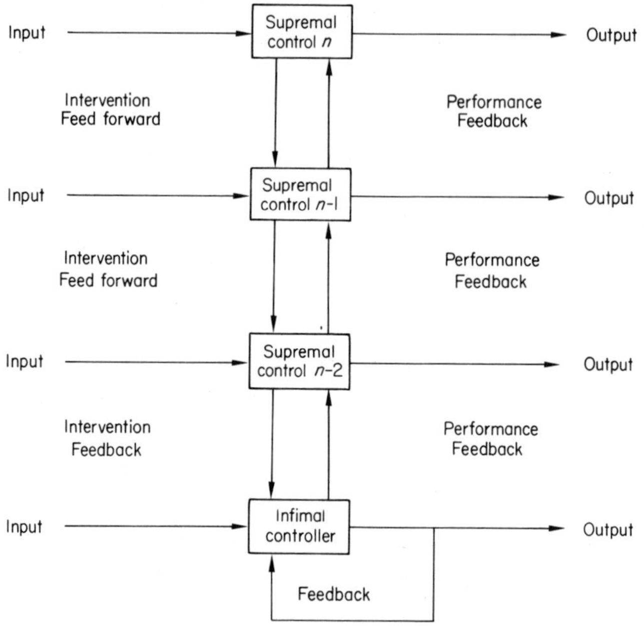

Fig. 11.5. A representation of the principle of hierarchical control. At any primary (infimal) level of control the relation between disturbance (input) and response (output) involves the contribution of information signals to higher (supremal) levels of control (performance feedback) and the reception of signals at these higher levels of control (intervention feedforward), as well as a local feedback onto the control of information about the consequences of its own output. This intervention of higher levels of control serves to relate the simple reflex relation between disturbance and response to the organism as a whole. (From Sitaraman and Rao, personal communication).

general are capable of phenotypic adaptive changes. Thus the primary disturbance sensors, their afferent pathways to the CNS, the neuronal complexes at the central nervous interfaces between afferent and efferent pathways, and the first-order and second-order endocrine glands, all being cellular structures, are themselves being modified in response to changes in their immediate environments.

Indeed, every nervous pathway between sensor and effector constitutes a specialized response of one cell to the influence of another at the synaptic junction between them. There is evidence that changes in the responsiveness of the post-synaptic neurone occur as a result of repeated synaptic activity, and it would seem reasonable to suggest that the phenomena of accommodation, improvement in the precision of motor actions with practice, and perhaps even of memory, are manifestations of the capacity of cells to alter their function in response to alterations in their immediate environments.

This concept of synaptic events means, in effect, that there is no fundamental difference between rapid neuronally transmitted influences of one cell on another and the slower humorally transmitted influences. In both cases there are gaps between sequences of cellular functions which are bridged by chemical substances liberated from one cell and acting on another. In both cases the primary or principal action of the change in chemical environment seems to be on the structure and functions of the cell membrane of the responding cell. In both cases the continued or repeated release of the chemical from the one cell into the environment of the other causes prolonged changes in the responding cell which constitute, in the whole organism, processes of acclimation. The difference is in the distance that the chemical substance travels between the releasing and the responding cell. Since the word *hormone* is derived from a Greek word for 'I excite', there is no semantic difficulty in regarding synaptic transmitter substances as *local hormones*. There is also no biological difficulty in regarding synaptic transmission and changes in transmission as specializations of the responsiveness of cells to their immediate environments.

11.9 REFERENCES

1 Adolph E.F. (1964) Perspectives of adaptation: some general properties. In *Handbook of Physiology* (ed. D. B. Dill), Section 4, Adaptation to the Environment, pp. 27–35.

2 Bernard C. (1878) *Lecons sur les phenomenes de la vie*. Balliére, Paris.

3 Bligh J. (1973) *Temperature Regulation in Mammals and Other Vertebrates*, pp. 228–302. North-Holland, Amsterdam.

4 Cannon W.B. (1929) Organization for physiological homeostasis. *Physiol. Review* **9**, 399–431

5 Eagan J.C. (1963) Introduction and terminology. *Fed. Proc.* **22,** 930–2.

6 Edelman I.S. & Ismail-Beigi F. (1974) Thyroid thermogenesis and active sodium transport. *Recent Progress in Hormone Research* **30,** 235–54.

7 Hart J.S. (1957) Climatic and temperature induced changes in the energetics of homeotherms. *Rev. Can. Biol.* **16,** 133–74.

8 Heroux O., Depocas F. & Hart J.S. (1959) Comparison between seasonal and thermal acclimation in white rats. 1. Metabolic and insulative changes. *Can. J. Biochem. Physiol.* **37,** 473–8.

9 Hochachka P.W. & Somero G.N. (1973) *Strategies of Biochemical Adaptation.* Saunders, Philadelphia.

10 Prosser C.L. (1964) Perspectives of adaptation: theoretical aspects. In *Handbook of Physiology* (ed. D. B. Dill), Section 4, Adaptation to the Environment. pp. 11–25.

Prelude to Chapter 12

There is an unfortunate tendency to regard the organ level of organization as the only level at which animals are adapted to their environment. And there is also a tendency to regard the cellular and sub-cellular levels of organization as fixed entities, possibly related to the environment which prevailed during the early evolution of life, but otherwise unrelated to present-day conditions. Microbiologists were probably the first to realize the extent to which cells are adapted to their environment, for obvious reasons, and some of the ideas which they developed have now permeated biochemistry and animal physiology. We have abundant evidence for the cellular and chemical basis of a variety of adaptations in many different animals. The cellular adaptations which occur in the lifetime of animals are vital for survival, and have immense interest. The following chapter deals with a number of examples, in cells, tissues and organs. They demonstrate the versatility and complexity of cellular organization, especially in those animals which appear to be careless in maintaining their 'milieu interior' constant during periods of environmental change.

Chapter 12
Cellular adaptation to the environment

M.SMITH

12.1 INTRODUCTION

It has been said with some justification that the living cell is inherently an unstable and improbable organization, maintaining its structure and function only through the constant use of energy. This fragility, which is also seen in its general susceptibility to changes in the external environment, does not occur by chance. It arises from the fact that all cells have to perform conflicting functions in order to survive. Their prime function is to maintain constant an intracellular environment substantially different from that of its surroundings for, without this, metabolism ceases and the cell decays. This regulation cannot, however, be brought about by making the plasma membrane permanently impermeable, since it is by this route that the cell receives nutrients essential for its future growth and development. It may not be too much of an exaggeration to suggest that cells have to adapt continually to strike a balance between these conflicting requirements. Exposing cells to markedly different environments will shift this equilibrium more than one might normally expect, but the methods used to maintain homeostasis under both conditions will be essentially similar. Before describing these methods in detail, however, it is perhaps worthwhile having a brief look at one or two developmental changes in cellular function, since these are in many ways similar to those encountered when cells adapt to changing environments.

Oocytes taken from *Xenopus* during an early stage in their development are relatively permeable to ions. They have a low membrane resistance, but this increases considerably towards the end of maturation. The mechanism causing this increase is unknown, but the effect is to protect the embryo against osmotic shock during its early development in pond water. First cleavage of the fertilized oocyte is associated with a temporary fall in resistance and hyperpolarization of the cell membrane. These changes coincide with the transient appearance of newly synthesized membrane at the bottom of the cleavage furrow. Later, as more cells form, it can be shown that the membrane at the inner surface of these cells is highly permeable to potassium, while that facing the external environment remains impermeable [45]. Cellular sodium content, but not activity, falls as the embryo develops and there is a tendency for cellular potassium to increase. The importance of potassium in activating protein synthesis and the inhibitory effect of sodium, tested in a cell-free system, has been convincingly demonstrated by Lubin [25]. One might suppose that small fluctuations in the cellular sodium to potassium ratio could activate the synthesis of a new type of membrane, but there is no proof of this at the present time.

An intercellular cavity, formed after the initial cleavage, increases in size throughout the pregastrular stages of development. Fluid held within this cavity contains 100 mM sodium and 1 mM potassium. Several theories have been put forward to explain the formation of this fluid, the most likely one being that sodium actively transported from the cells into the intercellular space pulls water after it, the speed of blastocoel formation being governed by the passive permeability of the outer cell membrane to water [45].

The conclusions that can be drawn from this work are threefold. First, that there are conditions where a manipulation of passive permeability will be sufficient to give a cell immediate protection against changes in the environment (the mature oocyte). Second, that the insertion of a sufficient number of sodium pumping sites into a cell membrane will allow that cell to control its Na^+ concentration, even though it is now in communication with an alien environment through a low resistance pathway (the embryo). Thirdly, that the joining together of cells to form a tissue will set up asymmetries, both in membrane properties (high and low potassium permeabilities in the same cell membrane) and in the composition of the external environment (pond water on one side and 100 mM Na on the other). It is this organized manipulation of pump and leak properties in cell membranes and the ability to modify biochemical pathways within the cell, which together constitute the phenomenon of adaptation.

12.2 ADAPTATION OF SINGLE CELLS

12.2.1 The bacterial cell

Bacteria in general tolerate wide variations in environmental osmotic pressure, remaining alive both in distilled water and in concentrated salt solutions. They can maintain an osmotic pressure difference between cytoplasm and the external environment of up to 20 atmospheres. This tolerance results in part from the dual nature of the bacterial cell wall. The outer wall acts as a rigid structure giving shape to the bacterium and mechanical support for the inner cytoplasmic membrane. Digestion of the wall with lysozyme leads to the formation of vesicles, called protoplasts, having all the properties of the intact cell except a resistance to osmotic swelling [35]. This proves that it is the outer wall and not some property of protoplasmic cohesion, which confers protection against osmotic damage.

Kepes [17] has calculated that duplication of cells each hour requires the consumption of carbon at a rate equal to about 3% of the dry weight of cells per minute. To maintain this growth rate the bacterial cell must be continually able to detect, transport and metabolize, a great number of different nutrients. Carriers for amino acids are permanently present in the cytoplasmic membrane; carriers for other substrates being made as and when they appear in the external environment. This type of adaptive response is called enzyme induction.

Induction and repression of bacterial enzymes

The bacterial cell synthesizes enzymes capable of metabolizing the substrate in addition to the membrane carrier, the complete system being referred to as a permease [3]. The first permease to be analysed in detail was that dealing with the transport and metabolism of lactose in *E. coli* [15]. The complete series of events associated with the induction of the lactose permease is shown in Fig. 12.1.

The DNA of *E. coli* contains a regulator gene (R) which is transcribed to form mRNA coding for the synthesis of a repressor protein. This repressor protein binds to an operator region (O) of the DNA molecule, stopping transcription of the structural genes for three separate proteins. It is these three structural genes which are known collectively as the lac operon. Small amounts of β-galactoside, coming into the cell by diffusion or on a small amount of carrier, bind to the repressor protein causing it to be released from the operator region. This frees the structural genes for transcription. A polycistronic mRNA molecule is then formed, coding for all proteins specified by the operon. This is then translated and the cell begins to rapidly transport and metabolize large amounts of β-galactoside. The whole process takes about two minutes to complete.

The synthesis of some substances by the bacterial cell can also be repressed by adding them to the culture medium. The organization of enzyme repression by the bacterial cell, which is in many ways similar to that of enzyme induction, will not be described here. It functions, along with induction, as a means of increasing the efficiency with which the cell operates.

Spore formation

Bacteria in culture normally exist in a state of exponential growth in medium

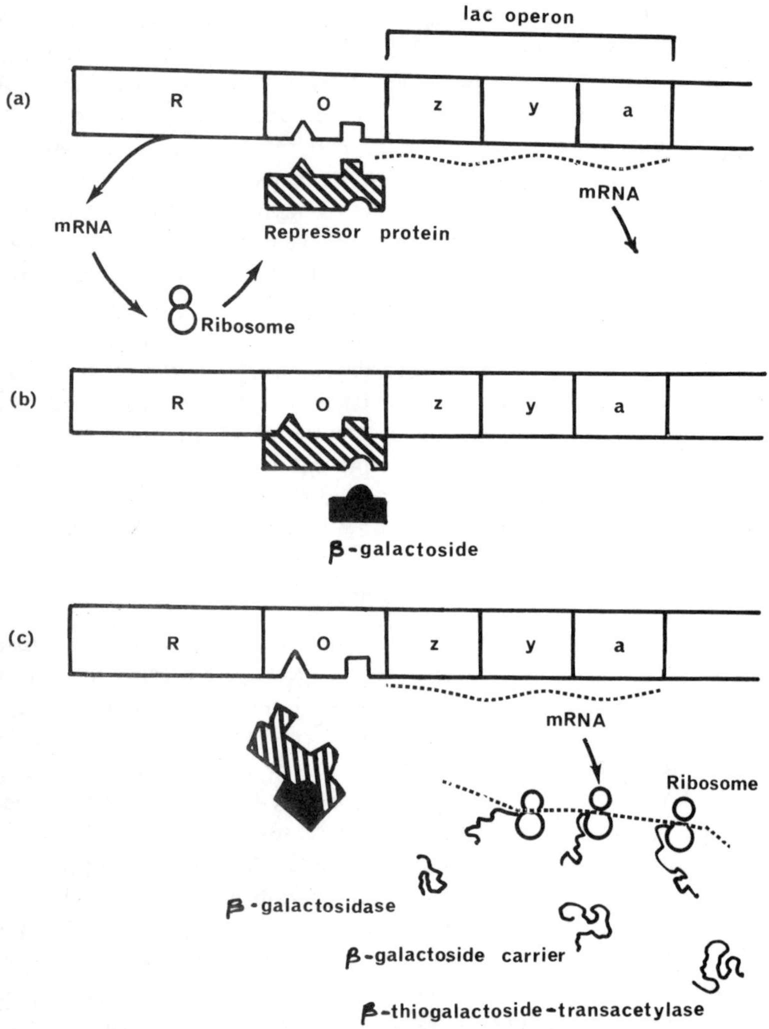

Fig. 12.1. Stages in the induction of the lac operon in *E. coli* leading to the synthesis of lactose permease. (a) The regulator gene (R) is transcribed to form a repressor protein which binds to the operator gene (○) stopping transcription of the lac operon. (b) β-Galactoside binds to the repressor protein changing its conformation so that it no longer binds to the operator gene. (c) The repressor protein separates from the operator gene allowing transcription of the z, y and a regions of the lac operon. Polycistronic mRNA is then translated to produce the final proteins.

providing an unlimited amount of nutrients. Under natural conditions, however, the bacterial cell will spend prolonged periods of time under conditions of partial or total starvation. The immediate response of bacteria to starvation is to synthesize proteases. The exact mechanism leading to this synthesis is not known. They provide free amino acids in the cell for the synthesis of new enzymes and, hydrolyse any extracellular protein which may be present. If this should prove inadequate in providing the cell with sufficient substrates to maintain growth, proteases continue their intracellular hydrolysis to provide additional amino acids, which are then used for spore formation.

The morphological changes occurring during sporulation are shown in Fig. 12.2. Stage O shows the vegetative cell growing normally. Stage 1 is associated with the formation of chromatic filaments. Protein turnover increases at this time and proteases are produced together with some antibiotics and ribonucleases. Stage 2 is characterized by the formation of a spore septum and the separation of chromosomes. A spore protoplast is formed from this extended septum in stage 3. This is associated with the production of a heat-resistant catalase, a glucose dehydrogenase and an alkaline phosphatase. The function of these enzymes is unknown but they seem to be important, for bacteria lacking the ability to make these enzymes are also poor producers of spores. Material

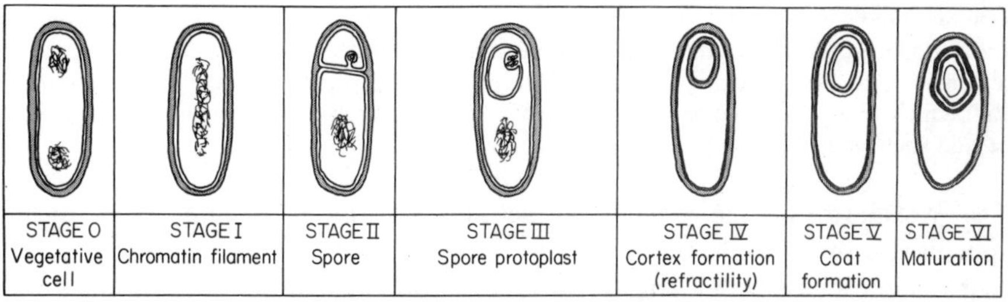

Fig. 12.2. Morphological events associated with sporulation in *Bacillus* spp. This is a composite diagram incorporating information obtained by various authors with different types of aerobic spore-forming Bacilli. The time scale is about 8 hours. (From [30].)

is laid down between the two membranes of the protoplast in stage 4, dipicolinic acid is formed which protects the spore from heat damage. The formation of an outside coat in stage 5 confers further resistance to damage from heat, while in stage 6 the coat becomes laminated and the spore dehydrates. The final spore is extremely resistant to damage. It can remain viable in an unfavourable environment for many years.

It is not possible to reverse the process of sporulation once it has started and cells are said to become committed to sporulate at a certain stage in their development. This process is interesting, for it suggests that sporulation is associated with the production of mRNA molecules more stable than those usually found in the vegetative cell. The sequential development of commitment, described in detail for *B. subtilis* [51], is shown in Fig. 12.3.

The addition of actinomycin D, a specific inhibitor of transcription, allows one to time the synthesis of new mRNA molecules and to relate this to the time of mRNA expression. Adding actinomycin D, 90 minutes after the onset of sporulation stops the development of spore resistance to various chemicals (stage 4), but not the synthesis of alkaline phosphatase, even though alkaline phosphatase has not been synthesized at the time of actinomycin addition.

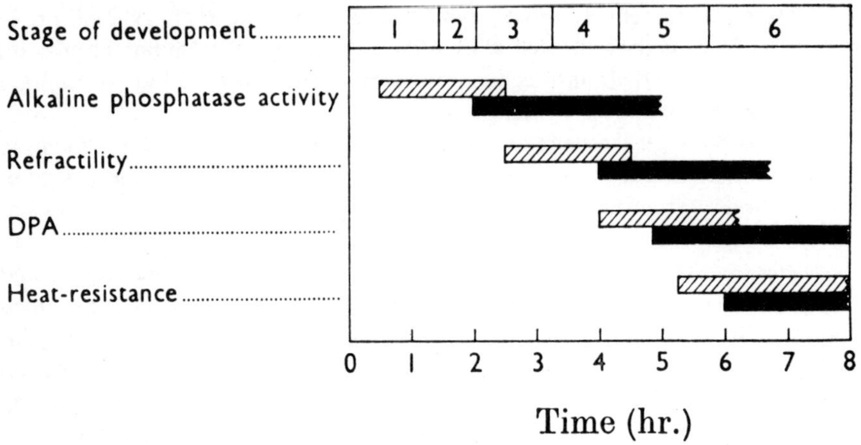

Fig. 12.3. Composite diagram illustrating events connected with sporulation. Hatched rectangles indicate intervals during which cells acquire the potential ability to carry out the process concerned. This is the period during which that process becomes resistant to actinomycin D. The black rectangles indicate the period of expression of the potential ability. Refractility refers to an increased ability of the spore to survive the normally lethal effects of certain chemicals. DPA, deposition of dipicolinic acid. (From [51].)

The resistance of the system to actinomycin D at certain times during sporulation implies that the required mRNA has already been synthesized, but that it is present in an inactive form. Sporulation appears to be controlled both by a change in transcription leading to the formation of stable mRNA molecules and by a control of mRNA activation leading to translation.

The bacterial spore germinates when the environment again becomes favourable for growth. This aspect of adaptive control, which is not discussed here, has been reviewed recently by Gould [10]. The processes leading to spore formation and germination in bacteria are, in many ways, similar to those found in yeasts and slime moulds. The comparative aspects of adaptive changes in primitive organisms have been described and compared with those of bacteria by Mandelstam [31].

12.2.2 The lymphocyte

Membrane-environment interactions

So far we have been describing the reaction of a cell to its environment in terms familiar to molecular biologists. When studying the mammalian lymphocyte we can see changes taking place directly on the membrane surface. This has been made possible by the original finding that antibodies, raised to serum immunoglobulin and made fluorescent by chemical reaction with fluorescein isothiocyanate, will bind to the cell surface in sufficient quantities to be seen under ultraviolet light [40]. By these means it was shown that the initial binding of antibody was spread diffusely over the cell surface. This was a transient phenomenon, however, fluorescent patches quickly formed and these then moved together to form a cap over the Golgi pole of the cell. Capping was rapidly followed by pinocytosis. The formation of the cap, but not of the initial patch, was shown to be an energy-dependent process [53]. The binding of a substance to more than one site seems to be essential if the subsequent reorganization of membrane surface is to take place. The binding of univalent immunoglobulin (i.e. half the complete molecule) to lymphocyte membranes produces only a diffuse fluorescence. The lymphocyte membrane shows a single specific interaction between surface immunoglobulin and antibody, but it also contains the histocompatibility antigen and receptors for histamine, insulin, growth hormone, the activated C_3 component of complement and several different mitogens. Those interested in a more general description of receptor-ligand interactions are referred to a recent review by Cuatrecasas [6].

Aggregation of membrane proteins by the binding of ligands is now known to occur in other cells besides the lymphocyte and a general theory of membrane structure, the fluid mosaic model, has been put forward to account for this phenomenon [44]. Plasma membranes are considered to exist as fluid phospholipid bilayers in which float a number of proteins having specificities for a wide variety of different ligands. The binding of a ligand to its particular receptor protein can cause lateral movement within the plane of the membrane leading to aggregation with similar complexes. This leads to the formation of patches of aggregated protein which act as a signal to the cell from the outside environment. The response of the lymphocyte to such a signal is to initiate a complicated series of biochemical events leading to the eventual transformation of the resting cell into one which synthesizes and secretes antibody proteins.

Transformation

Only a very small proportion of the total lymphocyte population undergoes transformation following challenge with specific antigens. Mitogens (agents which cause a wide variety of cells to undergo mitosis) cause a much more general response. This has led to their widespread use as transforming agents. The assumption is that biochemical changes induced by mitogens will closely resemble those induced under more normal circumstances. The following is, therefore, mainly a description of changes induced by the binding of mitogens (phytohaemagglutinin and concanavalin A) to mixed populations of thymus and bone-derived lymphocytes.

Mitogen-induced aggregation of proteins normally leads to capping and endocytosis of membrane as described above, but it is only the initial aggregation of surface proteins which is necessary for transformation to occur [11]. Several biochemical changes occur within minutes of the formation of these micro-aggregates and it is not yet possible to distinguish the sequence in which these changes take place. Present opinion would suggest, however, that calcium plays an important role in the initiation of transformation. Reducing the concentration of calcium in the outside environment below 10^{-4} M inhibits transformation without affecting mitogen binding and the introduction of a calcium ionophore (A23187) into the membrane causes morphological transformation in the absence of mitogen [29]. Binding of mitogen is quickly followed by a 10- to 50-fold increase in the cellular concentration of cyclic GMP and this may act as an intracellular messenger between membrane and nuclear DNA [12]. The aggregation of membrane proteins by multivalent ligands probably leads to the formation of polar channels which increase the permeability of the cell membrane to calcium [29]. Free intracellular calcium may activate the synthesis of cyclic GMP or act directly to modify transcription of nuclear DNA.

Other changes in lymphocyte biochemistry occurring within 30 minutes of mitogen binding include an increased permeability to a variety of metabolites, an increased permeability to potassium, an increased incorporation of phosphate into monophosphoinositide, a stimulation of glycolysis and an increased incorporation of long-chain fatty acids into phospholipids. There is also an increased acetylation of histones in the nucleus, followed by an increased phosphorylation of nuclear proteins and new synthesis of RNA. The incorporation of tritiated thymidine into nuclear DNA is considerably greater some 40 hours later and transformation is then considered complete. The resulting blast cell is considerably larger than the resting lymphocyte, many polysomes are present and the cell shows increased pinocytotic activity. The precise control of transformation at the genetic level remains to be elucidated.

12.2.3 Cooperativity between cells

We have already described how the coming together of cells during development allows certain asymmetries of transport to become established. The following sections describe how cells in tissues modify their integrated function in response to environmental changes. There are, however, some circumstances where single cells also interact with each other to produce changes in cellular function. Since the environment of a cell contains other cells, and since this environment will also change with time, it seems worthwhile describing, briefly, some of these cell-to-cell interactions.

The cooperation of cells through the release of humoral factors is now well established for the lymphocyte. The antibody response of many antigens depends on an interaction between the thymus derived (T) and the non-thymus derived (B) cell, with the T cell 'helping' the B cell to produce antibodies. This effect depends, in part, upon the release of some factor by the T cell. This was shown in experiments where T cells were first grown in culture and the cell free medium then used to help the B cell respond to mitogen [1]. A second hypothesis is that T cells bind antigens, concentrating them so that they may form an antigenic bridge between T and B cells. Both mechanisms probably act together to facilitate B cell transformation. The role of macrophages in collecting antigens for the B cell to respond to is also well established. This aspect of cell interaction has been reviewed by Unanue [54].

Another type of cell-to-cell interaction involves the cellular exchange of either nucleotides, enzymes capable of metabolizing nucleotides, or of RNA capable of coding for the synthesis of these enzymes. The experiments involve the use of wild-type and variant cell strains of hamster fibroblasts [39]. These variant strains are either deficient in inosine pyrophosphorylase (IPP^-) or thymidine kinase (TK^-). Tritiated hypoxanthine is incorporated into nucleotides of wild-type cells but hardly at all into the IPP^- variant. Mixing the two cell lines together in equal proportions causes the label to be incorporated equally into

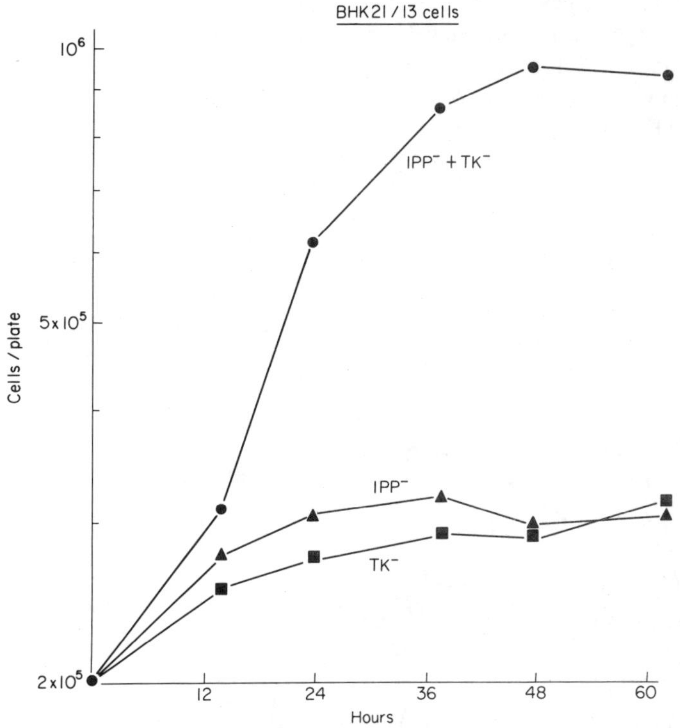

Fig. 12.4. Growth of IPP^- and TK^- Hamster fibroblast cells separately and in mixed (1:1) culture, in medium containing hypoxanthine, aminopterin and thymidine. (From [39].)

both populations. Identical experiments can be performed with tritiated thymidine using wild-type and TK^- cells. Again the mixing of wild-type cells with the enzyme deficient variant causes the nucleotide to become incorporated into both types of cell. An elegant experiment showing cooperation between IPP^- and TK^- cells is shown in Fig. 12.4.

IPP^- and TK^- cells, cultured separately in aminopterin containing medium to block synthesis of IMP and TMP but with hypoxanthine and thymidine present, show only limited growth. The mixed culture grows well in this medium, maintaining a doubling rate equal to that of the wild-type cell. Cell-to-cell transfer may occur across cytoplasmic bridges, through low resistance junctions, or by the mutual ingestion of pieces of different cells by a process similar to phagocytosis. The finding that cellular transfer can take place raises the possibility, in theory at least, that RNA may move between cells. If this does occur it could have great relevance to many different types of adaptive phenomena.

12.3 ADAPTATION OF CELLS IN TISSUES

The multicellular organism encounters all the problems of a single cell in responding to changes in the external environment. It differs only in its complexity of organization and development. This raises its own problems of communication, but it does mean that adaptation of a single tissue can, on occasion, enable the whole organism to survive. A diagrammatic way of illustrating this is shown in Fig. 12.5.

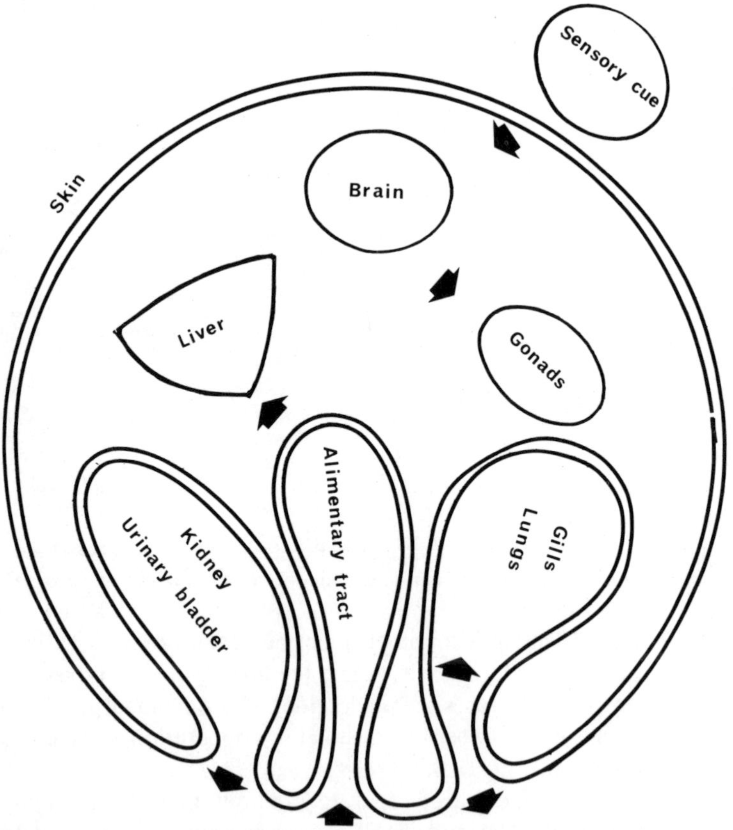

Fig. 12.5. Representation of a multicellular organism as a single cell. Tissues take the place of cell components; epithelial tissues substitute for the plasma membrane and the liver substitutes for intracellular metabolic enzymes. The problem of communication between the environment and cells held deep within the body is solved through the use of hormones released under neuronal control.

In this case the whole organism has been portrayed as a single cell. The epithelial tissues are considered analogous to the plasma membrane. They act as a barrier to the environment but retain the capacity to adapt to it when this proves necessary. The alimentary tract and liver are together taken to be analogous to the permease of a bacterial cell. They respond to feeding and starvation by the induction and repression of many different types of enzyme. The problem of communication in the multicellular organism is solved both neuronally and by the secretion of hormones. There is no analogy here with single cells though they too are capable of responding to hormonal stimulation.

The epithelial tissues are, by their position in relation to the rest of the organism, best able to appreciate a change in the external environment. Adaptation of their function in response to this change might be such that homeostasis is preserved throughout the rest of the organism. One would not then expect any further change in cellular function. Sometimes, however, adaptation in epithelial tissues will not be successful, either because the change in environment is too severe or because it is not amenable to control at this level of organization, e.g. a change in body temperature in poikilotherms. In these cases the endodermal tissues must also adapt if the organism is to survive.

Many of the adaptive responses in multicellular organisms are under hormonal control, hormones being liberated either directly by a change in blood composition or neuronally as a result of changes in sensory input to the brain. This allows endodermal tissues to react without experiencing directly the effects of a change in external environment. The following sections provide examples of some of these changes, using a number of different external stimuli to elicit adaptive responses.

12.3.1 Epithelial tissues

Skin

It has long been known that the amphibian skin can remove sodium from its environment. There is now good morphological evidence to suggest that it is the outermost layer of cells in the *stratum granulosum* which is performing this function. Placing frogs in distilled water stimulates sodium transport, both by release of vasotocin from the neurohypophysis and by an increase in the circulating level of aldosterone. Vasotocin stimulates adenyl cyclase to produce cyclic AMP and this then increases, in some ill-defined way, the ease with which sodium enters the skin. Aldosterone only acts after a delay of two to three hours. It is thought to produce its effect by a stimulation of DNA-dependent RNA synthesis, though the original evidence for this, which was obtained with toad urinary bladder, has been disputed recently [22].

Changing the environment of a frog or toad to one which is rich in sodium depresses the release of vasotocin and aldosterone and the absorption of sodium falls accordingly. This inhibition of sodium transport becomes more pronounced over a period of several days, and it is then not possible to restore sodium transport fully by the injection of either vasopressin (acting like vasotocin) or aldosterone [4, 14]. Further information on the nature of this long-term adaptation can be gained by measuring the kinetics of sodium uptake in skins taken from *Bufo viridis* fully adapted to fresh water or saline. The rapid uptake of sodium follows Michaelis–Menten kinetics in both cases with the apparent affinity of the uptake process for sodium remaining unchanged by adaptation (calculated K_m values 12·0 and 11·8 mM). There is, however, a three to four-fold fall in the rate at which sodium enters the skin (Katz & Smith, unpublished observations). Confirmation that this is due to a regulation of entry and not exit processes comes from the finding that amiloride, a specific inhibitor of sodium entry, causes marked inhibition of transport in skins taken from fresh-water-adapted toads, but only a small inhibition in the salt-adapted animal. It seems, to be the number and not the nature of the sodium entry sites which is being modified by adaptation to saline. The exact way in which this change is organized has yet to be determined. (See also Chapter 5).

Gills

Euryhaline fish survive in environments of different salinities ranging from fresh to sea water. The skin of these fish remains virtually impermeable to ion movements, electrolyte balance being controlled mainly through changes in gill functions. Gill structure is itself complicated by the fact that it has to perform a number of different functions. The epithelium contains three distinct types of cell, the epithelial or pillar cell, whose primary function is to exchange respiratory gases between blood and environment, the goblet cell and the mitochondria rich or chloride cell. The structure of a typical chloride cell is shown in Fig. 12.6 [41]. It is this cell which is thought to be responsible for the active transport of sodium and chloride ions. The cell contains a complicated system of microtubules, numerous mitochondria and an apical crypt, which is only seen in the sea-water-adapted cell. Chloride ions can be located histochemically both in the crypt and in the microtubular system of these cells. Both the number of chloride cells and the diameter of the microtubular system within each cell increase on adaptation to sea water. These results provide further morphological evidence for the direct involvement of chloride cells in the active secretion of chloride.

The gills of the sea-water-adapted fish also excrete sodium, but this excretion is not linked directly to that of chloride. Part of the sodium efflux is balanced by an influx of potassium in the sea-water-adapted gill. The situation in gills of fresh-water-adapted fish is more complex. In this case sodium and chloride ions are absorbed by the gill epithelium, part of the sodium absorption being in exchange for ammonium and hydrogen ions, part of the chloride absorption being in exchange for bicarbonate. The relative importance of these multiple exchange mechanisms to the overall electrolyte balance of the fish has been analysed in detail by Maetz [27].

The euryhaline fish in sea water maintains a concentration of sodium in its blood considerably lower than that of its environment. One might expect, by

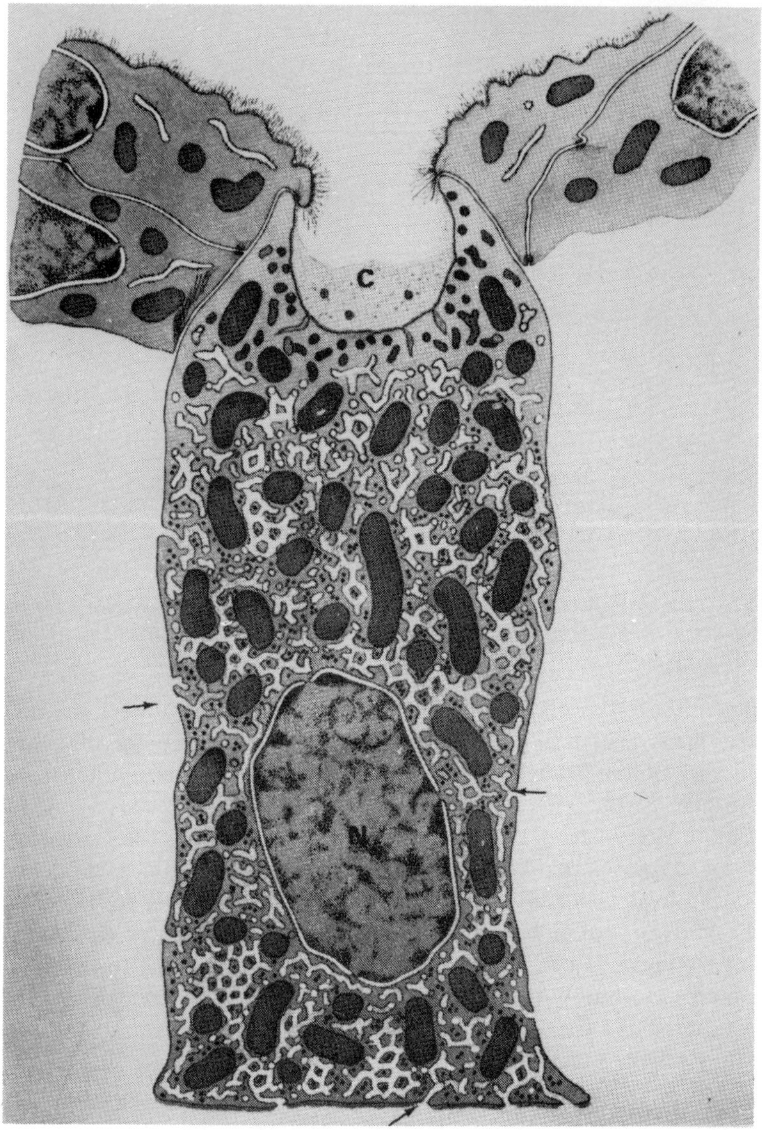

Fig. 12.6. Schematic representation of a typical salt-water-adapted chloride cell in fish gill. N, nucleus; C, apical crypt; arrows indicate connection between the microtubular system and the plasma membrane of the basal and lateral surfaces; dark ovals represent mitochondria. (From [41].)

analogy with the frog skin, that such a condition would be accompanied by a fall in the permeability of the gill epithelium to sodium, but the reverse is true. The bidirectional flux of sodium is some two to three hundred times greater in the sea-water-adapted fish. Placing a sea-water-adapted fish into fresh water causes an immediate fall in sodium efflux. This is shown for the eel in Fig. 12.7. The mechanism by which sodium efflux is rapidly reduced is not understood. An

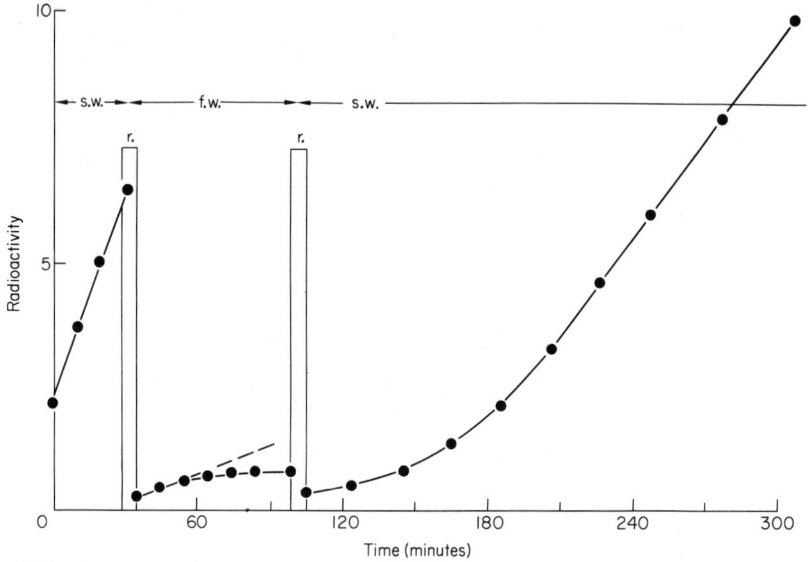

Fig. 12.7. Demonstration of an initial and a secondary regulation of sodium efflux by the eel gill measured during a prolonged period in fresh water and upon subsequent return to sea water. (From [27].)

exchange diffusion mechanism for sodium situated in the gill epithelium would produce this type of result [36], but then so would a change in diffusional permeability to sodium brought about by alterations in the trans-epithelial electrical gradient [49].

Of more interest from the point of view of adaptation is the further decrease in sodium efflux seen to take place thirty to sixty minutes after the initial transfer from salt to fresh water. Figure 12.7 shows a typical response for the eel. In this case the efflux of sodium begins to tail off after only 30 minutes' contact with the new environment. If the fish is replaced in sea water at this time, the sodium efflux increases, but not to the pre-adaptation level. During the next sixty minutes the efflux of sodium then increases slowly to approach the rate found in the fully adapted sea-water fish. A readaptation to sea water has taken place. Although these changes are quick in onset they represent only the beginning of the adaptive process. Full adaptation to different media may take several days to complete. The immediate fall in sodium efflux following transfer from sea water to fresh water is more dramatic than the secondary regulation. It is, however, this secondary inhibition of sodium efflux which is vital for the fish's survival. The rapid fall in sodium efflux is shown to a variable degree by both stenohaline and euryhaline fish, but it is only the euryhaline species which show the delayed adaptive response to the environment.

All epithelial tissues are in a constant state of renewal and any adaptive change which takes more than a few days to complete will be partly expressed through the presence of new cells. This rate of cellular renewal depends upon the adaptive state of the organism, being increased considerably during adaptation to sea water. There are also obvious changes in function occurring within hours of a change in environment. These must be organized within the existing cell population, with or without help from secreted hormones. An attempt to describe adaptation of gill function, both in terms of cellular and molecular renewal, is shown in Fig. 12.8.

Three possible ways of inducing molecular changes during adaptation from fresh water to sea water are considered. Each of these possibilities assumes protein synthesis of membrane carriers to be repressed in the fresh-water-adapted state. This assumption is based on the finding that inhibitors of protein synthesis, injected into fish at the time of transfer to sea water, *accelerate* the speed at

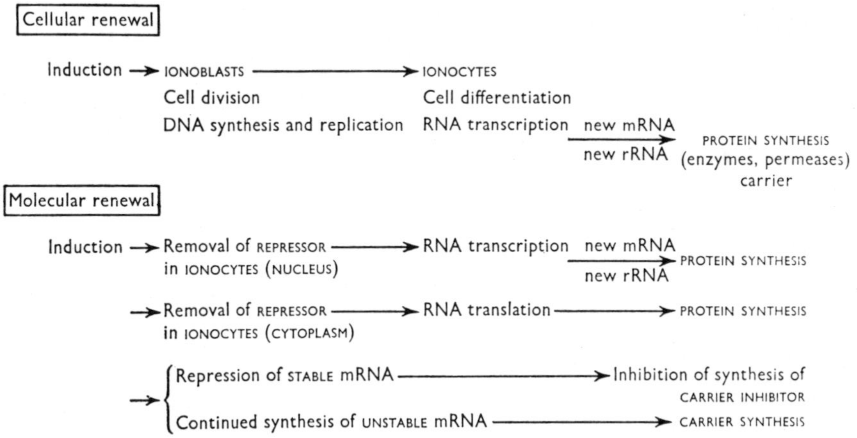

Fig. 12.8. Different ways of regulating gill function during adaptation of fish to sea water. Cellular renewal and molecular renewal should be regarded as working in parallel rather than constituting alternative pathways for expression of the final adaptive response. (From Maetz [26]).

which adaptation takes place [28]. This type of anomalous response would be produced if the mRNA for membrane carriers had a longer half-life than that for the postulated inhibitor. Cortisol probably initiates adaptive changes in gill function by stimulating the synthesis of sodium pump sites (the Na-K ATPase) and a prolactin-like hormone possibly controls the synthesis of a repressor for this enzyme. The hormonal state of the fish would, presumably, also determine the functional properties of newly synthesized cells. The function of cellular renewal would then be to perpetuate changes organized initially in the original epithelium.

These postulated mechanisms for adaptive control cannot be tested with anything like the rigour applied to bacterial systems. Neither do they explain how transport reverses on adaptation to sea water. A change in carbonic anhydrase activity also takes place in gill epithelium during adaptation to sea water. The molecular organization of this change and its relevance to active chloride transport has yet to be defined.

Intestine

The ability of the intestine to transport electrolytes and to absorb and metabolize ingested nutrients is at least one order of magnitude greater than that found for other tissues. These functions are carried out by a rapidly changing cell population. The entire epithelium renews itself every two to three days. This represents a replacement of about 10^9 mucosal cells per day for the young rat, that is about 4% of the total number of cells in the body [23]. The energy expended in maintaining these high rates of cellular renewal and transport must be considerable. The situation is in some ways similar to that found in bacteria, growth and function both being dependent upon a constant supply of nutrients. One might predict from this that the intestinal mucosa would show some of the versatility of the bacterial cell in responding to changes in its external (in this case lumenal) environment. Evidence has been presented recently to suggest that this is so, at least as far as disaccharidases and glycolytic enzymes are concerned [42, 52].

Changes in intestinal function taking longer than two or three days to complete have not been considered here except where they complete a series of earlier adaptive changes. This omission is justified by an inability to distinguish, with certainty, long-term adaptive changes from those caused by alterations in intestinal morphology. Even short periods of fasting can affect intestinal structure. This is shown for the rat intestine in Table 12.1. An overnight fast has no effect

Table 12.1. The morphological features and lipid content of the small intestine of fasted and fed rats. Rats were fasted for 15 hours prior to experiment. Results give mean values ± S.D. of 10 observations. (From [34]).

Observation	Fasted	Fed
Body weight (g)	204 ± 27	214 ± 25
Intestinal wet weight		
Total small intestine (g)	5·015 ± 0·514	6·122 ± 0·572
Mucosa (% total)	39 ± 4·8	48 ± 4·8
Dry weight (% total)	23·6 ± 1·2	23·0 ± 1·4
Lipid content (mg g^{-1})	41·8 ± 5·2	41·8 ± 5·8
Intestinal length (cm)	124·8 ± 7·8	126·0 ± 7·7

on body weight, lipid content or on the length of the intestine, but the actual weight of the intestine and the amount of mucosal tissue fall significantly. The DNA content of the intestine in the fed group of rats is also greater, suggesting that more cells are present in the mucosa of fed animals. This increase in cell mass is associated with an increase in the transport of glycine and 3-o-methyl glucose [34]. A rough calculation would suggest that the mucosa of the fed rat contains 8×10^8 more cells than the fasted mucosa. The increase in transport probably reflects this increase in total cell population.

Starving animals for longer periods of time causes a further loss of mucosal tissue and a decreased rate of cellular renewal. This is associated with an *increased* transport rate for different sugars. It has also been possible to show the active transport of L-glucose using intestines from semi-starved rats [38]. The situation is complicated with short-term fasting producing different effects from long-term starvation. These long-term changes in transport and metabolism probably result from adaptive changes taking place within the mucosa, but the changes in morphology make quantification of these findings extremely difficult.

The function of the intestinal epithelium is basically twofold, to sustain itself and to pass on material essential for the growth and development of the whole animal. Many aspects of this latter function are under hormonal control. One

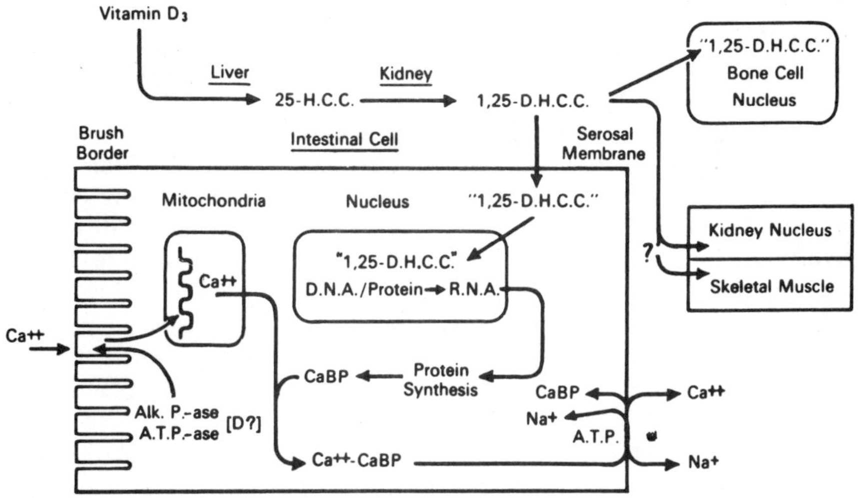

Fig. 12.9. Scheme of vitamin D action compiled from previous work on rats and chicks. (From [19].)

example is the control of calcium transport through the action of 1,25-dihydroxycholecalciferol (1,25-D.H.C.C.), a kidney metabolite of vitamin D_3. The permeability of the intestinal epithelium to calcium is normally low. Variations in the amount of calcium ingested produce only minimal changes in blood levels. As soon as blood calcium falls, however, a series of counter-balancing measures comes into operation leading to an increased absorption of calcium. The first effect seen on reducing blood calcium is an increase in parathyroid hormone release. This acts on the bone to mobilize calcium and on the kidney, where it stimulates the synthesis and release of 1,25-D.H.C.C. The metabolic pathways leading to the formation of 1,25-D.H.C.C. and its subsequent action on intestinal mucosa, is shown in Fig. 12.9.

Vitamin D_3 is first hydroxylated in the liver to form 25-hydroxycholecalciferol. This steroid is then transported to the kidney in a protein-bound form, where a second hydroxylation takes place to produce 1,25-D.H.C.C. It is this second hydroxylation, carried out by a kidney mitochondrial hydroxylase, which is thought to be stimulated by the presence of parathyroid hormone. 1,25-D.H.C.C. leaves the kidney to become localized preferentially in the nuclei of bone, kidney and intestinal cells. In the case of the intestinal cell there appears to be a receptor protein for 1,25-D.H.C.C. present in the cytoplasm. The nucleus also contains a protein of the same size which can bind 1,25-D.H.C.C. [21]. Whether this protein is itself a repressor of mRNA synthesis has yet to be determined. The presence of 1,25-D.H.C.C. in the nucleus leads to the formation of new mRNA molecules coding for the synthesis of a calcium binding protein (CaBP). There is some discussion as to how CaBP, which constitutes nearly 3% of the total supernatant protein from mucosal homogenates, acts to increase calcium transport. Wasserman and Corradino [55], quoting evidence for CaBP location in the brush border region of the epithelial cell, suggest that it aids calcium entry. Kodicek [19] sees CaBP as a competitor with mitochondrial protein for the binding of free calcium ions, the Ca-CaBP complex then being dissociated at the site of the calcium pump, presumably because the pump has an even higher affinity for calcium. The relation between CaBP and calcium transport is intimate, but certain discrepancies between the rate of formation of CaBP and changes in calcium transport need to be explained before one can define its function fully. Other steroids are known to change both enzyme activities and functional properties of intestinal mucosa. Some of these changes are localized within the brush border region of the epithelial cell [7, 18, 37].

An alteration in body temperature produces a more general adaptive response in the intestine. This can be seen in hibernating animals, where both the active transport and the passive permeability to ions decrease [9]. It can also be seen in fish kept at different environmental temperatures, where both the transport of electrolytes and non-electrolytes show adaptive changes [48]. An example of some of these changes is shown for the goldfish in Fig. 12.10.

Increasing the environmental temperature from 15 to 30°C causes an immediate, actinomycin D resistant, increase in protein synthesis. This is followed, some 10 hours later, by a second surge in protein synthesis. This second increase, which is much bigger than the first and which takes place together with an increase in RNA synthesis, is abolished by the previous injection of actinomycin D. The ability of glucose to support a transmucosal potential difference changes 15 to 20 hours after raising the body temperature. Glucose initially increases the potential (that is the permeability of the brush border membrane to sodium) at incubation temperatures around 15°C. After adaptation, however, this effect can only be produced at incubation temperatures greater than 30°C [46]. Sodium transport across the intestine also adapts 15 to 20 hours after the initial switch in body temperature. Sodium transport is partly dependent on the presence of glucose and one might expect the adaptation of a glucose response to cause this change in sodium transport. This is unlikely to be the complete answer, however, for regulation of sodium transport also takes place with the same time course in goldfish gallbladder in the absence of glucose [5]. Na-K ATPase activity remains high as sodium transport adapts, but it falls significantly some 10 to 20 days

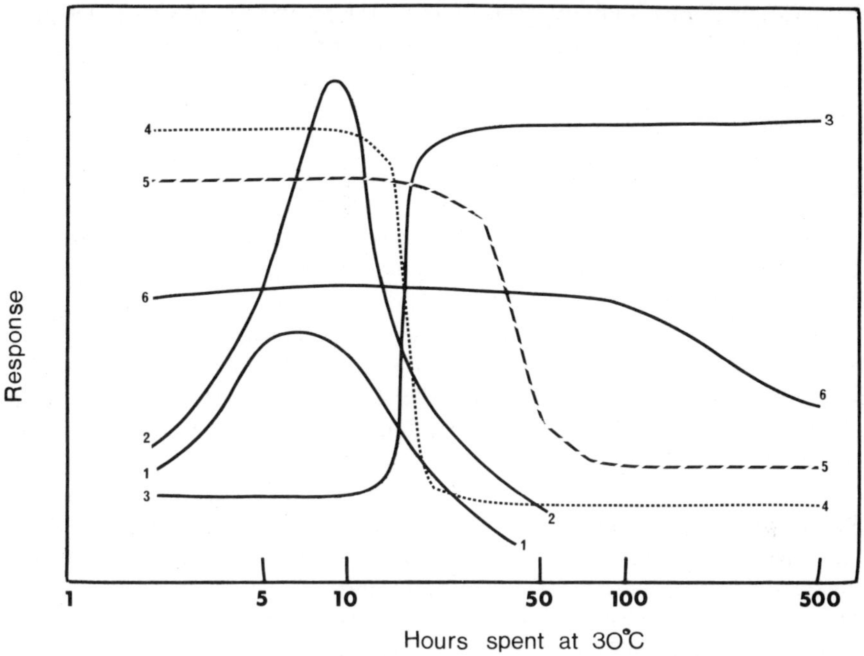

Fig. 12.10. Time course for adaptive changes taking place in goldfish intestine following a 15°C rise in environmental temperature. 1, RNA synthesis; 2, Actinomycin D sensitive protein synthesis; 3, Lowest temperature at which glucose stimulates sodium entry into the mucosal cell; 4, sodium transport; 5, change from $C_{22:6}$ to $C_{18:0}$ in mucosal membrane phospholipids; 6, Na-K ATPase activity of mucosal microsomal fractions. Composite figure derived from results referred to in the text.

later. The first adaptive response seems to be a regulation of passive sodium entry into the mucosal cell. This is consistent with results obtained on the gall-bladder showing a *decreased* intracellular sodium concentration and an increased potassium concentration at the time when sodium transport is first regulated [5]. The final change in Na-K ATPase activity is very probably associated with the production of new cells, cellular renewal in the fish intestine being much slower than in the mammal.

The membrane phospholipids of 15°C-adapted goldfish intestines contain large amounts of long chain, unsaturated, fatty acids ($C_{22:6}$ and $C_{20:4}$). The proportion of saturated fatty acids (mainly $C_{18:0}$) increases at high environmental temperatures [16]. The time course for this change (32–48 hours) is again different from that for sodium transport.

The lessons to be learnt from this type of analysis are twofold, firstly, that cellular adaptation to the environment can involve qualitative changes in function (the temperature at which glucose increases the brush border permeability to sodium), as well as the more usual quantitative changes. Secondly, that different time courses exist for different adaptive changes. One might suppose that the earliest recorded changes are the most important for survival. If this is so, then the control of passive sodium permeability in the goldfish intestine will be more important than any delayed alteration in sodium pumping capacity.

12.3.2 Endothelial tissues

Liver

Reversible enzyme induction and repression in response to changes in circulating blood levels of sugars and amino acids have been reported for the liver. The adaptive changes which take place here are probably organized in the same way as in bacterial systems, but they take longer to complete. Several genes can be involved in the transcription of single multi-enzyme systems in higher animals. This constitutes another difference from the bacterial cell, where a single stretch of DNA codes for the whole permease system. A list of some of the inducible enzymes found in liver is given in Table 12.2 [24].

The systems studied in most detail are those involving induction of threonine dehydrase, which can increase in concentration as much as 300 times when the amino acid concentration in blood increases, and tryptophan pyrrolase, which is under dual control from tryptophan and cortisone. The synthesis of many other liver enzymes can be increased by the presence of steroid hormones, particularly cortisone. Actinomycin D will abolish these inductive effects, showing

Table 12.2. Some inducible enzymes in the liver. (From [24]).

Enzyme	Inducing agent	Repressing agent
Glycerol phosphate dehydrogenase (mitochondrial)	Thyroxine	
Malic enzyme		Fasting
Phosphoenolpyruvate carboxykinase	Cortisone Fasting	
Pyruvate carboxylase	Cortisone Fasting	
Serine deaminase	Glucagon, hydrocortisone, some amino acids	Glucose Serine
Serine dehydratase	Some amino acids	Glucose
Serine phosphate phosphatase		Serine
Threonine dehydrase	Some amino acids	
Tryptophan pyrrolase	Cortisone Tryptophan α-Methyltryptophan	
Tyrosine transaminase	Cortisone, insulin, glucagon	Growth hormone

that the changes in enzyme activity represent real changes in the ability of the cell to synthesize proteins.

The function of the liver is closely allied to that of the intestine. Enzymes in both tissues show adaptive changes in the presence of steroids and glycolytic enzymes can be induced in both tissues by the prior administration of different carbohydrates [52]. The ability of the intestine to metabolize, as well as transport, substrates has been consistently underestimated in the past. Much could be gained from a comparative study of these two tissues in the future.

Muscle and brain

Nerve and muscle fibres normally exist in an environment where the supply of nutrients remains reasonably constant, the liver removing most of the amino acids and sugars from the hepatic portal system. One would not therefore expect to see adaptive changes similar to those reported for liver. There are, however, at least two instances where nerve and muscle fibres show adaptive changes in response to alterations in the external environment. The first is caused by a change in osmolarity in the circulating blood, brought about by an incomplete regulation of electrolyte balance during transfer of animals to environments of different salinity. The second is caused by a change in body temperature.

Changes in blood osmolarity that arise when crustacea are transferred from fresh water to sea water cause an immediate decrease in cell volume. This effect takes place throughout the body. Adaptive changes, initiated by the change in blood osmolarity, cause the levels of free amino acids to increase within cells, so that the osmolarity of cellular fluid again approaches that found in blood. The possible mechanisms for these changes have been described elsewhere (Chapter 5).

Changing the body temperature of poikilotherms will cause an immediate disorganization of cellular transport and metabolism. The primary aim of adaptation must be to re-establish order out of chaos. It should be emphasized, however, that this does not *necessarily* mean a complete return to the pattern of organization seen to operate at the previous environmental temperature. Failure to appreciate this point could lead to a misinterpretation of the functional significance of these adaptive changes. Adaptation involves both a reconstitution of cell membranes and a restructuring of metabolic enzymes. Mention has already been made of the changes in lipid composition which follow a change in environmental temperature. These changes, which are also found in brain and muscle phospholipids, follow a definite pattern, the long-chain unsaturated fatty acids substituting for the short-chain saturated fatty acids, as the environmental temperature decreases. The aim of such changes is said to be to maintain membrane fluidity, so that it will continue to conduct current and generally carry out the transport functions assigned to it. Some of these functions are mediated through the action of membrane-bound enzymes. The properties of these enzymes are likely to be determined by the nature of the surrounding phospholipids. This applies to plasma membrane Na-K ATPase, which continues to operate at low temperatures in cold-adapted fish [47] and to mitochondrial membranes, where a change in phospholipid composition probably affects the efficiency of oxidative phosphorylation [2]. It is not known how these changes in membrane composition come about. It could involve *in situ* substitution of one fatty acid acyl group for another or the synthesis of new phospholipid membranes.

The cytoplasmic membrane contains the gates by which substrates enter cells. Establishing control of these gating mechanisms ensures that substrates necessary for the survival of the organism, will again be presented for metabolism, in an ordered fashion. The metabolic enzymes, however, will each be responding differently to the change in environmental temperature, their rates of catalysis

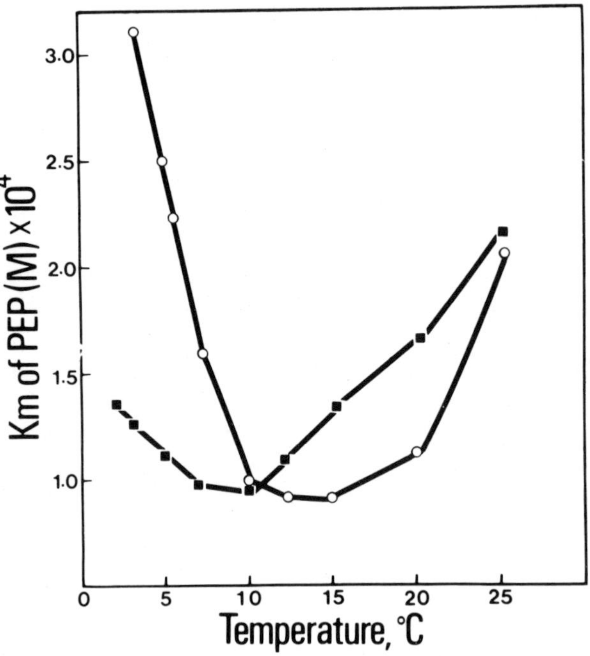

Fig. 12.11. The influence of temperature on the apparent Michaelis constant (K_m) of phosphoenol pyruvate (PEP) for pyruvate kinase enzymes from warm- and cold-acclimated trout. ■: cold-adapted pyruvate kinase; ○: warm-adapted pyruvate kinase. (From [50].)

depending on their individual energies of activation. A further regulation of enzyme concentrations would, theoretically, complete adaptation and there is evidence to show that such regulation takes place. Evidence for a more qualitative change in enzyme function is presented, for trout muscle pyruvate kinase, in Fig. 12.11 [50].

The apparent affinity (K_m) of the warm-adapted pyruvate kinase for its substrate reaches a minimum, that is highest affinity for substrate, at an incubation temperature similar to that of its natural environment. The K_m increases rapidly at lower incubation temperatures. Pyruvate kinase, isolated from trout adapted to low temperatures, no longer shows this increase in K_m. The temperature of highest affinity for substrate now lies at about 10°C; again very close to the environmental temperature of the fish. Similar U-shaped affinity-temperature curves, which change on adaptation, have now been described for muscle fructose diphosphatase and lactate-dehydrogenase; for brain cholinesterase and choline acetyltransferase; for liver isocitrate dehydrogenase and citrate synthase. The ubiquitous nature of this adaptive response needs explanation. It has been suggested that the change in K_m enables an enzyme to maintain a constant reaction rate at different environmental temperatures [13]. Even assuming this to be desired objective, it is difficult to see why one needs more than one enzyme to achieve it. Any enzyme whose K_m increased in proportion to the environmental temperature would maintain constant reaction rates, provided the substrate concentration also remained constant. It might be more profitable to ask why enzymes need to operate with maximal binding efficiency for substrate. We already know that enzymes prepared from poikilotherms tend to be more unstable than those prepared from mammals. We also know that enzymes resist denaturation more readily when they are bound to substrates. Adaptive changes leading to the production of enzymes having high affinities for substrates may be essential, not for maintaining reaction rates constant, but for preserving their own integrity.

Gonads

Development of the gonads in birds is often initiated by an ability to sense changes in the external environment. These environmental cues are numerous and varied. Rainfall in a normally arid region, a sudden abundance of food, a change in environmental temperature or an increased ability to find materials suitable for nest building, have all been known to act as sensory stimuli leading to the release of gonadotrophins. One of the most widely used environmental cues at mid and high latitudes is the seasonally dependent change in daylength. Birds begin to release gonadotrophins from the hypophysis once the daylength exceeds a critical limit. The gonads then develop and breeding follows at times most suited to the future survival of the young. The cellular response to the environment in such situations can be considered to exist at two levels, in the brain, where the incoming signal is first recognized by the animal and in the gonads, which act as a target site for the neuronally discharged hormones.

The relation between time of exposure of the bird to light and release of gonadotrophins is not a simple one. Exposing birds to fixed periods of light will trigger the release of hormones during one part of the day but not at others. This variable sensitivity of the brain to a constant stimulus suggests that some form of circadian function is present. This was shown to be true for the white-crowned sparrow in recent experiments summarized in Fig. 12.12 [8].

The birds had been kept previously under conditions where release of gonadotrophins was suppressed (8 hours light, 16 hours dark, 8L 16D). The control levels of luteinizing hormone (LH) were determined under these conditions. The birds were then placed in the dark, to be removed at known times afterwards for one 8-hour period of light. Blood samples were again taken and assayed for

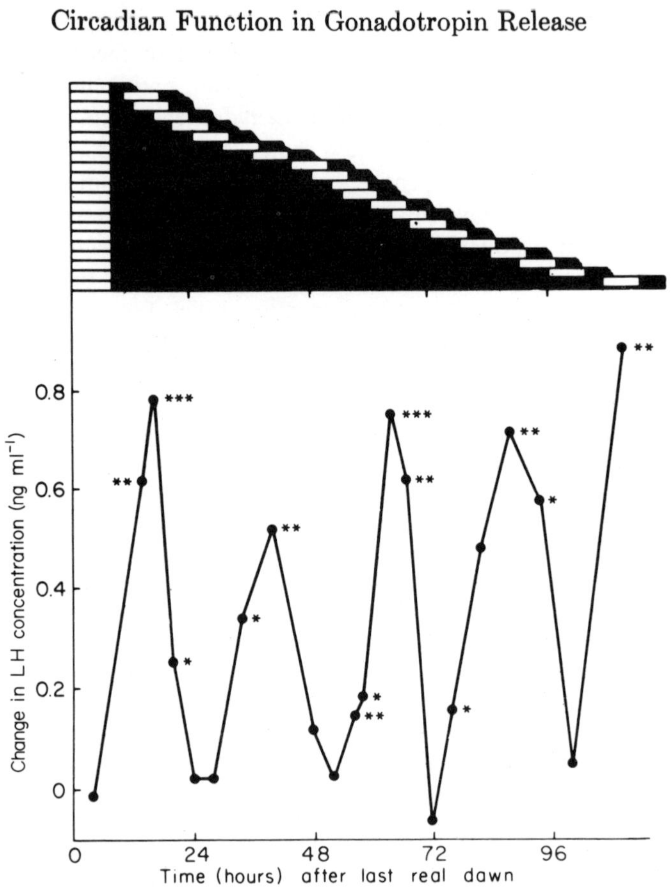

Fig. 12.12. The effect of an 8-hr photoperiod given at various intervals after entry to darkness on plasma LH concentration in White-crowned Sparrows. The white and black bars at the top illustrate the various treatments. Birds were previously maintained on 8L and 16D and a pre-experimental blood sample was taken for all birds early in the last 8-hr light period. The post-experimental sample was taken 7–16 hr after the end of the test photoperiod. The ordinate shows the change in plasma LH concentration between these two samples that resulted from a particular treatment. (From [8].)

LH. The results show regular periods when light could stimulate the release of LH. Greatest effects were produced by light given 12, 36, 60, 84 and 108 hours after the last dawn. Little or no release was seen with treatments given 0, 24, 48, 72 or 96 hours after the beginning of the experiment. This circadian rhythm disappeared after a period of several days. The level of LH remained high, suggesting that the original induction of release switched on a process which then remained functioning for long periods of time. The circadian oscillator within the brain which is responsible for this type of response must be related to some cellular process, but its anatomical location and biochemical mode of operation is completely unknown.

Gonadotrophins released from the pituitary affect the gonads in three different ways. They stimulate general growth and maintain tissue structure; they stimulate the formation of spermatozoa and ova and they increase the biosynthesis of steroid hormones. Newly synthesized steroid hormones then modify the further release of gonadotrophins, probably by controlling the synthesis and secretion of specific releasing factors in the hypothalamus and pituitary. The action of LH on testosterone production in the testis and progesterone synthesis in the corpus luteum appears to be mediated primarily through the action of cyclic AMP. LH stimulates the production of cyclic AMP in both tissues [21, 33] and cyclic AMP, added to incubation media containing slices of testis or corpus luteum, stimulates the production of testosterone or progesterone [32, 43]. Cyclic AMP is thought to act by the initial activation of a phosphorylase which breaks down glycogen to form glucose-6-phosphate. Metabolism of glucose-6-phosphate through the pentose phosphate pathway increases the amount of NADPH available, which then acts as a critical co-factor in the biosynthesis of steroids from cholesterol.

The ability of LH to stimulate the production of cyclic AMP in the gonads provides only one example of how different polypeptide hormones produce their effects. The initial binding of the hormone to the target cell provides the specificity of response; the cyclic AMP then acts as a common intracellular messenger. The ability of higher organisms to use hormones in this way enables cells to respond to changes in the external environment without directly experiencing these changes for themselves. The level at which this operates for gonadal development is one of the most sophisticated, the cellular response being triggered early to coincide at some future date with the critical change in external environment.

12.4 CONCLUSIONS

The fact that cells adapt to their environment can only be appreciated once that environment has changed. I am assuming here, for the purpose of argument, that the presence of hormones in the vicinity of a cell will also constitute a change in external environment. This method of detecting adaptation, which is of course unavoidable, produces two unfortunate consequences. First of all it tends to obscure the fact that cells, kept under unchanging conditions, still have to balance their transport and metabolism to maintain constant an internal environment different from that of its surroundings. Secondly it leads one to assume that adaptation is only completely successful when cellular metabolism returns to a level similar to that found in the previous steady state. I have tried to suggest in the foregoing discussion that adaptive changes in cells are more likely to be accomplished by changing the pattern of a previously organized balance than by the initiation of some completely new phenomenon called adaptation. The new balance for the cell will involve changes in transport and metabolism. The final pattern may correspond closely to the previous one, but this is not essential. It follows that a knowledge of how cells normally balance pumps against leaks, how they utilize ion gradients as energy sources and how they distribute high energy phosphates along different metabolic pathways, will all provide useful knowledge which will enable one to decide why certain changes take place on adaptation. We have now progressed beyond the mere cataloguing of adaptive changes to a point where explanations of their functions can be specified in detail.

The organization of adaptive changes at the molecular level is best understood in bacteria. This is because of the large number of genetic variants available for study and also because the bacterial cell is relatively simple compared with a multicellular organism. It is not clear how far one can use information gained from bacteria to explain how changes take place in higher organisms. The pattern of changes seems to be similar in many instances, but the detailed organization may be different. It still seems worthwhile, however, emphasizing those features of adaptation which are common to all cells. An epithelial cell may have special problems in providing substrates for the rest of the organism besides itself, and one would expect to see differences in adaptive response because of this specialized function, but the methods used to change transport across the cell are likely to be similar to those involved in regulating the normal passage of solutes across membranes.

12.5 REFERENCES

1 Andersson J., Möller G. & Sjöberg O. (1972) B lymphocytes can be stimulated by concanavalin A in the presence of humoral factors released by T cells. *Eur. J. Immunol.* **2,** 99–101.

2 Caldwell R.S. & Vernberg F.J. (1970) The influence of acclimation temperature on the lipid composition of fish gill mitochondria. *Comp. Biochem. Physiol.* **34,** 179–91.

3 Cohen G.N. & Monod J. (1959) Bacterial permeases. *Bact. Rev.* **21,** 169–94.

4 Crabbé J. (1964) Stimulation by aldosterone of active sodium transport across the isolated ventral skin of amphibia. *Endocrinology* **75,** 809–11.

5 Cremaschi D., Smith M.W. & Wooding F.B.P. (1973) Temperature-dependent changes in fluid transport across goldfish gallbladder. *J. Membrane Biol.* **13,** 143–64.

6 Cuatrecasas P. (1974) Membrane receptors. *Ann. Rev. Biochem.* **43,** 169–214.

7 Doell R.G. & Kretchmer N. (1964) Intestinal invertase: precocious development of activity after injection of hydrocortisone. *Science, N.Y.* **143,** 42–4.

8 Follett B.K., Mattocks P.W. Jr. & Farner D.S. (1974) Circadian function in the photoperiodic induction of gonadotrophin secretion in the white-crowned sparrow, *Zonotrichia leucophrys gambelii. Proc. Nat. Acad. Sci. U.S.A.,* **71,** 1666–9.

9 Gilles-Baillien M. (1970) Permeability characteristics of the intestinal epithelium and hibernation in *Testudo hermanni,* Gmelin. *Arch. Int. Physiol. Biochim.* **78,** 327–38.

10 Gould G.W. (1969) In *The Bacterial Spore* (eds G. W. Gould & A. Hurst), pp. 397–444. Academic Press, New York & London.

11 Greaves M.F. & Bauminger S. (1972) Activation of T and B lymphocytes by insoluble phytomitogens. *Nature, New Biol.* **235,** 67–70.

12 Hadden J.W., Hadden E.M., Haddox M.K. & Goldberg N.D. (1972) Guanosine 3′:5′-cyclic monophosphate: A possible intracellular mediator of mitogenic influences in lymphocytes. *Proc. Nat. Acad. Sci.* U.S.A. **69,** 3024–7.

13 Hochachka R.W. & Somero G.N. (1972) Biochemical adaptation to the environment. In *Fish Physiology* (Eds. W. S. Hear & D. J. Randall), pp. 100–156. Academic Press, New York & London.

14 Hornby R. & Thomas S. (1969) Effect of prolonged saline-exposure on sodium transport across frog skin. *J. Physiol., Lond.* **200,** 321–44.

15 Jacob F. & Monod J. (1961) Genetic regulatory mechanisms in the synthesis of proteins. *J. Molec. Biol.* **3,** 318–56.

16 Kemp P. & Smith M.W. (1970) Effect of temperature acclimatization on the fatty acid composition of goldfish intestinal lipids. *Biochem. J.* **117,** 9–15.

17 Kepes A. (1964) The place of permeases in cellular organization. In *Cellular Functions of membrane transport* (ed. J. F. Hoffman), pp. 155–69. Prentice-Hall, New Jersey.

18 Koldovsky O. & Sunshine P. (1970) Effect of cortisone on the developmental pattern of the neutral and the acid *β*-galactosidase of the small intestine of the rat. *Biochem. J.* **117,** 467–71.

19 Kodicek E. (1974) The story of vitamin D from vitamin to hormone. *Lancet* **1,** 325–9.

20 Kuehl F.A. Jr, Patanelli D.J., Tarnoff J. & Humes J.L. (1970) Testicular adenyl cyclase: stimulation by the pituitary gonadotrophins. *Biol. reprod.* **2,** 154–63.

21 Lawson D.E.M. & Emtage J.S. (1974) Localization and function of 1,25-dihydroxycholecalciferol in chick intestine. *Biochem. Soc. Spec. Publ.* **3,** 75–90.

22 Leaf A. & Sharp G.W.G. (1971) The stimulation of sodium transport by aldosterone. *Phil. Trans. Roy. Soc. Lond. B.* **262,** 323–32.

23 Leblond C.P. (1965) The time dimension in histology. *Am. J. Anat.* **116,** 1–28.

24 Lehninger A.L. (1970) In *Biochemistry. The molecular basis of cell structure and function.* Worth, New York.

25 Lubin M. (1964) Cell potassium and the regulation of protein synthesis. In *Cellular Functions of membrane transport* (ed. J. F. Hoffman), pp. 193–211. Prentice-Hall, New Jersey.

26 Maetz J. (1970) Mechanisms of salt and water transfer across membranes in teleosts in relation to the aquatic environment. *Mem. Soc. Endocrinol.* **18,** 3–29.

27 Maetz J. (1971) Fish gills: mechanisms of salt transfer in fresh water and sea water. *Phil. Trans. Roy. Soc. Lond. B.* **262,** 209–49.

28 Maetz J., Nibelle J., Bornancin M. & Motais R. (1969) Action sur l'osmorégulation de l'anguille de divers antibiotiques inhibiteurs de la synthèse des protéines ou du renouvellement cellulaire. *Comp. Biochem. Physiol.* **30,** 1125–51.

29 Maino V.C., Green N.M. & Crumpton M.J. (1974) The role of calcium ions in initiating transformation of lymphocytes. *Nature* **251,** 324–7.

30 Mandelstam J. (1969) Regulation of bacterial spore formation. *Symp. Soc. gen. Microbiol.* **19,** 377–401, Cambridge University Press, London.

31 Mandelstam J. (1971) Recurring patterns during development in primitive organisms. *Symp. Soc. exp. Biol.* **25,** 1–26, Cambridge University Press, London.

32 Marsh J.M. & Savard K. (1966) The stimulation of progesterone synthesis in bovine corpora lutea by adenosine 3′,5′-monophosphate. *Steroids* **8,** 133–48.

33 Mason N.R., Marsh J.M. & Savard K. (1962) An action of gonadotropin *in vitro*. *J. Biol. Chem.* **237,** 1801–6.

34 McManus J.P.A. & Isselbacher K.J. (1970) Effects of fasting versus feeding on the rat small intestine. Morphological, biochemical and functional differences. *Gastroenterology,* **59,** 214–21.

35 McQuillen K. (1956) Capabilities of bacterial protoplasts. In *Bacterial Anatomy*, 127–49, *Sixth Symposium of the Society for General Microbiology*. Cambridge University Press, London.

36 Motais R., Garcia Romeu F. & Maetz J. (1966) Exchange diffusion effect and euryhalinity in teleosts. *J. gen. Physiol.* **50,** 391–422.

37 Moog F. (1953) Developmental adaptations of alkaline phosphatases in the small intestine. *Fedn. Proc. Fedn Am. Socs exp. Biol.* **21,** 51–66.

38 Neale R.J. & Wiseman G. (1968) Active transport of L-glucose by isolated small intestine of dietary-restricted rat. *J. Physiol. Lond.* **198,** 601–11.

39 Pitts J.D. (1971) Molecular exchange and growth control in tissue culture. In *Growth Control in Cell Cultures. Ciba Found. Symp.* (eds G. E. W. Wolstenholme & J. Knight), pp. 89–105. Churchill Livingstone, Edinburgh & London.

40 Raff M.C., Sternberg M. & Taylor R.B. (1970) Immunoglobulin determinants on the surface of mouse lymphoid cells. *Nature, Lond.* **225,** 553–4.
41 Ritch R. & Philpott C.W. (1969) Repeating particles associated with an electrolyte-transport membrane. *Exptl. Cell Res.* **55,** 17–24.
42 Rosenweig N.S. & Herman R.H. (1968) Control of jejunal sucrase and maltase activity by dietary sucrose or fructose in man. A model for the study of enzyme regulation in man. *J. clin. Invest.* **47,** 2253–62.
43 Sandler R. & Hall P.F. (1966) Stimulation *in vitro* by adenosine-3′,5′-cyclic monophosphate of steroidogenesis in rat testis. *Endocrinology* **79,** 647–9.
44 Singer S.J. & Nicolson G.L. (1972) The fluid mosaic model of the structure of cell membranes. *Science,* **175,** 720–31.
45 Slack C. & Warner A.E. (1973) Intracellular and intercellular potentials in the early amphibian embryo. *J. Physiol. Lond.* **232,** 313–30.
46 Smith M.W. (1966) Influence of temperature acclimatization on sodium-glucose interactions in the goldfish intestine. *J. Physiol., Lond.* **182,** 574–90.
47 Smith M.W. (1967) Influence of temperature acclimatization on the temperature-dependence and ouabain-sensitivity of goldfish intestinal adenosine triphosphatase. *Biochem. J.* **105,** 65–71.
48 Smith M.W. (1972) Temperature adaptation of transport properties of poikilotherms. In *Hibernation and Hypothermia, perspectives and challenges* (eds F. E. South, P. J. Hannon, J. S. Willis, E. T. Pengelley & N. R. Alpert), pp. 216–37. Elsevier, Amsterdam.
49 Smith P.G. (1969) The ionic relations of *Artemia salina* (*L*). II. Fluxes of sodium, chloride and water. *J. Exp. Biol.* **51,** 739–57.
50 Somero G.N. (1972) Molecular mechanisms of temperature compensation in aquatic poikilotherms. In *Hibernation and Hypothermia, perspectives and challenges* (eds F. E. South, J. P. Hannon, J. S. Willis, E. T. Pengelley & N. R. Alpert), pp. 55–80. Elsevier, Amsterdam.
51 Sterlini J.M. & Mandelstam J. (1969) Commitment to sporulation in *Bacillus subtilis* and its relationship to development of actinomycin resistance. *Biochem. J.* **113,** 29–37.
52 Stifel F.B., Rosenweig N.S., Zakim D. & Herman R.H. (1968) Dietary regulation of glycolytic enzymes. I. Adaptive changes in rat jejunum. *Biochim. Biophys. Acta* **170,** 221–7.
53 Taylor R.B., Duffus W.P.H., Raff M.C. & de Petris S. (1971) Redistribution and pinocytosis of lymphocyte surface immunoglobulin molecules induced by anti-immunoglobulin antibody. *Nature, New Biol.* **233,** 225–9.
54 Unanue E.R. (1972) The regulatory role of macrophages in antigenic stimulation. *Advances in Immunology* **15,** 95–165.
55 Wasserman R.H. & Corradino R.A. (1971) Metabolic role of vitamins A and D. *Ann. Rev. Biochem.* **40,** 501–32.

Prelude to Chapter 13

Temperature and heat flow feature in any discussion of environmental physiology, and it is legitimate to ask whether this is because heat production and flow are particularly important aspects of the relation between organism and environment, because heat production, heat loss and body temperature are particularly easy things to measure, or because of the narrow view, taken so often, that the environment has only meteorological components. The answer, surely, is that the liberation and flow of kinetic energy is fundamental to the phenomenon of life.

If we exclude the cold- and heat-resistant spore-forming bacteria, and the unicellular inhabitants of hot springs it is generally true to say that a living organism can survive only while its constituent cells and fluids have temperatures within a range of approximately 0° to 45°C. Below 0°C death is usually the result of ice-crystal formation, and above 45°C death is often the result of cell protein and phospholipid disorganization (see Chapter 20).

Temperature is an expression of the kinetic energy of the molecules, atoms and ions of which matter is composed. This heat may come from within the body as a result of metabolic processes (chemical changes) by which the chemical energy of foodstuffs is liberated and appears as kinetic energy or heat; it may also come from outside the body as a result of heat flow down a thermal gradient or by radiative transfer.

Most chemical reactions are temperature dependent, and have Q_{10} values of 2–3—that is to say the rate of chemical processes increase 2–3 times for every 10°C rise in temperature. The uncontrolled accumulation of heat within an animal body would result in a run-away effect on body temperature: a rise in body temperature would cause a further rise in heat production which would cause a further rise in body temperature. . . . This process would soon destroy the animal.

The unimpeded flow of heat down an energy gradient from the organism to the environment results in a tissue temperature only slightly above, and wholly dependent on, the ambient temperature. Thus, a fall in ambient temperature to below 0°C would also destroy the animal.

In cold-blooded aquatic organisms, for example, in which there is little or no control over the heat flow to the environment, and little or no opportunity to choose a 'preferred' thermal environment, body temperature will vary seasonally with that of the environment, and activity might be expected to vary with the changes in body temperature That some such temperature-conforming animals can maintain fairly constant levels of activity despite slow (seasonal) changes in environmental and body temperatures is evidence of changes in cellular functions in relation to temperature. Similarly, some organisms can tolerate ambient and body temperatures at one season which would be fatal at another and this again is evidence of seasonal changes in cellular functions in relation to temperature.

The biological advantages of maintaining a body temperature near to the upper lethal level is that it affords a high rate of activity. This requires a high level of heat production (*Tachymetabolism*), a resistance to the flow of heat away from the animal to the environment, and the ability to vary both heat production and heat loss in immediate response to changes in the thermal relations between the animal and the environment. These functions are discussed in Chapter 20. The degree of these responses is not fixed, however. There are daily and seasonal changes in the capacity to produce heat, and in the capacity to aid or hinder heat loss, and these changes are consistent with the daily and seasonal changes in the environment.

Chapter 13
Thermal adaptation in the whole animal

H. POHL

13.1 INTRODUCTION

Temperature is one of the critical environmental factors limiting animal life and its distribution on earth. The range of body temperature which is permissive for activity, development and reproduction of animals is between 0 and 45°C although several highly specialized species can live either temporarily in a frozen or supercooled state or permanently in warm springs of 50°C. During the course of evolution, structural and functional organization have enabled animal species either to conform to the outside thermal environment (*conformers*), or to be permanently or temporarily independent of variations of environmental temperature conditions (*regulators*) [31]. Distribution of animal life has therefore been (and may still be) extending from the more uniform temperature conditions of land and water within the Tropics toward the poles into areas with more or less extreme climatic conditions (continental, desert or arctic climate).

Animals are generally adapted either to tolerate a wide variation of environmental temperature (*eurythermal*) or to live within a restricted range of thermal conditions (*stenothermal*). By definition, every species or subspecies (race) is physiologically adapted to its natural environment [33]. Each species or subspecies can therefore be characterized by its adaptive responses to temperature which can be either genetically determined (*genetic adaptation* [45]) or acquired by environmental conditions (*acclimatization*).* These may vary on a daily, tidal, seasonal or latitudinal basis and are often associated with particular phases or stages of a life cycle.

It is not the aim of this chapter to give a complete picture of all possible forms of adaptive adjustments to either cold or heat in various groups or classes of animals. The major object will be to outline and exemplify the main principles by which animals, both poikilothermic and homeothermic, aquatic and terrestrial, adapt to variations in the thermal environment during life time.

13.2 MODES OF THERMAL ADAPTATION

13.2.1 Resistance and capacity adaptation

Adjustments to long-term and to seasonal changes in climatic conditions may involve behavioural, morphological or physiological processes. Morphological and behavioural adjustments are initiated, accompanied or followed by functional changes at central nervous, organ and cellular levels. These can be described as *resistance adaptation* or *capacity adaptation* [30].

Resistance thermal adaptation refers to the survival limits of a whole organism as well as of functions on the suborganic level (see Chapter 12), and is conventionally demonstrated by a *tolerance polygon* (Fig. 13.1). The figure shows the temperature limits for survival of a fish, the sockeye salmon (*Oncorhynchus nerka*) of the Pacific coast, which has been studied in fresh water by Brett and co-workers [17]. The two lines labelled 'upper and lower lethal temperature' represent the incipient lethal temperatures at which 50% of the sample can survive indefinitely continued exposure. The two outer lines show the temperatures which kill 50% of the sample at the indicated length of time (1000 or 100 min, respectively). The graph also shows the selected (*preference*) temperature of this species at various acclimation temperatures. The size of the polygon and its relative position within the two coordinates is a characteristic of this species.

Capacity thermal adaptation is measured as any rate function of an animal under various environmental temperatures. This indicates the capability of an animal to adjust metabolically for changes in temperature. The interaction of both types of adaptive responses, resistance and capacity adaptation, has not been studied extensively and may open interesting aspects for future research.

* If an animal is studied under the influence of one controlled environmental factor, the term *acclimation* is conventionally used in order to distinguish between naturally induced (acclimatization) and artificially induced (acclimation) changes [45].

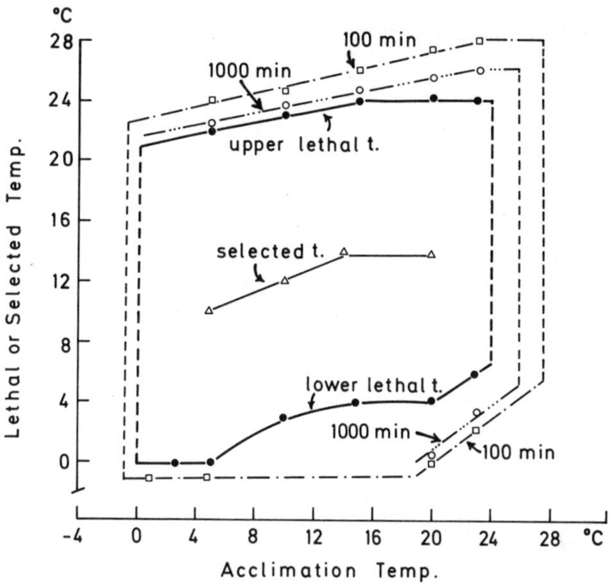

Fig. 13.1. Upper and lower lethal temperatures (tolerance polygon) and selected (preference) temperature of the sockeye salmon (*Oncorhynchus nerka*), in fresh water, in relation to acclimation temperature. The inner polygon represents the temperature tolerance at which 50% of the sample survives on unlimited time of exposure. The two outer polygons refer to 1000 and 100 mins of exposure, respectively. Modified from [17].

13.2.2 Types of metabolic compensation

In poikilothermic animals, especially aquatic forms but also in terrestrial insects, metabolic compensation is the principal mechanism of adjustment to fluctuating thermal conditions [32, 37].

The two general schemes (Fig. 13.2) are described in order to demonstrate different types of compensatory adjustments of rate functions in poikilothermic animals. Both schemes differ mainly in the way the measurements are made.

On the upper left diagram of the figure (Fig. 13.2A), 5 types of responses of rate functions (for instance, respiration) are shown [30]. When a poikilothermic animal which has been maintained (acclimated) at a particular temperature (T_1) is transferred to a higher temperature (T_2), its metabolic rate increases to a new level (solid line A_1A_2). This is a direct response to the new temperature. If the animal is maintained at this new temperature for days or weeks, compensation normally occurs in that its metabolism either gradually returns to the level it held before at T_1 (ideal or perfect compensation; Type 2), or to some new level. It may also overcompensate (supraoptimal compensation; Type 1), or maintain a level above that of the direct response (inverse compensation; Type 5). No subsequent change (Type 4) indicates that the animal does not compensate or acclimate for changing temperature. Whether the animal has been acclimated to the new temperature (T_2) or not, can be tested by returning it to the original temperature (T_1). When its metabolic rate has been stabilized at the higher acclimation temperature, metabolism falls below the level originally held at T_1 (solid line B_1B_2).

In the above scheme, the animals are being tested at only two acclimation temperatures and the compensatory responses can be studied at steady state and during the course of acclimation (see below). The second scheme which has been developed by Prosser [31], describes 5 types of acclimatory responses which are based on the relative position and the slopes of the rate-temperature (R–T) relations of animals which have been acclimated to different temperatures and measured over a range of test ambient temperatures (Fig. 13.2; diagrams B 1–5).

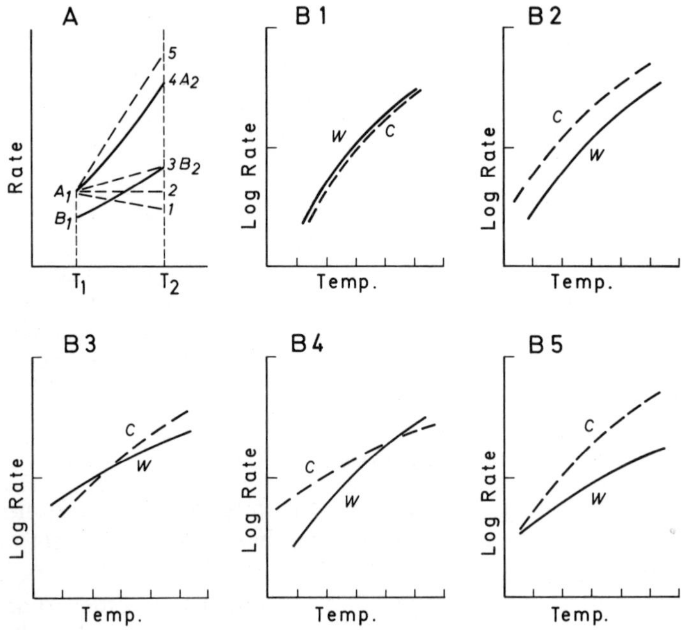

Fig. 13.2. Types of capacity thermal adaptation. A: Rate function measured at two test ambient temperatures. Acclimation temperature for curve $A_1A_2 = T_1$; for curve $B_1B_2 = T_2$ (from Precht *et al.* [30]). B1–5: Patterns of acclimation of rate functions measured at different test temperatures. *W* for warm-acclimated animals; *C* for cold-acclimated animals. From [32].

When there is no acclimation, the R–T curves coincide for animals maintained at different temperatures (Type B1). If the R–T curve is higher or lower in one group but does not cross the other(s), this type of acclimation is termed *translation type* (Type B2). If one curve rotates about a midpoint, which means that the slope changes, the response is called *rotation type* (Type B3). In many experimental data, a combination of the translation and rotation types of responses has been observed which allows the distinction of two further types (translation and rotation type; Types B4 and B5). These types of compensatory responses are characterized by the intersection of the R–T curves of the different acclimation groups at either the higher or the lower end of the temperature scale.

For each of these types, numerous examples have been described [27, 32, 34,

37); although it is often difficult to distinguish clearly between different types, particularly between Types B3 and B4 or B5. Some categories are characteristic of particular enzyme reactions and activities [27, 31].

The two schemes which have been developed primarily for responses of poikilothermic animals (*ectotherms*), are, in a more general sense, applicable also for homeotherms (*endotherms*). Contrary to the direct and positive relation between rate function and tissue or environmental temperature (conventionally given as Q_{10} of the Van't Hoff–Arrhenius plot) in poikilotherms, the metabolic rate of homeotherms is, within a broad range of environmental temperature reversely related to ambient or peripheral (skin) temperature. Homeotherms regulate their body temperature against a thermal gradient between the body and the environment by adjusting various rate functions which are associated

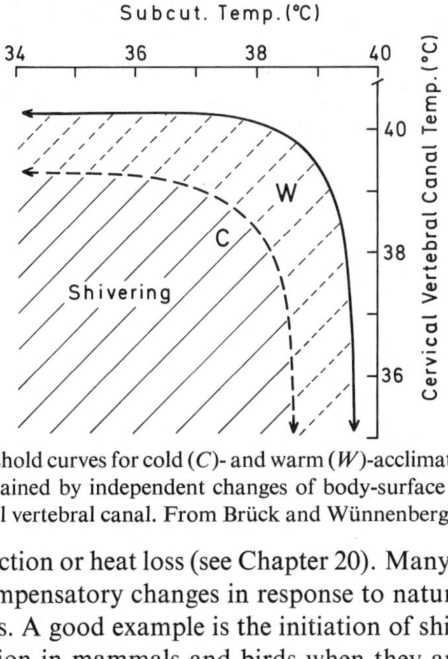

Fig. 13.3. Shivering threshold curves for cold (*C*)- and warm (*W*)-acclimated guinea-pigs (4 to 8 weeks of age). Values obtained by independent changes of body-surface temperature and the temperature of the cervical vertebral canal. From Brück and Wünnenberg; modified from [23].

with either heat production or heat loss (see Chapter 20). Many of these functions show considerable compensatory changes in response to naturally or artificially changing temperatures. A good example is the initiation of shivering, which is a thermal defence reaction in mammals and birds when they are exposed to low ambient temperatures, and which is activated by the influence of input signals from the thermosensors in the central body and at the periphery (see Chapter 20). The threshold curves for elicitating shivering have been measured in guinea-pigs of the age of 4 to 8 weeks by independent heating and cooling of the body surface and the cervical vertebral canal (Fig. 13.3) [23]. Over the total range of determination, the threshold curve of the animals reared in the cold (cold-acclimated) lies below that of animals reared in the warmth (warm-acclimated) which is a 'translation response' (Type B2, Fig. 13.2).

13.2.3 Time course of thermal adaptation

The time course of compensatory adjustments after transferring an animal from one acclimation temperature to another can be studied by measuring rate functions, like respiration or excretion rate, at intervals after the transfer. Acclimation to heat (see Section 13.4) can be complete within 24 hours [11]. Acclimation to cold (see Section 13.3) reaches steady state within 20 days in most animal species, both poikilothermic and homeothermic, but can also be achieved within one day in some species [6, 8, 11, 21]. The time necessary for gain or loss of acclimation can be very similar, as, for instance, in the insect *Blatella germanica* [8]. If a reduced ambient (and body) temperature induces cold torpor (below 15°C in this species), no further acclimation takes place.

Another important parameter in the study of thermal adaptation is the time pattern of exposure to cold or heat which is required for complete acclimation or acclimatization. The pattern can be a single-step change in temperature, a steadily increasing or decreasing temperature, or intermittent changes in temperature as they naturally occur during daily or seasonal cycles. All of these different patterns exert acclimatory influences on animals, for example, by changing survival rate or thermoregulatory functions [23]. Cyclic changes in climatic conditions have been of particular relevance for the evolution of daily (*circadian*) and seasonal (*circannual*) rhythms which are related also to behavioural, morphological and physiological thermal adaptations (see Chapter 15).

13.2.4 Non-thermal influences on thermal adaptation

Although temperature is the dominant factor which activates most thermal adjustments, other environmental factors, light, humidity, oxygen pressure, salinity of water, etc., are of considerable importance [34]. Diet, age, body size, and even increased physical fitness by exercise can also modify the acclimatory responses to temperature in animals [23, 34]. For example, in a slug (*Arion circumscriptus*) it has been shown that body weight influences the changes in oxygen consumption during cold- and warm-acclimation [11]. In larger individuals the compensatory changes in metabolic rate during acclimation to cold were greater than in smaller individuals, when rates of metabolism were measured at the same experimental temperature. Similar size-dependent compensatory changes have been found in insects and arachnids [11] and may occur also in vertebrates.

Besides the difference in metabolic acclimation between individuals of the same species, different types of acclimation responses, according to Precht's and Prosser's classification, have also been found at various stages of the life cycle of an individual or during ontogenetic development [37].

Light as an effective stimulus for thermal adaptation needs special consideration [2, 21]. For example, a photoperiodic stimulus can cause the development of the brown adipose tissue, which is a thermogenetic organ involved in metabolic acclimatization to cold in small mammals, and especially in hibernators [56, 59]. Seasonal acclimatization is a gradual process with a rhythmic component. This may be an endogenous rhythmicity as with other seasonally changing behavioural and physiological functions (see Chapter 15). Photoperiod acts only as a timing factor (*Zeitgeber*). It synchronizes rhythmic modifications in the neuro-endocrine system with the seasonally changing environment; thus preparing the animals for defence against heat or cold before a change in the environmental temperature itself becomes effective [21].

13.3 ADAPTATION TO COLD

13.3.1 Behavioural mechanisms

(a) Invertebrates

The locomotory behaviour of invertebrates when the temperature of the environment is suddenly changed may be directed or undirected (shock). Unicellular organisms (ciliates) and higher invertebrates (ants and locusts) aggregate at a particular selected temperature (*preference temperature*). Mosquito larvae (*Aedes communis*), for instance, aggregate in the warmest part of a pool and travel clockwise around the pool during the day according to the position of the sun [11]. Directed orientation to the sun (positive phototaxis) and the selection of suitable micro-habitats is particularly necessary for the survival of insects at northern latitudes. These creatures need radiant solar energy to sustain the active phase of their life cycles during the arctic and antarctic summer [11].

Temperature preference may vary with different stages in the life cycle of an individual: for instance, during certain instar larval stages, before pupation and in the adult. Larvae of the housefly (*Musca domestica*) feed at preferred temperatures between 30° and 37°C, but pupation in the ground occurs at 15°C [11]. The preferred range of temperature and the threshold for spontaneous movements can be modified by acclimation or acclimatization. Herter, who pioneered the studies on temperature preferences in animals by means of a temperature gradient apparatus, observed clustering of ants (*Formica rufa*) at 23·5°C after acclimation to 3–5°C. Ants acclimated to 25–27°C clustered at 32°C [11]. Similar examples from other insect species have been reported since [34, 39]. In the crayfish *Orconectes immunis*, which has been studied in a temperature gradient under natural light conditions, the preferred temperature showed a daily cycle which was associated with the daily rhythm of activity and rest [51].

Many activities of insects and other invertebrates, such as feeding at favoured localities, burrowing during periods of inactivity and basking in the sun are under the control of endogenous *c.* 24 h-rhythms (circadian rhythms). Many congeneric insect species, for example carabids, are either day-active (*diurnal*) or night-active (*nocturnal*) according to their dependence on temperature and (or) humidity [77]. The survival value of these rhythms lies primarily in the anticipation of events that may be harmful for an organism [40]. For example, the eclosion of many insect species from pupae is rigidly controlled by endogenous timing mechanisms (endogenous clocks) that permit delicate structural, physiological and behavioural modifications to occur at the most favourable environmental conditions [71].

(b) Poikilothermic vertebrates

Poikilothermic vertebrates, both aquatic and terrestrial forms, also select temperatures which are optimal for their various activities. Several species of fish which have been acclimated to different temperatures, differ in their preference temperatures and in other functions, such as cruising speed or shock reaction [15]. The animal performs best at a particular temperature when it has been acclimated to that temperature [16]. Using the data of McCrimmon [16] this can be demonstrated in two species of fish, the Atlantic salmon (*Salmo salar*) and

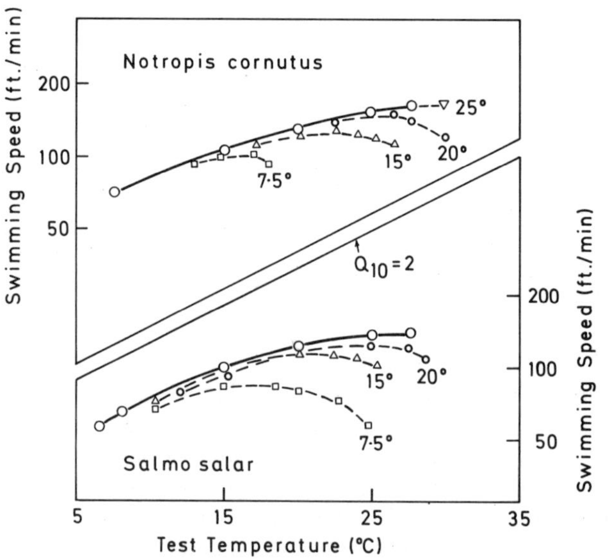

Fig. 13.4. Influence of temperature on cruising speed of young Atlantic salmon (*Salmo salar*) and the minnow (*Notropis cornutus*) in relation to acclimation temperature. The dashed lines connecting symbols refer to measurements of acclimated fish at various indicated acclimation temperatures. Solid lines connect values of fish acclimated to the respective test temperature. Data from McCrimmon; after [16].

the minnow (*Notropis cornutus*) (Fig. 13.4). The influence of thermal history on performance is shown in the upper temperature range: the decrease in performance with increasing ambient temperature is directly related to acclimation temperature. The effect of acclimation on the temperature preferendum has been mostly studied in fishes; the responses are diverse, however, and both positive and slightly negative correlation coefficients occur [15]. In fish, the *final preferendum*, the temperature at which acclimation temperature and preferred temperature are identical, may indicate the temperature in nature at which a species will be found during its active season or the optimum temperature for activity [15, 16]. In reptiles, the temperature preferenda show good agreement with the body temperature during activity in nature [16].

Basking in the sun is one of the principal behavioural mechanisms by which terrestrial poikilotherms, especially reptiles, regulate body temperature. Lizards are known to shuttle between sun and shade in order to maintain a preferred body temperature [12, 36]. Reptiles may prefer a body temperature that is optimal for one particular state of activity, but they may also be active at a particular time of day at non-preferred temperatures [36]. The significance of daily rhythms has been demonstrated by Heath in the lizard *Phrynosoma solare*. The animal emerges from the soil, where it rests during the night, before the temperature of the surrounding air increases. An endogenous circadian rhythm allows ectothermic animals to secure a safe nocturnal shelter without losing time for activity in the sun during the next morning [12].

(*c*) *Homeothermic vertebrates*

Homeothermic vertebrates, particularly small mammals, use behavioural mechanisms mainly to conserve heat rather than to gain heat. Nest-building, burrowing, curling or huddling are the principal means to reduce heat loss to the environment. Activity, which in a broad sense includes many functions controlled by different internal drives and motivations, for example nest building, can also be affected by acclimation [3]. It is still not completely explored in which way different forms of activity contribute to temperature regulation (for instance, by producing heat), although specific movements may reduce heat loss [3].

The ways in which behavioural mechanisms may contribute in order to achieve optimal temperatures have been studied in mice, rats and pigs. These animals learned to press a switch to obtain radiant heat [21, 42, 43]. The experiments on pigs (*Sus scrofa*) by Baldwin and Ingram demonstrated very clearly that the reinforcement behaviour was not only dependent on light or temperature, but primarily on the phases of the daily (circadian) cycle of activity and rest. In both, pigs and mice the rate of reinforcement was affected by acclimation [42].

13.3.2 Morphological mechanisms

Acclimatory changes in structure are mainly to the integument (including extremities and appendages). These changes are to the texture, pigmentation, quality and quantity of hair and feathers or subcutaneous fat, which alter the penetration, absorption and reflection of long- and short-wave radiation [21, 28, 29]. They can be classified as resistance adaptations to temperature and to harmful ultra-violet radiation. Capacity adaptations mostly involve changes in organ weight and structure [19, 20].

The ability to change pigmentation of the skin is well developed in amphibians and reptiles. The extent to which these changes relate to thermoregulation rather than to protection against predators, is not readily discernible. This may depend on the phase of the daily activity cycle of the particular species [12, 36]. The desert iguana (*Dipsosaurus dorsalis*) is dark only for brief periods in the morning while basking to absorb radiant energy while the ambient temperature is still low [28, 36]. In the horned lizard (*Phrynosoma solare*), the degree of pigmentation relates to body size. Larger individuals are darker than smaller ones, probably because of their smaller surface area-to-body mass ratio and hence a slower rate of heat gain per unit mass [46].

A common feature of most mammals and birds is that they change their pelage or plumage from summer to winter and vice versa. In mammals, the insulative property of the fur is proportional to its thickness [21]. Winter fur of wild mice, rats, hares and other mammals is different from summer fur in both quantity (number of hair fibres per unit surface area) and quality (which may be estimated by trapped air) [21]. The absolute change in thickness is greater in large mammals; it varies between about 10% in mice and about 50% in bear and wolf [21]. In birds, feathers are primarily adapted for flight; therefore only small changes in plumage can occur in response to heat and cold [25]. Only in larger species, for instance in the willow ptarmigan (*Lagopus lagopus*), do seasonal plumage changes contribute substantially to temperature regulation by varying the overall thermal conductance and the lower critical temperature at which insulative (vasomotor) regulation changes to metabolic regulation [81].

In addition to seasonal changes in pelage and plumage, morphological modifications in organ weight (for example, the heart) and in insulating tissues (subcutaneous fat) occur in response to cold acclimation or acclimatization [19, 20, 25]. Rats which have been reared in the cold have shorter tails. This reduction in surface area conserves heat [50].

Most structural modifications that protect invertebrates against cold relate to particular stages during development. Conspicuous examples are the pupae of insects which permit overwintering in a state of quiescence. This and similar stages in lower invertebrates are under neuro-endocrine control and are influenced or initiated by seasonally changing environmental factors (see Chapter 15).

13.3.3 Physiological mechanisms

(*a*) *Invertebrates*

Physiological adjustments to cold during the life cycle of invertebrates can be divided into 3 categories: (i) changes which increase cold tolerance (resistance adaptation); (ii) metabolic changes which allow activity at low temperature (capacity adaptation); and (iii) changes which permit the reduction of metabolic rate to a lower level (state of quiescence or torpor).

The capability of a species to acclimate or acclimatize to cold reflects the past thermal history and the latitude of its habitat [27]. This can be illustrated by two subspecies of the copepod *Euterpina acutifrons* from the Atlantic coasts of Brazil (24°S lat.) and of South Carolina (35°N lat.) [80]. Both populations of the small (dimorphic) males show the same general pattern of thermal acclimation: a greater range of metabolic compensation at low temperature than at high temperature (Fig. 13.5). The more southern population has a lower metabolic rate at

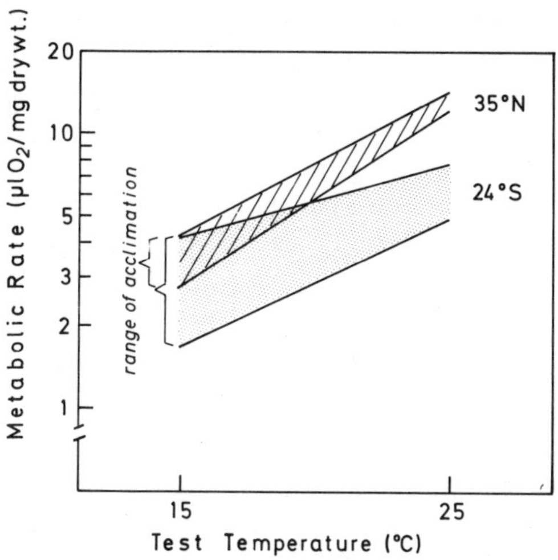

Fig. 13.5. Range of acclimation of metabolic rate in two populations of small males of the copepod *Euterpina acutifrons* living at the Atlantic coast of South Carolina (35°N lat.) and of Brazil (24°S lat.). The animals were acclimated to either 15° or 25°C and each group was tested at both temperatures. The cross-hatched and stippled areas refer to the total ranges of possible acclimation in the two geographic populations. From [80].

the higher temperature reflecting better adaptation to its mean habitat temperature. Species living in arctic climate with little temperature variation are less able to modify their physiological responses than are species living under more variable climatic conditions. An example is the endemic antarctic crustacean *Euphausia superba*. Its maximum motor activity occurs at −1·8°C which is the freezing point of sea water. At 4°C, 100% of the population dies within 24 hours [27]. The range of tolerance is a characteristic of each state of development of a species. In the pupae of the pyralid moth, *Anagasta kühniella*, the mortality rate is affected not only by temperature and the duration of acclimation, but also by age [11].

Many invertebrates respond to a lowered temperature with metabolic compensation. The influence of acclimation has been measured in many species, both aquatic and terrestrial [8, 11, 37]. In the slug *Arion circumscriptus*, for instance, metabolic rate decreases 1 to 1·5% per degree increase in acclimation temperature between 5 and 25°C [11]. Seasonal acclimatization has also been reported, for example, in the tropical earthworm *Megascolex mauritti*. Metabolic rate at the same ambient temperature was higher during winter than during summer. In addition, the relation between metabolism and body weight varied with season [11].

Temporary quiescence is a well-known phenomenon during various states of development in insects and other invertebrates. It normally occurs as seasonal dormancy (diapause or hibernation) (see Chapter 15).

(*b*) *Poikilothermic vertebrates*

The existence of fish in arctic waters the temperature of which never rises more than 1°C above zero, has puzzled physiologists. The concept of cold adaptation which implies that arctic fish have a higher metabolic rate than congeneric species living in warmer waters, has been criticized mainly on the grounds that high metabolic rate requires high energy input and reduces the ability to increase metabolism above this already high standard level (scope of activity) [14, 60]. In a recent survey, Holeton presented metabolic data from 11 species of fishes which live in the shallow waters of Resolute Bay in northern Canada at water temperatures around −1·7°C for most of the year. The rate of oxygen uptake of most arctic species was found to be well below the levels generally considered indicative of cold-adaptation. Important findings were: (i) that it normally takes several hours from the beginning of capture until respiratory gas exchange of a fish has reached equilibrium; and (ii) that the degree of spontaneous activity varies widely among different species [60]. Wells, a pioneer in this field, had already suggested that metabolic compensation is largely effected by changes in locomotion [17]. The optimum temperature, at which metabolism is highest, and the range of temperature tolerance of fish can be altered by acclimation [16]. Since the supply of oxygen limits the range of maximal activity, metabolic compensation involves changes in the mechanisms of oxygen uptake and transport. In the goldfish (*Carassius auratus*), differences in hemoglobin concentration and the number of hemoglobin components have been found to be related to different acclimation temperatures [61].

Resistance adaptation as well as capacity adaptation to cold is well documented in reptiles [12, 36]. The critical temperature minimum (CTm) at which coordinate locomotory movements are lost, has been determined in 29 Australian lizards and 4 snakes (involving 13 genera) by Spellerberg [75]. During summer, the CTm varied between 2·2 and 9·8°C. Acclimation to one degree below the CTm shifted the critical temperature minimum in each species to a lower temperature within 24 hours. A steady state was reached within 10 days. The lowest recorded temperature at which the locomotor responses could still be observed in the cold acclimated animal was −0·52°C. The variability of the CTm due to acclimation or acclimatization allows compensation for changes in environmental temperature throughout the year, even for short-term changes. A circadian variation in CTm has also been found under natural and artificial day–night conditions as well as at constant illumination and temperature. This is evidently endogenous (Fig. 13.6) [76]. In general, metabolic compensation constitutes only a part of total adaptation to cold in amphibians and reptiles. Behavioural mechanisms and physiological adjustments which are associated with the reduction of metabolic processes (cold torpor) are superior for survival in cold environments [5, 12, 36].

(*c*) *Homeothermic vertebrates*

Birds and mammals, as well as some reptiles during particular states of life, are able to maintain relatively constant body temperature. These animals have achieved a high level of homeostatic control of body temperature by regulating

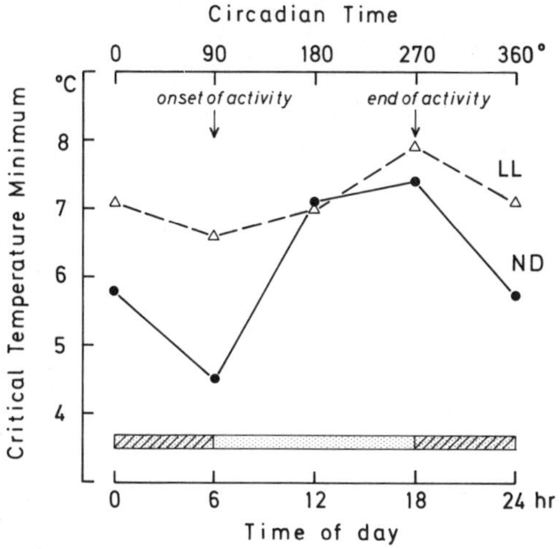

Fig. 13.6. Critical temperature minimum (CTm) of the lizard *Lacerta sicula* as a function of time. ND (lower time scale): animals kept under natural daylight condition and temperatures (10–33°C); LL (upper time scale): animals kept under constant light (*c.* 50 lux) and temperature (26°C). Data from [76].

heat production and heat loss [2, 4]. Species that live in a cold environment during at least parts of their lives, have developed means of changing metabolic processes (for instance the ability to switch to non-shivering thermogenesis), vascularization and vasomotor control and the tolerance of peripheral tissues to cold [20, 21]. Irving has called attention to the fact that metabolic adjustments of animals living in cold climates are limited since they require period of rest and of social activities to the same extent as do animals that inhabit warmer regions: 'The decisive difference in resisting cold lies in the mechanisms for conserving heat' [62; p. 94]. The crucial factor which limits insulative adaptation is body size. Smaller mammals and birds rely primarily on metabolic adjustments, while larger species in both groups of animals adjust to cold mainly by changes in insulation [19, 73, 81].

An animal's overall thermal conductance can be described mathematically by a model that relates total conductance (or its reciprocal total insulation) to the rate of heat loss per degree change in ambient temperature [19, 20, 69, 72]. This model is based on Newton's law of cooling as modified by Fourier to apply to the heat exchange between a body of known surface and the surrounding air [65]. If body temperature remains constant, heat production may be substituted for heat loss. The following simple equation applies

$$H = C_t\,(T_b - T_a)$$

where H is heat loss per surface area (or heat production), C_t is the overall (total) thermal conductance or heat transfer coefficient, T_b is mean body temperature and T_a ambient temperature.

This model is graphically shown as Type I in Fig. 13.7. Overall thermal conductance (C_t) refers to the slope of the curve or line which relates heat production (metabolic rate) to ambient temperature. If C_t remains constant over the range of ambient temperature tested, the straight line representing heat loss or heat production intersects the temperature scale at mean body temperature (T_b). B and B' represent the lower critical temperature, measured at the temperature scale, for warm- and cold-acclimated or summer- and winter-acclimatized

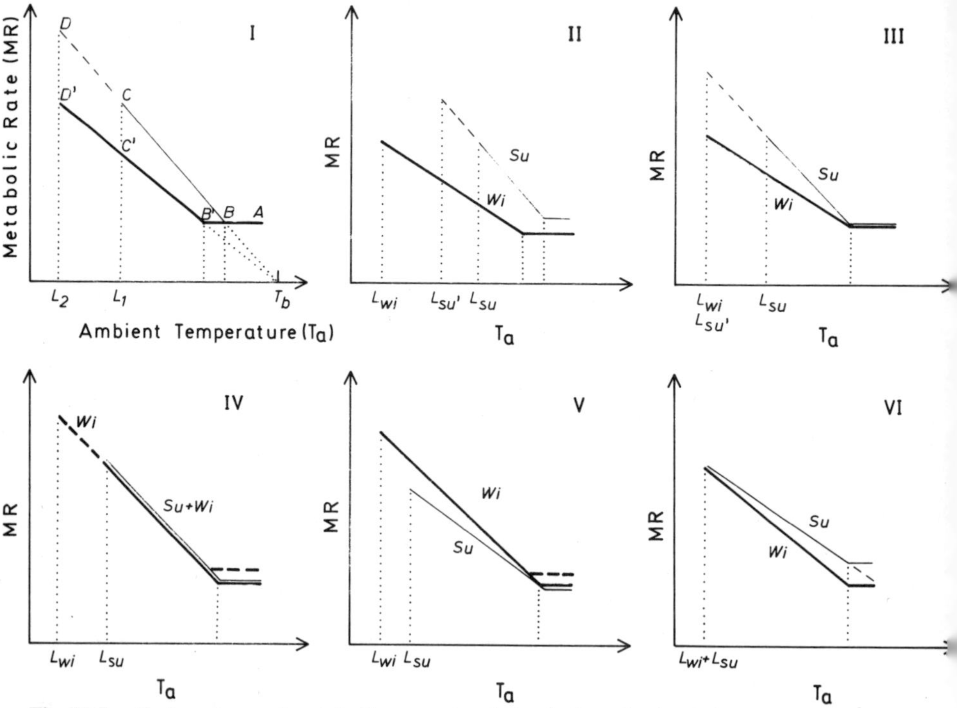

Fig. 13.7. Various types of metabolic versus insulative acclimatization in homeotherms. Basic model (Type I) from Hart [19]. Extension of the low temperature limits from L_1 to L_2 may be carried out through insulative or metabolic adjustment. Insulative acclimatization implies a lowering of the critical temperature from B to B' and a change in slope from BC to $B'C'D'$, so that the energy expenditure is not greater at L_2 (D') than at L_1 (C). Metabolic acclimatization implies an extension of the line BC to BCD, with greater energy expenditure at L_2 (D) than at L_1 (C). Types II–VI show modifications of the basic model as derived from empirical data (see text). Su = summer-acclimatized animals; Wi = winter-acclimatized animals.

animals, respectively, below which heat production increases. AB or AB' is the metabolically neutral temperature zone at which only insulative (physical) regulation occurs. C or C' and D or D' indicate the maximal level of heat production at the temperature limits (L_1 or L_2) for the respective acclimation temperatures or seasons. It must always be borne in mind, however, that both endogenous and exogenous factors (including methods of determination) can modify the responses. The most obvious variations are day–night (circadian) differences [41, 72].

Summer and winter differences in the lower critical temperature without and with differences in basal or resting metabolic rate (Types I and II), are typical for large mammals (e.g. porcupine, fox, hare (see Fig. 13.9), seal [19–22]) and for relatively large birds (willow ptarmigen [81]). These differences are due principally to changes in insulation of fur or feathers. Differences like those of Type III have been found mainly in birds, for instance in the great tit (*Parus major*) [58]. Seasonal modifications that can only be measured when the animals are exposed to very low temperatures include increased capacity for producing heat during winter or cold and (or) extended time for maintenance of high heat production (Type IV). Examples have been described for small mammals (deermice) and several species of small birds [21]. Type V has been recently observed in a small passerine bird (*Acanthis flammea*) that lives in subarctic conditions during winter [73]. The enhanced capacity of this 14 gram-bird to produce heat (measured while resting during the day) may reflect its ability to metabolize almost as much energy during short daily photoperiods in subarctic winter as during long photoperiods in summer [21]. Birds that do not possess the ability to acclimate metabolically or by changing thermal conductance, or which show seasonal differences like that of Type VI, as for instance the blackcap warbler (*Sylvia atricapilla* [66], cannot withstand winter at northern latitudes. These birds normally migrate to warmer climate (see Chapter 15).

(*d*) *Heterothermic vertebrates*

Most homeotherms are poikilothermic during the early time of life. Infant mammals or nestling birds can withstand low body temperature that would kill them when they have fully developed control of body temperature [1]. For instance, the mountain white-crowned sparrow (*Zonotrichia leucophrys oriantha*) when taken out of the nest and exposed to 6°C for 10 min, cools down to 20°C without harmful effects until the age of 3 days. At the age of 7 days, the bird becomes fully homeothermic [70].

Daily torpor is a characteristic of many small rodents and insectivores (bats) and also of some birds. It saves energy or conserves food reserves during unfavourable environmental conditions. The pocket mouse (*Perognathus californicus*) can enter torpor and arouse immediately thereafter at an ambient temperature of 15°C with an expenditure of energy only 55% of that required to maintain a high body temperature over the same period [78]. Small birds, like hummingbirds or African sunbirds (*Nectarinia* spp.) that live at high altitude up to 4500 metres, reduce metabolism (and hence body temperature) during their rest period [13, 49]. The poor-will (*Phalaenoptilus nuttallii*) can lower its body temperature down to 8·5°C at an air temperature of about 5°C [13].

In some small mammals, for instance the deermouse, *Peromyscus leucopus* [54] or the Djungarian dwarf hamster, *Phodopus sungorus* [53], daily torpor only occurs during winter. Winter dormancy (in bears) and true hibernation which require deep changes in the whole organism are considered in Chapter 15.

13.4 ADAPTATION TO HEAT

13.4.1 Behavioural mechanisms

(*a*) *Invertebrates*

Animals which are not specially adapted for life in high water or air temperatures avoid high temperatures even when body temperature can be actively lowered by physiological mechanisms [11]. Burrowing is the most successful behavioural adaptation in terrestrial annelids, molluscs and arthropods. A remarkable behavioural adjustment against overheating and dessication can however be observed in some semi-aquatic forms that live in the tidal zone along coasts. During low tide, these animals would be exposed to high solar radiation. Tidal migrators, like the sand beach amphipod *Synchelidium* sp. move up and down the beach with rising and falling water. The amphipod's tidal activity rhythm has characteristics comparable to those of circadian rhythms. The rhythm will persist for weeks and even months in the laboratory far from sea and the concurrent environmental stimuli with a period which deviates from 24 hrs 51 min (that is twice the normal period of the tidal cycle). Endogenous timing allow these crustaceans to be independent of environmental stimuli such as concurrent waves which are unreliable indicators of the critical phase of the tide [52].

Similarly, day–night (circadian) rhythms are involved in many activities of desert insects [10]. Most of these species are active only during the night or emerge from the pupal state at dusk when temperature and water conditions are most favourable [9, 40].

(*b*) *Poikilothermic vertebrates*

Among poikilothermic vertebrates, reptiles are the most characteristic inhabitants of hot desert climate. The thermal preferendum of reptiles is not greatly modified by acclimation and must therefore be considered a genetically determined characteristic of a species [35, 36].

A distinct temporal programme of activities related to temperature regulation can be observed in the marine iguana *Amblyrhynchus cristatus* from the Galapagos Islands. This reptile orients its body to the sun or away from it according to its thermoregulatory need [82]. The daily cycle of thermoregulatory behaviour is illustrated for sub-adult males, young animals and for the breeding colony during the time of harem formation (Fig. 13.8). During the early morning after returning from feeding at sea, the iguanas bask in the sun with flat posture in order to gain maximal heat. After warming up they re-enter the breeding colony. During midday, an elevated basking posture facilitates regulation of heat gain and heat loss. This results in a relatively constant body temperature of 38°C in adult iguanas over an air temperature range between 24 and 53°C. Heat loss can be increased by exposing parts of the body to the cold wind stream from sea.

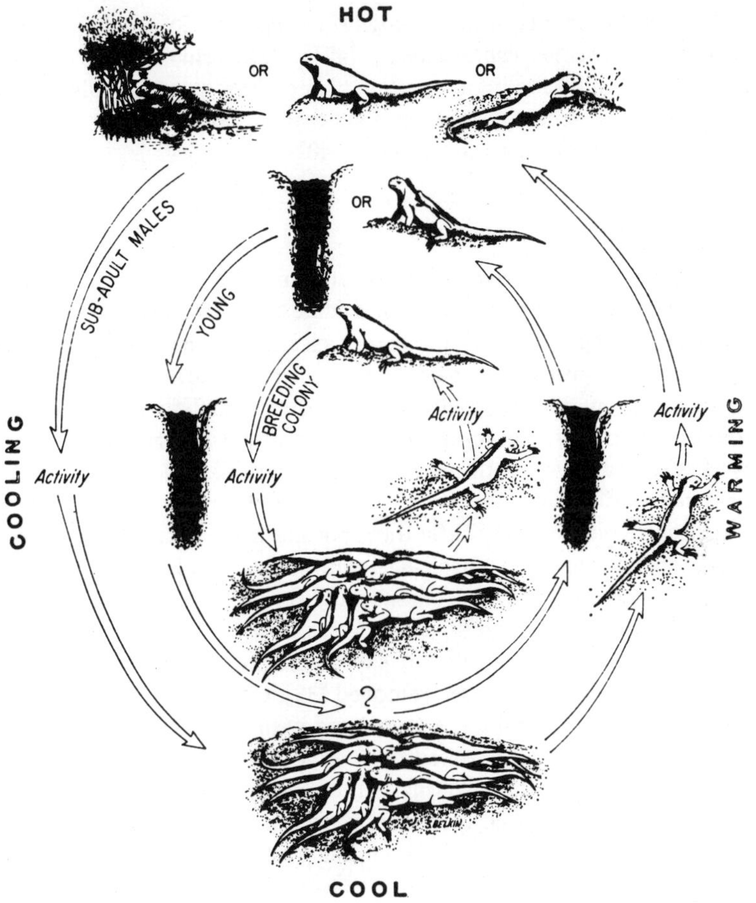

Fig. 13.8. The daily cycle of temperature related behaviour of 3 types of Galapagos marine iguana sub-groups (sub-adult males, young animals and breeding colony) during the time of harem formation. From [82] with permission.

After sunset, when ambient temperature falls, the iguanas cluster together with their heads directed towards the centre [36, 82].

(*c*) *Homeothermic vertebrates*

Small mammals, which have large surface areas in relation to body mass, gain heat more rapidly when exposed to the sun in desert climate than do larger mammals. Most small desert species therefore spend the day in burrows (for example kangaroo rats and jumping mice), and become active at night. Diurnal species, like the desert antelope squirrel (*Ammospermophilus leucurus*) retreat into their burrows when the climatic conditions become stressful as during the middle of the day [24]. Birds also seek shade. This behaviour has been explicitly demonsrated in the cactus wren (*Campylorhynchus bruneicapillus*) [74] and in the roadrunner (*Geococcyx californianus*) [47]. Daily rhythms are particularly marked in desert and savannah species which endure large day–night variations in temperature, but such rhythms are a general characteristic of most mammals and birds in all climatic circumstances [9, 40].

13.4.2 Morphological mechanisms

Most invertebrates which live in desert climate or in areas with hot summers, spend the warmest part of the year in a state of dormancy (estivation or diapause), either as eggs, larvae, pupae or as adults. The associated structural changes may be considerable particularly when estivation involves a state of extreme dessication. These modifications are related chiefly to the low humidity or drought conditions. Some animals, for example desert snails, can remain inactive for several years until the next heavy rainfall [11].

Some morphological adaptations which enable animals to withstand heat stress are genotypic and vary little during a life time. Changes in fur or in the length of appendages during heat acclimation are mostly considered to be the converse of those during cold acclimation [22].

Fur or feathers can serve as a barrier against heat gain as well as against heat loss. The body temperature of sheep increases during exposure to solar radiation after the fleece has been removed [38]. Changes in colour or glossiness of fur have also been found to be associated with differences in heat resistance. South African cattle with sleek summer coats have lower body temperatures than have animals with dark woolly winter coats [21]. However, because of its higher reflectivity of infra-red radiation, the dense coat of black sheep is a better insulator than the thinner coat of brown sheep [38]. The property of mammalian pelt or avian plumage in absorbing or reflecting radiant energy is different for short and long wavelength [29]. Infra-red emissivity and convective heat loss from differently coloured pelts or plumage have been found to be related only to the temperature difference between the hair or feather surface and the environment [55]. Thus, it must be assumed that different mechanisms (colour, density, glossiness) act in a complementary or compensatory way to minimize radiative heat gain or facilitate heat loss [68].

13.4.3 Physiological mechanisms

(*a*) *Invertebrates*

The principal physiological adaptations of animals living in hot climate are: (i) a lowering of metabolism, (ii) an increase in evaporation, and (iii) estivation or diapause. Terrestrial invertebrates exposed to high ambient temperature are threatened at the same time by dessication. Thus, heat and water balance are closely related, particularly in those animals that lack a protective integument.

Both the incipient upper lethal temperature and the tolerable duration of exposure to a high ambient temperature have been used as criteria for heat tolerance. Generally, the upper lethal temperature is changed less by acclimation to heat than is the lower lethal temperature by acclimation to cold. This may be because the optimum temperature is usually very close to the upper lethal temperature [33]. Metabolic compensation has been studied in some tropical invertebrates, including molluscs, crustaceans and other arthropods. Animals acclimated to about 34°C had a 10 to 15% lower metabolic rate than animals acclimated to 20°C when both groups were measured at 20°C. At 34°C ambient temperature, the difference between the two acclimation groups increased to about 30% [11].

Estivation or diapause occur widely among invertebrates living in desert environments. Prolonged dormancy may result from either the direct effects of the environment or may be a phase in the normal life cycle of an animal. Its control by endogenous and exogenous factors are considered in Chapter 15.

(*b*) *Poikilothermic vertebrates*

Within genetic limits, many poikilothermic vertebrates can modify their ability to withstand high temperature to various extents by acclimatory changes. The upper limit of heat tolerance has been determined by measuring the incipient *upper lethal temperature* or the *critical temperature maximum* (CTM) which was first introduced by Cowles and Bogert [5, 36]. Animals were exposed to rapid heating of 1°C per minute or slow heating of 1°C or less per day. In the guppy (*Lebistes reticularis*) and in another tropical fish (*Tilapia mossambica*), the CTM depended on the temperature of acclimation, while the upper lethal temperature was not modified by acclimation [16]. This indicates that upper lethal temperature and CTM are independent criteria for determining temperature tolerance.

The average rate of thermal acclimation in fish has been found to be more than 1°C per day and a 1°C change in acclimation temperature which may allow adjustments to even brief changes in ambient temperature in the field [15, 16]. It is noteworthy that the highest acclimatory effect in one species was induced by a 24-hr cyclic fluctuation in ambient temperature. Fry concluded that the effective acclimation temperature may be the daily maximum rather than the daily mean [16].

A daily rhythm of the CTM has been demonstrated in the eastern painted turtle (*Chrysemys picta*) which is comparable to that already mentioned for the critical temperature minimum (CT_m) in section 13.3.3 [36]. Significant effects of photoperiod or season on the CTM have been found in fishes [6, 15, 16], amphibians [67] and in reptiles [16]. In the painted turtle, a difference in photoperiod between 8 and and 16 hours of light per day was equivalent of a 4°C difference in acclimation temperature [16].

The range of acclimation is as important as the rate of acclimation for successful occupation of climate with relatively large daily or seasonal temperature variations. In North America, high altitude forms of amphibia are similar to low altitude forms at higher latitudes in terms of their ability to acclimate. Species of restricted geographical range have little ability to acclimate [5].

Metabolic compensation has been explicitly demonstrated in species of all 3 classes of poikilothermic vertebrates [5, 16, 17, 36]. In lizards and turtles, long-term exposure to about 35°C resulted in a reduction of metabolic rate at both low and high ambient temperatures (translation type; see section 13.2) as compared to the metabolic rates of animals acclimated to about 15°C. Other species only partially compensated metabolically [12, 36]. Important variables in the mechanisms involved in acclimatory metabolic compensations are heart-stroke volume, O_2-carrying capacity, or the O_2-saturation of blood [78].

(c) *Homeothermic vertebrates*

Physiological adaptations to heat in warm-blooded animals are primarily augmentative adjustments to processes of heat loss. These can be changes in sensible (or non-evaporative) heat loss effected by changes in the conductance of peripheral tissues or insensible (or evaporative) heat loss effected by changes in active sweating or panting. Acclimatory modifications to heat loss have been described in domestic and wild birds [13]. The most obvious differences occurred in the panting response of turtledoves (*Streptopelia turtur*): panting was initiated at higher ambient temperature when the birds had been acclimated to heat [18]. This change in the panting threshold, which has also been found in other species, was associated with a reduced metabolic rate (lower heat load) [7, 13]. Yellow buntings (*Emberiza citrinella*) and ortolans (*E. hortulana*) had decreased metabolic rates at 32·5 and 36°C ambient temperatures, respectively, after they had been maintained at high temperatures for several weeks. This decline did not occur, however, when the birds were exposed to lower temperatures (10–14°C) for 8 hours each day during the acclimation period [13]. This and other observations indicates that metabolic adjustments to heat are not significant in birds when naturally acclimatized.

The effect of acclimation to heat on thermoregulatory mechanisms of mammals has been studied mostly in the larger species. The metabolic rate of the macaque (*Macaca mulatta*), was diminished after prolonged exposure to 35°C compared with those of control monkeys (25°C) and of cold-acclimated (5°C) monkeys [48]. A greater heat resistance which was associated with a reduction in metabolic rate was also found in smaller species, for instance in the golden hamster (*Mesocricetus auratus*) [22].

Seasonal acclimatization in the level of the thermoneutral metabolism, the upper critical temperature, and in evaporative heat loss has been found in the desert cottontail (*Sylvilagus audubonii*) (Fig. 13.9; right diagram [57]). During summer, the zone of thermoneutrality was shifted to higher temperatures, the resting metabolic rate was lower in the upper temperature range, and evaporative heat loss increased at a slower rate with increasing ambient temperature as compared to winter. It is instructive to compare these marked effects with the insignificant effects on the same parameters in a related species, the varying

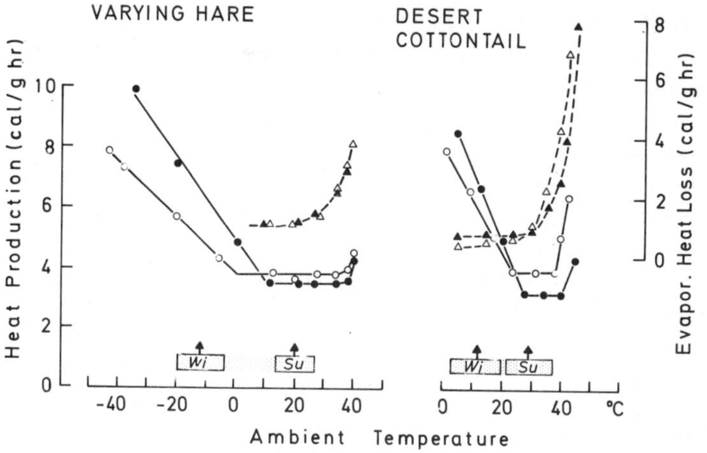

Fig. 13.9. Heat production and evaporative heat loss of desert cottontail (*Sylvilagus audubonii*) and varying hare (*Lepus americanus*) in relation to ambient temperature during summer (closed symbols) and winter (open symbols). Left ordinate (circles): average heat production; right ordinate (triangles): average evaporative heat loss. The bars and arrows along the abscissa refer to the average range and the means of summer and winter temperature at the respective localities where the animals were maintained. Data for varying hare from [22]; data for desert cottontail from [57].

hare (*Lepus americanus*) [22], which is an inhabitant of continental and subarctic climate (Fig. 13.9; left diagram). The significant seasonal changes in the hare obviously lie on the cold side of the temperature range.

The ability of several small rodents to decrease metabolic rate or to increase body temperature (heat storage) without corresponding increase in metabolic rate at high ambient temperature must be considered adaptations to desert life, which can be modified by acclimation [22]. Similar adjustments seem to occur in large mammals (for example calves and pigs) exposed to hot environments. The reduction in metabolic rate was associated with lower food intake and (or) endocrine changes, for instance in thyroid activity [38].

Heat loss from naked appendages has been found to account for a considerable amount of total heat loss in rat, muskrat and beaver [22]. In the rat, the critical temperature for increasing vasodilation in the tail is greatly influenced by acclimation temperature. Tail temperature of rats acclimated to 20°C increased sharply at 26°C ambient temperature, while in rats acclimated to 30°C no vascular response occurred over the tested range of ambient temperature up to 36°C [22]. During heat acclimation in sheep, changes in various physiological functions have been measured: increased water intake, reduced urine volume, higher sodium retention, increased rate of respiratory water loss, and others [21, 38].

13.5 CONCLUSIONS

Phenotypic adaptation (acclimation) of animals to cold or heat has been studied mostly by exposing individuals to controlled temperature conditions for long periods. This is the usual experimental way of determining the range of physiological variations which can occur in a species or race within its genetic capabilities. On the other hand, the study of naturally induced acclimatization—essentially seasonal effects—relates the effects of a single environmental factor to those which occur in more natural circumstances [21]. Although some species do not acclimate to temperatures beyond those representing the normal seasonal temperature range, the capacities for successful acclimatization may require the ability to adapt to temperatures beyond those within the range of variation in a particular habitat [27]. It must be realized that the adaptive variations which occur in animals when exposed to a single controlled environmental factor (for instance: temperature) may not be the same as those which occur when the same individuals are exposed to naturally changing climatic conditions, with or without temperature changes. The influence of various competing environmental factors in the adaptive responses in animals is not fully understood. It is, however, evident that one environmental factor (e.g. photoperiod) can take over—by genetic selection—the role of a factor to which a specific function has been primarily adaptable (e.g. temperature). Generally, differences between acclimation and acclimatization have been found to be less marked in poikilotherms than in homeotherms [34]. This may reflect the different degrees of complexity of thermoregulatory responses of the poikilotherms and homeotherms to changes in the environment.

The genetic potential of a species or race for variation of physiological, morphological and behavioural functions determines its eco-geographic distribution. Natural selection has often tended to favour genetic strains of a species that react in a different way or degree to the environment [11, 33]. If a genetic variation occurs in the direction of some profitable adaptation to a new environment or food resource, it can succeed and result in the evolution of a new subspecies or race, only if it does not compromise the adaptation of the species to other ecological factors. Further studies of the interactions between organisms and their environment at both whole animal and cellular levels are essential [33]. A recent example of the development of new geographic races on the basis of physiological and morphological variation is the house sparrow (*Passer domes-*

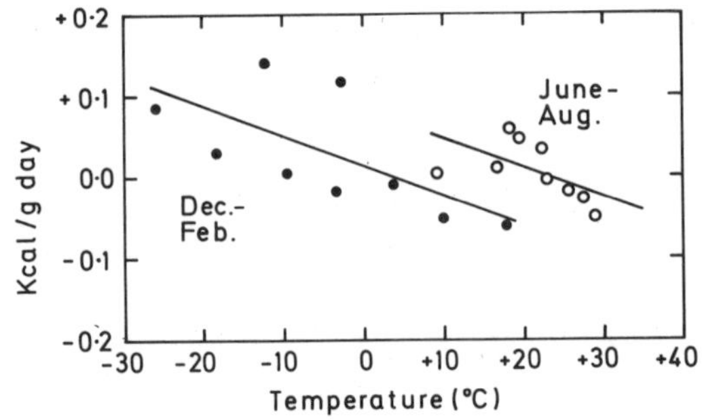

Fig. 13.10. Difference between measured and expected rates of basal metabolism of house sparrows (*Passer domesticus*) during summer and winter in relation to the mean temperature at various geographic localities in North America. From [64].

ticus) [44, 63, 64]. Adaptive adjustments to climatic conditions (including seasonal changes) in various parts of North America, have led to the differentiation of new sub-species which live at distinct localities with widely different climate. The difference between measured and expected rates of basal metabolism in different geographically separated populations of house sparrows has been shown to be a function of the average summer and winter temperature at the respective localities (Fig. 13.10 [64]).

As already pointed out in the preceding sections, behavioural mechanisms play a major role in adaptation to cold and heat. Modifications of behaviour allow animals to cope with environmental stress as well as to explore new environments. It has been suggested that the origin of temperature regulation was by behaviour, as it may still be occurring in reptiles and primitive mammals [26, 33]. Thus, besides physiological and morphological adaptation, behavioural adjustments to the thermal environment may be considered important steps in the sequence of events that favour speciation as well as a higher degree of internal control against outside influences.

Acknowledgement

I gratefully acknowledge critical comments by Drs J. Aschoff and G. Heldmaier.

13.6 REFERENCES

Part 1: Books and reviews

1 Adolph E.F. (1963) How do infant mammals tolerate deep hypothermia? In *Temperature—Its Measurement and Control in Science and Industry* (ed. J. D. Hardy) Vol. 3, Part 3, pp. 511–15. Reinhold, New York.

2 Aschoff J. (1971) Temperaturregulation. In *Physiologie des Menschen* (eds O. H. Gauer, K. Kramer & R. Jung) Bd. 2, pp. 43–116. Urban & Schwarzenberg, Munich, Berlin, Vienna.

3 Barnett S.A. & Mount L.E. (1967) Resistance to cold in mammals. In *Thermobiology* (ed. A. H. Rose) pp. 410–77. Academic Press, New York & London.

4 Bligh J. (1966) The thermosensitivity of the hypothalamus and thermoregulation in mammals. *Biol. Rev.* **41,** 317–67.

5 Brattstrom B.H. (1970) Amphibia. In *Comparative Physiology of Thermoregulation* (ed. G. C. Whittow) Vol. 1, pp. 135–66. Academic Press, New York & London.

6 Brett J.R. (1956) Some principles in the thermal requirements of fishes. *Quart. Rev. Biol.* **31,** 75–87.

7 Calder W.A. & King J.R. (1974) Thermal and coloric relations of birds. In *Avian Biology* (eds D. S. Farner & J. R. King) Vol. 4, pp. 259–413. Academic Press, New York & London.

8 Clarke K.U. (1967) Insects and temperature. In *Thermobiology* (ed. A. H. Rose) pp. 293–352. Academic Press, New York & London.

9 Cloudsley-Thompson J.L. (1961) *Rhythmic Activity in Animal Physiology and Behaviour*. 236 pp. Academic Press, New York & London.

10 Cloudsley-Thompson J.L. (1964) Terrestrial animals in dry heat: arthropods. In *Handbook of Physiology*, Sect. 4 (ed. D. B. Dill) pp. 451–65. Amer. Physiol. Soc. Washington, D.C.

11 Cloudsley-Thompson J.L. (1970) Terrestrial invertebrates. In *Comparative Physiology of Thermoregulation* (ed. G. C. Whittow) Vol. 1, pp. 15–77. Academic Press, New York & London.
12 Cloudsley-Thompson J.L. (1971) *The Temperature and Water Relations of Reptiles.* 159 pp. Merrow, Watford, Herts.
13 Dawson W.R. & Hudson J.W. (1970) Birds. In *Comparative Physiology of Thermoregulation* (ed. G. C. Whittow) Vol. 1, pp. 223–310. Academic Press, New York & London.
14 Dunbar M.J. (1968) Ecological Development in Polar Regions; A Study in Evolution. 119 pp. Prentice-Hall, New Jersey.
15 Fry F.E.J. (1964) Animals in aquatic environments: fishes. In *Handbook of Physiology*, Sect. 4 (ed. D. B. Dill) pp. 715–28. Amer. Physiol. Soc. Washington, D.C.
16 Fry F.E.J. (1967) Responses of vertebrate poikilotherms to temperature. In *Thermobiology* (ed. A. H. Rose) pp. 375–409. Academic Press, New York & London.
17 Fry F.E.J. & Hochachka P.W. (1970) Fish. In *Comparative Physiology of Thermoregulation* (ed. G. C. Whittow) Vol. 1, pp. 79–134. Academic Press, New York & London.
18 Gelineo S. (1964) Organ systems in adaptation: the temperature regulating system. In *Handbook of Physiology*, Sect. 4 (ed. D. B. Dill) pp. 259–82. Amer. Physiol. Soc. Washington, D.C.
19 Hart J.S. (1957) Climatic and temperature induced changes in the energetics of homeotherms. *Rev. Canad. Biol.* **16,** 133–74.
20 Hart J.S. (1963) Physiological responses to cold in non-hibernating homeotherms. In *Temperature—Its Measurement and Control in Science and Industry* (ed. J. D. Hardy) Vol. 3, Part 3, pp. 373–406. Reinhold, New York.
21 Hart J.S. (1964) Geography and season: mammals and birds. In *Handbook of Physiology*, Sect. 4 (ed. D. B. Dill) pp. 295–321. Amer. Physiol. Soc. Washington, D.C.
22 Hart J.S. (1971) Rodents. In *Comparative Physiology of Thermoregulation* (ed. G. C. Whittow) Vol. 2, pp. 1–149. Academic Press, New York & London.
23 Hensel H., Brück K. & Raths P. (1973) Homeothermic Organisms. In *Temperature and Life* (eds H. Precht, J. Christophersen, H. Hensel & W. Larcher) pp. 503–761. Springer-Verlag, Berlin, Heidelberg, New York.
24 Hudson J.W. & Bartholomew G.A. (1964) Terrestrial animals in dry heat: estivators. In *Handbook of Physiology* Sect. 4 (ed. D. B. Dill) pp. 541–50. Amer. Physiol. Soc. Washington, D.C.
25 Irving L. (1972) Arctic Life of Birds and Mammals including Man. In *Zoophysiology and Ecology* (eds D. S. Farner *et al.*) Vol. 2, 192 pp. Springer-Verlag, Berlin, Heidelberg, New York.
26 Johansen K. (1962) Responses to heat and cold in lower mammals (a review). *Int. J. Biometeor.* **6,** 3–28.
27 McWhinnie M.A. (1967) The heat responses of invertebrates (exclusive of insects). In *Thermobiology* (ed. A. H. Rose) pp. 353–73. Academic Press, New York & London.
28 Norris K.S. (1967) Color adaptation in desert reptiles and its thermal relationships. In *Lizard Ecology—a Symposium* (ed. W. W. Milstead) pp. 162–299. University of Missouri Press, Columbia.
29 Øritsland N.A. (1968) Energy significance of absorption of solar radiation in polar homeotherms. In *Antarctic Ecology Symposium* pp. 464–70. Cambridge University Press, London.
30 Precht H., Laudien H. & Havsteen B. (1973) The normal temperature range. In *Temperature and Life* (eds H. Precht, J. Christophersen, H. Hensel & W. Larcher) pp. 302–99. Springer-Verlag, Berlin, Heidelberg, New York.
31 Prosser C.L. (1958) The nature of physiological adaptation. In *Physiological Adaptation* (ed. C. L. Prosser) pp. 167–80. Amer. Physiol. Soc. Washington, D.C.
32 Prosser C.L. (1962) Acclimation of poikilothermic vertebrates to low temperatures. In *Comparative Physiology of Temperature Regulation* (eds J. P. Hannon & E. Viereck) pp. 1–44. Arctic Aeromedical Laboratory, Fort Wainwright, Alaska.
33 Prosser C.L. (1965) Levels of biological organization and their physiological significance.

In *Ideas in Modern Biology* (ed. J. A. Moore) Proc. XVI Int. Congr. Zool., Vol. 6, pp. 357–90. The Natural History Press, Garden City, New York.
34 Prosser C.L. & Brown F.A. Jr. (1961) *Comparative Animal Physiology* (2nd edition). 688 pp. W. B. Saunders Comp., Philadelphia, London.
35 Schmidt-Nielsen K. & Dawson W.R. (1964) Terrestrial animals in dry heat: desert reptiles. In *Handbook of Physiology*, Sect. 4 (ed. D. B. Dill) pp. 467–80. Amer. Physiol. Soc. Washington, D.C.
36 Templeton J.R. (1970) Reptiles. In *Comparative Physiology of Thermoregulation* (ed. G. C. Whittow) Vol. 1, pp. 167–221. Academic Press, New York & London.
37 Vernberg F.J. & Vernberg W.B. (1970) Aquatic invertebrates. In *Comparative Physiology of Thermoregulation* (ed. G. C. Whittow) Vol. 1, pp. 1–14. Academic Press, New York & London.
38 Whittow G.C. (1971) Ungulates. In *Comparative Physiology of Thermoregulation* (ed. G. C. Whittow) Vol. 2, pp. 191–281. Academic Press, New York & London.
39 Wigglesworth V.B. (1965) *The Principles of Insect Physiology* (6th rev. edition). Dutton, New York.

Part 2: Other references

40 Aschoff J. (1964) Survival value of diurnal rhythms. *Symp. Zool. Soc. Lond.* **13,** 79–98.
41 Aschoff J. & Pohl H. (1970) Rhythmic variations in energy metabolism. *Fed. Proc.* **29,** 1541–52.
42 Baldwin B.A. & Ingram D.L. (1968a) The effects of food intake and acclimatization to temperature on behavioral thermoregulation in pigs and mice. *Physiol. & Behavior* **3,** 395–400.
43 Baldwin B.A. & Ingram D.L. (1968b) Factors influencing behavioral thermoregulation in the pig. *Physiol. & Behavior* **3,** 409–15.
44 Blem C.R. (1974) Geographic variation of thermal conductance in the house sparrow (Passer domesticus). *Comp. Biochem. Physiol.* **47**A, 101–8.
45 Bligh J. & Johnson K.G. (1973) Glossary of terms for thermal physiology. *J. appl. Physiol.* **35,** 941–61.
46 Bogert C.M. (1959) How reptiles regulate their body temperature. *Sci. Amer.* **200,** 105–20.
47 Calder W.A. (1968) The diurnal activity of the roadrunner, Geococcyx californianus. *Condor* **70,** 84–5.
48 Chaffee R.R.J. & Allen J.R. (1973) Effects of ambient temperature on the resting metabolic rate of cold- and warm-acclimated Macaca mulatta. *Comp. Biochem. Physiol.* **44**A, 1215–25.
49 Cheke R.A. (1971) Temperature rhythms in African montane sunbirds. *Ibis* **113,** 500–6.
50 Chevillard L., Portet R. & Cadot M. (1963) Growth rate of rats born and reared at 5° and 30°C. *Fed. Proc.* **22,** 699–703.
51 Crawshaw L.I. (1974) Temperature selection and activity in the crayfish, Orconectes immunis. *J. comp. Physiol.* **95** A, 315–22.
52 Enright J.T. (1963) The tidal rhythm of activity of a sand-beach amphipod. *Z. vergl. Physiol.* **46,** 276–313.
53 Figala J., Hoffmann K. & Goldau G. (1973) Zur Jahresperiodik beim Dsungarischen Zwerghamster Phodopus sungorus Pallas. *Oecologia* (*Berl.*) **12,** 89–118.
54 Gaertner R.A., Hart J.S. & Roy O.Z. (1973) Seasonal spontaneous torpor in the white-footed mouse, Peromyscus leucopus. *Comp. Biochem. Physiol.* **45** A, 169–81.
55 Hammel H.T. (1956) Infrared emissivities of some arctic fauna. *J. Mammal.* **37,** 375–8.
56 Heldmaier G. & Hoffmann K. (1974) Melatonin stimulates growth of brown adipose tissue. *Nature Lond.* **247,** 224–5.
57 Hinds D.S. (1973) Acclimatization of thermoregulation in the desert cottontail, Sylvilagus audubonii. *J. Mammal.* **54,** 708–28.
58 Hissa R. & Palokangas R. (1970) Thermoregulation in the titmouse (Parus major L.). *Comp. Biochem. Physiol.* **33,** 941–53.

59 Hoffman R.A., Hester R.J. & Towns C. (1965) Effect of light and temperature on the endocrine system of the golden hamster. *Comp. Biochem. Physiol.* **15,** 525–33.
60 Holeton G.F. (1974) Metabolic cold adaptation of polar fish: fact or artefact? *Physiol. Zool.* **47,** 137–52.
61 Houston A.H. & Cyr D. (1974) Thermoacclimatory variation in the haemoglobin system of goldfish (Carassius auratus) and rainbow trout (Salmo gairdneri). *J. Exp. Biol.* **61,** 455–61.
62 Irving L. (1966) Adaptation to cold. *Sci. Amer.* **214,** 94–101.
63 Johnston R.F. & Selander R.K. (1964) House sparrows: rapid evolution of races in North America. *Science, Wash.* **144,** 548–50.
64 Kendeigh S.C. & Blem C.R. (1974) Metabolic adaptation to local climate in birds. *Comp. Biochem. Physiol.* **48**A, 175–87.
65 Kleiber M. (1972) Body size, conductance for animal heat flow and Newton's law of cooling. *J. Theor. Biol.* **37,** 139–50.
66 Klein H. (1974) The adaptational value of internal annual clocks in birds. In *Circannual Clocks* (ed. E. T. Pengelley) pp. 347–91. Academic Press, New York & London.
67 Mahoney J.J. & Hutchison V.H. (1969) Photoperiod acclimation and 24-hour variations in the critical thermal maxima of a tropical and a temperate frog. *Oecologia* (*Berl.*) **2,** 143–61.
68 Marder J. (1973) Body temperature regulation in the brown-necked raven (Corvus corax ruficollis)—II. Thermal changes in the plumage of ravens exposed to solar radiation. *Comp. Biochem. Physiol.* **45**A, 431–40.
69 McNab (1970) Body weight and the energetics of temperature regulation. *J. Exp. Biol.* **53,** 329–48.
70 Morton M.L. & Carey C. (1971) Growth and the development of endothermy in the mountain white-crowned sparrow (Zonotrichia leucophrys oriantha). *Physiol. Zool.* **44,** 177–89.
71 Pittendrigh C.S. (1960) Circadian rhythms and the circadian organization of living systems. *Cold Spr. Harb. Symp. Quant. Biol.* **25,** 159–84.
72 Pohl H. (1969) Some factors influencing the metabolic response to cold in birds. *Fed. Proc.* **28,** 1059–64.
73 Pohl H. & West G.C. (1973) Daily and seasonal variation in metabolic response to cold during rest and forced exercise in the common redpoll. *Comp. Biochem. Physiol.* **45**A, 851–67.
74 Ricklefs R.E. & Hainsworth F.R. (1968) Temperature dependent behavior of the cactus wren. *Ecology* **49,** 227–33.
75 Spellerberg I.F. (1972) Temperature tolerances of Southeast Australian reptiles examined in relation to reptile thermoregulatory behaviour and distribution. *Oecologia, Berl.* **9,** 23–46.
76 Spellerberg I.F. & Hoffmann K. (1972) Circadian rhythm in lizard critical minimum temperature. *Naturwissenschaften* **59,** 517–18.
77 Thiele H.U. & Weber F. (1968) Tagesrhythmen der Aktivität bei Carabiden. *Oecologia, Berl.* **1,** 315–55.
78 Tucker V.A. (1965) The relation between the torpor cycle and heat exchange in the California pocket mouse Perognathus californicus. *J. Cell. Comp. Physiol.* **65,** 405–14.
79 Tucker V.A. (1966) Oxygen transport by the circulatory system of the green iguana (Iguana iguana) at different body temperatures. *J. Exp. Biol.* **44,** 77–92.
80 Vernberg W.B. & Moreira G.S. (1974) Metabolic-temperature responses of the copepod Euterpina acutifrons (Dana) from Brazil. *Comp. Biochem. Physiol.* **49**A, 757–61.
81 West G.C. (1968) Seasonal differences in resting metabolic rate of Alaskan ptarmigan. *Comp. Biochem. Physiol.* **42**A, 867–76.
82 White F.N. (1973) Temperature and the Galapagos marine iguana—insights into reptilian thermoregulation. *Comp. Biochem. Physiol.* **45**A, 503–13.

Prelude to Chapter 14

Life may have originated in a totally anoxic environment. The formation of oxygen in the atmosphere was considered in detail in Chapter 3. Although the first formation of free oxygen perhaps 3×10^9 years ago was probably achieved by the photolysis of water vapour, it was the photosynthetic property of blue-green algae and the burial of a proportion of the organic matter containing reduced carbon which resulted in a rapid rise in the partial pressure of atmospheric oxygen. Thus, to some large extent, the 'contamination' of the atmosphere with free oxygen may be considered as one of the first biologically-induced pollutions of the environment to which life had to become adapted.

The suggestion is made in Chapter 3 that the appearance of the eucaryotic cell, and later of the metazoa probably reflects the rise in the level of atmospheric oxygen. All living unicellular eucaryotes are either obligate aerobes or dependent on obligate aerobes: their metabolic processes are directly or indirectly dependent on the availability of free oxygen.

It is also pointed out in Chapter 3 that free oxygen initially exerted an effect as a solute in surface waters. The high ultra-violet radiation made land surfaces hostile environments for the eucaryotic cell before the formation of a protective ozone layer. This had occurred by the end of the Silurian period, 4×10^8 years ago, and colonization of the land then became possible.

In the following Chapter, it is emphasized that life progressed from the open sea to shallow fresh water and then to land through an increasing partial pressure of oxygen. The subsequent, and relatively recent, migration of animals to high altitudes, at which the partial pressure of oxygen is greatly reduced, involves the reversal of this long evolutionary history of life.

The evidence presented in Chapter 14 is that the eucaryotic cell is genotypically adapted to an environment with a high oxygen content, and that there is little indication of genotypic adaptations of organisms native to high altitudes to low partial pressures of oxygen. The adaptations that do occur are apparently phenotypic acclimatizations to the various environmental stresses of high altitudes. There is no evidence of physiological embarrassment when an organism native to a high altitude is abruptly transferred to sea level.

This may be because there has not yet been time enough for the emergence of genetic adaptations to high altitude environments, but the natural distribution of animal life at high altitude may depend more on the availability of food supplies than on the partial pressure of oxygen. Thus the stress of hypobaric hypoxia imposed on organisms at the altitudes at which there are adequate food supplies may be insufficient to effect the selection of adaptive mutants.

High altitude physiology centres upon the effect on the organism of the low oxygen tension. For the occasional visitor to high places, this is, indeed, the principal cause of his discomfort. For the resident, the environmental stress is more complex. A high intensity of ultra-violet radiation, seasonal extremes of temperature and other meteorological conditions, the inadequacy of food supplies, and a reduced capacity of an ageing body to respond adequately to these stresses, may all be significant and interacting environmental influences on organisms at high altitudes. The most severe medical problems of native man at high altitudes seem to be closely related to malnutrition and to the effects of growing old. The pathological effects of high altitude on transported domestic species may not be due to hypoxia alone: an additive effect of low oxygen tension and cold exposure on pulmonary artery pressure may be the factor that leads to physiological deterioration. Thus it is clear, that in future, studies of both fundamental and applied physiology of man and other animals at high altitude must be related to the full impact of the environment on the organism.

Chapter 14
High altitude adaptations in the whole animal

C. MONGE AND J. WHITTEMBURY

14.1 INTRODUCTION

The role of oxygen in shaping evolution has not been described as well as, for example, that of osmotic pressure as an influence in natural selection [89]. Since oxygen enters most organisms by passive diffusion through oxygen-tension gradients, it is important to note that the solubility and therefore the partial pressure of oxygen in fresh water at equilibrium with the atmosphere is greater than that of sea water, and that atmospheric air at sea level contains the highest natural concentration of oxygen and therefore the highest natural partial pressure of oxygen. Thus with the evolutionary progression of life from salt water to fresh water to air, the diffusional supply of oxygen to tissues has progressively increased. This may have had an important influence on the subsequent evolution of the tachymetabolic birds and mammals from the bradymetabolic fishes, amphibians and reptiles.

The density of the atmosphere, and therefore the total pressure and the partial pressure of oxygen in the atmosphere, decreases as the height above the sea increases. This means that as terrestrial organisms have migrated from sea level and established themselves at increasingly higher altitudes, the availability of oxygen to the tissues has progressively decreased. Thus adaptation to low partial pressures of oxygen involves the reversal of a long evolutionary progression in the opposite direction.

Compared with the time-scale of life (*c.* 3×10^9 years) and of terrestrial life (*c.* 2×10^8 years), the invasion of high altitude environments by complex multicellular vertebrate forms of life has occurred only relatively recently. It is not surprising, therefore, that there is little evidence of genetic adaptation to the low oxygen tension of high altitude environments. In the mammals, about which more is known than of other classes of vertebrates, it would seem that adaptations to high altitude are phenotypic (acclimatory), not genotypic, since species native to high altitude environments encounter no physiological difficulties when moved to sea level.

Because adaptation to high altitude is predominantly phenotypic, and because there are stressful components of high altitude environments other than the low partial pressure of oxygen, especially the low air temperature, high intensity of solar radiation and shortage of food, the duration of exposure to high altitude, and the influence of these other environmental factors must be taken into account in the interpretation of studies of the physiological responses to high altitude.

14.2 THE ENVIRONMENT

There is no standard definition of what constitutes a high altitude environment. The land surface rises progressively from sea level to a maximum height of 8700 m. As altitude increases the partial pressure of oxygen diminishes, but the stress of any given altitude is affected by latitude, and by more local circumstances such as the extent of shelter from prevailing winds. Air temperature and the direction, intensity and spectral distribution of the radiation energy flux vary greatly between day and night, and with the latitude. Another important environmental factor at high altitude is the availability of food. Both plant and animal food stuffs become increasingly scarce as altitude increases, and the possibility that under-nutrition is contributory to any chronic condition at high altitude, must be considered.

For a study of the physiological effects of P_{O_2} alone, simulation in decompression chambers is the experimental ideal, for when studies are made in natural high-altitude environments, the other complicating environmental factors must be eliminated. On the other hand, for studies of the adaptations of organisms to natural high-altitude environments, the concentration of attention on the effects of the low P_{O_2}, may give rise to deceptive and erroneous conclusions.

14.3 ANIMAL DISTRIBUTION AT HIGH ALTITUDE

Despite the adverse circumstances of high altitude environments, animals and man have become established in almost all the high mountain ranges of the world: the Andes [66, 72], the Himalayas [59, 90], the Alps, the Rocky Mountains [30] and others.

Invertebrates and lower vertebrates are well able to tolerate very low atmospheric pressures. Insects occur at altitudes of 6000 m in the Himalayas [59, 90], and some amphibians and reptiles can survive rapid exposures to simulated altitudes of 23 km [39]. Mammals, by contrast, can tolerate only moderate altitudes, and it may be postulated that mammals, which have an oxygen requirement some 4–5 times that of a lower vertebrate of the same body size and at the same tissue temperature (see Chapter 20), have been unable to adapt, either phenotypically or genotypically, to the very low partial pressures of oxygen which the invertebrates and lower vertebrates can survive.

The steep escarpment between the coastal desert and the high Andes renders the Andes particularly suitable for high altitude acclimatization (natural phenotypic adaptation) studies, because of the possibility of rapid transition. Furthermore the geological, zoological and anthropological histories of the South American continent including the Andes, are well documented. South America became isolated from the continental mass about 60 million years ago. Since then its indigenous fauna evolved in isolation, and have become distinctly different from those of other continents. The Andes were formed during major disturbances to the Earth's crust about 18 million years ago, and the exploitation of this newly formed high-altitude terrain was an ecological and physiological challenge to the South American fauna. Then about 10 million years ago, a weak land link formed between the South and North American continents, and some limited two-way migration occurred across this central American isthmus.

The earliest occupation of South America by man can be dated at about 10 thousand years ago, and there is evidence of his early occupation of territories at altitudes above 3000 m [16, 50]. However, the introduction of European domestic animals to the Andean pastures did not occur until 500 years ago when the Inca dynasty was conquered by the Spaniards.

The Himalayas are less densely populated by man and his domesticated mammals than are the Andes, but the Himalayas are much older and have been occupied longer, so there has been more time for genetic adaptations to occur. Thus despite their remoteness the Himalayas would be the better place to look for phylogenetic adaptations. (See note added in press, p. 303)

14.4 INVERTEBRATES AND LOWER VERTEBRATES

Insects of the orders *Thysanura* and *Collembola*, which are considered to be the most primitive of contemporary insects, have been found on rocks covering Himalayan glaciers at altitudes of 5300 to 5800 m. As there is no plant life at this altitude, these insects probably live off blown debris [59, 90]. In the Andes, fish (trout) occur in great numbers in Lake Titicaca and other lakes and rivers at altitudes of 4000 m, and toads of the genus *Telmatobius* have developed a totally aquatic life in the high Andean lakes.

14.4.1 Birds

Many species of birds live in the high mountains, but it seems that few, if any, are irreversibly adapted to the rarified atmosphere, for some species make frequent visits to sea-level environments. The Andean condor (*Vultur gryphus*), for example, may feed at the sea-shore and return to the high peaks in the same day. The Andean gull (*Larus serranus*) also flies to and fro between the Andean plateaus and the desert coastal plains and the Amazonian jungle, which is not far above sea level [46]. Darwin's rhea (*Pterocnemus pennata barapacensis*) and the Andean goose (*Chloephaga melanoptera*) are also typical Andean birds.

14.4.2 Mammals

South American camelids native to the Andes include the undomesticated guanaco (*Lama guanicoe*) and vicuña (*Lama vicugna*) which occur at 1000 to 5300 m and 4200 to 5500 m respectively, and the domesticated llama (*Lama glama*) and alpaca (*Lama pacos*) which are husbanded at altitudes of 2000 to 4000 m and 4300 to 4700 m respectively.

Several species of rodents occur in quite large numbers at high altitude [72]. They are most useful as experimental animals as some species occur only in high altitude habitats, while others occur at all altitudes between their highest habitats and sea level [67]. Of the latter group, the guinea-pig (*Cavia porcellus*) is a domesticated species, and the cavy (*Cavia tschudii*) is an undomesticated species.

The Himalayan yak (*Bos grunniens*) can be found at 6000 m, and Megatherium fossil remains have been found in the Peruvian Andes at 4500 m [27, 40]. The Peruvian punas (Andean plateaux) hold 15 to 20 million sheep which graze at altitudes of 4000 to 5000 m. Brown Swiss cattle can be successfully husbanded at altitudes of up to 4000 m, but the Holstein breed can only tolerate somewhat lower grazing land. Dogs are common in the high Andes, but cats are rather scarce.

14.5 ADAPTATION TO LOW AMBIENT OXYGEN TENSION (Po_2)

Figure 14.1 is a flow diagram of the path oxygen takes from ambient air to cell mitochondria. Adaptation to low Po_2 consists of changes in the primary biochemical processes of energy expenditure and oxygen utilization at the intracellular level, and in the mechanisms concerned in the transport of oxygen to the mitochondrial sites of these processes. Polycythemia—an increase in red blood cell numbers, and therefore in the oxygen-carrying capacity of the blood—is perhaps the most important of these mechanisms, but most mammals respond to high altitudes with an increase in the ventilatory rate. This has been observed in dogs [51], sheep, cattle and yaks [48] and llamas [13]. Although the basal

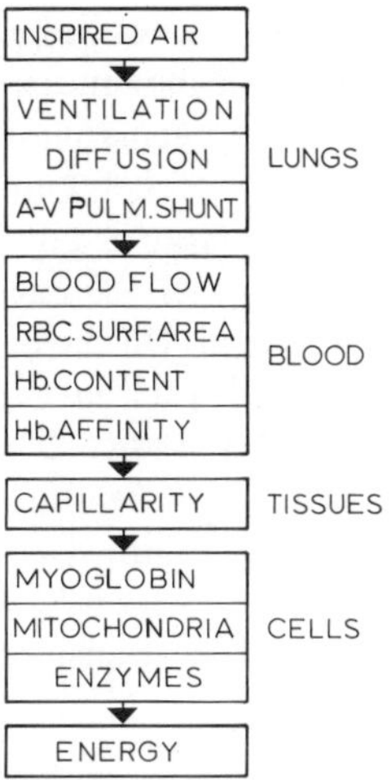

Fig. 14.1

ventilatory rate is higher in humans born and bred at high altitudes, they show a diminished sensitivity to a hypoxic stimulus [85, 49, 84]. As the incidence of chronic mountain sickness also increases with age, a decrease in pulmonary ventilation may be the primary reason for the sickness in natives of high altitude environments [86]; and because of this inadequate pulmonary ventilation, the alveolar partial pressure of CO_2 (Pa, CO_2) rises to close on 40 mmHg [63, 62] which is the normal value for mammals at sea level. The ventilatory response of cattle when taken to high altitude may also be inadequate [33], and they develop a pathological condition (Brisket disease) which is similar to that of mountain sickness in man, and which may also lead to heart failure [38].

When man moves up to a high altitude environment, adaptation has been found to involve both a higher ventilatory rate and an increased pulmonary diffusion [100], but in llamas [5] and dogs [3], both of which are well established in high altitude habitats, the pulmonary alveolar-arterial diffusion gradient is lower in those living in the Andes than at sea level. An interesting difference in the oxygenation of the blood pulmonary capillaries has been noted in the llama and sheep [4]; during an acute exposure to low barometric pressure, llamas had a higher arterial oxygen pressure than did sheep. The llama is evidently better able to optimize the transport of oxygen from the alveolus to the blood in the lungs.

Polycythemia has long been considered an important adaptive response to high altitude. The increased haemoglobin concentration augments the oxygen-carrying capacity of the blood and helps maintain the Po_2 gradient between capillaries and cells [42, 75]. Practically all exotic domestic mammals introduced into the Andes by the Spanish conquistadors develop polycythemia in this hypoxic environment [64].

This response also occurs in man and has been extensively studied [43, 60,

81, 28, 78]. Nevertheless, experiments on dogs [34, 87, 88] show that blood O_2 transport, when studied as a function of the haematocrit, is maximal at an erythrocyte concentration of about 40%, a normal figure for dogs. After acclimatization to low barometric pressure, this maximum is increased slightly to 46%. These studies indicated that with higher haematocrit values there is a diminished blood flow because of the increase in viscosity. Thus, the potential advantage of the increased O_2-carrying capacity is largely negated by the reduced blood flow. Since viscosity is a logarithmic function of the haematocrit [103], only a slight haematocrit increment seems to be useful. On the basis of a mathematical analysis of O_2 transport, Crowell and Smith [21] have concluded that the optimum haematocrit corresponds to a blood viscosity 2·7 times greater than that of plasma. The data of Pirofsky [73] and Whittembury *et al.* [103] show that both at sea level and at high altitude the optimum haematocrit for human beings is about 42%, a figure close to normal at sea level. In fact, an excessive polycythemia in man at high altitude has been considered contributory to chronic mountain sickness [63].

The haematocrit value does not increase in all mammals at high altitudes. The Andean camelids (llama, vicuña and alpaca) and rodents (chinchilla and viscacha) do not show this response [36, 35, 80, 61]. Some rodents whose native habitat is the Andes show no changes in haematocrit when moved to or raised at sea level [70, 69]. In the case of camelids, the large number of very small red cells (microcytosis), the relatively high haemoglobin concentration in the cells, and the relatively high oxygen affinity, may be advantageous in high altitudes but are not necessarily specific adaptations to high altitudes as they occur also in the low-altitude desert camelids of Africa [9].

The elliptical shape of the red cells of camelids may also be useful but has not been studied. Microcytosis is of definite importance in increasing red-cell oxygenation rate. Figure 14.2 drawn from the data of Holland and Forster [41], shows the correlation between the reaction velocity constant (k'_c) and the reciprocal of the red-cell radius (l/r) when the cell is assumed to be spherical. We have calculated the linear regression line and plotted l/r values available for llamas and vicuñas [5, 36]. Camelids share with sheep and goats the advantage of

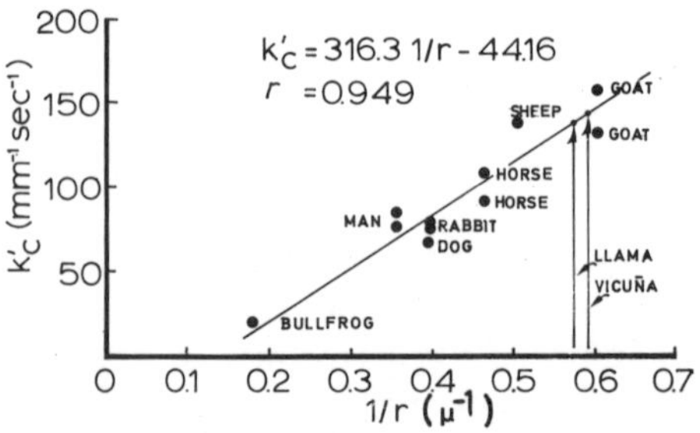

Fig. 14.2. Velocity constant of red-cell oxygenation (k'_c) as a function of the red-cell radius reciprocal (l/r), assumed to be spherical. Plotting and dots according to [41]. Values for llama and vicuña from [5] and [36].

a higher oxygenation rate. At the same haematocrit values blood viscosity in the alpaca and man are comparable [103].

Bullard *et al.* [15] have shown that certain rodents (the golden-mantled ground squirrel and yellow-bellied marmot) although native to a region approximately 3800 m, do not present marked polycythemia but have high red cell and plasma volumes relative to body weight. The authors suggest that red-cell volume increase may be an initial response and that an expansion of plasma volume may represent a secondary adaptation. The adverse effects of an increased haematocrit would thus be reduced but at the expense of an increase in total volume.

Since polycythemia does not occur in several species which inhabit high altitude environments we may conclude that a high haematocrit is not an essential adaptive response to altitude.

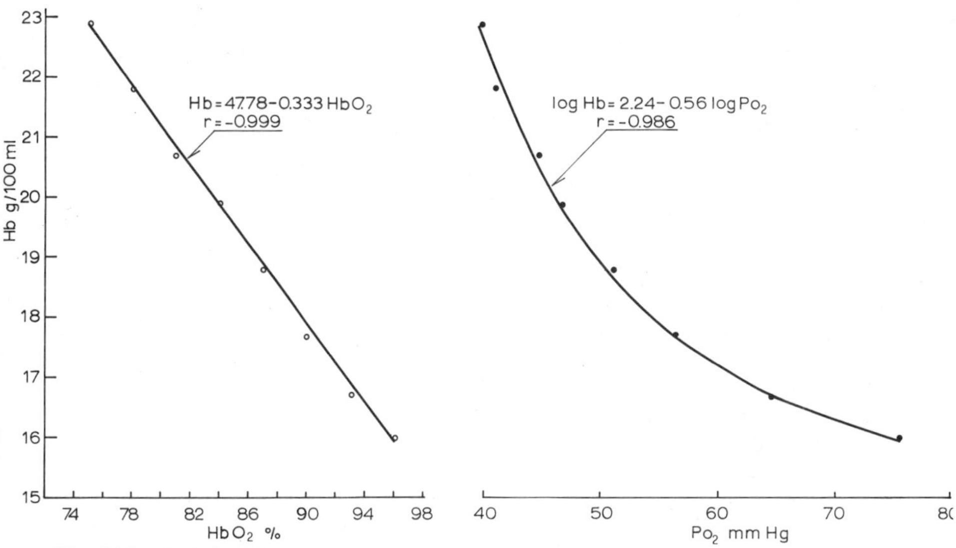

Fig. 14.3. Relationship between hemoglobin concentration and hemoglobin oxygen saturation (on the left) and blood O_2 pressure (on the right). Notice the very high correlation between Hb and HbO_2% and between log Hb and log Po_2. From [43] and [1].

Despite many studies of hypoxic polycythemia, the cause of the increase in red-cell formation rate is not known. Weil *et al.* [102] found a poor correlation between red-cell mass and Pa,O_2 and a better one with Sa,O_2. On this basis, they postulated that Sa,O_2 rather than Pa,O_2 is the trigger mechanism. However, a good linear correlation does not constitute definite evidence. Thus, Fig. 14.3 has been constructed with data from Hurtado *et al.* [43] and Aste and Hurtado [1] regarding highland natives living permanently at different altitudes. It shows an excellent correlation between Sa,O_2 and Hb concentration and between log Pa,O_2 and log Hb concentration. The factor or factors triggering polycythemia responses remain elusive. Unfortunately, the erythropoetin assay is still a difficul technical problem [29].

Although an increased blood flow is a typical response to acute exposure to hypoxia this is not common in altitude—acclimatized mammals. Thus, a normal cardiac index has been found in the acclimatized Andean man [32, 101, 94] and dog [3]. The limited advantages of increasing blood flow in the acclimatized animal are well explained by Luft [55]. In some high altitude Peruvian rodents Morrison and Elsner [68] found higher resting heart rates than in sea-level species. After two months' residence at sea level, the animals were taken back to 4500 m. No significant heart rate increase was then observed. Species native to sea-level habitats, however, showed a higher heart rate when taken to high altitude. The authors suggest that in this respect high altitude species are genetically adapted to their environment.

The affinity of haemoglobin for oxygen has received considerable attention. Haemoglobin of man at high altitude has less affinity than that from man at sea level [1, 45]. Most investigators have considered this shift in the O_2 dissociation curve to the right to be a convenient adaptive response favouring O_2 unloading at the tissue level. In contrast to this view, and on the basis of comparative physiological studies, other investigators [64, 19, 20, 14, 65] have called attention to the fact that the haemoglobins of animals naturally acclimatized or adapted to a hypoxic environment have more rather than less O_2 affinity.

Schmidt-Nielsen and Larimer [83] have shown that P_{50} (mmHg O_2)—a measure of Hb affinity for O_2—is correlated with body weight according to $P_{50} = a\ W^{-b}$ type of function. In the upper part of Fig. 14.4 we have plotted data of several investigators [42, 14, 83, 24]. It can be seen that sea-level mammals present a clearly different correlation from that of species like the Andean camelids (llama, vicuña, alpaca) and rodents (chinchilla, viscacha). Burrowing squirrels, whose subterranean habitats may have a low $P\text{O}_2$, approximate the high altitude correlation line. The grey squirrel, which does not face hypoxic challenges, is close to the sea-level regression line. The Himalayan yak, however, resembles the sea-level group although it has greater affinity than its sea-level relative, the domestic cow. High-altitude-adapted man seems to be exceptional, not only because of his poor ventilatory response to a hypoxic stimulus, but also because his haemoglobin has less rather than more affinity for oxygen. This diminished affinity found in acclimatized man and also in sea-level mammals when acutely exposed to a hypoxic environment [8, 10, 97] cannot be considered advantageous in itself.

2,3 Diphosphoglycerate (2,3 DPG), and ATP to a minor extent, strongly influence Hb affinity for O_2 [18, 11]. Humans acclimatized to high altitude have an increased amount of 2,3 DPG in red cells (25), which is lost on return to sea level [52]. Reynafarje and Rosenmann [82] have described a correlation between red cell 2,3 DPG concentration and body weight in mammals. Using a log–log scale we have plotted these data on the lower part of Fig. 14.4. The similarity between this plot and that for P_{50} as a function of body weight is striking. The same authors found that sheep and cattle have no red cell 2,3 DPG. The order Artiodactyla lacks 2,3 DPG [20] but alpacas and llamas are exceptions to this rule [82]. This finding adds a new dimension to the remarkable blood properties of the camelid family.

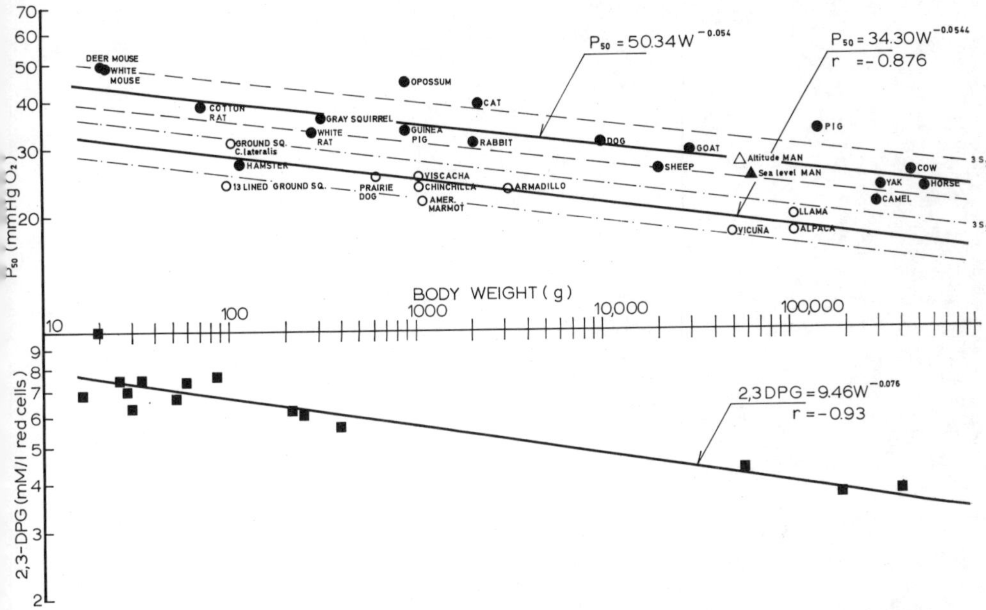

Fig. 14.4. Haemoglobin affinity (P_{50}) and concentration of 2,3 dyphosphoglycerate in red cells (2,3 DPG) as a function of body weight. Both scales are logarithmic. In the upper part of the figure, closed circles correspond to sea level mammals and open circles to either high altitude or burrowing mammals. Regression lines are shown plus and minus three standard deviations. Plotting is based on [83], [14], [24] and [42]. Notice the lack of overlapping between the two groups. In the lower part of the figures data are from [82].

Haemoglobin carbamoylation increases blood oxygen affinity in rats [26]. Animals treated in this way could survive exposure to low barometric pressure, which caused a high mortality in control rats. Results were interpreted as indicating that increased rather than decreased affinity is of adaptive value. The O_2 dissociation curve has adaptive value because of its shape [75, 55] rather than its shift to the right or to the left. At high altitude, in animals with marked sigmoid curves, O_2 conductance is facilitated by the fact that haemoglobin acts on the steep part of the curve. Oxygen can then be released with slight changes in Po_2. There is, however, a close relation between the curve shape and body weight. We have drawn Fig. 14.5 on the basis of the abundant collection of curves in Schmidt-Nielsen and Larimer's article [83]. The curves for small animals approach straight lines. Therefore a property of apparent adaptive value at high altitude is not present in small animals although numerous small rodents are adapted to high altitude. The difficulty of interpreting acclimatization on the basis of a single parameter is again manifested.

14.5.1 Tissues

Despite adaptive changes at high altitude in the ventilatory and diffusion properties of the lungs, the O_2-carrying capacity and oxygen affinity of the mixed

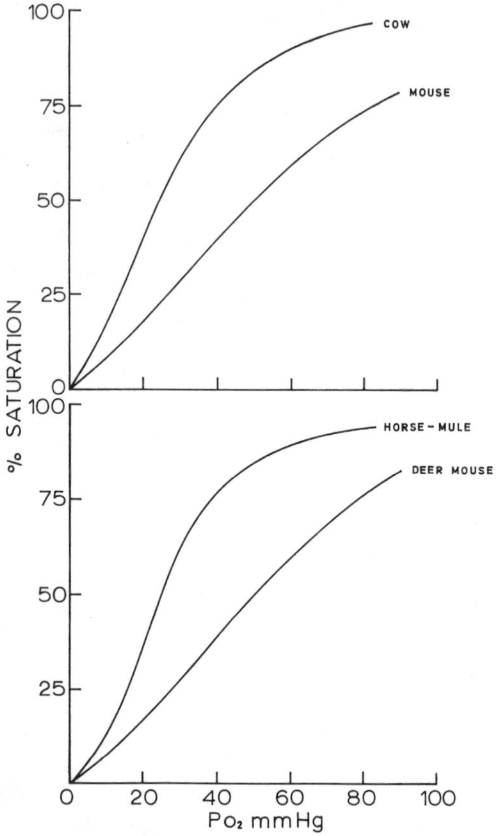

Fig. 14.5. Blood oxygen dissociation curves for small (mouse and deer-mouse) and large (cow and horse-mule) mammals. From [83].

venous blood O_2 pressure ($P\bar{v},O_2$) is usually lower than at sea level. Since $P\bar{v},O_2$ represents an approximation to tissue pressure, it has long been postulated that the tissues themselves somehow contribute to an improved O_2 conductance. Fig. 14.6 [adapted from 5, 14 and 42] shows a comparative study of llama, ground squirrel and man. At sea level (upper part of the figure), it is seen that between llamas and man there is a difference in the O_2 gradients between Pa,O_2 and $P\bar{v},O_2$. Through polycythemia and by lowering Hb affinity for O_2, man maintains a high tissue O_2 pressure. As we have seen, however, these are not necessarily useful adaptive responses *per se*. In llamas, normal tissue functions occur at low Po_2 even at sea level and are, therefore, truly adapted to hypoxia. We have seen that the llama does not need increased haematocrit value at high altitude. Banchero [5] found that its dissociation curve is also unchanged during exposure to high altitude. In the lower portion of the same figure it can be seen that the ground squirrel, a burrowing rodent—used to a hypoxic environment even at sea level—has an extremely low $P\bar{v},O_2$.

Krogh [47] described the relation between the Po_2 pressure gradient and the diffusion from a capillary into the surrounding tissue. The equation is:

$$T_o - T_R = \frac{P}{d}\left(1{\cdot}15\ R^2 \log\frac{R}{r} - \frac{R^2 - r^2}{4}\right)$$

where T_o and T_x represent oxygen tensions in the capillary and at a point in which $x = R$, respectively, P is the gas exchange or O_2 consumption; d is the diffusion constant for animal tissue; and r is the capillary radius. A greater

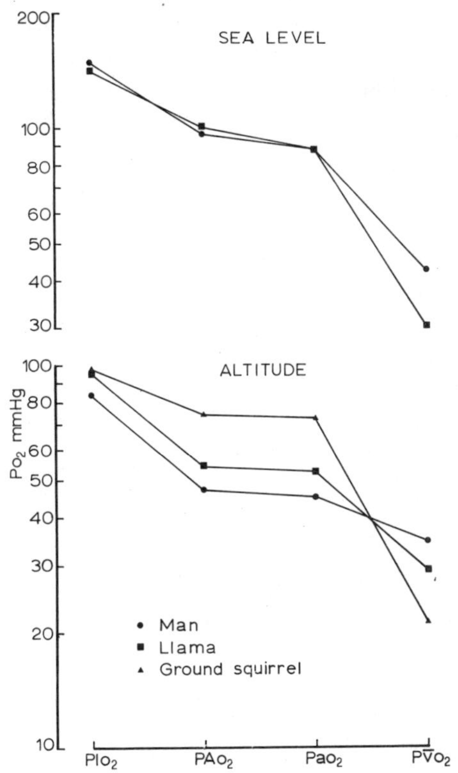

Fig. 14.6. Po_2 gradients ranging from inspired air (PI,O_2) to mixed venous blood ($P\bar{v}$,O)$_2$ In order to make slopes comparable the Po_2 is logarithmic. Plotting and data according to [5], [14] and [42].

muscle capillarity has been found in guinea-pigs native to the Peruvian mountains and dwelling at altitudes of 4500 m, than in guinea-pigs at sea level [99]. An increased muscle capillarity in rats occurred during a 5-week exposure to a simulated altitude of 6000 m [17]. A similar increase in capillary density occurred in the right ventricle of rats exposed several weeks to simulated altitudes of 3500 m [95]. Tenney and Ou [93] also confirmed an increased tissue capillarity in rats acclimatized during a 5-week period to simulated altitudes of 5600 m. using a 'tissue diffusing capacity' method based on CO uptake rate from subcutaneous gas pockets. Banchero *et al.* [2] measured muscle fibre diameters and respiratory parameters of dogs at 1600 m and after acclimatization during a 3-week period to 4800 m. We have calculated the Po_2 at the centre of the muscle fibre from their data using Krogh's cylinder equation. In Fig. 14.7 we have applied $T_o = P\bar{v},o_2$, in accordance with Tenney and Ou [93]. The most hypoxic part of a tissue is at the venous end of a capillary and the pressure at this level should be approximated by $P\bar{v},o_2$. It can be seen that a reduction in capillary radius (R) of dogs at high altitude causes the drop in fibre Po_2 due to their lower $P\bar{v},o_2$ to be reduced. A reduction of muscle fibre diameter seems to play a role in tissue adaptive response. Nevertheless, as Fig. 14.7 shows, the calculated values for R lie practically on the horizontal portion of the curve. Therefore, the advantages of this adaptive response are limited. Since the intercapillary distance is usually shorter than fibre diameters, the role of increased capillarity is also limited.

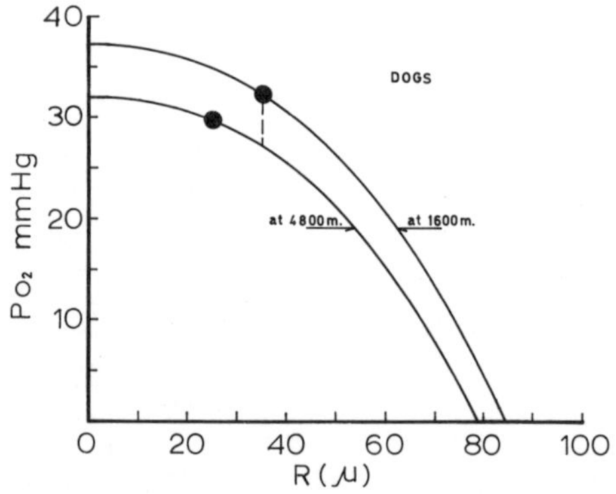

Fig. 14.7. Muscle fibre Po_2 calculated from muscle fibre radius (R) by means of Krogh's equation. Data from [2] from altitudes 1600 m and 4800 m for dogs. Plotting is according to [93]

14.5.2 Cells

An increased myoglobin in the muscles of Andean dogs has been considered an important adaptive response which facilitates oxygenation [44]. This increase in myoglobin also occurs in Andean guinea-pigs [91] and man [77]. Turek *et al.* [96] found heart myoglobin correlated with age rather than with weight. Using a weight correlation comparison they found an increase of the right ventricle myoglobin concentration in rats exposed to hypoxia and an unchanged concentration in rats born in hypobaria. Since laboratory rats develop marked polycythemia and severe cardiomegaly even at moderate altitude, reports of heart myoglobin concentrations have to be interpreted with caution.

Mammals at high altitude cannot avoid a drop in tissue Po_2 despite the efforts of the organism to increase the availability of oxygen to the tissues. However, at high altitude Andean man [42] [94], dogs [3], llamas [5] and rats [97] consume the same amount of oxygen as they do at sea level. This is also true of an individual organ, the kidney, in Andean man [76] and for isolated tissues from animals acclimatized to high altitude [53, 98, 31].

The absence of a lowering of oxygen consumption in the circumstance of low tissue Po_2 indicates biochemical adaptations in high-altitude animals. Different experimental approaches in different species have yielded results that are inconsistent with each other and difficult to interpret. Here discussion is largely limited to studies in animals born and living at high altitude.

In human sartorius muscle [77] and in the myocardium of high altitude guinea-pigs, rabbits and dogs [37], respectively, lactic dehydrogenase activity is no greater than that found in these tissues in animals kept at sea level. Apparently, anaerobic glycolysis plays no role in acclimatization to high altitude. Yet, the accumulation of lactic acid in the plasma of Andean natives after exercise is less than at exercise at sea level [42]. Lower liver lactate and higher liver, kidney and heart succinate was found in Andean guinea-pigs after 10-minute periods of acute anoxia than in control guinea-pigs from the coastal plain. These differences suggest a higher rate of tissue lactate utilization in succinic acid formation in the tissue of animals adapted to high altitude. There are similar differences in the tissue of lower animals and a cautious suggestion was made [23] that these findings may serve to explain the low accumulation of lactic acid in high-altitude natives after exercise.

In cattle there is an increased number of mitochondria in heart tissue at high altitude, but not in the liver [71]. Since heart muscles in high-altitude animals have to adapt both to hypoxia and to haemodynamic changes, this change in mitochondria concentration is not necessarily an adaptation to low Po_2. No changes in the number and size of cells and mitochondria were found in the liver, muscle, heart and brain of the high-altitude guinea-pig [12]. So far it has not been generally observed that acclimatization to high altitude results in morphological changes in cells or mitochondria.

Increases in the concentration of mitochondrial enzymes have been found in high-altitude animal tissues: an increase in electron transport and in cytochrome a_3 oxidase activity per mitochondria in the heart muscle of Andean cattle [71]; an increased succinic dehydrogenase activity in the liver of Andean guinea-pigs, rabbits and dogs [37]; an increased DPNH-oxydase and transhydrogenase activity in Andean natives [92] and an increase in mitochondrial oxygen consumption per unit of ADP concentration in the liver of Andean guinea-pigs [79]. In this last instance it was calculated that there was a 15% chemical energy increase per minute at high altitude and this increment was considered to be of adaptive value.

Thus there are biochemical indications of an increased aerobic capacity at the mitochondrial level at high altitude. This is mainly produced by an increased oxidative enzyme activity allowing the tissues to consume a constant amount of O_2 in the presence of a diminished O_2 concentration (low Po_2) in the cell environment.

14.6 CONCLUSIONS

Phenotypic adaptation to the natural environment (acclimatization) involves the integration of the many concurrent physiological responses. These are never complete because of the continuous changes in the environment which elicit continuous changes in the responses of the organism which can never achieve a steady state of complete integration [7]. Obviously, animals having the greatest genotypic capacity for phenotypic change will acclimatize best. The situation changes whenever the greater ability of some individuals to tolerate an adverse environment results in the selection of genotypic adaptations to this environmental circumstance. When this occurs adaptation resides not in the sum of several individual quantitative responses but resides in fixed qualitative changes.

We agree with Bullard [14] that any genetic selection of mammals by, and for, high-altitude environments is small. This may be because man and the domestic animals in their high-altitude habitats are still within their maximum phenotypic capacities to adapt, and because the stresses of these altitudes are not so hazardous to life as to result in the selection of mutants which favour survival. Perhaps the absence of vegetation, and therefore the first step in a nutritional chain, limits the altitude at which animal life can be sustained, and that in consequence, animals cannot live at altitudes at which the atmospheric environment *per se*, is sufficiently perilous to exert a selective influence on genotypes.

South American camelids, though considered to be high-altitude mammals appear not to be specifically adapted to high altitudes. They have a long history of sea-level residence, and though certain properties in their blood are excellent for life in high altitude they also occur in their sea level Asian and African relatives. The fact that burrowing mammals do so well in high altitude may be due to their genotypic adaptations to hypoxic subterranean conditions. Possible exceptions to this rule might be the small rodents studied by Morrison [67], which seem to be genotypically adapted to high altitude.

Despite the challenging aspects of such environments—man and animals are able to live at very high altitude. Indeed, old civilizations flourished in the Andean plateaux thousands of years ago. Although there is an apparent absence of genotypic adaptations, there has almost certainly been a natural selection of individuals with greater capacities for phenotypic adaptations to high-altitude environments.

The acclimatized animal seems able to tolerate other stresses besides hypoxia with an equal or higher capacity than his sea-level counterpart [63, 54]. Barbashova [6] considered that in this tolerance resides the true capacity to adapt to high altitude. The changes involved in an increased oxygen conductance were not considered by her to be of truly adaptive value.

When the phenotypic changes are inadequate, pathological changes take place. Chronic mountain sickness in humans, Brisket disease in cattle, right heart failure in sheep and in chickens [22] are consequences of inadequate ability to acclimatize.

Recently, it has been established that age is an important factor in the incidence of chronic mountain sickness in man [104]. Because of this, it has been pointed out that the hitherto unqualified statements on the capacity of human beings to live at very high altitudes of 4000 m or more need qualification [65]. This age factor has not been studied in other species dwelling in high altitude but in rats acclimatized during twenty-four days to intermittent experimental hypobaria, age was a limiting factor in their acclimatization capacity [58]. A reduction in longevity beyond the phase of fecundity is of no evolutionary significance; and in any case, for most animals, whether in natural environments or domesticated (except pets) old age is rare. Thus so long as the high altitude itself exerts no great influence on survival to sexual maturity, and has no adverse effects on fecundity in the young adult, the contribution of altitude effects on the time and cause of death will be without influence on heredity. However, there is evidence of premature death of cats at high altitude, and of the infertility of sheep. Thus strains of the cat and sheep which can survive and reproduce at high altitudes may well exhibit genotypic adaptations which have resulted from an intense natural selection.

Comparative studies of high-altitude physiology are illuminating. In some lower vertebrates, for example, the affinity of haemoglobin for oxygen increases when their natural habitat becomes less oxygenated [56, 74]. This agrees with findings of an apparent genotypic adaption in animals whose natural sea-level environment is hypoxic. Other sea-level mammals, by contrast, show a diminished haemoglobin affinity for oxygen when exposed to hypobaria. Therefore, the common belief that this response is of adaptive value should be reconsidered. Another example is that of mammals showing hypertrophy of the right side of the heart after acclimatization to hypoxia. This has been attributed to the need for increased perfusion in the lung's upper poles. Since this response is also present in birds [57]—the respiratory anatomy of which is very different from that of mammals—this hypothesis also merits reconsideration. Clearly studies of comparative and evolutionary physiology are contributing much towards the comprehension of high-altitude acclimatization and adaptation problems.

Note added in press

A recent paper (G. Morpurgo *et al.*, 1976, *Proc. Nat. Acad. Sci., USA*, **73**, 747–51) on adaptation of Sherpas in the Himalayas confirms previous reports of only mild polycythemia, the absence of chronic mountain sickness and an increased haemoglobin oxygen affinity among these people. These observations are in line with the blood characteristics of other high altitude mammals, and suggest a natural selection to high altitude among the Himalayans not seen in Andean human populations.

14.7 REFERENCES

1 Aste-Salazar H. & Hurtado A. (1944) The affinity of hemoglobin for oxygen at sea level and high altitudes. *Am. J. Physiol.* **142,** 733–43.

2 Banchero N. (1974) Capillary density of skeletal muscle in dogs exposed to simulated altitude. *Proc. Soc. Exptl. Biol. and Med.* **148,** 435–9.
3 Banchero N., Cruz J. & Bustinza J. (1975) Mechanism of O_2 transport in Andean dogs. *Resp. Physiol.* **23,** 361–70.
4 Banchero N. & Grover R.F. (1972) Effects of different levels of simulated altitude on O_2 transport in llama and sheep. *Am. J. Physiol.* **222,** 1239–45.
5 Banchero N., Grover R.F. & Will J.A. (1971) Oxygen transport in the llama (*Lama glama*). *Resp. Physiol.* **13,** 102–15.
6 Barbashova Z.I. (1964) Cellular level of adaptation. In *Handbook of Physiology*. Section 4. Adaptation to the Environment (eds D. B. Dill, E. F. Adolph & C. G. Wilber) pp. 37–54. Williams & Wilkins, Baltimore.
7 Barcroft J. (1934) *Features in the architecture of physiological function*, pp. 172–215. Cambridge University Press, London.
8 Barker J.N. (1957) Role of hemoglobin affinity and concentration in determining hypoxia tolerance of mammals during infancy, hypoxia, hyperoxia and irradiation. *Am. J. Physiol.* **189,** 281–9.
9 Bartels H., Hilpert P., Barbey K., Betke K., Riegel K., Lang E.M. & Metcalfe J. (1963) Respiratory functions of blood of the yak, llama, camel, Dybowsky deer, and African elephant. *Am. J. Physiol.* **205,** 331–6.
10 Baumann R., Bauer Ch. & Bartels H. (1971) Influence of chronic and acute hypoxia on oxygen affinity and red cell 2,3 diphosphoglycerate of rats and guinea pigs. *Resp. Physiol.* **11,** 135–44.
11 Benesch R. & Benesch R.E. (1967) The effects of organic phosphates from the human erythrocyte on the allosteric properties of hemoglobin. *Biochem. Biophys. Research Commun.* **26,** 162–7.
12 Brahim A. (1967) *Contenido de ácido desoxiribonucleico en tejidos de cobayos del nivel del mar y de las grandes alturas.* Tesis, Bachiller. Universidad Nacional Mayor de San Marcos, Lima.
13 Brooks III J.G. & Tenney S.M. (1968) Ventilatory response of llama to hypoxia at sea level and high altitude. *Resp. Physiol.* **5,** 269–78.
14 Bullard R.W. (1972) Vertebrates at altitudes. In *Physiological Adaptations. Desert and Mountains* (eds M. K. Yousef, S. M. Horvath & R. W. Bullard) pp. 209–25. Academic Press, New York & London.
15 Bullard R.W., Broumand C. & Meyer F.R. (1966) Blood characteristics and volume in two rodents native to high altitude. *J. Appl. Physiol.* **21,** 994–8.
16 Cardich A. (1960) *Investigaciones prehistóricas en los Andes Peruanos. Antiguo Perú, Espacio y Tiempo* (ed. Mejía Baca) p. 89. Lima.
17 Cassin S., Gilbert R.D. & Johnson E.M. (1966) Capillary development during exposure to chronic hypoxia. *Brooks A. F. Base. Techn.* No. 66–16.
18 Chanutin A. & Curnish R.R. (1967) Effect of organic phosphates on the oxygen equilibrium of human erythrocytes. *Arch. Biochem. Biophys.* **121,** 96–102.
19 Chiodi H. (1962) Oxygen affinity of the hemoglobin of high altitude mammals. *Acta Physiol. Latinoam.* **12,** 208–9.
20 Chiodi H. (1970/71) Comparative study of the blood gas transport in high altitude and sea level camelidae and goats. *Resp. Physiol.* **11,** 84–93.
21 Crowell J.W. & Smith E.E. (1966) Mathematical determination of the optimal haematocrit. *The Physiologist* **9,** 161.
22 Cueva S., Sillau H., Valenzuela A., Plog H. & Cardenas W. (1970) Hipertensión pulmonar, hipertrofia cardiaca derecha y Mal de Altura en pollos parrilleros. In *Cuarto Boletín Extraordinario* (eds M. Moro & E. R. Zaldivar) pp. 142–6. Centro de Investigacion I.V.I.T.A. U.N.M. de San Marcos, Lima.
23 De Silva E. & Cazorla A. (1973) Lactate, α-GP and Krebs cycle in sea-level and high-altitude native guinea pigs. *Am. J. Physiol.* **224,** 669–72.
24 Dhindsa D.S., Hoversland A.S. & Metcalfe J. (1971) Comparative studies of the respira-

tory functions of mammalian blood. VII. Armadillo (*Dasypus novemcinctus*). *Resp. Physiol.* **13,** 198–208.

25 Eaton J.W., Brewer G.J. & Grover R.F. (1969) Role of red cell 2,3 diphosphoglycerate in the adaptation of man to altitude. *J. Lab. Clin. Med.* **73,** 603–9

26 Eaton J.W., Skeleton T.D. & Berger E. (1974) Survival at extreme altitude: protective effect of increased hemoglobin oxygen affinity. *Science* **183,** 743–4.

27 Engel F. Personal communication.

28 Faura J., Ramos J., Reynafarje C., English E., Finne P. & Finch C.A. (1969) Effect of altitude on erythropoiesis. *Blood* **33,** 668–76.

29 Fisher J.W. (1972) Erythropoietin: Pharmacology, Biogenesis and Control of Production. *Pharmacol. Rev.* **24,** 459–507.

30 Folk G.E. Jr (1966) *Introduction to Environmental Physiology.* Lea & Febiger, Philadelphia.

31 Frehn J.L. & Anthony A. (1961) Respiration of liver slices from normal and altitude-acclimatized rats. *Am. J. Physiol.* **200,** 527–9.

32 Grollman A. (1930) Physiological variations of the cardiac output of man. VII. The effect of high altitude on the cardiac output and its related functions: an account of experiments conducted on the summit of Pike's Peak, Colorado. *Am. J. Physiol.* **93,** 19–40.

33 Grover R.F., Reeves J.T., Will D.H. & Blount S.G. Jr. (1963) Pulmonary vasoconstriction in steers at high altitude *J. Appl. Physiol.* **18,** 567–74.

34 Guyton A.C. & Richardson T.Q. (1961) Effect of hematocrit on venous return. *Circulation Research* **9,** 157–64.

35 Hall F.G. (1937) Adaptation of mammals to high altitudes. *J. Mammalogy* **18,** 468–72.

36 Hall F.G., Dill D.B. & Barron E.S.G. (1936) Comparative physiology in high altitudes. *J. Cell Comp. Physiol.* **8,** 301–13.

37 Harris P. (1971) Some observations on the biochemistry of the myocardium at high altitude. In *High Altitude Physiology* (eds R. Porter & J. Knight) pp. 125–9. Ciba Foundation Symposium. Churchill Livingstone, Edinburgh & London.

38 Hecht H.H., Kuida H., Lange R.L., Thorne J.L. & Brown A.M. (1962) Brisket disease. II. Clinical features and hemodynamic observations in altitude-dependent right-heart failure of cattle. *Am. J. Med.* **32,** 171–83.

39 Hock R.J. (1964) Animals in high altitudes: reptiles and amphibians. In *Handbook of Physiology.* Section 4, Adaptation to the Environment (eds D. B. Dill, E. F. Adolph & C. G. Wilber) pp. 841–2. Williams & Wilkins, Baltimore.

40 Hoffstetter R. (1970) Vertebrados cenozoicos y mamíferos cretásicos del Perú. *Acta IV Congr. Latin. Zool.* **2,** 971–83.

41 Holland R.A.B. & Forster R.E. (1966). The effect of size of red cells on the kinetics of their oxygen uptake. *J. Gen. Physiol.* **49,** 727–42.

42 Hurtado A. (1964) Animals in high altitude: Resident man. In *Handbook of Physiology.* Section 4, Adaptation to the Environment (eds D. B. Dill, E. F. Adolph & C. G. Wilber) pp. 843–60. Williams & Wilkins, Baltimore.

43 Hurtado A., Merino C. & Delgado E. (1945) Influence of anoxemia on the hemopoietic activity. *Arch. Int. Med.* **75,** 284–323.

44 Hurtado A.A., Rotta A., Merino C. & Pons J. (1937) Studies of myohemoglobin at high altitudes. *Am. J. Med. Sci.* **194,** 708–13.

45 Keys A., Hall F.G. & Barron E.S.G. (1936) The position of the oxygen dissociation curve of human blood at high altitude. *Am. J. Physiol.* **115,** 292–307.

46 Koepcke M. (1964) *Las aves del Departamento de Lima* (ed. M. Koepcke) p. 59. Lima.

47 Krogh A. (1918/19). The number and distribution of capillaries in muscles with calculations of the oxygen pressure head necessary for supplying the tissue. *J. Physiol., Lond.* **52,** 409–15.

48 Lahiri S. (1971) Genetic aspects of the blunted chemoreflex ventilatory response to hypoxia in high altitude adaptation. In *High Altitude Physiology* (eds R. Porter & J. Knight) pp. 103–12. Ciba Foundation Symposium. Churchill Livingstone, Edinburgh & London.

49 Lahiri S., Kao F.F., Velásquez T., Martínez C. & Pezzia W. (1970) Respiration of man during exercise at high altitude: highlander vs. lowlander. *Resp. Physiol.* **8,** 361–75.

50 Lanning E.P. (1965) Early man in Peru. *Scientific American* **223,** 68–76.

51 Lefrançois R., Gautier H. & Pasquis P. (1968) Ventilatory oxygen drive in acute and chronic hypoxia. *Resp. Physiol.* **4,** 217–28.

52 Lenfant C., Torrance J., English E., Finch C.A., Reynafarje C., Ramos J. & Faura J. (1968). Effect of altitude on oxygen binding by hemoglobin and on organic phosphate levels. *J. Clin. Invest.* **47,** 2652–6.

53 Lipin J.L. & Whitehorn W.V. (1950) Role of changes in metabolism in acclimatization of albino rats to reduced barometric pressure. *Fed. Proc.* **9,** 79.

54 Lozano R., Torres C., Marchena C., Whittembury J. & Monge C.C. (1969) Response to Metabolic (Ammonium Chloride) Acidosis at Sea Level and at High Altitude. *Nephron* **6,** 102–9.

55 Luft U.C. (1972) Principles of Adaptations to Altitude. In *Physiological Adaptations. Desert and Mountains* (eds M. K. Yousef, S. M. Horvath and R. W. Bullard) pp. 143–56. Academic Press, New York & London.

56 McCutcheon F.H. & Hall F.G. (1937) Haemoglobin in the amphibia. *J. Cell and Comp. Physiol.* **9,** 191–7.

57 McGrath J.J. (1971) Acclimation response of pigeons to simulated high altitude. *J. Appl. Physiol.* **31,** 274–6.

58 McGrath J.J., Prochazka J., Pelouch V. & Ošťádal B. (1973) Physiological response of rats to intermittent high-altitude stress: effects of age. *J. Appl. Physiol.* **34,** 289–93.

59 Mani M.S. (1962) *Introduction to High Altitude Entomology.* Methuen, London.

60 Merino C.F. (1950) Studies on blood formation and destruction in the polycythemia of high altitude. *Blood* **5,** 1–31.

61 Miller P.D. & Banchero N. (1971) Hematology of the resting llama. *Acta Physiol. Latinoam.* **21,** 81–6.

62 Monge C.C., Lozano R. & Carcelén A. (1964) Renal excretion of bicarbonate in high altitude natives and in natives with chronic mountain sickness. *J. Clin. Invest.* **43,** 2303–9.

63 Monge M.C. & Monge C.C. (1966) *High altitude diseases.* Charles C. Thomas, Springfield, Illinois.

64 Monge M.C. & Monge C.C. (1968) *Adaptation of Domestic Animals* (ed. E. S. E. Hafez) pp. 194–201. Lea & Febiger, Philadelphia.

65 Monge C.C. & Whittembury J. (1974) Increased hemoglobin-oxygen affinity at extremely high altitudes. *Science* **186,** 843.

66 Morrison A. (1974) *Land Above the Clouds* (ed. C. Willock). Librerías A. B. C., Lima, Peru.

67 Morrison P. (1964) Wild animals at high altitudes. Effects of barometric pressure on survival. In *The Biology of Survival. Symp. Zool. Soc., London* **13,** 49–55.

68 Morrison P. & Elsner R. (1962) Influence of altitude on heart and breathing rates in some Peruvian rodents. *J. Appl. Physiol.* **17,** 467–70.

69 Morrison P.R., Kerst K., Reynafarje C. & Ramos J. (1963) Hematocrit and hemoglobin levels in some Peruvian rodents from high and low altitudes. *Int. J. Biometeor.* **7,** 51–8.

70 Morrison P.R., Kerst K. & Rosenmann M. (1963) Hematocrit and hemoglobin levels in some Chilean rodents from high and low altitude. *Int. J. Biometeor.* **7,** 45–50.

71 Ou L.C. & Tenney S.M. (1970) Properties of mitochondria from hearts of cattle acclimatized to high altitude. *Resp. Physiol.* **8,** 151–9.

72 Pearson O.P. (1951) Mammals in the highlands of Southern Peru. *Bull. Museum Comp. Zool.* (*Harvard College*) **106,** 117–74.

73 Pirofsky B. (1953) The determination of blood viscosity in man by a method based on Poiseuille's law. *J. Clin. Invest.* **32,** 292–8.

74 Prosser C.L. & Brown F.A. Jr (1962) Respiratory functions of body fluids. In *Comparative Animal Physiology* p. 217. Saunders, Philadelphia & London.

75 Rahn H. (1966) Introduction to the study of man at high altitudes: Conductance of O_2

from the environment to the tissues. In *Life at High Altitudes*, pp. 2–6. Panamerican Health Organization, No. 140.

76 Rennie D., Lozano R., Monge C.C., Sime F. & Whittembury J. (1971) Renal oxygenation in male Peruvian natives living permanently at high altitude. *J. Appl. Physiol.* **30,** 450–6.

77 Reynafarje B. (1962) Myoglobin content and enzymatic activity of muscle and altitude adaptation. *J. Appl. Physiol.* **17,** 301–5.

78 Reynafarje C. (1970) Control humoral de la eritropoyesis en la altura. *Arch. Inst. Biol. Andina* (Lima) **3,** 252–9.

79 Reynafarje B. (1971) *Mecanismos moleculares en la adaptación a la hipoxia de las grandes alturas*. Tesis Doctoral. Universidad Nacional Mayor de San Marcos, Lima.

80 Reynafarje C., Faura J., Paredes A. & Villavicencio D. (1968) Erythrokinetics in high-altitude adapted animals (Llama, alpaca, vicuña). *J. Appl. Physiol.* **24,** 93–7.

81 Reynafarje C., Lozano R. & Valdivieso J. (1959) The polycythemia of high altitudes: Iron metabolism and related aspects. *Blood* **14,** 433–55.

82 Reynafarje B. & Rosenmann M. (1971) Niveles de 2,3 difosfoglicerato en el eritrocito de mamíferos. *Arch. Inst. Biol. Andina. (Lima)* **4,** 67–73.

83 Schmidt-Nielsen K. & Larimer J.L. (1958) Oxygen dissociation curves of mammalian blood in relation to body size. *Am. J. Physiol.* **195,** 424–8.

84 Severinghaus J.W. (1972) Hypoxic respiratory drive and its loss during chronic hypoxia. *Clinical Physiol.* **2,** 57–79.

85 Severinghaus J.W., Bainton C.R. & Carcelén A. (1966) Respiratory insensitivity to hypoxia in chronically hypoxic man. *Resp. Physiol.* **1,** 308–34.

86 Sime F., Monge C.C. & Whittembury J. (1975) Age as a cause of Chronic Mountain Sickness (Monge's Disease). *Int. J. Biometeor.* **19,** 93–8.

87 Smith E.E. & Crowell J.W. (1963) Influence of hematocrit ratio on survival of unacclimatized dogs at simulated high altitude. *Am. J. Physiol.* **205,** 1172–4.

88 Smith E.E. & Crowell J.W. (1967) Role of an increased hematocrit in altitude acclimatization. *Aerospace Med.* **38,** 39–43.

89 Smith H. (1951) Comparative Physiology of the Kidney. In *The Kidney Structure and Function in Health and Disease*. pp. 520–74. Oxford University Press, Oxford & New York.

90 Swan L.W. (1961) The ecology of the high Himalayas. *Scientific American* **205,** 68–78.

91 Tappan D.S. & Reynafarje B. (1957) Tissue pigment manifestation of adaptation to high altitudes. *Am. J. Physiol.* **190,** 99–103.

92 Tappan D.V., Reynafarje B., Potter V.R. & Hurtado A. (1957) Alterations in enzymes and metabolites resulting from adaptation to low oxygen tensions. *Am. J. Physiol.* **190,** 93–8.

93 Tenney S.M. & Ou L.C. (1970) Physiological evidence for increased tissue capillarity in rats acclimatized to high altitudes. *Resp. Physiol.* **8,** 137–50.

94 Torrance J.D., Lenfant C., Cruz J. & Marticorena E. (1970/71) Oxygen transport mechanisms in residents at high altitude. *Resp. Physiol.* **11,** 1–15.

95 Turek Z., Grandtner N. & Kreuzer F. (1972) Cardiac hypertrophy, capillary and muscle fiber density, muscle fiber diameter, capillary radius and diffusion distance in the myocardium of growing rats adapted to a simulated altitude of 3500 m. *Pflügers Arch.* **335,** 19–28.

96 Turek Z., Ringnalda B.E.M., Grandtner M. & Kreutzer F. (1973) Myoglobin distribution in the heart of growing rats exposed to a simulated altitude of 3500 m in their youth or born in the low barometric chamber. *Pflügers Arch.* **340,** 1–10.

97 Turek Z., Ringnalda B.E.M., Hoofd L.J.C., Frans A. & Kreuzer F. (1972) Cardiac output, arterial and mixed venous O_2 saturation, and blood O_2 dissociation curve in growing rats adapted to a simulated altitude of 3500 m. *Pflügers Arch.* **335,** 10–18.

98 Ullrick W.C., Whitehorn W.V., Brennan B.B. & Krone J.G. (1956) Tissue respiration of rats acclimatized to low barometric pressure. *J. Appl. Physiol.* **9,** 49–52.

99 Valdivia E. (1958) Total capillary bed in striated muscle of guinea pigs native to the Peruvian mountains. *Am. J. Physiol.* **194,** 585–9.

100 Velásquez T. (1956) Maximal diffusing capacity of the lungs at high altitudes. *School of Aviation Medicine*. Rept 56–108. U.S.A.F. Randolph Field, Texas.
101 Vogel J.A., Hansen J.E. & Harris C.W. (1967) Cardiovascular response in man during exhaustive work at sea level and high altitude. *J. Appl. Physiol.* **23,** 531–9.
102 Weil J.V., Jamieson G., Brown D.W. & Grover R.F. (1968) The red cell mass-arterial oxygen relationship in normal man. *J. Clin. Invest.* **47,** 1627–39.
103 Whittembury J., Lozano R., Torres C. & Monge C.C. (1968) Blood viscosity in high altitude polycythemia. *Acta Physiol. Latinoam.* **18,** 355–9.
104 Whittembury J. & Monge C.C. (1972) High altitude, haematocrit and age. *Nature* (London) **238,** 278–9.

Prelude to Chapter 15

By tradition, physiology is an experimental science concerned with the study of the functions of contemporary organisms. The individual functions of cells, structures, organs and systems are deduced from studies made under controlled conditions in which the interactions of the many concurrent activities of the living system are reduced to a minimum. This is essential if one is to get clear and repeatable responses to particular disturbances such as the stimulation of a nerve, the injection of a chemical substance or a change in the physical environment. The understanding of physiology requires an intellectual synthesis of these isolated pieces of information so as to give the illusion, at least, of knowing how the entire organism responds to changes in its external and internal environments so that it may stay alive and to reproduce.

This emphasis on laboratory experimentation under controlled conditions has led to an acute awareness of both gross and subtle differences in the functions of different species, but physiologists in general have been slow to appreciate the cyclic changes in functions which occur within a species during the course of a nychthemeron (a period of day and night) and in the course of each year. Those authoritative statements in students' textbooks about the 'normal' levels of chemical and physical properties of body tissues and body fluids are often based on measurements made on medical students at, say, 10.00 hr. Misunderstandings and mis-diagnoses occur when these 'standards' are related to measurements made in the casualty ward in the middle of the night. Franz Halberg, who coined the term **circadian** to describe the approximately 24-hourly rhythmicity of many bodily functions even when all external time-clues (*Zeitgeber*) are denied the subject, has emphasized the need to record the nychthemeral rhythmicity of all bodily functions in both health and disease if errors in clinical judgement are to be avoided.

Annual rhythmicities still receive tardy recognition by some 'traditional' physiologists who may even regard seasonal changes as exceptional rather than general because they are not evident in laboratory-bred white rats! Many zoological physiologists, by contrast, are of the opposite opinion: that the processes of adaptation of organisms to seasonal changes in the environment involve changes in virtually every aspect of bodily functions. This is certainly borne out by the findings of zoologists in the U.S.S.R. who have captured Siberian rodents at all seasons of the year and then examined a whole range of bodily functions under the controlled laboratory conditions that would satisfy the traditional physiologist. With hibernating species the profound and predictable changes in functions with the seasons are well documented and readily accepted. The generality of seasonal changes in non-hibernants should also be acceptable: we all know that we adapt to summer heat and winter cold, and that we feel particularly stressed not by the heat of the summer or by the cold of the winter, but by sudden spells of unseasonal weather for which we are physiologically unprepared.

Since the whole of physiology relates to the capacity of organisms to make appropriate and adequate responses to disturbances; since a characteristic of living cells, systems and organisms is that they can adapt phenotypically (acclimate) to changes in the environment, and since the whole organism is involved in these processes, it is not surprising that, when looked for, seasonal changes can be found at all levels of function. The cosy world of the laboratory-bound physiologist with his standard preparations, and an annual cycle marked only by terms and vacations, has gone. Life is a dynamic phenomenon, changing in synchrony with the seasons, and physiology is the study of this dynamic equilibrium in a system in which the capacity to respond to stresses is being continuously adjusted to the nature and the severity of those stresses. Since both the environmental stresses and the physiological responses are multifactorial, these single adaptive changes (= *acclimation*) have also to be studied in an artificially simplified environment in the laboratory and then related to natural environmental circumstances which elicit complex changes in functions (= *acclimatization*).

Chapter 15
Seasonal changes in the whole animal

HERMANN POHL

15.1 INTRODUCTION

Variations in daylight, temperature or precipitation associated with seasons are among the predominant cyclic environmental factors that influence animals throughout their lives. The range of these variations depends on latitude, altitude and local climatic conditions. Seasonal changes in structure and function occur in animals in almost all life-zones, but they are more prevalent at middle and high latitudes than at lower ones.

Seasonal changes in animals have been considered as 'acquired' (phenotypic) but they are, for the most part, not entirely the result of direct influences of the environment on the animal. They are based on the interaction of various environmental effects (light, temperature, nutritional and social) with endogenous rhythmic components, including seasonal rhythms [1, 11, 20]. Changes in either light, temperature or nutrition have been the ultimate (evolutionary) causes (*ultimate factors*) for the occurrence of functional changes at times of the year when they are most advantageous to survival of a species [3, 83], but the actual timing factors (*proximate factors*) may be quite different from the ultimate ones. The seasonal change in daylength must be considered a principal proximate factor in the timing of seasonal changes in mid- and high-latitude species [15].

Most seasonal modifications involve profound physiological adjustments with concomitant changes in morphology and behaviour. It is therefore necessary for an animal to 'anticipate' forthcoming seasons and to begin appropriate physiological preparations in advance of changes in the ultimate environmental factors [1]. An important prerequisite for such anticipation is the ability of the animal to measure time [8].

The primary emphasis of this chapter will be on the rhythmic nature of seasonal changes in animals. In the first part, the general principles of annual time measurement and of the temporal control of seasonal changes in animals, will be described. In the second part, some selected seasonal phenomena will be cited as illustrations of the principles previously outlined.

15.2 EXOGENOUS VERSUS ENDOGENOUS CONTROL OF SEASONAL CHANGES

A change in any behavioural, morphological or physiological function of an animal at a particular time of year can be the result of either a direct (causal) or indirect (releasing or synchronizing) effect of the environment on the animal. Generally, 3 types of temporal control of seasonal changes can be distinguished:

1 A seasonally changing environmental factor which may be a change in intensity or duration of light, temperature, precipitation, oxygen supply, nutrition or social factors may directly and solely influence or cause a change in a specific animal function.

2 A seasonally changing environmental factor may initiate or release a specific functional change, the temporal characteristics of which are endogenous, and which may subsequently cause or release a change of another function.

3 A particular functional change may be initiated endogenously by an internal 'clock' which is synchronized and set in proper phase with the annual solar cycle by environmental stimuli (*Zeitgebers*). This implies that the particular function also changes periodically in the absence of the Zeitgeber but with a period length of approximately one year (*circannual* rhythm), rather than exactly one year (annual), provided that the internal and external conditions *per se* are permissive.

The first type of temporal control may—in its strict sense—be rare in animals. Poikilotherms, for example fish, are active only at particular water temperatures, and thus seasonal changes in the temperature of the water can directly influence the level and duration of activity. In most birds living at middle and high latitudes, the seasonal changes in daylength (photoperiod) directly effect their activity time [18]. In all such cases, however, it is possible that this direct response to an environmental variable only 'masks' other seasonal functions or responses which have their own endogenous temporal properties (cf. Section 15.4.1).

So far the second type has been found to be the most universal and common principle of the temporal control of seasonal changes in animals [8, 15]. Seasonal variation in reproductive functions, growth, social behaviour or acclimatization (see Chapter 13) have been shown to be released or 'triggered' by environmental stimuli, especially changes in daylength or temperature or both. Several examples of photoperiodically controlled responses, for instance the initiation of diapause in insects or the beginning of breeding and migration in birds will be considered in the following sections (15.4.3, 4 and 6). The principal characteristics of this type of control are: (i) mechanisms which provide the temporal sequence of internal changes and events, and (ii) mechanisms which measure time by using periodic information of the environment as a 'calendar' for proper timing of these changes (see Section 15.3.1) [14, 15].

The third type of control has probably evolved independently but may interact with the second type. The animal has its own circannual clock which has only to be 'rephased' once a year in order to be synchronized with its seasonal environment (Section 15.3.2). Seasonal animal events like the beginning of homeward migration of birds that winter close to the Equator and breed in the Arctic, or the spontaneous awakening of hibernating mammals several metres deep in the ground, occur at the right time during the year because of the existence of an endogenous circannual clock. In both cases no distinct environmental stimuli may have affected the animals at the time the events normally occur. Besides the conspicuous adaptive significance of endogenous temporal control in some species, as for instance in the two examples just mentioned [19, 33], this third type of control seems to be a quite general phenomenon in animals since it has also been found in species which are usually not exposed to a constant or unpredictable environment during some part of the year [45, 79].

15.3 PRINCIPLES OF ANNUAL TIME MEASUREMENT

15.3.1 Photoperiodic time measurement

The variation of day (or night) length is the most reliable temporal information about seasons at middle and high latitudes. More than a century ago, it was suggested that plants and animals use this information for controlling seasonal functions [8]. Marcovitch (1924) first discovered that in animals daylength effects the appearance of oviparous females in plant lice (aphides), and at the same time Rowan found that changes in daylength (photoperiod) control seasonal migration and reproduction in birds [8]. About 10 years later, Bünning proposed that an innate daily (circadian) rhythm of photosensitivity is causally involved in the mechanisms by which organisms measure annual time through changes in daylength [8]. It has been assumed that both plant and animal functions are influenced by light only during particular phases of their circadian

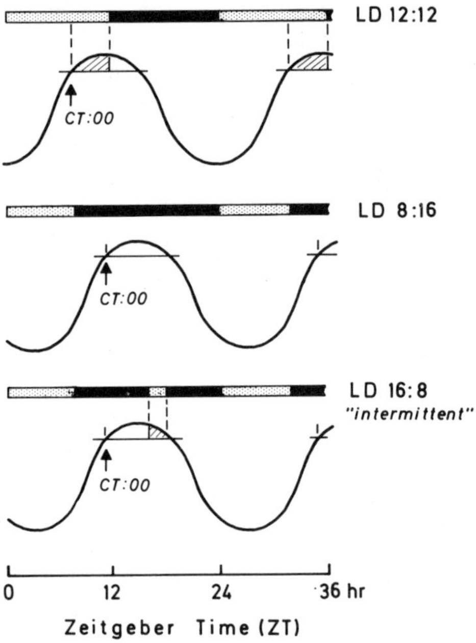

Fig. 15.1. Model of *external coincidence* for measurement of daylength under 3 photoperiodic conditions. An underlying circadian oscillation is divided into a photo-sensitive phase (above threshold) and an insensitive phase (below threshold). If light coincides with the sensitive phase (cross-hatched area), photoperiodic induction occurs. The time scale refers to *Zeitgeber time* (ZT) or *environmental time*. The onset of the photo-sensitive phase is arbitrarily set at *circadian time* (CT) or *subjective time* zero. Adapted from [78].

rhythms. Only when the light fraction of the natural (or artificial) light–dark (LD) cycle either coincides with a light-sensitive phase, or is above a specific threshold sensitivity, does photoperiodic induction occur and cause the stimulation or inhibition of biological changes at the appropriate times of year (Fig. 15.1).

Two experimental techniques have been used to evaluate the mechanism of photoperiodic time measurement and the role of the circadian rhythm. Both were used first in plants but were later applied to animals—particularly to insects and birds [8, 27, 52].

In experiments of the first type (Fig. 15.2A), an artificial LD cycle with a period of 24 hrs and a constant light fraction were used. The dark fraction of the cycle was interrupted by light breaks of 1 or 2 hrs (or even of a few minutes) at different phases during the cycle. In this example, the percentage of diapausing larvae of the moth *Pectinophora gossypiella* (the pink bollworm) was measured. Larvae of the last instar were maintained for several cycles of 13 hrs of light and 11 hrs of darkness with a 1-hr light break occurring at different phases during the dark fraction. Diapause was totally inhibited when light fell in the dark fraction about 14 to 15 hrs after the beginning of the light time [39]. Experiments of this type have demonstrated that photoperiodic control of seasonal change is based on a difference in the sensitivity of the organism to light at various phases of a 24-hr rhythm.

The example of the second type of approach (Fig. 15.2B) is from a study on the house finch (*Carpodacus mexicanus*) [58]. Groups of birds were maintained at different artificial LD cycles with periods ranging from 12 to 72 hrs. The light fraction was held constant at 6 hrs in each cycle which resulted in dark fractions of 6 to 66 hrs duration. Testicular development only took place at cycles of 12, 36

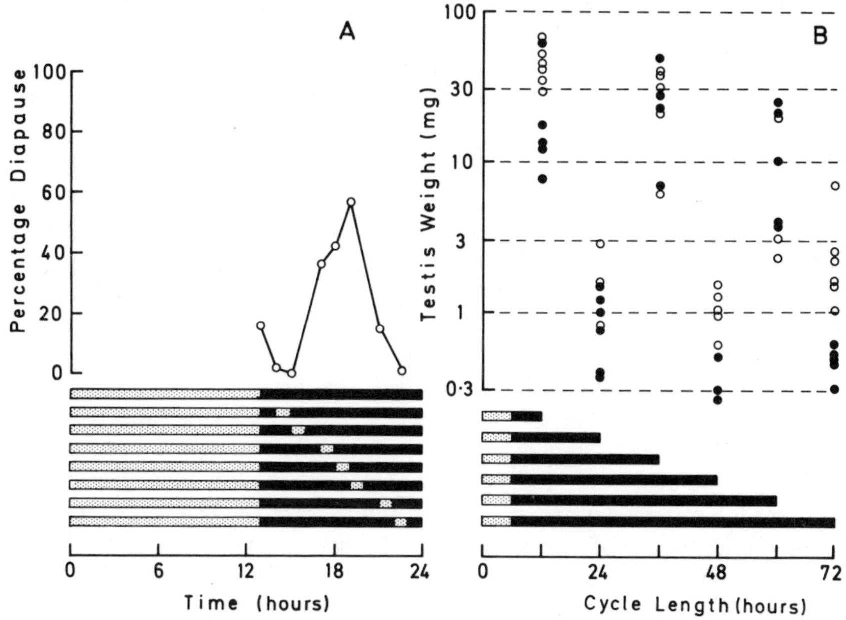

Fig. 15.2. (A) Percentage of diapausing individuals of the moth *Pectinophora gossypiella* at 12:12 hr light-dark cycles without and with 1 hr light breaks at different phases during the dark fraction. From [39]. (B) Testis weight of house finches (*Carpodacus mexicanus*) kept at light–dark cycles with different cycle lengths but a constant light fraction of 6 hr. The open and closed circles represent individuals from two independent sets of data. The data points (single means in A or groups of individuals in B) refer to the respective light–dark regimes shown at the bottom. From [58].

and 60 hrs, i.e. at LD cycles with periods differing by 24 hrs. This was unequivocal evidence that a circadian rhythm of photosensitivity with a period close to 24 hrs was basically involved in photoperiodic induction. The experiment further demonstrated that neither the duration of light time nor of dark time *per se* was decisive, but merely the *critical phase* at which the light coincided with the birds' circadian rhythms of responsiveness to light.

Bünning's hypothesis of photoperiodic time measurement (i.e. the external coincidence model [78]) explains most of the evidence of the involvement of a circadian rhythm. It has been shown, however, that, besides its inducing effects on seasonal functions, the photoperiod also influences the phase relations between the circadian system and the external *Zeitgeber* (phase-controlling effect) [41, 76]. In other words, the *photoperiodically inducible phase* of the circadian rhythm may not be *locked* to a particular phase of the environmental cycle but may vary in its phase relation in response to changes in duration and intensity of light. The light-sensitive phase might therefore be related to circadian time or subjective time rather than to (arbitrary) Zeitgeber time or environmental time (cf. Fig. 15.1) [78]. A dual role of changes in light can also be seen in other functional differences. For examples, differences in the reception mechanisms (retinal or extra-retinal light perception); differences in the sensitivity threshold and action spectra which have been shown to differ also for retinal and extra-retinal receptors; and differences (structural and physiological) in the mechanisms that transmit light information to the neuroendocrine system [6, 30].

The circadian clock is composed of a multiplicity of oscillators (multi-oscillatory system) that control various metabolic functions at organ and cellular levels [42, 75]. These components have distinct phase relations and temporal order within the organisms. Thus, *internal coincidence* of various circadian rhythms or clocks within the animal may be necessary for photoperiodic induction [76]. A particular hypothesis is that two independent circadian clocks, which are differently responsive to light, control the same (or different but related) physiological functions: a so-called *light-on* (or dawn) oscillator and a *light-off* (or dusk) oscillator [13, 59, 77]. If photoperiodic induction depends only on a specific steady-state relation of constituent oscillations, it seems plausible that factors other than light (e.g. temperature or even social factors) may also effect the phase relations, and hence, induce seasonal changes [77].

For precise timing of seasonal events, the measurement of daylength must involve the discrimination between increasing and decreasing photoperiod. This could be achieved either directly by the measurement of direction changes or indirectly by a combination of two measurements which initiate different physiological responses, the sequence and duration of which are temporally *programmed* in the animal [8]. However, environmental factors (light intensity, temperature, rainfall) may influence or modify these responses. In insects, extreme changes in temperature have been found to interfere with or even disrupt the photoperiodic control of diapause, and temperature control can substitute for photoperiodic control [8].

The possibility that time measuring systems other than the circadian clock may be involved in photoperiodic control of seasonal functions cannot be excluded. In some insect species [8, 67], for instance, observations have been interpreted as due to *hourglass*-like mechanisms which measure dark or light fractions by different photochemical reactions [27, 76].

15.3.2 The circannual clock

The existence of an endogenous annual clock has long been discussed [7, 8, 55], but it was not until 1963 that Pengelley and Fisher presented conclusive evidence of a *true* circannual rhythm in a hibernating mammal [74]. The following 3 criteria would verify—by analogy to circadian rhythms—the endogenous nature of annual or seasonal rhythms [33]:

1 The rhythm should persist under constant conditions, i.e. without any relevant annual stimulus (*Zeitgeber*) from the environment.

2 The interval (period) between identical or corresponding phases of the rhythm should deviate from exactly 12 months or 365 days.

3 A differential sensitivity to the synchronizing *Zeitgeber* (photoperiod, temperature, etc.) should be on an annual or seasonal basis.

As an example of circannual rhythms that both persist under seasonally constant conditions and deviate in their period length from 12 months, the rhythms of migratory activity (*Zugunruhe* [84]) and moult of a palearctic warbler (*Phylloscopus trochilus*) are illustrated (Fig. 15.3A) [54]. The bird was raised by hand and kept under a constant artificial LD cycle of 12 hrs of light and 12 hrs of darkness at about 20°C for 28 months. Nightly activity, which is a

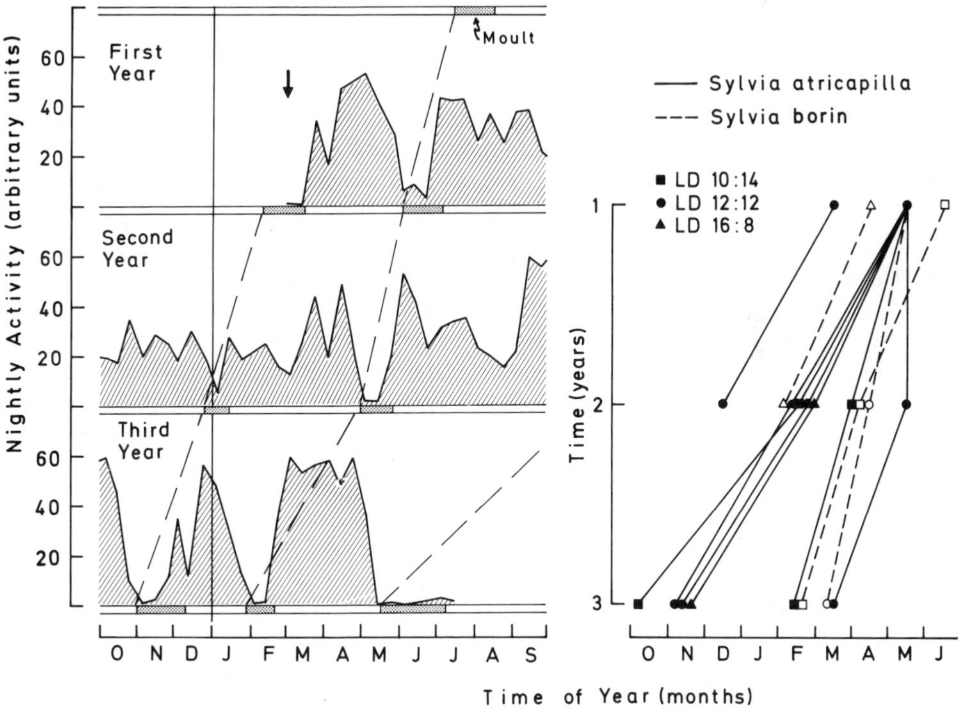

Fig. 15.3. Left diagram. Nightly activity (*Zugunruhe*) and moult schedules of a willow warbler (*Phylloscopus trochilus*) kept at a constant 12:12 hr light–dark cycle and constant temperature (21°C) for 28 months. From [54]. Right diagram: Maximal testis weights of 3 garden warblers (*Sylvia borin*) and 7 blackcaps (*S. atricapilla*) in relation to their position on the time scale (abscissa) in 3 consecutive years under different constant photoperiodic conditions (see different symbols). Testis weight was determined by laparotomy at 1 to 3 months' intervals. From [19]. In both diagrams, lines connect corresponding phases of rhythmic functions of individuals.

characteristic of caged migratory birds at the times of migration [84] was recorded continuously by microswitches under the perch, and the state of moult was determined at regular intervals. From the beginning of the experiment, peaks of nightly activity and moult alternated in about the same bi-modal pattern as in warblers kept under natural changes in daylength at the breeding area of the population. Minimal activity during the night, which was associated with moult, occurred about 2 months earlier in consecutive years. Similar results on groups of warblers of the genus *Sylvia* (*S. borin* and *S. atricapilla*) that were held under different constant photoperiods, showed circannual rhythms of various seasonal functions, such as *Zugunruhe*, body weight (pre-migratory obesity), moult and testis size (Fig. 15.3B) [7, 19]. In some individuals the rhythms persisted under constant conditions for as long as 6 full cycles.

The influence of temperature on circannual rhythms was studied in hibernating ground squirrels (genus *Spermophilus*) by Pengelley and colleagues [33]. Although a slight but consistent dependence of the period length—measured between successive onsets of hibernation (cf. Fig. 15.8)—on temperature (between 0 and about 35°C) was found, a change in period length of less than 10% over a 10°C change in temperature can be regarded as lacking specific temperature-dependence.

By searching for relevant environmental stimuli (*Zeitgebers*) which will synchronize circannual rhythms with seasons, an annual rhythm of sensitivity has been found to changes in both light and temperature. These may be considered the principal seasonal *Zeitgebers*. In the starling, *Sturnus vulgaris*, a change from a 12:12 hr LD cycle to constant dim light of about 1 lux had different effects on testis size at different times of the year [56]: maximal enlargement of the testis occurred in early spring; the opposite effect (decrease in size) occurred in summer. In late summer and autumn, a change in the light conditions had no effect on the testis size (cf. Section 15.4.3). In the golden-mantled ground squirrel, *Spermophilus lateralis*, a change in environmental temperature from 35° to 0°C induced hibernation with different time lags (from 3 to 200 days) depending on the phase of the annual cycle of body weight when temperature was changed. In this case, the seasonal change in body weight reflected changes in the preparatory state of the animal for hibernation [74, 31] (cf. Section 15.4.5).

All these properties support, or are at least consistent with, the hypothesis that innate circannual rhythms are the basis for a *circannual clock* serving as a 'temporal matrix' of events that occur in the external environment during the course of the year. Recent studies on seasonal rhythms of various physiological and behavioural functions in migratory birds have shown that under certain environmental conditions the phase relations between particular functions can change [7]. This is particularly conspicuous in such functions as, for example, migratory activity (*Zugunruhe*) and moult which have always been considered as mutually exclusive events (cf. Section 15.4.6 and Fig. 15.10). The loss of *internal coincidence* between distinct phases of circannual rhythms (or of various clocks) can lead to the temporal dissociation or desynchronization of rhythmic components controlling different metabolic pathways. Thus, it can be argued that rigid control of internal temporal order of various circannual rhythms or clocks can provide the manifestation of overt rhythms over many cycles under seasonally constant environmental conditions.

15.4 SELECTED SEASONAL PHENOMENA

15.4.1 Seasonal effects on circadian rhythms

The significance of a specific daily (circadian) pattern of activity has been related to various factors in the environment, of which climatic stress (see Chapter 13),

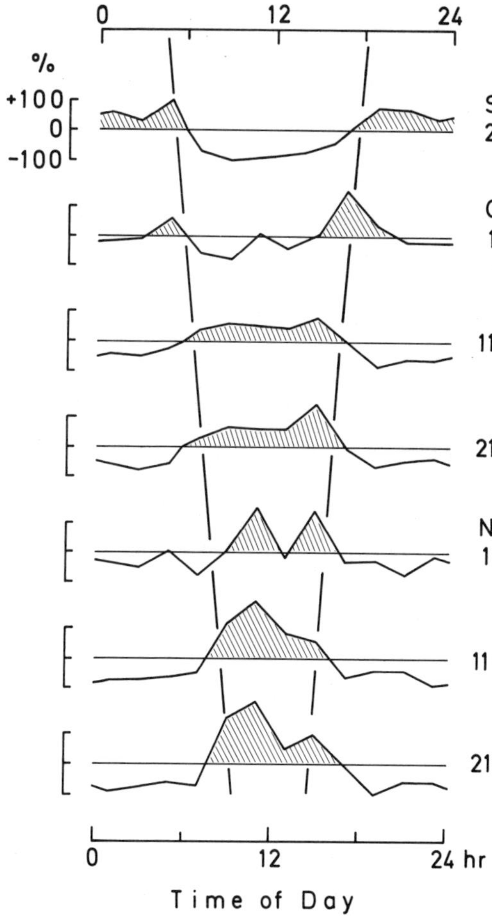

Fig. 15.4. Change from night to day activity in sculpins (*Cottus gobio*) under natural light conditions at the Arctic Circle. Each curve shows the percent deviations of 2-hr values from the 24-hr means averaged from several fishes over a 10-day period. Locomotor activity was measured through breaking of an infra-red light beam by the swimming fish. The converging lines indicate the 5-lux limits. [40].

the availability of food and the protection from predators are the most obvious [42]. In all classes of animals, special adaptations to either diurnal or nocturnal life have evolved, and in many habitats congeneric species have occupied ecological niches which differ in their spatial as well as temporal properties [11, 64].

Seasonally changing patterns of daily activity are widespread in many classes of animals from insects to mammals. In some arctic insect larvae, fishes, birds and mammals, daily activity rhythms desynchronize or disappear during midsummer when differences in light intensity become imperceptable [50, 73, 85]. A seasonal change from nocturnal activity in summer to mostly diurnal activity in winter was first observed in voles (*Microtini*) but occurs also in several species of fish (Fig. 15.4) [40, 49, 73]. A latitudinal influence on the circadian activity pattern during midsummer was observed in the mayfly (*Baetis rhodei*) in central and northern Europe. At latitudes of 51 and 60°N, the sampling number of flies in a stream drift showed a distinct peak at midnight. At 67°N lat., only a weak daily pattern occurred while the light intensity in the stream remained above 100 lux during midsummer [73].

It is well known that during the breeding season the different species of songbirds in a particular habitat begin singing at distinct times before, during or after sunrise. These species-specific differences can be related to different light

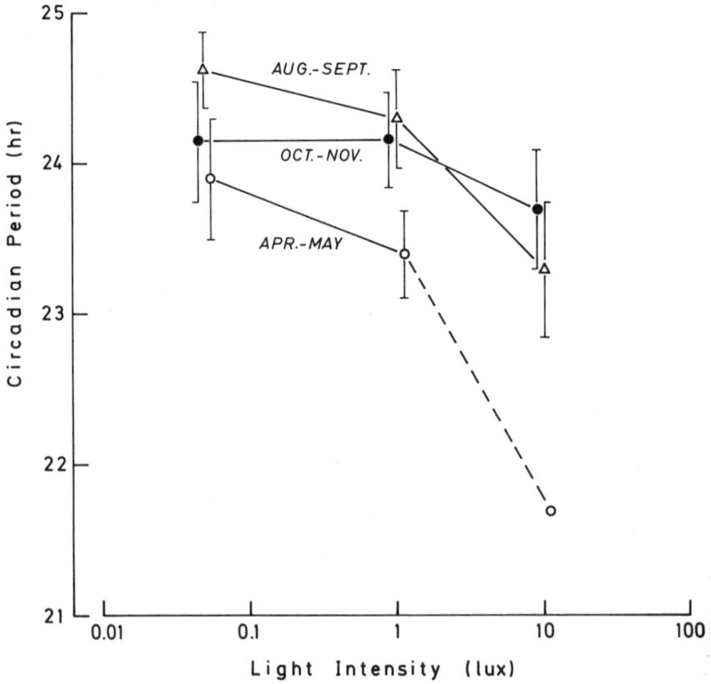

Fig. 15.5. Mean duration of circadian period of locomotor activity rhythms of 5 to 7 redpolls (*Acanthis flammea*) measured in constant illumination at 10°C, in relation to light intensity at different times of the year. The vertical lines are ±one standard deviation. Birds measured at 0·05 lux during August were in heavy moult. From [81]; including new unpublished data.

sensitivity thresholds or different innate phase relations between a bird's circadian rhythm of activity and the natural light–dark cycle. The beginning and end of daily activity of birds in relation to sun time or dawn and dusk however change during the year, especially in species that live in areas with extreme seasonal changes in daylight, as for instance in the Arctic [43].

An experiment with a small passerine bird (*Acanthis flammea*) which inhabits arctic and subarctic regions during summer and winter, showed that a seasonally changing sensitivity of the circadian system to light must be considered among the factors primarily responsible for seasonal changes in daily activity in relation to light or darkness (Fig. 15.5) [81]. Birds of a northern breeding population were subjected to constant illumination of various intensities at different times of the year, i.e. at different phases of the birds' annual cycles. The period length of the free-running circadian rhythm of cage activity was determined after a 2 weeks' exposure to each light intensity. During summer moult the birds had significantly longer circadian periods than during autumn or spring when the periods were shortest. Under natural light conditions, moulting birds of the same species begin activity later with respect to dawn than during other times of the year and especially than during the breeding season. These observations are consistent with the hypothesis proposed by Aschoff that the circadian period determines the phase relations between an animal's circadian activity rhythm and the natural light–dark cycle [41]. External factors (e.g. temperature) as well as internal factors (e.g. reproductive state) can, however, influence these relations [57, 81].

15.4.2 Metabolism and food preference

The metabolic energy required by animals for activity and growth depends on the process involved and the time of the year. In poikilothermic animals, the metabolic rate is a function of environmental temperature unless they are specifically adapted or acclimatized to temperature (see Chapter 13). Thus, mobility and productive processes (reproduction, growth, etc.) are restricted to times when biotic factors (e.g. food supply) and abiotic factors (e.g. temperature) are at optimum level. In homeothermic animals a major portion of the total energy expenditure during the year is required for maintenance of a high and regulated body temperature. The influence of season on quantitative and qualitative aspects of energy metabolism has been investigated mostly in homeotherms, and most particularly in birds [9, 38]. Quantitative aspects relate mainly to the amount of energy required for various activities, the rate of energy flow through an individual or a whole population. Qualitative aspects refer to metabolic efficiency and dietary selection [38]. The occurrence of a species in a particular environment, its abundance and the timing of all functional changes and events during a yearly cycle depend ultimately on the amount of energy it can mobilize at a specific time of year [65]. The following two examples illustrate several of the features involved.

The seasonal patterns of abundance and diversity of insectivorous birds on the arctic tundra, which are related primarily to seasonal cycles of insect prey, are among the most conspicuous of seasonal adaptations [62]. Measurements of energy cost for temperature regulation and breeding activities (egg laying, incubation, feeding young, etc.) in various species of sandpipers (genus *Calidris*) have shown that the precise timing of energy-demanding processes determines reproductive success and survival [38]. Because of the short time available for reproduction, which extends over only 25 days from establishing territories until complete incubation, and the high metabolic costs (about 2·5 times the standard resting rate [26]), energy must be mobilized at a high rate in adults engaged in various reproductive activities [38]. To secure successful raising of sandpiper chicks, the hatching of the eggs must coincide with the peak of emergence of

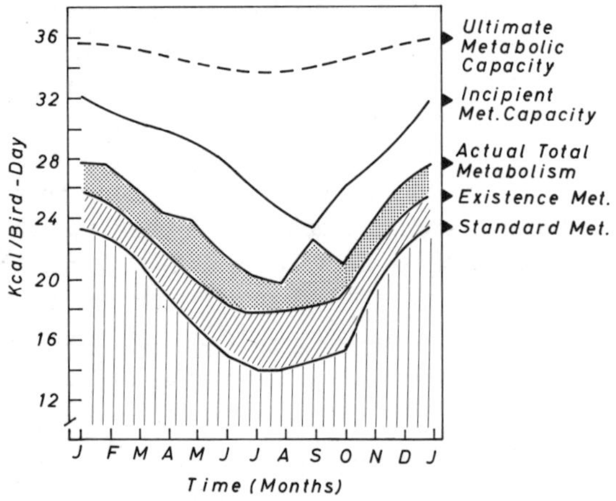

Fig. 15.6. Monthly variation of energy metabolism of the house sparrow (*Passer domesticus*) throughout the year. (Savings due to nightly roosting habits are not included in the graph.) Details in the text. After [65].

adult insects which in turn is dependent on the time of snow melt. Hence, the increasing temperature at the breeding sites triggers off the reproductive activities of the birds concomitantly with the maximum availability of food [62].

Permanent residency of birds at middle and high latitudes is another example which shows how animals adapt to seasons in order to cope with large fluctuations in environmental conditions. The energy budget of the house sparrow (*Passer domesticus*) has been extensively studied during several decades by Kendeigh and his students [65]. The recent review of their work gives an almost complete picture of seasonal changes in energy metabolism attributed to various activities as well as the total flow of energy during the year (Fig. 15.6). The diagram shows the mean monthly variation in the energy metabolism of the house sparrow from the population living in central Illinois (*c.* 40°N lat.). Standard metabolism which varies between 14 kcal per day (0·68 W) and bird in summer and 23·5 kcal (1·14 W) in winter, represents daytime metabolism of inactive birds at the respective daylengths and mean monthly temperatures and include tissue metabolism for temperature regulation and the heat increment of feeding. Existence metabolism is defined as the metabolic requirement of a bird living in a cage without additional productive activity. The curve of the actual total metabolism includes the additional energy costs of the locomotor activity of free-living birds (searching for food, short-distance flights, social interaction, etc.) and for productive activities (reproduction, moult, etc). The *incipient metabolic work capacity* is the amount of energy mobilized at the lower limits of tolerance at the particular months. The difference between this level of metabolism and the actually measured total metabolism gives the *latent metabolic work capacity* which is the energy readily available for exceptional, productive and thermoregulatory demands. The curve representing the *ultimate metabolic work capacity* relates only to the winter- or cold-acclimatized animal during severe cold-stress. From the total yearly energy expenditure of a 28 gram sparrow which amounts to *c.* 8750 kcal (36·6 MJ), nearly 50% must be attributed to the basal metabolic rate; about 20% to energy used for temperature regulation; about 12·5% each for the heat increment through specific dynamic action of food digestion and for locomotor activity, and only about 5% for reproduction and moult.

With changing energy demands during the year, alterations occur in food [38, 46]. Many granivorous birds are known to rely on high protein diet (insects) when feeding their young. The tree sparrow (*Spizella arborea*) changes from an insectivorous to granivorous diet. Associated with this there are profound seasonal changes in specific enzymes and digestive or assimilative functions [38]. In the bearded tit (*Panurus biarmicus*), adaptive seasonal modifications in the gizzard from summer to winter have been found to be associated with changes in food preference [82]. Evidently these seasonal changes in metabolic functions and dietary selection are controlled by circannual rhythms as are many other seasonally changing functions of animals [46, 80].

15.4.3 Reproduction

(a) Timing and synchrony

The majority of animals reproduce annually at a time determined by particular environmental circumstances [1, 3]. A continuous ability to reproduce is rare in wild populations and occurs mainly in species in tropical habitats. In many of these populations, however, either only the males are continuously sexually prepared, or individuals reproduce once or twice a year at different times according to particular schedules. This means that all reproductive stages can be found within a single population at a particular time of year [24]. In tropical birds as well as in a crayfish (*Orconectes pellucidus*) that lives in caves, reproductive cycles of less than a year (between 5 and 12 months) have been observed. This is indicative of endogenous control of breeding in the absence of seasonal environmental cues [2, 63]. In *colony breeders* on tropical islands, social factors may be responsible for synchronizing individuals to breed at the same time [24].

In constant or in unpredictable environments, social factors, such as simultaneous swarming or the synchronous activity of sexually mature males and females, as well as intra- and inter-specific competition, should be considered as important evolutionary causes of innate rhythms of reproduction with periods of less than or approximately one year.

Exposure to predators of unprotected eggs or un-experienced young must be regarded the most critical point in the reproductive sequence of species which require precise timing [70]. The more extreme the seasonal variations in the environment—which is most obvious in Arctic and desert circumstances—the shorter is the time of reproduction of a species in a particular habitat [44]. Reproductive cycles, including the development of offspring, are therefore more synchronous among different species living in the same environment than among populations of a single species in quite different environments [44].

(*b*) *Photoperiod and temperature*

The most comprehensive studies of exogenous factors which influence or control reproductive cycles have been done on vertebrates, particularly fish [37] and small birds [16, 28], but also in reptiles [4, 29] and mammals [15, 20, 34]. One prominent feature of annual reproductive cycles is the alternation of an active (*progressive*) and an inactive (*preparatory* or *refractory*) phase which has been clearly demonstrated in reptiles and birds [16, 52, 69]. During the refractory phase which follows gonadal regression, the reproductive system is unresponsive to such environmental stimuli as changes in photoperiod or temperature or both. Photo- and thermo-refractoriness must both be considered specific adaptations to environmental conditions. A protracted refractory phase may prevent gonadal development at the 'wrong' time of the year. This is important in trans-equatorial migratory birds, for instance, that are subjected to relatively long or even increasing photoperiods after arrival at their wintering habitats. A short refractory period, by contrast, is advantageous to birds which inhabit semi-arid regions. These birds are prepared to breed within a few days at most times of the year when the environmental conditions are permissive, for instance, after a heavy rainfall [24].

In poikilothermic animals photoperiodic regulation of reproduction is greatly influenced by temperature [4]. In two species of lizards (*Anolis carolinensis* and *Lacerta sicula*), daylength and temperature both effect testicular recrudescence, but the sensitivity of the reproductive system to each of these factors varies seasonally [51, 69]. In *L. sicula campestris*, the transition from the *regenerative* (preparatory) phase to the early progressive phase of the male reproductive cycle is associated with a gradually decreasing threshold (or increasing *reaction-readiness*) to photoperiodic stimuli: in late autumn, the most effective photoperiod is 20 hrs; towards the end of the winter 12 hrs or less of light exposure will induce a response [51]. According to the general principles outlined in Section 15.3.2, a periodically changing sensitivity to environmental stimuli is essential for exogenous timing of an internal circannual clock. In both species, testicular development begins spontaneously in the spring, even at low body temperature and independently of the photoperiodic conditions, which indicates an endogenous periodic component [51, 68]. Similarly, interacting exogenous effects have been found in the control of gametogenesis, nest-building and spawning behaviour of fish [37] and of the ovarian cycle in invertebrates: molluscs, crustaceans and insects [12, 15].

(*c*) *Mammals and birds*

In large mammals with long gestation times, for example: deer, sheep and goats, copulation occurs in autumn or winter which allows birth of young in spring and early summer while the environmental conditions are optimal [1, 20]. Innate seasonal rhythms of reproduction and associated functions (e.g. rutting time and antler growth in deer) have been found in several species [20, 53, 60]. In some of these, the synchronizing effect of photoperiod predominates; in others day-length merely accelerates oestrus or promotes gonadal regression [34, 61]. In several mustelid species photoperiod controls the delayed implantation of the fertilized ovum. Long photoperiods shorten the gestation time by reducing the duration of delayed implantation [15].

The significance of the pineal gland in mediating photoperiodic control of reproductive function has been extensively studied in the golden hamster (*Mesocricetus auratus*) [35]. During short days in winter, the pineal gland is maximally active and the reproductive organs involute. The gonads, however, spontaneously regenerate in spring if short photoperiods are experimentally maintained. During long summer days, the pineal function is inhibited and the gonads are reproductively competent. At this time, the reproductive organs are refractory to the normally inhibitory influence of darkness and the activity of the pineal gland. From these findings it is evident that the annual cycle of reproduction in the hamster has both endogenous and exogenous components.

In birds, photoperiodic regulation of reproduction has been found chiefly among species inhabiting middle and high latitudes throughout the year but also in trans-equatorial migrants [15, 17]. In more than 50 avian species, mostly passeriformes, it has been shown that changes in daylength control the male reproductive cycle. Long days induce testicular recrudescence, short days terminate the refractoriness of the testes to photoperiodic stimulation. In addition to its initiating or releasing effects, a given photoperiod is *essential* for the development of the male gonads. A certain amount and duration of light is demanded in some species to secure full enlargement of the testes [16]. In the female reproductive cycle only the initial phase of ovarian development is controlled by light. Complete development and oviposition require additional environmental and social stimuli, for example: the presence of the male, nesting material, and others [24].

A circannual rhythm of testis size has been demonstrated in two species of palearctic warblers (*Sylvia borin* and *S. atricapilla*) which were hand-raised from the age between 2 and 9 days and kept under different constant photoperiods and constant temperature for 3 years (cf. Fig. 15.3B) [7]. The periodicity of the rhythm varied between 9 and 11 months in individuals, independently of the duration of the photoperiod. It is noteworthy that a circannual rhythm was present in both species, although one (*S. borin*) is a trans-equatorial migrant and the other (*S. atricapilla*) migrates mainly within the temperate zone between about 30° and 60°N latitudes [7]. In this context, it is remarkable that circannual rhythms as well as photoperiodic stimulation of reproduction have been found in species that are all-year residents in areas around the Equator [28, 48], although both mechanisms may have evolved under different environmental conditions and under different selection pressures. It is, therefore, not surprising that both photoperiodic time measurement and the circannual clock operate in a co-ordinated way in some species. This double strategy which provides precise correspondence between the bird's seasonal activities and the changing environment during the year, may well be an essential prerequisite for proper timing of reproduction and related functions in long-distance migrants.

15.4.4 Insect diapause

A great variety of adaptive mechanisms allow insects to occupy almost all geographic and climatic zones including those with extreme seasonal variations in temperature, light and humidity. Insects can generally exist in two states: a high energy *open* state and a low energy *closed* state [10]. The closed or inactive state, called diapause, is a seasonal adaptation that can occur during winter and summer when environmental conditions become harsh because of cold, heat, drought or famine. In this state metabolism is greatly reduced, heat or cold resistance is increased, and processes related to growth and formation are suspended. In many insect species with only one generation per year, diapause represents a normal phase of the life cycle and may be at any developmental stage: in the ovum, larvae, pupae or in the imago. It permits the continuity of life and ensures the synchronization of particular developmental stages with the seasons to which they are adapted [12]. This becomes particularly conspicuous in areas with a typical vernal rain fauna. In these semi-arid regions insects and many other invertebrates remain inactive during the greater part of the year [11].

The main characteristic in the regulation of diapause is the anticipation of adverse climatic or nutritional conditions. This can be seen particularly in species, such as the silkworm *Bombyx mori*, in which environmental factors, acting on the organism during a very early sensitive phase of embryonic development, determine whether females will produce eggs that are capable of undergoing diapausing state [15].

Among many ecological factors that can be regarded as the ultimate causes of diapause, photoperiod and temperature both act as proximate factors which promote or inhibit diapause in either *long-day* or *short-day* types of insects. In the *long-day* type of development which is widespread among insects, short days up to a critical daylength induce diapause (Fig. 15.7a). In the *short-day* type, the reverse situation occurs in that diapause can only be initiated by long

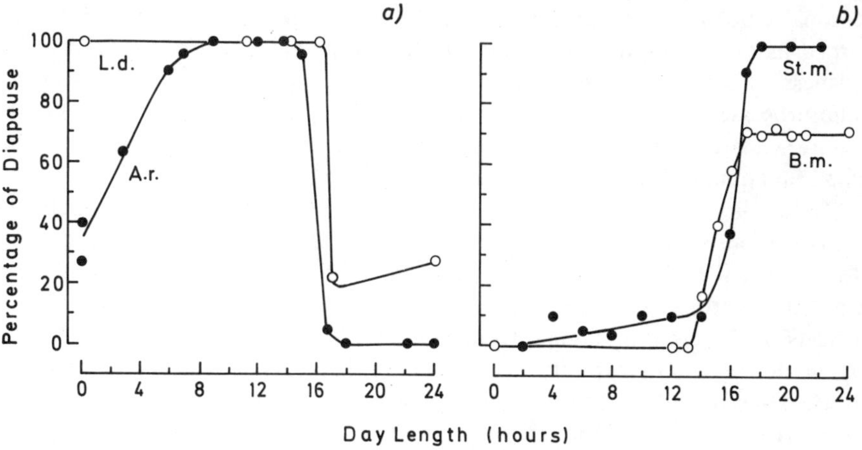

Fig. 15.7. Percentage of diapausing insects in relation to photoperiod. (a) *long-day type* species: *Leptinotarsa decemlineata* (L.d.) and *Acronycta ruminis* (A.r.); (b) *short-day type* species: *Stenocranus minutus* (St. m.) and *Bombyx mori* (B.m.). Data from Danilevsky *et al.*, Müller and Kogure (after [12]).

days (Fig. 15.7b). As in other light-mediated seasonal functions, the photoperiod which is effective in promoting diapause varies extensively among species and even among populations as a function of latitude. In other words, the same day length may serve as a different information for species or populations living at different latitudes [12]. Although in many species the length of the light or dark portion of a natural or artificial LD cycle is essential for either inducing or terminating diapause [27, 39], changing daylight has also been found to be effective, as for instance in the nymph of the dragonfly, *Anax imperator* [15].

The effect of temperature may be illustrated by two examples. In the caterpillar of the pine-moth *Dendrolimus pini*, preparation for diapause is most quickly achieved when the temperature is within the range preferred during active state. At lower temperatures (10 to 12°C) diapause occurs after 60 days, whereas at 23°C only 30 days are required. The temperature during induction also influences the duration of diapause [12]. In the larvae of the noctuid butterfly *Acronycta ruminis*, the short-day effect which normally initiates diapause in association with low temperature (which is a characteristic of most insects), is abolished by heating to 38°C for 3 hrs each day [10].

As might be expected in relatively short-lived animals such as insects, photoperiodic time measurement has the main controlling influence on seasonal changes like the transition from active to inactive life which occur only once or twice during the life span. Temperature represents a permissive factor that can even supersede photoperiod as the stimulus for initiating or terminating diapause, particularly if it acts at a particularly sensitive phase during development.

15.4.5 Seasonal torpidity in mammals

Seasonal torpidity in mammals which includes hibernation (an adaptation to seasonal cold) and estivation (an adaptation to seasonal drought) can be regarded as analogous to diapause of insects in terms of two common characteristics: (i) both phenomena represent a state of inactivity with reduced metabolic processes and increased independence of the environment, and (ii) both require a state of preparation which involves a multiplicity of appropriately timed functional changes at organ and cellular level [23, 31].

The ability to change from an homeothermic to an heterothermic state on a seasonal basis has evolved in several species of different phylogenetic groups of mammals [22]. Respiration and heart rate are temporarily reduced and body temperature drops to a lower level which is homeostatically regulated and which protects the hibernating animal from freezing [23, 31]. Hibernators and estivators do not remain in torpidity for the whole cold or dry season but periodically arouse either daily or in intervals of days or weeks depending on the species, on the internal state of preparation, and on external conditions, especially temperature [5, 23].

In ground squirrels (genus *Spermophilus*), chipmunks (genus *Eutamias*), dormice (genus *Eliomys*) and hedgehogs (genus *Erinaceus*), the readiness to hibernate and associated seasonal changes in functions, such as body weight (pre-hibernation fattening), food and water intake or locomotor activity, have been found to recur periodically under constant conditions of photoperiod and temperature, with the retention of the particular characteristics of different species [31, 33, 47, 60]. The cyclic changes in body weight reflect the state of preparation for hibernation (Fig. 15.8). Thus the circannual rhythms of body weight

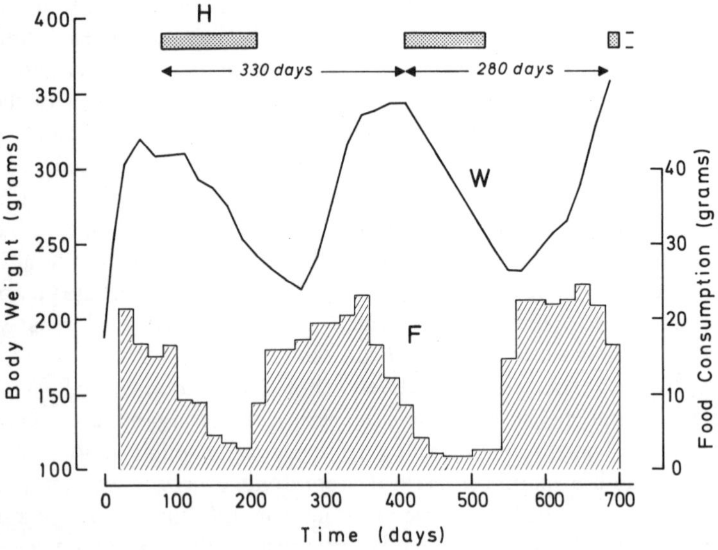

Fig. 15.8. Circannual rhythm of body weight (W), food intake (F) and hibernation (H) of a golden-mantled ground squirrel (*Spermophilus lateralis*) kept at a 12:12 hr light–dark cycle and 22°C for about 2 years. Food intake and body weight data were averaged over 20 days. Adapted from [74].

and hibernation seem to be intimately coupled. It has been found, however, that the manifestation of either rhythm can occur in the absence of the other. When the increase in body weight which normally precedes the onset of hibernation, was prevented by restricted access to food, ground squirrels (*S. lateralis*) hibernated at the same time as their conspecifics to which food was provided *ad libitum* and which reached their normal peak of body weight [33]. When both food and water were rationed for about 2 months during either the ascending or descending phase of the annual weight cycle, and the animals were frequently disturbed so as to prevent hibernation, the post-dietary weight did not return to the initial level but to a level determined by the underlying circannual rhythm [31, 60].

Environmental factors, such as daylength, temperature or shortage of food have been found to lengthen or shorten the active or the inactive phases of the circannual rhythm but the period between corresponding phases (e.g. the onset of hibernation) was not appreciably altered by any of these factors in ground squirrels [60]. In other hibernators, for instance the dormouse *Glis glis*, changes in photoperiod exerted a marked influence on the annual cycle of hibernation and related functions, like changes in body weight [31]. In the dormouse, the annual tendency to hibernate could be completely reversed within a year after a phase shift of the annual light cycle by 180 degrees (i.e. an interchange of light conditions prevailing at the same latitudes at the two hemispheres), while in the ground squirrel *S. tridecemlineatus* the rhythm maintained its original phase [72].

According to our present knowledge, the degree of endogenous control of seasonal torpidity in mammals seems to be different in various species, even among the Marmotini group of rodents. Within the genera *Spermophilus* (*Citellus*) and *Eutamias*, differences in the manifestation of circannual rhythms of functions related to hibernation and their degree of flexibility—determined by the amount of phase-shifting through external stimuli—could be related (i) to the specific external conditions prevailing at a particular habitat (including latitudinal and altitudinal differences), and (ii) to the specific physiological and behavioural features of the particular species. The latter may include differences in body size and in food habits (e.g. fattening or hoarding) [33, 60, 71].

15.4.6 Migration and related phenomena

Among the ultimate (evolutionary) causes for seasonal migration in animals, conditions favouring reproduction must be considered as a primary one. In the spring birds return several thousand miles following fixed routes to their breeding grounds at middle and high latitudes. Penguins and seals swim great distances to their breeding sites on shores and islands in either the northern or southern hemisphere, and salmons and eels migrate to their spawning places in streams or the open sea. Even insects, for instance the monarch butterfly (*Danaus plexippus*), make long latitudinal flights between winter and summer (breeding) habitats. In other species, for example large ruminating mammals (caribou, bison or antelopes) which inhabit the tundra, steppe or savannahs with extreme seasonal variation in temperature or precipitation or both, seasonal fluctuations in the availability of food are the principle reasons for long migratory movements. Likewise, many pelagic animals migrate at certain times of the year either vertically (e.g. marine crustaceans) or horizontally (e.g. whales) in search of better feeding places [21, 32, 36].

The seasonal appearance of birds on their arctic breeding grounds clearly demonstrates the times at which the conditions for reproduction are most favourable in this area (Fig. 15.9A), and the dates of their arrival and egg laying indicate the need for precise timing of migration and of physiological and behavioural changes related to various reproductive activities (Fig. 15.9B) [25].

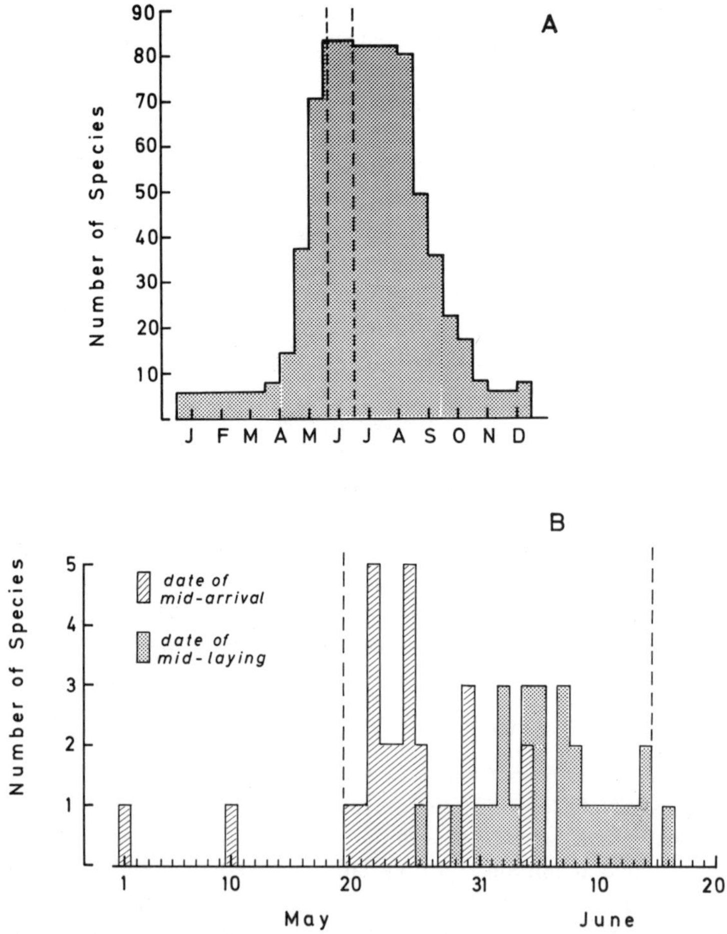

Fig. 15.9. (A) Seasonal occurrence of bird species at Ogoturuk Creek, Alaska (lat. 69°N) at two-week intervals throughout the year. From Williamson *et al.*, after [25]. (B) Dates of mid-arrival and mid-laying of 25 bird species at Anaktuvuk Pass, Alaska (lat. *c.* 68°N). From records made during several years of observation. Data from Table 5.1 in [25]. In both diagrams the vertical broken lines mark the same time interval.

As already mentioned in the previous sections, circannual rhythms are particularly pronounced in birds that migrate long distances, especially trans-equatorial migrants [18]. The ecological significance of internal control of annual periodicity in these birds is obvious [19]. Besides the timing of the gonadal cycle (cf. Section 15.4.3), the initiation and termination of the spontaneous

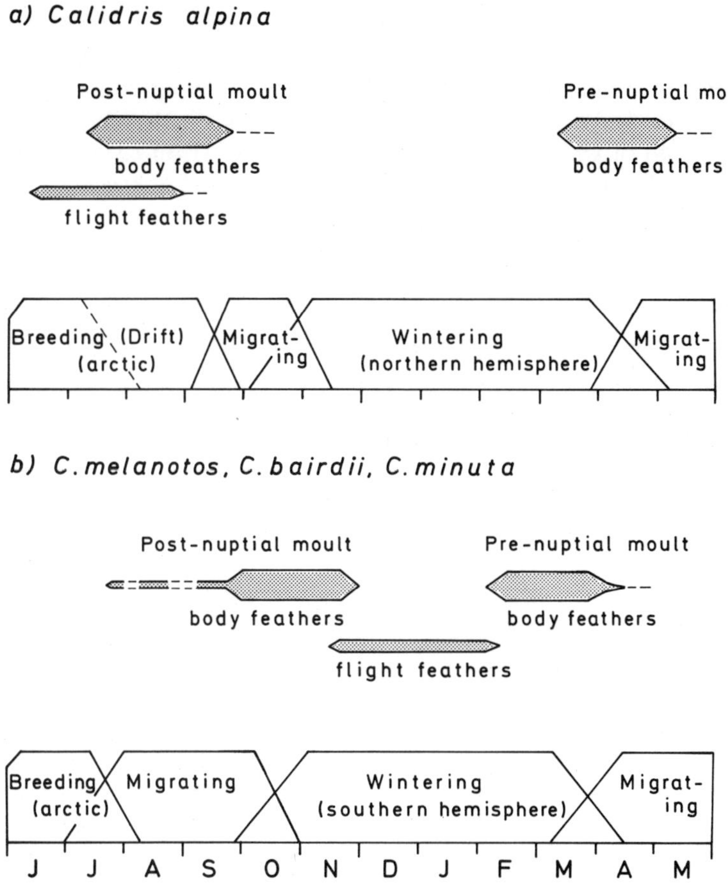

Fig. 15.10. Moult schedules of 4 Calidris-sandpipers breeding in the Arctic and wintering either north (upper diagram) or south (lower diagram) of the Equator, in relation to other major events of their annual cycles. From [62].

internal 'drive' for migration, which can be determined by directional movements [66] and by the amount of nightly activity (*Zugunruhe*), are endogenously programmed [19, 55].

The interrelations between different annual functions related to migration (in birds) are illustrated by the results of a comparative study on various species of sandpipers (genus *Calidris*) that breed on the arctic tundra but return to either north temperate or south temperate latitudes for wintering [62] (Fig. 15.10). The graph shows that the bi-modal seasonal pattern of moult differs in its phase relation to either the reproductive cycle or the seasonal migration according to the specific time and energy demands of migratory flight. In *C. alpina* which winters in north temperate regions, the post-nuptial moult of body feathers is almost complete when the birds start to migrate south, while in trans-equatorial migrants the onset of the heavy post-nuptial moult appears at the end of migration and moult continues through the summer in the southern hemisphere. The moult of flight feathers even occurs with a phase difference of 180 degrees (6-months) in the north and south temperate wintering species. Similarly, phase differences in annual moult schedules in relation to migration have been found under natural and constant photoperiodic conditions in 4 species of palearctic warblers, two of which (*Phylloscopus trochilus* and *Sylvia borin*) winter to the south of the Equator and the other two (*P. collybita* and *S. atricapilla*) winter to the north [7, 19].

These findings have an important bearing on the significance of an endogenous annual clock which involves a multiplicity of circannual rhythms with varying phase relations but which are synchronized and maintained in a species-specific temporal order by external cues. This view stands opposite to a still-prevalent opinion that a circannual cycle derives from a chain of successive events with intrinsic time lags (e.g. *hourglass*-like interval timers) which are causally dependent on each other [14, 31].

15.5 RETROSPECT

Seasonal adaptation to environmental stress implies two main strategies. Animals either cope with their environment ('take it' strategy) or escape to more favourable climate and food sources ('leave it' strategy) [38]. The 'take it' strategy has been widely exploited within the animal kingdom, in terrestrial as well as aquatic species. Processes of acclimatization to cold, heat or drought, which include temporary states of inactivity or torpidity are the most common types of seasonal responses of animals which enable them to withstand adverse environmental conditions. The 'leave it' strategy has been evolved in a relatively few animal species that are able to cover large distances by air, land or water and which can carry sufficient fuel (energy reserves) for the journey. Both strategies demand a great variety of physiological, morphological and behavioural adjustments timed to occur at the appropriate seasons.

Natural selection has repeatedly favoured the establishment of temporal pattern in which the seasonal availability of food coincides with the fuel needs for productive activities and physical work [5]. Precise timing of seasonal events must have been under high selective pressure since animals invaded geographic areas with large seasonal variation in temperature, light, drought, snow cover and other climatic factors. Since annual timing mechanisms may have developed independently and convergently many times in various classes, orders, and genera, it is to be expected that they vary considerably in their functional details and precision of operation [15, 77]. Even among species of the same genus, different time-measuring systems have developed according to the particular ecological conditions to which a species is exposed during the year, or the extent to which an animal must be able to respond to unpredictable external influences.

Acknowledgement

I wish to thank Drs J. Aschoff and E. Gwinner for valuable comments.

15.6 REFERENCES

Part 1: Books and reviews

1 Aschoff J. (1955) Jahresperiodik der Fortpflanzung bei Warmblütern. *Studium Generale* **8,** 742–76.

2 Ashmole N.P. (1971) Sea bird ecology and the marine environment. In *Avian Biology* (eds D. S. Farner & J. R. King) Vol. 1, pp. 223–86. Academic Press, New York & London.

3 Baker J.R. (1938) The evolution of breeding seasons. In *Evolution. Essays on Aspects of Evolutionary Biology* (ed. G. R. Beer), pp. 161–77. Oxford University Press, Oxford.

4 Bartholomew G.A. (1959) Photoperiodism in reptiles. In *Photoperiodism and Related Phenomena in Plants and Animals* (ed. R. B. Withrow) pp. 651–67. Am. Ass. Adv. Sci. No. 55, Washington, D.C.

5 Bartholomew G.A. (1972) Aspects of timing and periodicity of heterothermy. In *Hibernation and Hypothermia, Perspectives and Challenges* (eds. F. E. South *et al.*) pp. 663–80. Elsevier, Amsterdam.

6 Benoit J. & Assenmacher I. (eds) (1970) *La photorégulation de la reproduction chez les oiseaux et les mammifères.* C.N.R.S. Editeur, Paris.

7 Berthold P. (1974) Circannual rhythms in birds with different migratory habits. In *Circannual Clocks* (ed. E. T. Pengelley) pp. 55–94. Academic Press, New York & London.

8 Bünning E. (1973) *The Physiological Clock* (3rd rev. edition) 258 pp. The English Universities Press, London: Springer-Verlag, Berlin, Heidelberg & New York.

9 Calder W.A. & King J.R. (1974) Thermal and caloric relations of birds. In *Avian Biology* (eds D. S. Farner & J. R. King) Vol. 4, pp. 259–413. Academic Press, New York & London.

10 Clarke K.U. (1967) Insects and temperature. In *Thermobiology* (ed. A. H. Rose) pp. 293–352. Academic Press, London & New York.

11 Cloudsley-Thompson J.L. (1961) *Rhythmic Activity in Animal Physiology and Behaviour.* 236 pp. Academic Press, New York & London.

12 Danilevskii A.S. (1965) *Photoperiodism and Seasonal Development of Insects.* 283 pp. Oliver & Boyd, Edinburgh & London.

13 Danilevsky A.S., Goryshin N.I. & Tyshchenko V.P. (1970) Biological rhythms in terrestrial arthropods. *Ann. Rev. Entomol.* **15,** 201–44.

14 Enright J.T. (1970) Ecological aspects of endogenous rhythmicity. *Ann. Rev. Ecology and Systematics* **1,** 221–38.

15 Farner D.S. (1961) Comparative physiology: photoperiodicity. *Ann. Rev. Physiol.* **23,** 71–96.

16 Farner D.S. & Lewis R.A. (1971) Photoperiodism and reproductive cycles in birds. In *Photophysiology*: current topics in photochemistry and photobiology (ed. A. C. Giese) Vol. 6, pp. 325–70. Academic Press, New York & London.

17 Farner D.S., Lewis R.A. & Darden T.R. (1973) Photoperiodic control mechanisms:

homoiothermic animals. In *Biology Data Book* (2nd ed.) Vol. 2 (eds P. L. Altman & D. S. Dittmer) pp. 1047–52. Fed. Amer. Soc. Exper. Biol., Bethesda, Maryland.
18 Gwinner E. (1975) Circadian and circannual rhythms in birds. In *Avian Biology* (eds D. S. Farner & J. R. King) Vol. 5, pp. 221–85. Academic Press, New York & London.
19 Gwinner E. (1975) Adaptive significance of circannual rhythms in birds. In *Physiological Adaptation to the Environment* (ed. F. J. Vernberg). Intext Educational Publ. New York.
20 Hart J.S. (1964) Geography and season: mammals and birds. In *Handbook of Physiology* Sect. 4 (ed. D. B. Dill) pp. 295–321. Amer. Physiol. Soc. Washington, D.C.
21 Hasler A.D. (1971) Orientation and fish migration. In *Fish Physiology* (eds W. S. Hoar & D. J. Randall) Vol. 6, pp. 429–510. Academic Press, New York & London.
22 Hoffman R.A. (1964) Terrestrial animals in cold: hibernators. In *Handbook of Physiology* Sect. 4 (ed. D. B. Dill) pp. 379–403. Amer. Physiol. Soc. Washington, D.C.
23 Hudson J.W. (1973) Torpidity in mammals. In *Comparative Physiology of Thermoregulation* (ed. G. C. Whittow) Vol. 3, pp. 97–165. Academic Press, New York & London.
24 Immelmann K. (1971) Ecological aspects of periodic reproduction. In *Avian Biology* (eds D. S. Farner & J. R. King) Vol. 1, pp. 341–89. Academic Press, New York & London.
25 Irving L. (1972) Arctic Life of Birds and Mammals including Man. In *Zoophysiology and Ecology* (eds D. S. Farner *et al.*) Vol. 2, 192 pp. Springer-Verlag, Berlin, Heidelberg, New York.
26 King J.R. (1973) Energetics of reproduction in birds. In *Breeding Biology of Birds* (ed. D. S. Farner) pp. 78–107. Nat. Acad. Sci, Washington, D.C.
27 Lees A.D. (1968) Photoperiodism in insects. In *Photophysiology* (ed. A. C. Giese) Vol. 4, pp. 47–137. Academic Press, New York & London.
28 Lofts B. & Murton R.K. (1973) Reproduction in birds. In *Avian Biology* (eds D. S. Farner & J. R. King) Vol. 3, pp. 1–107. Academic Press, New York & London.
29 Mayhew W.W. (1968) Biology of desert amphibians and reptiles. In *Desert Biology* (ed. G. W. Brown Jr.) Vol. 1, pp. 195–421. Academic Press, New York & London.
30 Menaker M. & Oksche A. (1974) The avian pineal organ. In *Avian Biology* (eds D. S. Farner & J. R. King) Vol. 4, pp. 79–118. Academic Press, New York & London.
31 Mrosovsky N. (1971) *Hibernation and the Hypothalamus.* 287 pp. Appleton-Century-Crofts Educational Division, Meredith, New York.
32 Orr R.T. (1970) *Animals in Migration*, 303 pp. MacMillan, New York.
33 Pengelley E.T. & Asmundson S.J. (1974) Circannual rhythmicity in hibernating mammals. In *Circannual Clocks* (ed. E. T. Pengelley) pp. 95–160. Academic Press, New York & London.
34 Perry J.S. & Rowlands I.W. (eds) (1973) The Environment and Reproduction in Mammals and Birds. *J. Reprod. Fert.*, Suppl. 19, 613 pp. Blackwell Scientific Publications, Oxford.
35 Reiter R.J. (1974) Circannual reproductive rhythms in mammals related to photoperiod and pineal function: a review. *Chronobiologia* **1**, 365–95.
36 Ricard M. (1969) *The Mystery of Migration.* Constable, London.
37 Schwassmann H.O. (1971) Biological rhythms. In *Fish Physiology* (eds W. S. Hoar & D. J. Randall) Vol. 6, pp. 371–428. Academic Press, New York & London.
38 West G.C. & Norton D.W. (1975) Metabolic adaptations of tundra birds. In *Physiological Adaptation to the Environment* (ed. F. J. Vernberg). Intext Educational Publ. New York.

Part 2: Other references

39 Adkisson P.L. (1964) Action of the photoperiod in controlling insect diapause. *Amer. Natur.* **98,** 357–74.
40 Andreasson S. (1973) Seasonal changes in diel activity of *Cottus poecilopus* and *C. gobio* (Pisces) at the Arctic Circle. *Oikos* **24,** 16–23.
41 Aschoff J. (1960) Exogenous and endogenous components in circadian rhythms. In *Cold*

Spr. Harb. Symp. quant. Biol. (ed. A. Chovnick) Vol. 25, pp. 11–28. Long Island Biol. Ass., Cold Spring Harbor, L.I., N.Y.

42 Aschoff J. (1967) Adaptive cycles: their significance for defining environmental hazards. *Int. J. Biometeor.* **11,** 255–78.

43 Aschoff J.E., Gwinner A. Kureck & Müller K. (1970) Diel rhythms of chaffinches *Fringilla coelebs* L., tree shrews *Tupaia glis* L. and hamsters *Mesoricetus auratus* Waterh. as a function of season at the Arctic Circle. *Oikos* Suppl. **13,** 91–100.

44 Baker J.R. (1938) The relation between latitude and breeding seasons in birds. *Proc. Zool. Soc. Lond.* **108** (A), 557–82.

45 Berthold P. (1973) Circannuale Periodik bei Teilziehern und Standvögeln. *Naturwissenschaften* **60,** 522–3.

46 Berthold P. & Berthold H. (1973) Jahreszeitliche Änderungen der Nahrungspräferenz und deren Bedeutung bei einem Zugvogel. *Naturwissenschaften* **60,** 391–2.

47 Daan S. (1973) Periodicity of heterothermy in the garden dormouse, *Eliomys quercinus* (L.) *Netherlands J. Zool.* **23,** 237–65.

48 Epple A., Orians G.H., Farner D.S. & Lewis R.A. (1972) The photoperiodic testicular response of a tropical finch, *Zonotrichia capensis costaricensis. Condor*, **74,** 1–4.

49 Erkinaro E. (1969) Der Phasenwechsel der lokomotorischen Aktivität bei *Microtus agrestis* (L.), *M. arvalis* (Pall.) und *M. oeconomus* (Pall.). *Aquilo Ser. Zool.* **8,** 1–31.

50 Erkinaro E. (1969) Free-running circadian rhythm in wood mouse (*Apodemus flavicollis* Melch.) under natural light–dark cycle. *Experientia* **25,** 649.

51 Fischer K. (1974) Die Steuerung der Fortpflanzungszyklen bei männlichen Reptilien. *Fortschritte der Zoologie* **22,** 362–90.

52 Follett B.K. (1973) Circadian rhythms and photoperiodic time measurement in birds. *J. Reprod. Fert.* Suppl. **19,** 5–18.

53 Goss R.J. & Rosen J.K. (1973) The effect of latitude and photoperiod on the growth of antlers. *J. Reprod. Fert.* Suppl. **19,** 111–18.

54 Gwinner E. (1967) Circannuale Periodik der Mauser und der Zugunruhe bei einem Vogel. *Naturwissenschaften* **54,** 447.

55 Gwinner E. (1972) Adaptive functions of circannual rhythms in warblers. *Proc. XVth Int. Orn. Congr.* pp. 218–36. E. J. Brill, Leiden.

56 Gwinner E. (1973) Circannual rhythms in birds: their interaction with circadian rhythms and environmental photoperiod. *J. Reprod. Fert.* Suppl. **19,** 51–65.

57 Gwinner E. & Turek F. (1971) Effects of season on circadian activity rhythms of the starling. *Naturwissenschaften* **58,** 627–8.

58 Hamner W.M. (1963) Diurnal rhythm and photoperiodism in testicular recrudescence of the house finch. *Science* **143,** 1294–5.

59 Hamner K.C. & Hoshizaki T. (1974) Photoperiodism and circadian rhythms: an hypothesis. *BioScience* **24,** 407–13.

60 Heller H.C. & Poulson T.L. (1970) Circannian rhythms—II. Endogenous and exogenous factors controlling reproduction and hibernation in chipmunks (*Eutamias*) and ground squirrels (*Spermophilus*). *Comp. Biochem. Physiol.* **33,** 357–83.

61 Hoffmann K. (1973) The influence of photoperiod and melatonin on testis size, body weight, and pelage colour in the djungarian hamster (*Phodopus sungorus*). *J. comp. Physiol.* **85,** 267–82.

62 Holmes R.T. (1966) Breeding ecology and annual cycle adaptations of the red-backed sandpiper (*Calidris alpina*) in northern Alaska. *Condor* **68,** 3–46.

63 Jegla T.C. & Poulson T.L. (1970) Circannian rhythms—I. Reproduction in the cave crayfish, *Orconectes pellucidus inermis. Comp. Biochem. Physiol.* **33,** 347–55.

64 Kenagy G.J. (1973) Daily and seasonal patterns of activity and energetics in a heteromyid rodent community. *Ecology* **54,** 1201–19.

65 Kendeigh S.C. (1972) Monthly variations in the energy budget of the house sparrow throughout the year. In *Productivity, Population Dynamics and Systematics of Granivorous Birds* (eds S. C. Kendeigh & J. Pinowski) pp. 17–44. Warszawa.

66 Kramer G. (1949) Über Richtungstendenzen bei der nächtlichen Zugunruhe gekäfigter Vögel. In *Ornithologie als biologische Wissenschaft* (eds E. Mayr & E. Schüz) pp. 269–83. C. Winter Universitätsverlag, Heidelberg.
67 Lees A.D. (1965) Is there a circadian component in the Megoura photoperiodic clock? In *Circadian Clocks* (ed. J. Aschoff) pp. 351–6. North-Holland, Amsterdam.
68 Licht P. (1967) Environmental control of annual testicular cycles in the lizard *Anolis carolinensis*—I. Interaction of light and temperature in the initiation of testicular recrudescence. *J. exper. Zool.* **165,** 505–16.
69 Licht P. (1967) Environmental control of annual testicular cycles in the lizard *Anolis carolinensis.*—II. Seasonal variations in the effects of photoperiod and temperature on testicular recrudescence. *J. exper. Zool.* **166,** 243–53.
70 Moreau R.E. (1950) The breeding seasons of African birds. *Ibis* **92,** 223–67 and 419–33.
71 Morrison P.R. (1960) Some interrelations between weight and hibernation function. In *Mammalian Hibernation* (eds C. P. Lyman & A. R. Dawe) *Bull. Mus. Comp. Zool.* **124,** 75–91. Cambridge, Mass.
72 Morrison P.R. (1964) Adaptation of small mammals to the Arctic. *Fedn Proc. Fedn Amer. Socs exp. Biol.* **23,** 1202–6.
73 Müller K. (1973) Circadian rhythms of locomotor activity in aquatic organisms in the subarctic summer. *Aquilo Ser. Zool.* **14,** 1–18.
74 Pengelley E.T. & Fischer K.C. (1963) The effect of temperature and photoperiod on the yearly hibernating behavior of captive golden-mantled ground squirrels (*Citellus lateralis tescorum*). *Can. J. Zool.* **41,** 1103–20.
75 Pittendrigh C.S. (1960) Circadian rhythms and the circadian organization of living systems. In *Cold Spr. Harb. Symp. quant. Biol.* (ed. A. Chovnick) **25,** pp. 159–84. Long Island Biol. Ass., Cold Spring Harbor, L.I., N.Y.
76 Pittendrigh C.S. (1966) The circadian oscillation in *Drosophila pseudoobscurra pupae*: a model for the photoperiodic clock. *Z. Pflanzenphysiol.* **54,** 275–307.
77 Pittendrigh C.S. (1972) Circadian surfaces and the diversity of possible roles of circadian organization in photoperiodic induction. *Proc. Nat. Acad. Sci. USA* **69,** 2734–7.
78 Pittendrigh C.S. & Minis D.H. (1964) The entrainment of circadian oscillations by light and the role as photoperiodic clocks. *Amer. Natur.* **98,** 261–94.
79 Pohl H. (1971) Circannuale Periodik beim Bergfinken. *Naturwissenschaften* **58,** 572–3.
80 Pohl H. (1971) Seasonal variation in metabolic functions of bramblings. *Ibis* **113,** 185–93.
81 Pohl H. (1974) Interaction of effects of light, temperature, and season on the circadian period of *Carduelis flammea. Naturwissenschaften* **61,** 406.
82 Spitzer G. (1972) Jahreszeitliche Aspekte der Biologie der Bartmeise (*Panurus biarmicus*). *J. Orn.* **113,** 241–75.
83 Thomson A.L. (1950) Factors determining the breeding season of birds: an introductory review. *Ibis* **92,** 173–84.
84 Wagner H.O. (1930) Über Jahres- und Tagesrhythmus bei Zugvögeln. *Z. vergl. Physiol.* 12, 703–24.
85 West G.C. (1968) Bioenergetics of captive willow ptarmigan under natural conditions. *Ecology* **49,** 1035–45.

PART V

IMMEDIATE HOMEOSTATIC OR SENSORY RESPONSE

Chapter 16
Rapid responses of organisms to environmental changes

J. BLIGH

16.1 INTRODUCTION

The underlying theme of this book is that the whole gamut of physiology relates, directly or indirectly, to the processes by which life has been, and continues to be, sustained in a changing environment. The three types of response to the environment—evolutionary, acclimatory and immediate or reflex—relate to three principal time scales of environmental change. The last section of this book deals with the third of these time scales: the moment-to-moment variations in some component of the environment of the whole organism or of its constituent cells, which elicit immediate responses.

A comprehensive account of the immediate responses of animals and animal cells to their environments is obviously quite impossible here, and quite unnecessary, since most of what is taught in orthodox courses of mammalian physiology bears on the processes by which external and internal environmental changes are sensed and acted upon to maintain the integrity of the organism. The exterosensors, including the special sensors, and skeletal muscle are concerned with sensing and responding to changes in the external environment. The enterosensors and effector systems such as those of respiration, excretion, circulation and digestion are related to maintaining the chemical and physical properties of the internal environment in a state that ensures proper functioning of the organism's constituent cells. Peripheral nerves are concerned with rapid communication between sensors and effectors, while the cells of the central nervous system, which lie between the afferent pathways from sensors and the efferent pathways to effectors, are concerned either with the autonomic control of the internal environment (homeostatic functions) or with ordering the appropriate responses of the organism to changes in the external environment.

16.2 BEHAVIOURAL AND AUTONOMIC RESPONSES TO ENVIRONMENTAL CHANGE

Behaviour is often regarded as something distinct from physiology but, since behaviour usually relates to responses to an environmental change, and always involves co-ordinated actions by many tissues of the body, such activities of an organism are clearly physiological.

The apparently 'purposeful' pattern of body movement which is called behaviour may be instinctive (genotypic) or learned (phenotypic). Generally speaking the behavioural patterns involved in courtship, mating, nest-building and parental care are instinctive and presumably the appropriate external or internal stimulus triggers off a sequence of central nervous events which are 'built in' and unlearned. The extent to which man retains instinctive components of reproduction and parenthood is, of course, a much debated question. Many behaviour patterns are acquired and involve a process of learning from experience: the young otter, for example, learns to swim in much the same way as man learns most of his behavioural responses apart from primitive ones such as sleeping, eating and aggression.

The main distinction between behavioural responses, both instinctive and acquired, and simpler reflex responses is that in higher animals the former involve movements of the whole organism. In the more highly developed multicellular animals behavioural responses to the environment involve complex patterns of muscular activity, co-ordinated by the nervous system. A patterned muscular response might thus be taken as the definitive characteristic of behaviour applicable to movement.

16.3 RELATIONS BETWEEN STIMULUS AND RESPONSE—THE ROLE OF THE CNS

Most multicellular organisms react to any sudden peripheral sensory input with an alerting response. In the higher animals, the alerting of the CNS allows it to identify the nature of the alarm, and to activate appropriate effectors. The effector response may be specific to the particular disturbance, or it may be a general defensive or protective response such as flight or aggression. The identification of the disturbance may depend on the specificity of the stimulated sensors (e.g. pain sensors or temperature sensors), or on the way in which the central nervous system interprets trains of impulses from sensors of a similar type (e.g. in the recognition of a visual pattern or a particular sound or smell) or from a combination of qualitatively different sensors (e.g. in the recognition of the significance of a combination of sensory stimuli).

The resultant effector activity may be determined by *fixed* pathways through the CNS from sensors to effectors. This is the case with simple non-learned reflexes such as constriction of the pupil of the eye in response to a bright light; ipsilateral flexion and contralateral extension of limbs in response to a sharp pain in an extremity; and the occurrence of peripheral vasodilatation and sweating in response to a high ambient or body temperature.

In other circumstances, the effector response depends on how the central nervous system interprets disturbance signals in the light of information it has stored about similar input patterns on previous occasions. Such responses are *conditioned reflexes* (conditioned by previous experience). Appropriate responses to specific disturbances are thus 'learned' by animals individually. The use of memory (the term is used here in its widest sense to mean information stored after a previous experience) to fit responses to disturbances does not necessarily involve consciousness of experiences, or their re-call to consciousness for recognition when repeated.

Obviously the complexity and the originality of the response to a disturbance depends on the rigidity or plasticity of the central nervous pathways between sensors and effectors. These, as discussed above, may be fixed genetically, or fixed by phenotypic conditioning, or be novel consequences of novel experiences. A genotypic response may be exceedingly complex, but except for minor variations within the gene pool, is stereotype for the species. Only by processes of conditioning or learning can the individual animal respond to a stereotype stimulus in a non-stereotypic way. The implication of a change in sensor-effector relations resulting from previous sensory input or experience, is that some modification has occurred at the central nervous interface between afferent and efferent pathways. How the passage of a signal affects neurones in such a way that the passage of a subsequent signal is modulated is still speculative. This effect could be initiated by the brief change in the synaptic environment which subserves the transfer of the electrical signals from one nerve cell to another, and may involve more permanent structural and functional changes in the cells. Apparently the effect of such changes, is to make it easier for impulses to traverse a 'conditioned' or 'acclimatized' synapse than an unconditioned one. Thus the phenotypic changes in the relations between disturbance and response, as well as the unconditioned immediate responses to disturbance, most likely depend, as does so much else in physiology, on the responses of individual cells to their local environments.

16.4 THE INTEGRITY OF SINGLE CELLS IN THE RESPONSES OF MULTICELLULAR ORGANISMS TO THE ENVIRONMENT

There is no fundamental difference between the sensing of changes in the external environment of the whole organism and the sensing of changes in the local environment of individual nerve cells. The awareness of the external environment, and of changes in it, stems from the responsiveness of specialized nerve endings to particular physical or chemical influences. The sensing of the internal environment similarly depends on the specific sensitivity of nerve endings to particular chemical or physical modalities. The activation of interneurones and of the final effector cells also depends on the sensitivity of part of the cell to specific

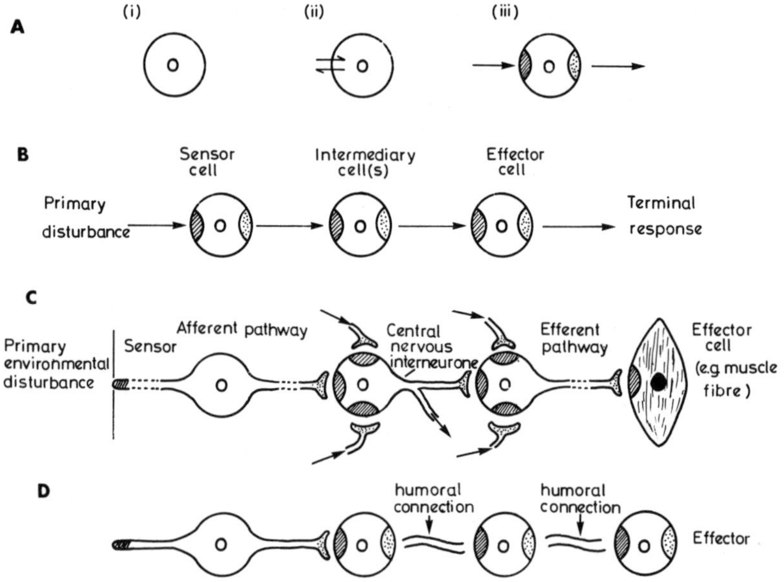

Fig. 16.1. An illustration of the principle of cell-environment interaction as the basis of the co-ordinated functions of multi-cellular organisms. (A) In the multicellular organism, the individual cell retains a large measure of autonomy and integrity (i), but can remain viable only by the continuous processes of chemical interchange with the environment (ii). A characteristic of specialized functions of cells is their particular sensitivity to environmental influences, often at specialized regions on the cell membrane, as indicated by the hatched area in (iii), and their discharge of particular cellular products into the environment, often from specialized regions of the cell membrane, as indicated by the stipled area in (iii). (B) The representation of the change of events between a primary disturbance and a terminal response in terms of the specialized capacity of cells to both sense and create environmental disturbances. (C) The extension of this principle to the neural pathway from primary sensor to a terminal effector, via the central nervous system. (D) An illustration of the fact that there is no fundamental distinction between the synaptic role of a 'detonator chemical transmitter', released by one cell, and sensed by an adjacent cell, and a 'modulator transmitter' released by one cell into the blood stream and sensed by a cell elsewhere in the organism.

environmental changes (Fig. 16.1). Thus every event in the neurones which form the pathways between sensors and effectors is the result of the responsiveness of individual cells to local environmental conditions and the capacity of individual cells to discharge substances which, by changing a local environment, act on other cells. In every instance special parts of the cell membrane are acting as sensors and transducers. The term 'sensors', as generally used by physiologists, seems to imply that such cells are more sensitive than other cells to changes in their environments. This is a dubious proposition. They differ only in that they respond to changes in the general external or internal environments rather than to much more localized changes that constitute the principal environmental influences on most other cells.

Examples chosen to illustrate, in more detail, the immediate responses of organisms to external or internal environmental disturbances (Chapters 17 to 20) were selected arbitrarily. Other editors would undoubtedly have chosen quite different examples. Chapter 17 of the book relates sensors of the external environment to feeding and the avoidance of predators. These activities are two of what may be regarded as the three most basic aspects of the life of an individual organism. The third is reproduction which was considered in Chapter 10. The discussion of buoyancy control (Chapter 18) will be new ground for those whose biological horizons have been largely confined to organisms with limbs and lungs. Apart from the intrinsic fascination of the ways in which buoyancy is achieved in marine organisms, this chapter should serve as a reminder that a great deal of specialization occurred during the evolution of life in an exclusively aqueous medium, and that means of overcoming gravity long predated the evolution of insects, birds and bats. The reason why this subject is often neglected (for instance, there is no mention of buoyancy in the index of J.Z. Young's 1955 edition of *Life of the Vertebrates*) may be that these mechanisms became obsolete in organisms which moved permanently on to dry land. Processes of colour change (Chapter 19), by contrast, are advantageous to organisms in atmospheric as well as aquatic environments. Thermoregulation (Chapter 20) is representative of homeostatic functions. Although life is a temperature-dependent phenomenon (being a complex system of chemical processes it could not be otherwise), the regulation of temperature at a particular point on the temperature scale is a comparatively recent biological innovation, made relatively easy in land animals by the lower thermal conductance of air than of water, and in certain aquatic animals, by special insulation. The advantage of thermoregulation at a high level in the range of thermal tolerance is in the avoidance of predators and the capture of prey. Temperature regulation is not a prerequisite of life. It is, however, a well studied and fairly well understood example of a homeostatic process by which the internal environment of the constituent cells of a multicellular organism can be buffered from changes in the external environment.

The more detailed treatment of these representative aspects of the short time-scale responses of organisms in the following chapters should serve to establish an attitude towards the study of physiology: that the functions of living things must always be considered in relation to the historical and contemporary circumstances of their being.

Prelude to Chapter 17

Factors of the environment which affect the animals inhabiting it are of two kinds: physical, and biotic. Physical factors include water, light intensity, temperature, pressure, and so on; while biotic factors consist of other living organisms. Some of these are predators, others are, for example, disease-causing parasites or competitors for food, breeding sites. The most intense competition occurs between individuals of the same species whose requirements are identical. Biotic factors are regarded by many ecologists as being density-dependent and therefore operating more forcibly to regulate animal populations when their densities are high than when they are low. Physical, or abiotic, factors, on the other hand, are assumed to be density-independent and therefore incapable of regulating animal populations. The validity of this assumption has, however, been much disputed.

Defences against endoparasites are mostly chemical and take the form of antibiotics, growth inhibitors, chemo-stimulants and so on. Ectoparasites are often countered by behavioural reactions such as scratching, mutual grooming, and instinctive acts that tend to hamper transmission from one host to another. Such aspects of environmental physiology are not considered in the present volume although they are clearly relevant, especially in view of the broad approach that we advocate. They have been excluded only on account of the need for brevity. Likewise, in the following chapter, sensory physiology in relation to food and predators has been discussed with respect to vision and chemoreception, especially in insects. This topic has been selected for detailed consideration but, as the authors point out, there are many other types of sensory receptor such as the infra-red receptors of pit vipers and some other snakes, the ultra-sonic system of bats, and the auditory receptors of a wide variety of animals, both invertebrate and vertebrate.

Sense organs are employed to detect friend or foe, prey or predator, as well as other biotic and physical factors of the environment. Associated with organs for the production of sound, scent (pheromones) and visual displays, sensory reception is essential for inter-communication. Indeed, as the first link in the chain of receptor, interneurone and effector, sense organs play an integral part in the animal control system.

Chapter 17
Sensory physiology in relation to food and predators

LESLEY J. GOODMAN AND JOHN A. PATTERSON

17.1 INTRODUCTION

An animal lives in an environment rich in potential sources of sensory information, but only certain aspects of this environment bear directly on the survival of the animal or of the species as a whole. The function of the sensory nervous system is to pattern the input which it receives from the receptor cells and sense organs, so that relevant aspects of the environment are enhanced at the expense of those aspects which are neutral or irrelevant in terms of survival. A central theme of sensory information processing is therefore one of selection and this process of selection functions not only at the level of the sensory nervous system but also in the operation of the receptor cells and in the design of sense organs.

This chapter illustrates some of the strategies which have evolved for the performance of this process of information selection. Apart from some general considerations concerning receptor cells and sense organs, we will refer predominantly to those aspects of sensory systems which are concerned with the identification of food and of predators.

17.2 RECEPTOR CELLS AND SENSE ORGANS

The fundamental input to the nervous system about the environment is from receptor cells which can transduce or translate the level of energy in the environment into events which can be manipulated by the nervous system. The environment contains three forms of energy—electromagnetic, chemical and mechanical in origin—which provides the basic environmental data for information selection. Most cells react to the application of each of these forms of energy, and this reflects the general irritability of the cell membrane. The important point about receptor cells is that in addition to a general responsiveness the cell possesses a markedly heightened sensitivity to one specific energy form. Receptor cells also have the ability to measure or encode, as a change in membrane potential, the intensity of the specific stimulus which falls on the cell and to transmit to other cells in the nervous system the information contained in the amplitude of the potential. Receptor cells are frequently classified according to the energy form to which they are sensitive. It is possible to speak therefore of chemoreceptors or mechanoreceptors. With electromagnetic energy the situation is more complicated because of the wide spectrum of forms of electromagnetic energy in the environment, so that no single design of receptor cell is highly sensitive to the whole of the range. Perhaps the most common form of receptor of this type are photoreceptors which can detect light. Other types are thermoreceptors, which are found in many animals and are sensitive to heat,

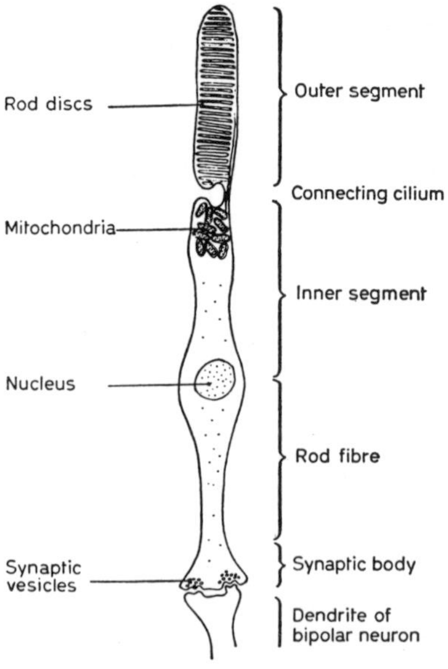

Fig. 17.1. Diagrammatic representation of a rod photoreceptor cell of the vertebrate retina. The rod discs of the outer segment are the result of repeated infolding of the cell membrane and carry the photopigment which captures photons in the transduction process. Reproduced from Smith, C.U.M. (1970) *The Brain—towards an understanding*, p. 152. Faber and Faber, London.

and the electroreceptors capable of detecting weak electrical fields which are possessed by some fish [23]. There is also evidence that some birds and insects are able to detect the earth's magnetic field, but the receptor cells have yet to be identified [35].

Special mechanisms have been developed by a number of receptor-cell classes to enable transduction to take place. Photoreceptors contain a photopigment which is situated on the large area of cell membrane formed by repeated folding of the cell surface, see Fig. 17.1. This photopigment can capture photons and initiate a process which results in a change in the membrane potential of the cell. Chemoreceptors possess putative 'receptor sites' on the cell membrane which can interact with molecules in the immediate environment of the cell and produce a

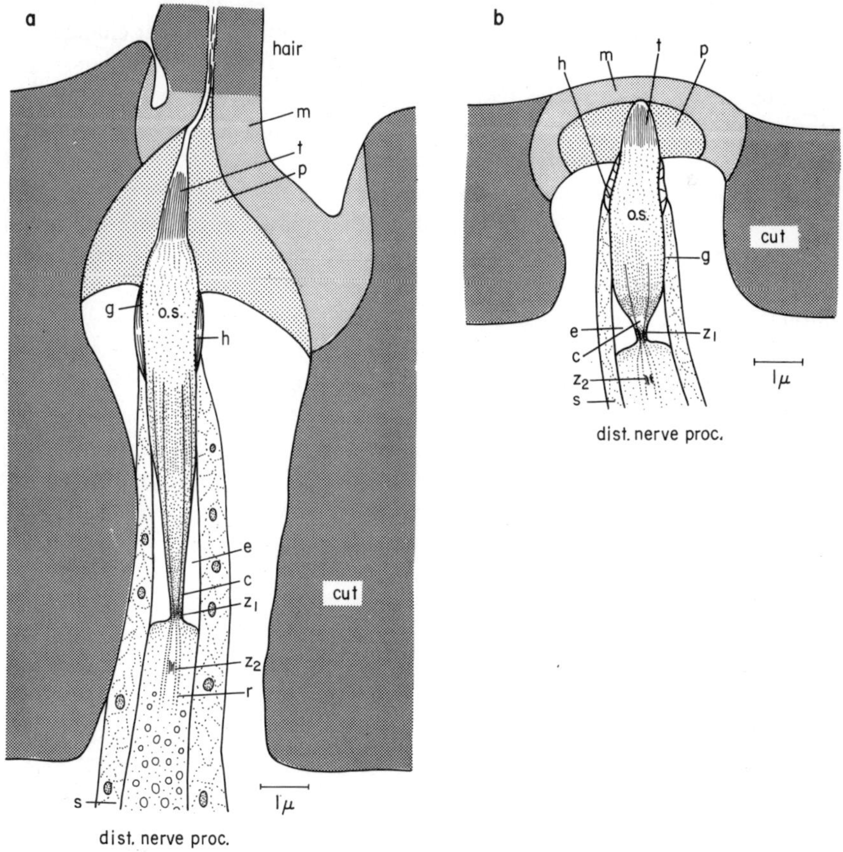

Fig. 17.2. Fine structure of two types of mechanoreceptor in the cuticle of the honey bee. (A) A fine trichoid sensillum from a cervical hair plate and (B) a campaniform sensillum on the head. c, ciliary structure; m, joint membrane in (A), cap membrane in (B); o.s. outer segment; p, cap; s, Schwann cell; r, root fibre; t, tubular body; cut, cuticle; z_1 z_2, centrosome-like structures. Reproduced from [33].

Deformation of the mechanoreceptive neuron is produced by movement of the hair relative to the body surface in (A) and by stresses in the cuticle producing a movement of the cap membrane in (B).

similar change in membrane potential, while mechanoreceptors seem to possess cell membranes which are especially sensitive to deformation.

The exact form of the energy actually transduced by the receptors, and its significance, can be influenced by the nature of any accessory and non-nervous structures which may surround the receptor cell, as for example when receptor cells are arranged in a sense organ. In mechanoreceptors the transduction process depends on the application of mechanical force to the dendrite of the receptor cell. Exactly which form of mechanical energy in the environment produces the deformation of the cell membrane depends on the physical situation of the mechanoreceptor in relation to the tissue which surrounds it. There are at least two types of mechanoreceptive sense organs on the body surface of insects: the campaniform sensillum and the trichoid sensillum [4, 33]. In the former, see Fig. 17.2B, the structure of the cuticular sense organ is such that changes in the stresses and strains in the cuticle result in bending of the mechanoreceptor dendrite. In the case of the trichoid sensillum a cuticular hair is capable of bending by virtue of an articulation situated at its base (Fig. 17.2A). Bending of the hair relative to the body surface produced by such agents as air currents or contact with the substratum or with other parts of the animal, produces bending or stretching of the mechanoreceptive dendrite situated at the base of the hair.

The vertebrate eye is a more complex sense organ. The presence of a light-proof backing to the photoreceptive cell layer and of an iris to regulate the amount of light entering the eye both contribute to the efficient operation of the eye. The lens is more important since it is able to organize the incoming light. The lens focuses an image of the visual environment onto the receptors and this allows the nervous system to build up a neural 'image' of the visual world. The muscles surrounding the eye can move the eye so that different parts of the visual world can be analysed, and also allow the eye to track objects moving in the visual environment. It is these features which make the vertebrate eye such a remarkable organ of distance perception.

17.3 NEAR AND DISTANCE PERCEPTION

We have seen something of the extent to which receptor cells and sense organs are able to select aspects of the environment for subsequent analysis by the sensory nervous system. We will now attempt to build up an idea of how the properties of receptor cells, sense organs and the sensory nervous system are united in the selection of food and the avoidance of predators, and to do this we will introduce the concept of near and distance perception.

If an animal is to act on information relating to the presence of food or of predators, there is clearly an advantage in detecting significant events when they are occurring at some distance from the animal. The greater the distance at which identification takes place, the longer the time which can be allowed for the production of suitable behaviour, with a resulting increase in the probability of a successful outcome. It is therefore possible to consider receptors and sense organs as contributing information to near or to distance perception.

All types of receptor cell can contribute information to the process of near perception since, ultimately, all receptors are only able to transduce the energy in their immediate vicinity. Distance perception, however, requires a certain arrangement of sense organs and a special property in the energy form transduced which together allow the nervous system to create a spatial display or 'picture' of the environment at a distance from the animal. The chief organs of distance perception are eyes and ears and it is characteristic that they occur in pairs. A pair of spatially separated sense organs is necessary since it is the parallax created by the arrival of energy from a single point in space at two spatially separated receptors which allows the nervous system to calculate the distance from the animal and the location of the source of the energy. The special feature of the energy form itself is that, for the accurate location of the source, the energy must pass through the environment from the source to the receptor in a straight line, or more accurately as a wave front radiating from the source. Such is the case with light and sound.

Ears are important in the location of food and of predators, especially when used in conjunction with echolocation as employed by bats [29] and cetaceans [17]. Similar mechanisms employing electrical discharges and electroreceptors are used by some fishes [23], notably gymnarchids, sternarchids and mormyrids. It is however the refracting eye of vertebrates which has received the most attention from physiologists and in the vertebrate visual system where the processes of sensory reception and integration in distance perception are best understood.

17.4 DISTANCE PERCEPTION: THE DETECTION OF FOOD AND PREDATORS BY THE VISUAL SYSTEMS OF FROGS AND TOADS

There is an array of about one million photoreceptor cells in the retina of the frog and each cell is capable of measuring the intensity of the light falling on it. Between these photoreceptors and the half million ganglion cells which connect the frogs retina to the brain, there are some $2\frac{1}{2}$–$3\frac{1}{2}$ million interconnecting cells, the anatomical connectivity and functional properties of which determine the form of the processed visual information which the ganglion cells transmit to the brain [21, 25] (see Fig. 17.3). Three distinct cell types are found in these interconnecting cells. Bipolar cells run through the retina from the level of the photoreceptors to the level of the ganglion cells. The other cell types, the amacrines and horizontal cells, have dendritic trees which spread out in the horizontal plane of the retina so that these cells interconnect many of the vertical columns formed by the photoreceptor, bipolar and ganglion cell layers. The amacrine cells do this near the ganglion cell layer, the horizontals nearer to the photoreceptors [8, 24].

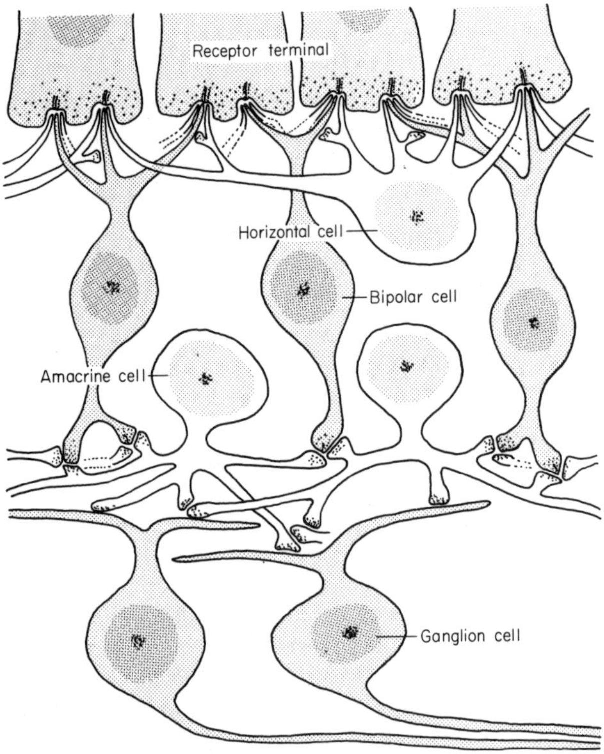

Fig. 17.3. A diagram of the cell types and cellular interconnections found in the retina of the frog. Reproduced from [25].

If the activity of a ganglion cell is recorded by inserting a fine microelectrode into the cell in the retina or close to a ganglion cell axon in the optic nerve, and a small spot of light in the visual field of the eye is used as a stimulus, then it is clear that the ganglion cell will only respond when the photoreceptors with which it is indirectly connected, are illuminated. This fraction of the total visual field of the eye forms the receptive field of the ganglion cell. The dimensions of this field are expressed as the number of degrees through which it is possible to move the stimulus and still obtain a response from the ganglion cell. The receptive field of a ganglion cell is of course much larger than that of a single receptor cell because of the horizontal connections between many photoreceptors and bipolar cells which are made by the horizontal and amacrine cells. Nor is the receptive field of a ganglion cell a simple affair which merely transmits to the brain the average intensity of the light falling on the receptor cells with which it is connected.

By switching a spot of light on and off in the centre of a ganglion cell receptive field, and recording the activity of the ganglion cell's axon in the optic nerve, Hartline [12] was able to demonstrate the presence of three different classes of ganglion cell, those excited by light-on (the 'centre-on' cells), by light-off (the 'centre-off' cells), and by both light-on and off (the 'on-off' cells). In addition the ganglion cell receptive field is known to have an inner region, where a stimulus will, for example, excite the cell, together with a surrounding region where the same stimulus will inhibit the cell [18]. In a later study, Lettvin, Maturana, McCullouch and Pitts [21] used stimuli in the form of movements of small targets on a grey background, with a visual contrast with the background provided by the relative lightness or darkness of the stimulating target. Using these more complex stimuli, Lettvin *et al.* [21] were able to classify ganglion cells into five types on the basis of the receptive field diameter and the preferred stimulus of each class. Each small part of the photoreceptor cell layer will contribute intensity information to each of these five types of ganglion cell. The type (1) ganglion cells correspond to Hartline's 'centre-on' cells and are stimulated by the presence of a contrast boundary in the receptive field. The type (3) cells detect the movement of a contrast boundary in the receptive field and correspond to Hartline's 'on-off' cells. Type (4) ganglion cells, which are the same as Hartline's 'centre-off' cells, together with the type (5) cells measure the general level of the light intensity prevailing in the receptive field. All this information is passed to the brain where a picture of the distribution and movement of areas of differing contrast can be built up. Perhaps the most significant class of ganglion cell revealed by Lettvin *et al.* are those of type (2). These are capable of detecting the movement in their receptive field of convex-ended objects which are darker than the background. The optimum dimensions of the stimulus for these cells were found to correspond well, in an idealized sense, with the dimensions of the insects on which the frog feeds, and type (2) cells were christened 'bug detectors' [21].

The idea that one class of cells in the frog's retina can provide all the information necessary to initiate prey capture behaviour is striking and the results of Lettvin *et al.*'s analysis are often quoted as an example of simple but adequate visual integration.

Lettvin *et al.*'s analysis does not, however, indicate how the animal is able to extract visual information about predators. As a result of working with different stimuli and a different but essentially similar animal, the toad, Ewert [10] arrives at a rather different interpretation of the events that occur in the retina. Ewert's analysis is extensive and includes events occurring in both the eye and the brain of the toad and the recognition of both prey and predator stimuli.

Ewert is careful to develop a full account of the behavioural responses of the toad to which the physiological evidence obtained from the brain and retina can be related. Ewert finds that toads respond with orienting and prey capturing activity to square objects moving in the visual field when they are 5–10 mm along each edge and 7 cm away from the animal. Under these conditions the object edge length on the retina subtends 4–8° of the visual field. Square objects of 30° edge length at the same distance produce avoidance reactions. The toad displays size constancy so that the actual size of the object is the important factor and not the angular dimensions which for any given object will vary with distance from the toad's eye. Ewert also shows that when a small square 2° in edge length is just sufficient to stimulate orientation, then extending the stimulus in the horizontal direction enhances the attraction of the stimulus for the toad, while extending it vertically enhances the repellance of the stimulus. Horizontal extension therefore corresponds to 'worm', while vertical extension corresponds to 'predator'.

On the basis of receptive field diameter, similar classes of retinal ganglion cell can be identified in the toad to those found in the frog. In the toad, however, cells of type (1), the sustained contrast detectors, are absent. The diameters of the

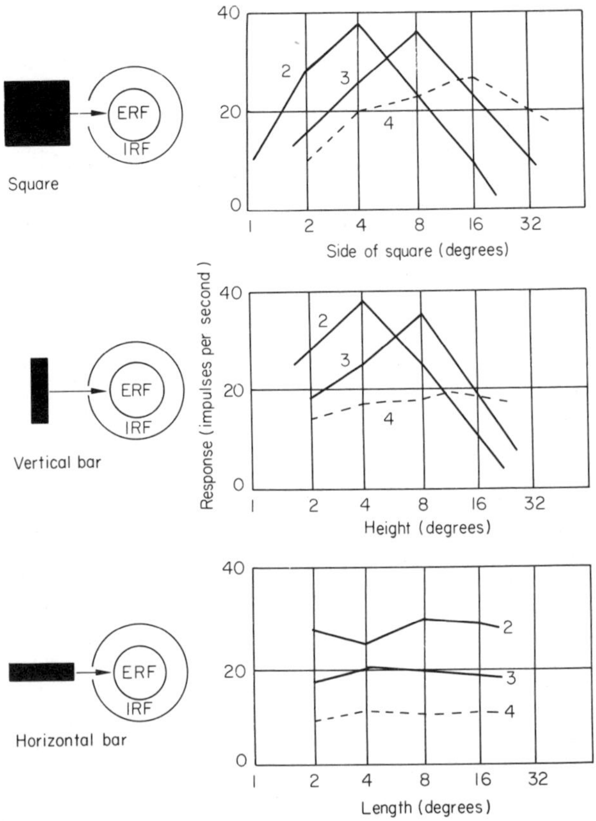

Fig. 17.4. The effects of different shapes and sizes of stimulus on the number of action potentials in the responses of ganglion cells of types (2), (3) and (4) recorded from the optic tectum of the toad. The three types of stimulus used are shown at left. The edge length of the stimulus was varied from 1° up to a maximum of 32°, measured as the angle subtended by the stimulus at the eye of the toad. ERF and IRF indicate the excitatory and inhibitory receptive fields of the ganglion cells. The ERF has a diameter of 4°, 8° and 12°–15° for type (2), (3) and (4) ganglion cells respectively. Note that the horizontal extension of a horizontally moving stimulus has little effect on the responses of the ganglion cells but that increasing the height of a horizontally moving vertical bar, or the edge length of a square produces curves shaped like an inverted 'V'. In these cases the greatest responses occur when the height of the bar or the edge length of the square equals the diameter of the ERF for each cell type. The data are modified after [10].

excitatory central regions of the type (2), type (3) and type (4) cells in the toad are 4°, 8° and 12°–15° respectively, and rather than studying the most effective type of stimulus for each class of cell as Lettvin *et al.* did for the frog, Ewert has concentrated on presenting the same moving stimuli to all classes of cell and has examined the different responses elicited by prey or predator stimuli.

The results of presenting the various types of stimulus to each of the retinal ganglion cell classes are summarized in Fig. 17.4. Extending a small square in the horizontal direction, that is, in the same plane as its motion, has relatively little effect on the responses recorded from each class of ganglion cell. Extending

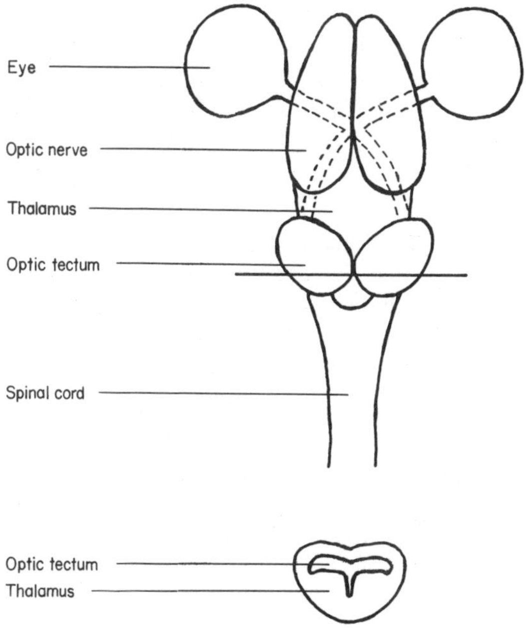

Fig. 17.5. Diagrammatic representation of (A), the external features of the toad's brain and of (B), a transverse section through the optic tectum and thalamus at the level indicated by the horizontal line in (A).

the square to form a vertical bar which is perpendicular to the direction of movement increases the response recorded from the cell until the edge length of the bar approximately equals the diameter of the excitatory region of the receptive field for each class of cell. Further extension so that the bar falls within the inhibitory surround of the receptive field produces a progressive reduction in the cell's response. There are, then, certain differences between the responses of these cells and the behaviour of the toad. The increased attraction of horizontally extended stimuli for the toad is not reflected in the responses of the cells and also the same responses are obtained from the ganglion cells with a narrow vertical bar as with a square of the same height. The cell confuses these two stimuli but the toad does not. The responses of the different classes of ganglion cells to the stimuli employed by Ewert are explicable on the basis of the different diameters of the receptive field for each class of cell and the relative strengths of the inhibitory surrounds. Presumably each class of cell can signal information about a different aspect of the stimulus other than size in a way which is comparable with the situation in the frog revealed by Lettvin *et al.* Ewert, however, suggests that there are no 'worm detectors' as distinct from 'enemy detectors' in the toad retina but that the differential analysis is performed in the brain, that is in the optic tectum, together with the pretectal region of the diencephalon and the thalamus (see Fig. 17.5).

Most of the ganglion cell axons terminate in the tectum, each in a different layer, where they form a projection of the visual environment such that each part of the tectum corresponds to a particular region of the total visual field. Ewert [10] finds that if a region of the tectum is stimulated electrically then the toad will turn so as to fixate with both eyes that region of the visual field which corresponds to the area of the tectum stimulated. The receptive fields of many of the cells of the tectum are larger than those of the ganglion cells from which they receive visual information, indicating that a convergence of input and an associated analysis has taken place comparable with that between receptor cells and ganglion cells in the retina. Some of the cells in the tectum, cells with excitatory receptive fields 10°–27° in diameter, are activated exclusively by moving objects. These cells are probably involved in the stimulus location system, the presence of which is shown by electrically stimulating the tectum. Deeper in the tectum are cells with much larger receptive fields which may cover the entire visual field in the front of the animal, the entire lower part of the visual field or the entire visual field on the other side of the animal. Other tectal cells, the type (1) and type (2) cells are probably concerned with detecting the 'prey' nature of the stimulus. These cells have excitatory receptive fields of 27° diameter and are excited mainly by stimuli extended in the direction of movement. In the type (1) cells extension perpendicular to the direction of movement has little effect on the response but in the type (2) cells perpendicular extension actually reduces the responses of the cell. Ewert considers these two classes of cell to be the triggering system for prey capture.

The thalamic pretectal region which lies ventral and anterior to the tectum is a second major destination for retinal ganglion cell axons. Electrical stimulation of this region elicits blinking, ducking, turning away or jumping, all of which may be considered as parts of avoidance behaviour. Ewert has identified four main types of thalamic neuron all of which have large receptive fields.

1 Cells with receptive fields 46° in diameter which respond to the movement of 'predator' objects extended perpendicularly to the direction of movement.

2 Cells with a receptive field about 90° in diameter responding to the movement of an object towards the toad.

3 Cells with a field about 45° in diameter responding to large stationary objects.

4 Cells responding to stimulation of balance receptors in the toad's ear, receptors which would be stimulated by evasive movements of the toad.

On the basis of these and other experiments, Ewert [10] considers the tectum to be concerned with prey recognition and the triggering of capture behaviour while the thalamic-pretectal region acts as a 'caution' system which both inhibits the tectum and activates avoidance behaviour. Experiments which study the behaviour of toads from which the tectum or the thalamic-pretectal region have been removed surgically both support and add to this idea. Toads in which the tectum is lacking do not show orienting behaviour to visual stimuli, neither do they exhibit avoidance behaviour. The implication is therefore that information is passed from the tectum, where orienting behaviour can be triggered by electrical stimulation, to the pretectum, where avoidance behaviour can be triggered by electrical stimulation. Removal of the pretectum, leaving the tectum intact, on the other hand, produces a marked release of orientation behaviour, which can now be elicited even by stimuli which the toad would normally identify as predatory in nature. This experiment indicates that the prey-capturing behaviour controlled by the tectum is under inhibitory influence from the pretectal region so that the animal will respond to prey stimuli only if they do not also activate the thalamic-subtectal system. Ewert has indeed been able to show in electrical recordings from type (2) tectal neurons that electrical stimulation of the thalamic-pretectal region inhibits the response of the type (2) neurons to moving stimuli. He has also shown that thalamic-pretectal units sensitive to movement can be excited by electrical stimulation of the tectum thus demonstrating the connection between thc tectum and the pretectum indicated by the surgical experiments.

In summary then Ewert [10] sees the operation of the retina and brain in the toad as selectively filtering the visual information transduced by the photoreceptors, so that the information passes through a series of 'windows'. Each retinal ganglion cell acts as a vertical window and detects extension perpendicular to the direction of movement. This process is repeated and amplified in the thalamic-pretectal region. Extension in a horizontal direction is detected by the horizontal window found in the type (1) tectal cells, and type (2) tectal cells perform a summation of the excitatory input from the tectal type (1) cells and the inhibitory input from the thalamic-pretectal cells. The summated output of the type (2) cells produces an orientation response of the toad if the output exceeds a certain threshold level of excitation. The identification of predator stimuli and the triggering of avoidance behaviour are processes which remain unclear, but it seems likely that cells in the thalamic-pretectal region summate information from the window filters situated in the retina and the optic tectum since the thalamic-pretectal region receives visual information from both these sources.

17.5 DISTANCE PERCEPTION: THE ROLE OF EYE MOVEMENTS IN THE VISUAL PROCESS

An object of suitable dimensions moving in the visual field of a toad will elicit orientation and prey-capture behaviour. The first part of this behaviour involves a movement of the toad's body which brings the stimulated region of the visual field to lie in the central part of the retina of both eyes, so that the 'prey' stimulus is brought into binocular fixation. The movement of the whole animal which accomplishes this can be called a fixation movement. If the 'prey' stimulus continues to move, the animal will make further movements so as to maintain the stimulus at the centre of both retinae, that is to keep the prey in front of the animal. These movements are called tracking movements. Movements of the whole body, of the head alone or of all or part of each eye are found to fulfil similar and additional functions in a wide variety of animals, and in all cases they constitute an important feedback system between the animal and its visual environment. Since any movement of the eye will change the image of the visual environment falling onto the photoreceptors, the movements of the eye, which are under the control of the animal's nervous system, can determine to a large extent which aspects of the environment the animal 'sees'. The effects of these eye movements fall into three main categories and are concerned with fixation of a part of the visual field, with stabilization of the visual field and with scanning of the visual field. Let us examine each of these in greater detail.

The fixation movements of the toad's body mentioned above result in the stimulated part of the visual field moving across the retina so as to lie over the central region. In comparison with other vertebrates the central region of the toad retina is not highly specialized. In many vertebrates, however, the central region is specialized to form an area centralis which possesses a much higher density of photoreceptors and associated neurons than the rest of the retina. This specialization reaches a peak in the fovea of mammals. These central regions are capable of a more detailed analysis of the visual environment than the remainder of the retina. In man the peripheral retina has, as a primary function, the detection of movement in the peripheral visual field. The occurrence of a movement in the peripheral visual field usually results in a very rapid fixation movement called a saccade which brings the stimulated region of the visual field to lie over the fovea where form and colour vision are most acute. This saccadic movement is produced by the extra-ocular muscles which surround the eye and is very rapid. A 10° movement takes only 45 milliseconds to complete and reaches a maximum velocity of 400°/second in man and represents one of the fastest contractions of which the body's musculature is capable [28]. Any further movement of the stimulus is compensated for by a tracking movement of the eye, again produced by the extra-ocular muscles, so that the stimulated region remains over the fovea. Similar fixation and tracking movements occur in mantids, which capture other insects for food, where the process is performed by movements of the head as a whole, the eyes themselves being immobile on the head [22]. It appears that in mantids too there is a specialized region of the insect's compound eye which is comparable to, and frequently called a 'fovea' [1]. In toads, man, mantids and many other animals, fixation and tracking movements serve to keep both eyes of the animal directed towards the stimulus so that binocular fixation can take place. Binocular fixation allows the nervous system to calculate the distance of the stimulus from the animal. This information is important in several aspects of behaviour, notably prey capture. The toad turns the whole body to move the eyes in order to fixate and track the prey, prey capture may only require the toad to approach sufficiently close to the prey for the tongue to be everted and the prey caught. In mantids, where fixation and tracking involve head-relative-to-the-body movements, the visual information as to the distance of the prey from the eyes must be integrated with mechanoreceptor information as to the relative position of head and body. This mechanoreceptive information is provided by sensory hairs arranged on plates of thickened cuticle on the neck of the animal. The way in which this mechanoreceptive information is combined with distance measurement to determine the timing, distance and direction of the prey-capturing strike of the raptorial prothoracic legs of the mantid has been studied in considerable detail by Mittelstaedt [26]. The integrative process is even more complex in animals such as mammals where the body, the head and each eye are all capable of independent motion and where eye movements are developed to the highest level of speed and complexity [28].

The second major role played by eye movements, that of stabilization, is concerned with compensating for the movement of the image of the visual environment across the photoreceptors produced by the locomotion of the animal, or under rather more unnatural circumstances, by the movement of the visual environment as a whole around the animal. If an animal is moving forward along the same line as the head–body axis, then the movement of the visual world will be least in the most anterior and most posterior regions of the visual field and greatest in the lateral region. Any movements of the eye, produced by movement of the eye alone or of the head can only compensate for the movement occurring in one part of the field because of the different velocities of image movement in different parts of the field. This consideration may be more important in those animals which do not possess a fovea or specialized area of photoreceptors, but in animals with a fovea or area centralis where visual analysis is most acute, the compensatory movements of the eye tend to stabilize the image of the visual world which falls on or is fixated by these regions. If the image of the visual world is continuously flowing past the animal, then the stabilization, produced by, as it were, tracking the movement of a part of the visual field, can only persist for a limited period of time before the eye, or the head, or both reach the physical limit of their movement. When this happens the eye is quickly returned to a new position near to the starting position of the tracking movement and the slower pursuit or tracking movement is repeated so that a different view or region of the continously changing environment is stabilized on the photoreceptors. This alternation of slow tracking movements and the fast saccadic returns is called an optokinetic nystagmus and can be demonstrated experimentally in a variety of ways.

If an animal is fixed in space and the visual environment is moved about it, as happens when an animal is placed in the centre of a striped drum and the drum is rotated about the animal, then an optokinetic nystagmus or the component movements can be readily demonstrated in many systems such as the eyestalk movements of the crab [2] (see Fig. 17.6A), the eyeball movements of primates and the head movements of locusts [32] and flies. If in a similar situation an

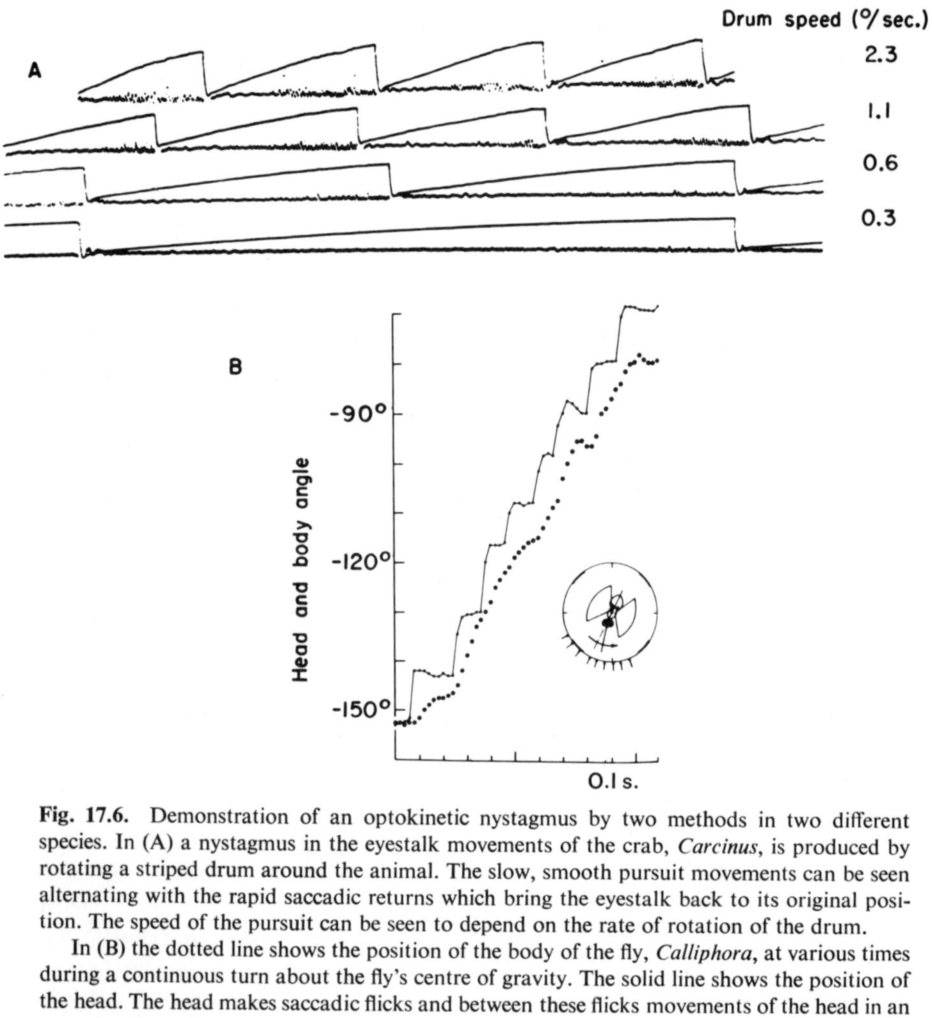

Fig. 17.6. Demonstration of an optokinetic nystagmus by two methods in two different species. In (A) a nystagmus in the eyestalk movements of the crab, *Carcinus*, is produced by rotating a striped drum around the animal. The slow, smooth pursuit movements can be seen alternating with the rapid saccadic returns which bring the eyestalk back to its original position. The speed of the pursuit can be seen to depend on the rate of rotation of the drum.

In (B) the dotted line shows the position of the body of the fly, *Calliphora*, at various times during a continuous turn about the fly's centre of gravity. The solid line shows the position of the head. The head makes saccadic flicks and between these flicks movements of the head in an opposite direction to the direction of the turning body stabilize a series of views of the visual environment on the eyes. These views are indicated by the arrows on the inset and the head relative to the body movements are comparable to those seen in the optokinetic nystagmus of the crab.

(A) is reproduced from [2]. (B) is reproduced from [20].

animal such as a flying fly is allowed to turn about its centre of gravity, while the visual environment remains stationary, then similar movements can be seen [20] (see Fig. 17.6B).

The data obtained from the crab, *Carcinus* [2], show clearly the smooth pursuit movements alternating with rapid returns and the way in which the rate of pursuit varies with different rates of movement of the visual environment, all of which are characteristic of optokinetic nystagmus. In the flying fly [20] on the other hand, the data show well how, though the animal's body is continuously turning, the head by virtue of the pursuit movements which it performs, is able to produce a series of different but stable views of the environment on the compound eyes between each of the saccadic flicks.

We can see therefore how the movements of eyes can bring regions of the visual field to lie over and to stay over certain parts of the photoreceptor array found in eyes and how movements of the visual field produced during the locomotion of the animal can be compensated for. What then of the remaining major category of eye relative-to-the-environment movements, those concerned with visual scanning? It is paradoxical that many of the visual systems which are so refined in producing fixation, tracking and optokinetic movements to stabilize regions of the visual field on the retina, should, once this stabilization has been accomplished, then proceed to deliberately move the eye so as to scan the image across the photoreceptors. Perhaps the explanation for visual scanning lies in the fact that photoreceptors, like most receptor cells, produce a proportionately larger response when a stimulus is presented or withdrawn than during the steady state conditions of stimulus presence or absence. It appears therefore that receptors are more sensitive to change than to steady states. Thus having stabilized the visual world on the photoreceptors, the application of a small, controlled movement to the visual image, by moving the eye, may greatly increase the rate of flow of information into the visual system and produce a concomitant improvement in the quality of the analysis achieved. This improvement in vision may well be especially important in, for example, phytophagous animals where the food source is not obligingly mobile as is normally the case in predatory animals. Therefore in many animals, particularly after a novel stimulus has been presented to the animal and fixation (if it occurs) has taken place, there may occur a scanning movement. This may be achieved in one of several ways.

In the primate eye there is a continuous tremor of the eye-ball, of 4–12 Hz frequency in man, which also accompanies object fixation. Ditchburn and Ginsborg [7] were able to completely stabilize images on the human retina by a number of techniques, the simplest of which involves mounting a small projector on a contact lens attached to the cornea. This can project an image of simple contrast boundaries onto the retina which remains in the same place regardless of any movements of the eyeball. Ditchburn and Ginsborg found that the detection of contrast boundaries becomes erratic in these conditions with parts of the subjective image fading and reappearing every few seconds. It appears that the tremor which occurs in normal vision causes the cells which detect the contrast boundaries to be continuously re-stimulated, making continuous perception of the contrast boundaries possible. Tremor is also found in the eyestalk movements of crabs in addition to the fixation, tracking and nystagmus movements described above [2], whereas in the primates each eye as a whole can move independently with respect to the visual environment. There are other ways of producing visual scanning which do not involve the independent movement of each eye. These are found in the movement of the head relative to the body seen in insects where again tremor or scanning can occur. In locust nymphs, Wallace

[34] also observed a form of scanning produced by flexing the pro- and meso-thoracic legs on one side of the body. In all these cases the eyes are moved in unison. Perhaps the most remarkable system involved in visual scanning is that in which the retina alone is moved relative to the static image created by the dioptrics of the eye. Movements of this type are found in the retinae of the principal eyes of salticid spiders [19], in the compound eyes of flies [27] and in the very simple visual system of the planktonic copepod, *Copilia* [11]. Land [19] has shown that the principal eyes of salticid spiders each have a retina, which when stimulated by the introduction into the visual field of a suitable target, moves so as to fixate the stimulus. The image of the stimulus is brought to the central region of the boomerang-shaped retina where the receptor cell density is ten times that of the rest of the retina. The retina then scans the image of the stimulus with a combination of side-to-side and torsional movements, with a frequency, for the side-to-side movements of 0·5–1·0 Hz. In addition to saccadic fixation and scanning movements the spider eye can also perform tracking, spontaneous and nystagmus movements which parallel those found in the movements of the whole eye found in primates.

We have seen already how the static features of sense organ design can filter or otherwise organize aspects of the environmental energy which receptor cells transduce. It is now possible to see how dynamic aspects of sense organ structure can control the nature of a sensory process, enhancing the abilities of the receptor cells and sensory nervous system in the task of information selection and processing.

17.6 CHEMORECEPTORS: DISTANCE PERCEPTION AND NEAR PERCEPTION

We have seen how the vertebrate eye acts as a distance receptor, and provides information which can determine whether an animal produces prey-capture or predator-avoidance behaviour. Once the prey has been caught, the final determination as to its suitability as food is frequently based on the function of receptors which provide information as to the chemical composition of the prey.

Chemoreceptors can also be involved in distance perception, notably as olfactory organs which are highly sensitive, to often very low concentrations, of airborne chemicals. One of the best known and most frequently cited examples of this is the orientation of the males of many moth species to the pheromones secreted by sexually mature females. The males possess olfactory sense organs on the antennae which can detect pheromone molecules in concentrations as low as 10^{-12}g/ml, as is the case for the silkworm moth *Bombyx* [30]. Female location is established by moving upwind in response to the pheromone. A similar involvement of antennal chemoreceptors in the perception of distant events is seen in other insects, for example locust nymphs which, when starved, will, if anything, march downwind when placed in an airstream. If the odour of freshly crushed grass is introduced into the airstream, then the nymphs turn and march upwind towards the source of the odour [16]. In many animals, whether predatory, herbivorous or omnivorous in habit, olfactory organs can operate in a similar way so as to locate food and avoid predators. These are not examples of true distance perception, however, since no spatial display of a distant environment is obtained as happens with visual and acoustic sense organs. Airborne chemicals are brought into the vicinity of the animal by the vagaries of air currents, while light and sound travel to the animals' sense organs as wave fronts enabling an accurate description of sources of the light and sound to be built up by the nervous system. Since the movements of chemical molecules do not possess this ability, no true distance perception of the chemical environment is possible. It is for this reason that the division of chemoreceptors into distance receptors—those of high sensitivity and concerned with olfaction and near receptors of moderate sensitivity and concerned with contact chemoreception or gustation—is somewhat arbitrary.

Chemoreception plays an important part in the recognition of food, mates, predators and of sites suitable for, for example, oviposition, and in the demarcation and recognition of territory. One area where a considerable knowledge of the chemoreceptive process has been achieved is in the study of the contact chemoreceptors on the tarsi of the legs and the labellum of the mouthparts of the fly *Phormia.*

17.7 NEAR PERCEPTION: THE CHEMORECEPTIVE SENSILLUM OF THE FLY

The feeding behaviour of flies is intimately associated with the chemoreceptive apparatus of the animal. The chemoreceptive sense organs involved in the feeding process are trichoid sensilla—small hairlike structures found on both the labellum of the mouth-parts and on the tarsi of the legs. Each hair contains up to five receptor cells surrounded by the trichogen and tormogen cells which are responsible for the secretion of the chitinous structures of the hair. One of the receptor cells has dendrites which terminate at the base of the hair and this is known to be a mechanoreceptor which monitors any movement of the hair with respect to the body surface [36]. The four remaining cells are all chemoreceptive in function and possess dendrites which pass up the central lumen of the hair almost to the tip, where a small pore, filled with viscous material connects the lumen of the hair with the exterior. Such a trichoid sensillum is illustrated in Fig. 17.7.

The behavioural analysis of the function of these chemoreceptors has depended on the fact that the application of certain chemicals to the sensilla will elicit proboscis extension and feeding while the application of another class of chemicals will inhibit this process, or if it is taking place, will cause feeding to stop and the proboscis to be retracted. Thus the function of the sensilla can be explored in terms of the acceptance or rejection thresholds of the various chemicals tested. The concept of threshold is frequently employed in the study of sensory physiology and behaviour, and designates the stimulus strength

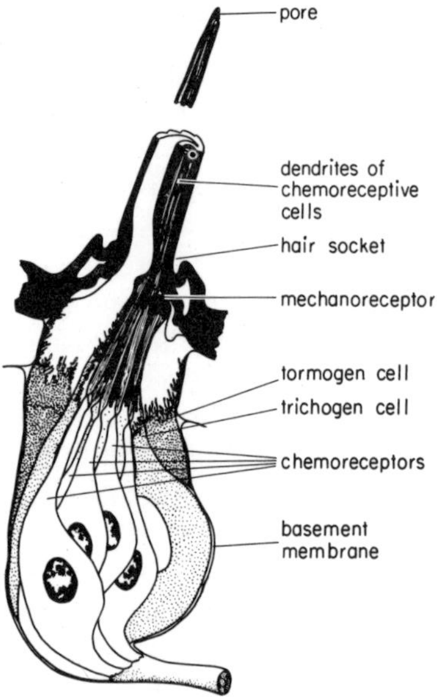

Fig. 17.7 Diagrammatic representation of a labellar chemoreceptive hair of the fly, *Phormia*, showing one mechanoreceptive and four chemoreceptive cells. The mechanoreceptor terminates at the base of the hair, where it is inserted into a socket in the body cuticle. The dendrites of the chemoreceptive cells continue to the apex of the hair terminating adjacent to the small pore which connects the lumen of the hair with the exterior.

which is just sufficient to elicit a physiological response in the cell under study or to produce a given piece of behaviour. In the case of acceptance thresholds it is the concentration of a chemical which is just sufficient to produce proboscis extension and/or feeding. Rejection can be studied in one of two ways. Either the substance to be tested can be mixed with a solution the strength of which is known to produce, for example, proboscis extension, and the concentration of the second chemical in the first can be increased with successive presentations until the application of the mixture to a tarsus fails to produce proboscis extension. The concentration of the second chemical is now just sufficient to inhibit the acceptance response which should be produced by the first chemical. The second method relies on the fact that the chemoreceptive information from all receptors is pooled centrally and that central summation occurs. In this case the stimulus which causes extension is applied to one tarsus and when extension has occurred a second chemical is applied to another tarsus. With successive presentations the concentration of the second chemical is then increased until its application to the second tarsus causes the retraction of the already extended proboscis. The concentration of the second chemical will then give a measure of the rejection threshold for that chemical.

Experiments of this nature have demonstrated that proboscis extension and feeding can be initiated by stimulating the labellar or tarsal sensilla with water or certain sugars or low concentration of salts, and in female flies at a certain stage of their adult life, with solutions containing proteins. The activity of the mechanoreceptor can also be important, for in a highly receptive fly simply bending a single labellar sensillum is a sufficient stimulus for the extension of the proboscis. Substances which are rejected by the fly are numerous and include salts (in high concentration), acids, alcohols, aldehydes, ketones, glycols and ethers (for review see [6]).

The acceptance and rejection threshold measurements have also provided information about the sensitivity of different parts of the chemoreceptive system to the same chemical [4] and have demonstrated the changes in sensitivity which accompany starvation and feeding [5].

The electrical activity of the cells within the sensillum can be studied in two ways. In one method a glass capillary is passed over the tip of the sensillum and the activity of the receptor cells is recorded by using as it were the pore in the tip of the hair, the fluid filled lumen and the dendrites themselves as an extension of the recording electrode. The neatness of the method lies in the fact that the recording electrode also provides the chemical stimulus in the form of the solution contained within the capillary. The major disadvantage of the technique is that it is not suitable for non-electrolyte solutions, such as sucrose, since these do not conduct electricity and must therefore be adulterated with a low concentration of electrolyte. In addition, evaporation from the tip of the capillary can complicate the exact measurement of the concentration of the stimulating chemical which is applied to the sensillum. A more sophisticated and technically trickier method involves puncturing the side wall of the hair so that a recording microcapillary can be inserted amongst the receptor-cell dendrites to record their electrical activity while a separate system delivers pure chemical stimuli in the form of solutions which may or may nor be electrolytes, to the tip of the hair.

Early theories [3] about the function of the different receptor cells in each sensillum were centred on the idea that some cells were involved purely with acceptance and others with rejection. When testing labellar chemoreceptors of *Phormia* with a series of salts, sugars, acids and alcohols, Hodgson and Roeder [15] found that one of the cells in the hair (the S receptor) was stimulated by sugars, while another cell (the L receptor) was stimulated by the non-sugars. The fact that the fly feeds on sugars suggested to the authors that the S receptor mediated feeding responses and the L receptor mediated rejection. Over a period of time, however, it became established that of the four cells, one is concerned with the detection of sugars [13], one with water [9], and two with salts [14, 31]—one sensitive to primarily monovalent anions (the anion receptor) and another to monovalent cations (the salt receptor). This meant that all four cells in each sensillum could be accounted for in terms of acceptance and that none is concerned solely with rejection, since water and sugars are accepted by thirsty and hungry flies respectively, and salts can be accepted in low concentrations, but are rejected in high concentrations. Rejection, therefore, is not determined peripherally by the chemoreceptors alone, but is a more complex and centrally determined function of the chemoreceptive system.

For each cell type the application of its appropriate stimulus results in the depolarization of the cell and the production of action potentials which are transmitted to the central nervous system. The frequency of the action potentials generally increases with increasing concentration of the chemical stimulus. The electrical responses of the various categories of cells is shown in Fig. 17.8. As the stimulus is applied there is usually a rapid, phasic response in the appropriate receptor cell, and this adapts after a few hundred milliseconds to a tonic level of firing which is higher than in the unstimulated cell and which depends on the concentration of chemical applied to the sensillum.

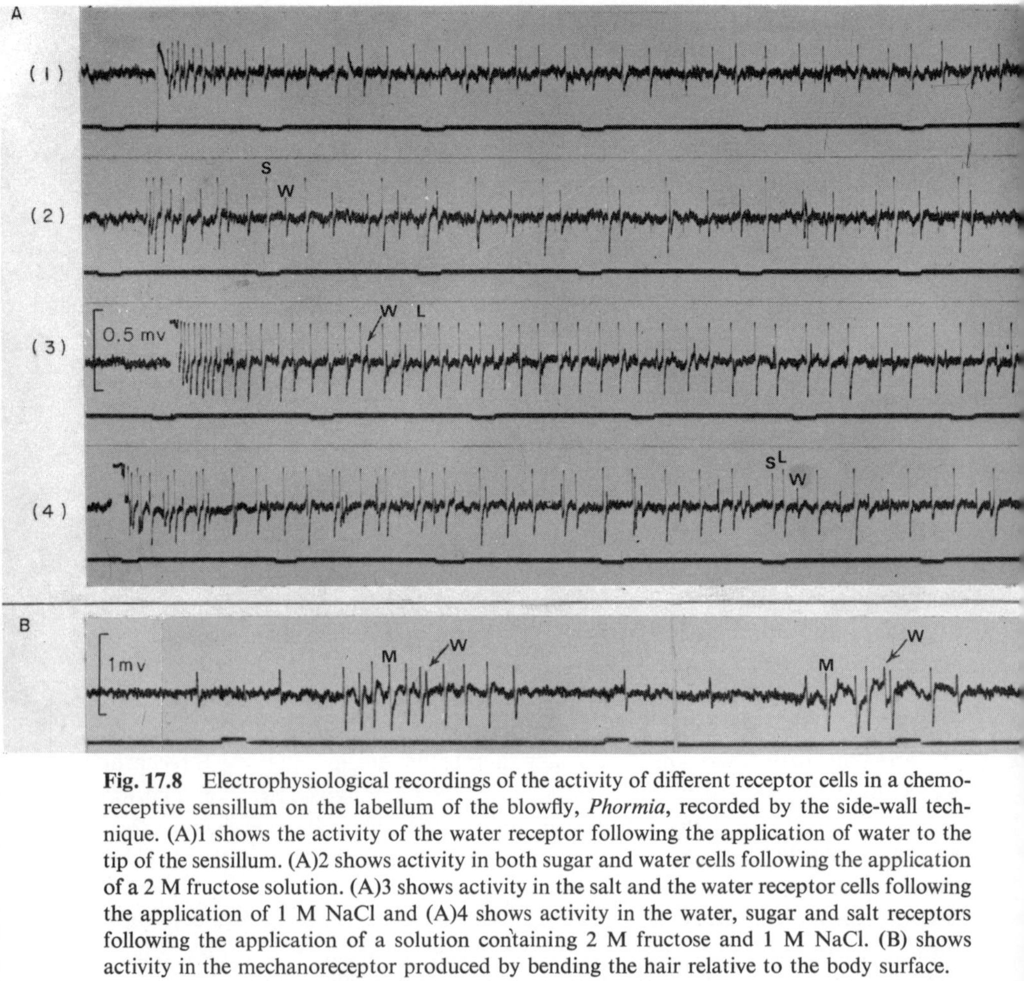

Fig. 17.8 Electrophysiological recordings of the activity of different receptor cells in a chemoreceptive sensillum on the labellum of the blowfly, *Phormia*, recorded by the side-wall technique. (A)1 shows the activity of the water receptor following the application of water to the tip of the sensillum. (A)2 shows activity in both sugar and water cells following the application of a 2 M fructose solution. (A)3 shows activity in the salt and the water receptor cells following the application of 1 M NaCl and (A)4 shows activity in the water, sugar and salt receptors following the application of a solution containing 2 M fructose and 1 M NaCl. (B) shows activity in the mechanoreceptor produced by bending the hair relative to the body surface.

Note that the rate of firing of the receptors is high immediately after the stimulus is applied, but that the rate adapts quickly to a lower level with the prolonged presence of the stimulus. W, S, L and M indicate action potentials produced by the water, sugar, salt and mechanoreceptor cells respectively, and the square wave pulses in the lower traces occur at intervals of 0·14 sec. These data have been rearranged from [9].

N.B. The activity of the fourth type of chemoreceptor cell—the anion receptor—the presence of which in chemoreceptive hairs of the blowfly has been demonstrated by Steinhardt (1965)—is not shown in these records.

It appears that one of each category of receptor cell is present in all of the sensilla which contain four chemoreceptive cells, although some labellar hairs contain only two or three cells. How then, with only four types of cell, is it possible for the animal to distinguish the subtleties of the chemical environment? The presence of a sugar and a water receptor will enable the fly to find food and drink but how are the wide range of rejected chemicals detected if the salt and anion cells are not concerned solely with rejection? In addition, the possession of only four classes of cell does not explain how insects such as locusts and grasshoppers, with essentially the same chemoreceptive apparatus, are able to obtain the chemoreceptive information to determine their often considerable feeding preferences in respect of the vegetation available in their environment. The process of discrimination does not seem to depend on the possession of a large number of receptor cells, each highly sensitive to a specific chemical. The answers seem to lie, as Dethier [6] has recently shown, in the spectrum of sensitivity of each of the four classes of cells. Dethier finds that the spectrum of sensitivity of each cell type is wider than perhaps originally thought, although the response of the cell will vary with both the actual chemical applied and with its concentration. Thus the sugar receptor is responsive not only to a wide range of sugars but also to cyclitols, some amino acids, certain glycosides, neutral salt solutions at high pH and to high concentrations of formic and acetic acids. The cation receptor can be stimulated by many salts, some acids, some amino acids,

Table 17.1. A comparison of the responses of salt, sugar and water receptor cells in three different labellar sensilla (C3, C11 and r2) of the blowfly *Phormia* to a variety of glycosides. The data are rearranged from [6] and illustrate the different response spectra obtained from different cells in the same sensillum and from the same cells in different sensilla. +, increase in frequency of impulses compared to unstimulated state; 0, no change in frequency, −, a suppression of the response to sugar or salt in the presence of the glycoside. Water was present in all solutions, and the water cell responded to water alone unless indicated by + or −.

	Response								
	Salt cell			Sugar cell			Water cell		
Compound	C3	C11	r2	C3	C11	r2	C3	C11	r2
Methyl glycoside (0·1 M)	+	0	+	+	+	+	0	0	0
Amygdalin (0·1 M)	0	0	0	0	0	0	0	0	0
Apiin (saturated)	0	+	+	0	0	0	0	0	0
Apomycin (saturated)	0	0	0	0	0	0	0	0	0
Heliotropin (saturated)	0	+	+	0	0	0	0	0	0
Salicin (0·1 M)	+	−	−	0	−	−	0	0	0
Sinigrin (0·1 M)	+	+	+	+	0	0	0	0	0
Tropaeolin (saturated)	+	+	+	0	0	+	+	0	+

and by some glycosides. The so-called anion receptor responds to many salts and to high concentrations of many acids such as 1 M valeric, formic and nitric acids. In addition, the activity of the water receptor can be enhanced by the glycoside, tropaeolin. When these spectra are studied for different labellar hairs Dethier finds that each sensillum possesses a slightly different spectrum. (See Table 17.1).

Here then is perhaps the clue to the wide powers of discrimination possessed by the fly. Discrimination is not achieved by the use of many different receptors, each only sensitive to a specific chemical, but rather there are many differences in the spectrum of sensitivity of each of the cells belonging to each class. It is not the analysis of each specific input to the central nervous system upon which discrimination is based but on the comparison of many slightly different but essentially similar inputs, in many ways a far more sophisticated process. A parallel may be drawn with the eye and with colour vision. The retina does not possess many receptor-cell classes each specifically tuned to one wavelength or colour of light. Instead usually three classes of cell are present, each class having a slightly different spectrum of wavelengths to which it is sensitive. Thus the input to the nervous system from cells with spectral peaks in the red, green and blue regions of the total light spectrum can be integrated by the nervous system to produce the subjective perception of many different individual colours. It would appear that an essentially similar process occurs in chemoreception.

17.8 REFERENCES

1 Barros-Pita J.C. & Maldonado H. (1970) A fovea in the praying mantis eye. II. Some morphological characteristics. *Z. vergl. Physiol.* **67,** 79–92.

2 Burrows M. & Horridge G.A. (1968) The action of the eye-cup muscles of the crab *Carcinus*, during optokinetic movements. *J. exp. Biol.* **49,** 223–50.

3 Dethier V.G. (1953) Summation and inhibition following contralateral stimulation of the tarsal chemoreceptors of the blowfly. *Biol. Bull. Woods Hole* **105,** 257–68.

4 Dethier V.G. (1976) *The Hungry Fly*. Harvard University Press.

5 Dethier V.G. (1966) Feeding Behaviour. In *Insect Behaviour*. Symp. Ent. Soc. London, No. 3. (P. T. Haskell) pp. 46–58.

6 Dethier V.G. (1974) The specificity of the labellar chemoreceptors of the blowfly and the response to natural foods. *J. Ins. Physiol.* **20,** 1859–69.

7 Ditchburn R.W. & Ginsborg B.L. (1952) Vision with a stabilised retinal image. *Nature, Lond.* **170,** 36–7.

8 Dowling J.E. & Boycott B.B. (1966) Organisation of the primate retina: electron microscopy. *Proc. Roy. Soc. B. 166* 80–111.

9 Evans D. & Mellon De F. (1962) Electrophysiological studies of a water receptor associated with the taste sensilla of the blowfly. *J. gen. Physiol.* **45,** 487–500.

10 Ewert J.P. (1974) The neural basis of visually guided behaviour. *Scientific American* **230,** 34–42.

11 Gregory R.L., Ross H.E. & Moray N. (1964) The curious eye of *Copilia. Nature, Lond.* **201,** 1166–68.

12 Hartline H.K. (1938) The response of single optic fibres of the vertebrate eye to illumination of the retina. *Am. J. Physiol.* **121,** 400–15.

13 Hodgson E.S. (1957) Electrophysiological studies of arthropod chemoreception II. Re-

sponses of labellar chemoreceptors of the blowfly to stimulation by carbohydrates. *J. Ins. Physiol.* **1,** 240–7.

14 Hodgson E.S., Lettvin J.Y. & Roeder K.D. (1955) The physiology of a primary chemoreceptor unit. *Science, Wash.* **122,** 417–18.

15 Hodgson E.S. & Roeder K.D. (1956) Electrophysiological studies of arthropod chemoreception. I. General properties of the labellar chemoreceptors of Diptera. *J. cell. comp. Physiol.* **48,** 51–76.

16 Kennedy J.S. & Moorhouse J.E. (1970) Laboratory observations on locust responses to windborne grass odour. *Ent. exp. & appl.* **12,** 487–503.

17 Kellog W.N. (1961) *Porpoises and Sonar.* University of Chicago Press, Chicago.

18 Kuffler S.W. (1953) Discharge patterns and functional organisation of mammalian retina. *J. Neurophysiol.* **16,** 37–68.

19 Land M.F. (1969) Movements of the retinae of jumping spiders (Salticidae: Dendryphantidae) in response to visual stimuli. *J. exp. Biol.* **51,** 471–93.

20 Land M.F. (1973) Head movement of flies during visually guided flight. *Nature, Lond.* **243,** 299–300.

21 Lettvin J.Y., Maturana H.R., McCulloch W.S. & Pitts W.H. (1959) What the frog's eye tells the frog's brain. *Proc. Inst. Radio Engrs.* (*N.Y.*) **47,** No. 11, 1940–51.

22 Levín L. & Maldonado H. (1970) A fovea in the praying mantis eye. III. The centering of the prey. *Z. vergl. Physiol.* **67,** 93–101.

23 Lissmann H.W. (1963) Electric location by fishes. *Scientific American* **208,** 53.

24 Maturana H.R., Lettvin J.Y., McCulloch W.S. & Pitts W.H. (1960). Anatomy and Physiology of vision in the frog (*Rana pipiens*). *J. gen. Physiol.* **43,** 129–76.

25 Michael C.R. (1969) Retinal processing of visual images. *Scientific American* **220,** 104–14.

26 Mittelstaedt H. (1957) Prey capture in mantids. In *Recent advances in invertebrate physiology*, pp. 51–71. University of Oregon Press, Oregon.

27 Patterson J.A. (1973) The eye muscle of *Calliphora vomitoria* L. I. Spontaneous activity and the effects of light and dark adaptation. *J. exp. Biol.* **58,** 565–83.

28 Robinson D.A. (1968) Eye movement control in primates. *Science, Wash.* **161,** 1219–24.

29 Sales G.D. & Pye J.D. (1974) *Ultrasonic Communication by Animals.* Chapman & Hall, London & New York.

30 Schneider D., Block B.L., Boeckh J. & Priesner E. (1967) Reaction of male moth to Bombykol. *Z. vergl. Physiol.* **54,** 192–209.

31 Steinhardt R.A. (1965) Cation and anion stimulation of electrolyte receptors of the blowfly *Phormia regina. Am. Zoologist* **5,** 651–2.

32 Thorson J. (1964) Dynamics of motion perception in the desert locust. *Science, Wash.* **145,** 69–71.

33 Thurm U. (1964) Mechanoreceptors in the cuticle of the Honey Bee: Fine structure and stimulus mechanism. *Science, Wash.* **145,** 1063–5.

34 Wallace G.K. (1959) Visual scanning in the desert locust (*Schistocerca gregaria*). *J. exp. Biol.* **36,** 512–25.

35 Wehner R. & Labhart T. (1970) Perception of the geomagnetic field in the fly *Drosophila melanogaster. Experientia* (Basel) **26,** 967–8.

36 Wolbarsht M.L. & Dethier V.G. (1958) Electrical activity in the chemoreceptors of the blowfly. I. Responses to chemical and mechanical stimuli. *J. gen. Physiol.* **42,** 393–412.

Prelude to Chapter 18

The density of the aquatic environment offers considerable resistance to movement but renders buoyancy an attractive option which several groups of animals have taken up. There are at least three selective advantages which common sense tells us buoyancy may confer on an animal. There is a saving in the energy cost of maintaining station in the water column, increased manoeuvrability, especially at low swimming speeds, and the ability to hover silently and motionless. The different buoyancy strategies adopted by siphonophores, fish and cephelapods are striking examples of the versatility of animals. The way the buoyancy mechanisms work, and the extent to which buoyancy is controlled on a day-to-day time scale, is the subject of the following chapter. A number of large gaps in our knowledge will become apparent to the reader, perhaps the chief of which is the energetic efficiency and speed of adjustment of the mechanisms in nature. As servo-systems, buoyancy devices are elegantly engineered to the environment in ways we little understand at present.

Chapter 18
Buoyancy

P. TYTLER

18.1 GENERAL CONSIDERATIONS

Buoyancy is the upthrust generated by the displacement of the ambient medium. Aquatic animals are considered to be neutrally buoyant when the resulting upthrust and weight of the animal are equal. An increase or decrease in the upthrust to weight ratio results in positive or negative buoyancy respectively. In a state of neutral buoyancy an animal can hover motionless in the water and so conserve a considerable amount of energy [3] and at the same time reduce conspicuousness. However since most animals contain a relatively high proportion of relatively dense structural tissue, neutral or positive buoyancy requires the development of buoyancy mechanisms which will provide the necessary upthrust to counteract the downthrust of the weight of the animal in water [2]. These buoyancy mechanisms can be divided into two general categories; they are either *static* or *adjustable*. Static buoyancy mechanisms usually involve a long-term reduction in the relative density of the animal, either by the inclusion of low-density metabolically derived substances, such as lipid [4, 6, 36] or ammonium ions or by the reduction in the density of structural tissues [21] and body fluids by the exclusion of relatively dense components such as protein, calcium and sulphate ions [23]. Alternatively the proportions of the structural tissues in the body may be reduced to achieve neutral buoyancy at the expense of strength and mobility [21]. Positively buoyant members of the plankton usually have static buoyancy mechanisms in the form of bubbles of gas or air on or within their bodies which they use to float at the surface of the water [53].

In the context of rapid adjustments to the environment the adjustable buoyancy mechanisms are most relevant. In most cases these involve the development of an internal gas-filled chamber. By changing the volume of the gas in the chamber the relative density of the whole organism can be altered to suit its requirements. The biological significance of the selection of gas-filled chambers is primarily twofold. The relative densities of the main gases used are so small that the upthrust they generate is practically equal to the weight of water they displace [2]. Also with the exception of carbon monoxide which will be considered separately all the gases are components of air which are absorbed and transported by and can be released from the blood. This, as will be discussed later, provides a mechanism of gaseous exchange between the medium and the buoyancy chamber and is used in most hydrostatic mechanisms to alter the volume of gas.

The development of adjustable buoyancy mechanisms is usually associated with regular vertical movements of many marine and freshwater animals. The most familiar and spectacular demonstration of which is the diurnal vertical movements of the deep scattering layers in oceanic waters [5]. The deep scattering layers are the stratified zones of sonic reverberations detected on ultrasonic echosounding recordings. The animals responsible for this phenomenon were found to contain flexible gas-filled chambers of such a size that the resonant frequency is similar to that used by the echosounding equipment (12–24 KHz). The evidence from midwater trawl catches and direct observations of these deep scattering layers from submersibles has indicated that mesopelagic lanternfish (Myctophidae) and siphonophores (Physonectae) are the principal members. At night they are found near the surface but around dawn they descend rapidly at 3·3 metres per minute until they level out in the early morning at depths between 300 and 500 metres, depending on the species and the environmental conditions. They remain at these depths during the day and begin their ascent to the surface in late afternoon, rising at 12 metres per minute. Smaller scale vertical migrations are found in many demersal animals such as codfish (Gadidae) [52] and cuttlefish (*Sepia officianalis*) [16] which migrate from the sea bed at dusk to a midwater depth several metres from the surface. Echosoundings of lakes also show that many freshwater fish and invertebrates perform diurnal vertical excursions. Also recent developments in the use of ultrasonic depth telemetry fish tags give clear evidence of short-term vertical movements to and from the surface over depths of 40 metres in marine fish [50].

The development of adjustable gas-filled buoyancy mechanisms has the potential of providing either the necessary upthrust for the ascent or for maintaining neutral buoyancy during vertical migrations. The problem of vertical movements is that the volume of gas is inversely proportional to the absolute pressure acting on it. The ambient pressure is directly related to depth and the pressure changes by one atmosphere for each 10 metre change in depth, 1 atm = 101·3 kNm^{-2}. At a depth of 50 metres the pressure is 5 atm or 6 atmospheres absolute, which includes the pressure of the atmosphere. In the case of vertical movements in either direction the relative pressure change ($\Delta p/P$ where Δp is the change in pressure and P is the initial pressure) is most relevant to changes in buoyancy. If one assumes the same initial volume, an upward movement of 200 metres from a depth of 600 metres ($\Delta p/P = 0{\cdot}33$) produces the same change in gas volume as a 10 metre ascent from 30 metres although the absolute distances moved are very different. It is also important to remember that although the initial volumes in both situations are the same, the volume at 600 metres (61 atmospheres absolute) contains about 15 times more gas molecules than at 30 metres (4 atm). Thus similar adjustments in volume and buoyancy at different depths can involve considerable differences in the number of molecules exchanged and consequently the energy cost of adjustment [3].

There appear to be two major evolutionary lines in the development of gas-filled hydrostatic organs each of which provide totally different solutions to the problems facing vertical migrants. In both fish and siphonophores upthrust is provided by a gas-filled flexible bladder in which the gas is in equilibrium with ambient pressures. Changes in volume are compensated either by the secretion of gas from a gas gland or by the venting or resorbing of excess gas through the aperture of a muscular sphincter in the bladder wall. Cephalopod molluscs on the other hand have developed rigid buoyancy chambers in which the gas is isolated from ambient pressures and buoyancy is adjusted by altering the proportions of gas and fluid in the chamber.

18.2 FLEXIBLE BUOYANCY CHAMBERS

18.2.1 The siphonophore float

The gas-filled floats of the siphonophores provide an interesting example of adjustable buoyancy mechanisms. The Portuguese Man-of-War, *Physalia physalis*, is probably the best known representative of this group and is predominately found floating on or near the surface [35]. On occasions individuals have been observed to sink below the surface and resurface several minutes later, indicating the presence of control over their buoyancy. The polyps of *Physalia* are suspended from a gas-filled bladder which floats on the surface of the sea and has the secondary function as a sail. The bladder consists of two layers: an outer thicker *pneumatocodon* which is separated from the inner *pneumatosaccus* by an extension of the gastro-vascular cavity and both layers contain muscle tissue which periodically contracts and causes the float to curl over on the surface of the sea and thus keeps the *pneumatocodon* moist and pliable. The musculature also appears to regulate the pressure of the gas within the float and may consequently adjust its buoyancy. At the trailing edge of the float there is an aperture guarded by a muscular sphincter, called the *pneumatophore* which when open during contraction of the musculature allows gas to be vented from the float.

The gas in the float contains concentrations of carbon monoxide of between 8 and 14% [55]. Carbon monoxide is both a respiratory and metabolic poison but its concentration in the float appears to be below the critical toxic level for the cytochrome systems of *Physalia* under atmospheric conditions. The gas is secreted from a specialized area of the *pneumatosaccus* called the gas gland [55, 56]. It appears that the source of the carbon monoxide is the β carbon radical of L-serine [56]. This single carbon fragment is transferred to folic acid to form tetrafolates from which carbon monoxide is eventually formed. The presence of high concentrations of folic acid and its derivatives in the gas gland tissue and the fact that aminopterin (a folic acid antagonist) reduces carbon monoxide synthesis in gas gland homogenates supports this suggestion [31]. The rate of synthesis is only 150 $\mu l\ h^{-1}$ at NTP which suggests that in *Physalia* adjustments in buoyancy are minor and occur over relatively long periods. The curious selection of carbon monoxide as a buoyancy agent rather than, for example, the less toxic carbon dioxide, may be related to its low solubility. It is 40 times less soluble in water than carbon dioxide and consequently diffuses more slowly through the thin moist *pneumatosaccus*. Carbon monoxide is generated by the organisms' metabolism whereas the buoyancy gases used by fish and cephalopods are derived from the atmosphere. The siphonophore system is a biochemical solution to a buoyancy problem and, as we shall see, that of fish is a physical strategy, using atmospheric gases available in its blood stream.

In contrast to *Physalia* there are numerous mesopelagic species of siphonophores which are known to perform vertical migrations. The physonectid *Nanomia bijuga* has been observed to move vertically to the surface at dusk at approximately 5 m min^{-1} [30]. This species has an apical float from which a cluster of swimming bells capable of considerable thrust are suspended. The structure of the float is essentially the same as that of *Physalia* but on a smaller scale. Analysis of the gas contained in the float has shown that carbon monoxide represents about 80–93% of the total gas volume. Thus at the maximum recorded depth of 300 m the P_{CO} will be nearly 30 atm! [41]. This is the highest 'concentration' of carbon monoxide found in a living system. The rate of CO production by the gas gland has not yet been measured but if neutral buoyancy is maintained at 300 m the rate must be greater than observed in *Physalia*. Clearly more research is required to measure the potential of CO production as a buoyancy mechanism and the tolerance of the tissues of this species to extremely high concentrations of toxic carbon monoxide.

18.2.2 The fish swimbladder

In bony fish (Order Teleostei) the adjustable buoyancy mechanism is the swimbladder [2, 32]. Since this group of fish is widely distributed throughout the water column and many species perform diurnal vertical migrations the gas contained within this flexible buoyancy chamber is subject to a wide range of absolute pressures and to rapid relative pressure changes. In the marine environment bony fish are found in all four depth zones (see Table 18.1) and functional swimbladders are completely absent from only the bathypelagic species which rely on static buoyancy mechanisms instead [38]. Swimbladders are also absent in some specialized groups, for example bottom-living flatfish, fast and perpetually swimming epipelagic scombroids and fish living in fast-flowing rivers. In these fish swimbladders offer no selective advantage in the niches which they occupy, in some cases its presence may be selectively disadvantageous [2].

Table 18.1. Representative species of the four main horizontal oceanic layers (37).

Depth (m)	Pressure (atm)	Layer	Species
0–150	1–16	Epipelagic	Sun-fish
150–1000	16–101	Mesopelagic	Lanternfish, melamphaids, stomiatoids, trichiuroids gonostomatids
1000–4000	101–401	Bathypelagic	Cyclothone, gonostomatids Xenodermichthys
Near the sea floor	Up to 400	Benthopelagic	Macruorids, eretmophorids, brotulids

The density of fish without swimbladders is about 1·07. Thus such a fish weighing 107 g will displace 100 cm^3 of water. Assuming the relative densities of sea water and fresh water to be 1·026 and 1·00 respectively then the weight of the fish in sea water will be 4·4 g (107–102·6 g) and in fresh water 7·0 g (107–100 g). By increasing the volume of the fish by 4·4 and 7·0 cm^3 by the presence of a gas-filled swimbladder neutral buoyancy in the marine and fresh water environments is effected [2]. Measurements of swimbladder volumes from marine and freshwater fish show general agreement with these theoretical figures.

During any vertical movement the resulting pressure change will be transmitted through the body of the fish to the flexible swimbladder wall which in some fish is so compliant that the gas within responds to the pressure change according to Boyle's Law [44]. In others the volume change during a pressure reduction is reduced by the tensile strength of the swimbladder wall [2]. Since a reduction in the ambient pressure to which the fish is adapted and at which it is neutrally buoyant will produce positive buoyancy and the tendency to accelerate upwards. Any constraint on this change will save the energy expenditure in swimming required to compensate for the upthrust generated by upward movements above the point of neutral buoyancy. In either case however the increased ambient pressure experienced during downward movements will, without compensation, result in a related reduction in buoyancy.

Benthopelagic fish are exposed to very high ambient pressures (see Table 18.1) so that the gas in the swimbladder contains a much greater volume of gas at STP than a similar sized epipelagic fish. Also the partial pressures of the components of the gas will be much higher than at atmospheric conditions. Thus deep-sea fish have to produce more gas and have to maintain it at higher partial pressures. Consequently the theoretical cost of maintaining neutral buoyancy at great depths is substantially greater than in epipelagic fish [38].

The potential of the swimbladder to maintain neutral buoyancy during short-term changes in pressure and long-term exposure to high ambient pressures provides an intriguing study in physiological adaptation to the environment.

Embryologically the swimbladder develops as a pouch from the foregut [26, 32, 51]. In some fish, *Physostomes*, the connection between the swimbladder and the gut is retained as the pneumatic duct, but in more advanced fish, *Physoclists*, the pneumatic duct has regressed and the swimbladder is closed. There is considerable variation in the shape and structure of the swimbladders of both *physostomes* and *physoclists* and there are many species which retain the pneumatic duct but in most other features closely resemble the *physoclists*. Also in some *physostomes*, for example herring (*Clupea harengus*) have a second duct leading from the posterior end of the swimbladder to the anus, the so-called *anal duct* [8]. The basic histological structure is similar in both main groups and retains many features of digestive tract from which it is derived. In the typical *physoclist* the swimbladder consists of four histologically discrete layers (Fig. 18.1D) [26].

The three inner layers resemble the mucosa and submucosa of the vertebrate digestive tract and are often referred to as the *tunica interna* in order to distinguish them from the outer layer, the *tunica externa*.

Since the adjustable buoyancy mechanisms are most highly developed and elaborate in the physoclists, it is considered appropriate to consider the organization of the closed swimbladder in most detail. Although the buoyancy control mechanisms of physoclists have been described by many authors the most recent advances in the understanding of the physiological mechanisms have been obtained by research on the eel *Anguilla vulgaris* which has a pneumatic duct but demonstrates many features more typical of physoclists especially in the mechanisms involved in inflating the swimbladder [46, 52].

For the maintenance of a constant gas volume or neutral buoyancy during variations in ambient pressure, mechanisms for inflating and deflating the swimbladder are obviously necessary. In physostomes with access to the water–air interface, air is swallowed at the surface and forced into the swimbladder through the pneumatic duct. Deflation is caused by passively venting the excess volume produced by reduction in pressure by way of the pneumatic or anal duct. Most physostomes possess a muscular sphincter at the distal end of the pneumatic duct although no sphincter has been described on the anal duct. Contraction of the sphincter in conjunction with contraction of the muscularis mucosae or the body musculature can result in a small reduction in gas volume in the swimbladder without release of gas [2]. Such changes in swimbladder volume provide a rapid

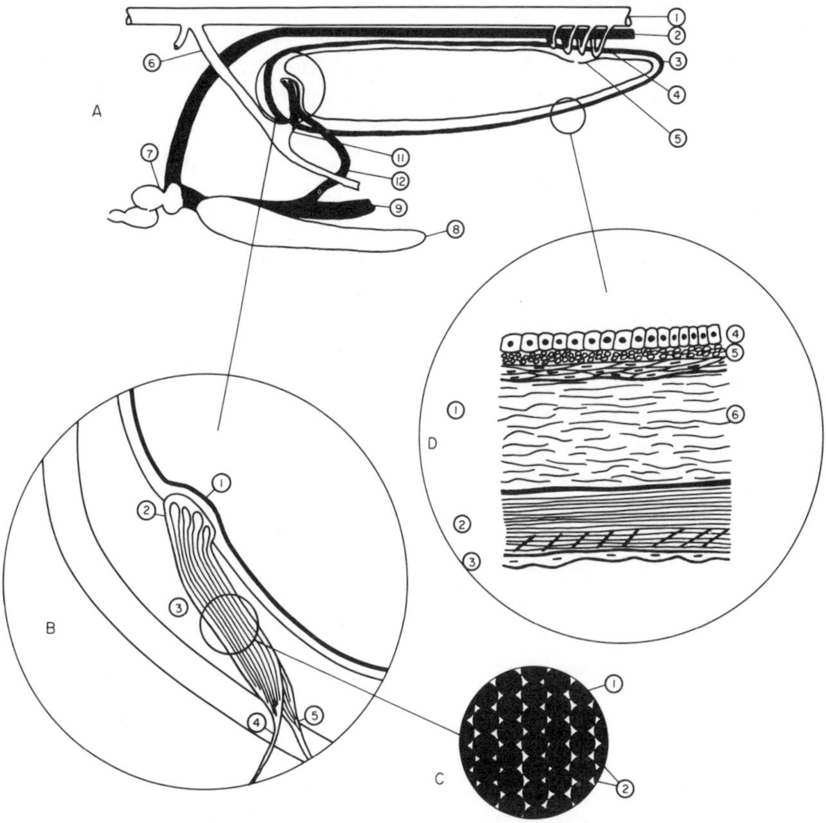

Fig. 18.1. The Physoclist swimbladder. (A) A diagram of the general structure and blood supply to the swimbladder of a typical physoclist. 1, dorsal aorta; 2, posterior cardinal vein; 3, swimbladder wall; 4, reabsorbant capillary tufts; 5, oval sphincter; 6, coeliac artery; 7, heart; 8, liver; 9, hepatic portal vein; 11, gas gland artery; 12, gas gland vein. (B) A detailed diagram of the rete mirabile and gas gland. 1, gas gland epithelium; 2, post rete capillary network; 3, rete mirabile; 4, gas gland artery; 5, gas gland vein. (C) A diagram of the arrangement of the afferent capillaries (2) and efferent capillaries (1) as seen in a cross section of a deep sea fish. (D) A diagram of the structure of the swimbladder wall. 1. The tunica interna which is composed of an epithelial layer (4), the muscularis mucosae (5), the submucosa (6) which consists of loose fibrous connective tissue carrying blood vessels, autonomic nerves and ganglion cells. 2. The tunic externa composed of dense collagenous connective tissue containing elastic fibres, varying amounts of smooth muscle and a peripheral layer of guanine crystals. 3. The serosa. From [27].

and convenient mechanism for fine adjustment in buoyancy and is used to good effect by many fresh-water fish [28]. In physostomes without ready access to the surface and physoclists with closed swimbladders the mechanisms for inflation result from the local reduction in the carrying capacity for dissolved gases of the blood flowing through the arterial blood vessels of the tunica interna of the swimbladder wall. The gases carried in the arterial blood of fish are in equilibrium with the water which is passed over the respiratory surfaces of the gills.

The partial pressures of the constituent gases dissolved in water are the same or less than that of surface water which is in equilibrium with atmospheric air [3].

If deep-sea fish are able to maintain neutral buoyancy at depth it is necessary to maintain a gas volume in the swimbladder of 5% of the volume of the fish. Consequently the gas in the swimbladder will have the same hydrostatic pressure as the surrounding water. At 990 metres for example the total gas pressure will be 100 atm. If we assume that the swimbladder gas has the same composition as air and ignore water vapour pressure then the partial pressures of the components will be 100 times the values for water surrounding the fish and its blood and tissues. This situation would lead to diffusion of gases from the swimbladder to blood, tissues and hence water in order to restore equilibrium. From measurements of the gas composition of swimbladders of various deep and surface living fish it has been calculated that the partial pressures of nitrogen, oxygen and carbon dioxide may exceed the values for atmospheric air [45, 47, 51]. In fact the partial pressure of nitrogen in swimbladders of some benthopelagic fish, for example *Macrourus sp.* caught at 1240 m, is as high as 10 atm which is about 12 times greater than atmospheric nitrogen [48]. The partial pressure of oxygen on the other hand may be as high as 176 atm which is 880 times greater than the Po_2 of atmospheric oxygen.

Three questions arise from these observations:

1 How are such high partial pressures of swimbladder gases produced?

2 How can the swimbladder retain the gas in spite of diffusion gradient across the swimbladder wall?

3 How can the tissue of the swimbladder tolerate or avoid the toxic effects of hyperbaric oxygen and the Pasteur effect?

The mechanisms responsible for the production of high partial pressures of the component gases of the swimbladder are not fully understood but a much clearer explanation is possible with the results from recent research [51]. The gas-producing apparatus of the swimbladder of physoclists and of the eel consists of glandular epithelium which is in intimate contact with the underlying rete mirabile (Fig. 18.1B) a complex capillary plexus. The glandular epithelium is a modification of the inner epithelium of the tunica interna of the swimbladder wall. In the eel the whole of the internal epithelium of the swimbladder wall consists of glandular tissue but in true physoclists it is localized to a patch or patches on the anterior ventral wall, which may consist of straight single layers of columnar epithelium or folded to form pouches. By a combination of elaborate folding and subsequent growing together the glandular epithelium of advanced physoclists may become a complex multi-layered gas gland with a system of intercellular ducts connecting the deeper layers with the lumen of the swimbladder [24, 26]. The whole inner surface of the epithelium facing the lumen of the swimbladder is coated with mucous which is thought to be secreted by the epithelium. Examination of newly-excised active glandular tissue will reveal the presence of tiny bubbles of gas contained within the mucous layer [46].

The rete mirabile is found in the loose connective tissue of the submucosal layer of the tunica interna [52, 53]. It consists of intermingled, parallel unbranched afferent and efferent capillaries which appose one another in such a way that the whole surface of each capillary is in intimate contact with adjacent capillaries (Fig. 18.1C). The afferent and efferent capillaries from a series of straight parallel hairpin loops the closed ends of which are imbedded in the glandular epithelium. There are between 88,000 and 250,000 such loops in the rete so that a cross-section of the rete of some species would reveal as many as 500,000 capillaries [45]. Although the volume of blood in the rete may be as small as 0·1 cm^3, the surface area of the walls of the capillaries within it can exceed 2600 cm^2. Since each afferent capillary is surrounded by at least 4 efferent capillaries there is an enormous surface area available for any diffusion caused by arterio-venous difference in solute for which the capillary walls are permeable.

It has been proposed that the release of gas from the glandular epithelium is produced by both reducing the affinity of haemoglobin for oxygen and reducing the solubility of the dissolved gases in the blood. Both mechanisms result in increasing the partial pressures of these gases in solution. In other words higher partial pressures of gas are required to maintain the same concentration of these gases in solution under these new circumstances. It has been demonstrated that the affinity for and carrying-capacity of blood of many fish is influenced by pH (the BOHR shift and ROOT effect) [51, 27]. By reducing the pH of the blood from the normal value of 7·8 in *Alphestes* sp. to 6·3 the P_{50} (partial pressure of oxygen required for 50% saturation of blood) changes from less than 1 atm to about 30 atm and even at partial pressures in excess of 80 atm the blood remained no more than 50% saturated. Thus even with 100% oxygen in the swim-bladder and a hydrostatic pressure euivalent to 800 m depth, blood at a pH of 6·3 in the rete can only reach 50% saturation. In other words oxygen can be unloaded from fully-saturated oxyhaemoglobin in the presence of high partial pressures of oxygen when the blood is acidified. Measurements of the blood entering and leaving the gas gland of the eel have shown that the efferent blood has a lower pH and higher lactic acid concentration than the afferent blood [51] (Fig. 18.2). The lactic acid appears to be secreted by the glandular epithelium even when exposed to Po_2 values up to 51 atm [12]. The fact that glycolysis and the production of lactic acid occurs at such high Po_2 values is a spectacular exception to the general rule that glycolysis in aerobic organisms predominates only under anaerobiosis; the so-called *Pasteur Effect*. The glucose 6-phosphate which is formed early in glycolysis is largely diverted to the hexose-monophosphate shunt. The resulting pentose phosphate may now enter the glycolytic pathway after being converted to glyceraldehyde 3-phosphate. This may explain the lack of Pasteur effect since in by-passing the step mediated by phospho-fructokinase the oxygen sensitive reaction is avoided [6]. The substrate for the lactic acid production is *not* now thought to be the glycogen granules found within the epithelium but more probably to blood glucose [12].

The total release of oxygen from oxyhaemoglobin by acidification, assuming complete deoxygenation, will increase the Po_2 of blood to 3 atm which is adequate for epipelagic fish but is inadequate for the deep-sea fish [51]. A drop in pH has also been shown to release N_2 from fish red cells perhaps by a change in the polar groups of the haemoglobin molecule [1]. In addition the secretion of lactic acid will, by increasing the concentration of solutes in the blood, reduce the solubility of the gases and thus increase their partial pressures in consequence [49, 51, 54]. This 'salting out' mechanism on its own is unlikely to raise the P_{N_2}, for example, to more than twice its atmospheric value [45]. It has been shown [52, 40] that the rete mirabile is a counter-current multiplier system which can produce P_{O_2} values of 2000 atm and P_{N_2} values of 23 atm. If it is initially assumed that the capillary walls of the rete are impermeable to hydrogen and lactate ions but will allow free diffusion of gases then the explanation of the multiplier mechanism is relatively simple. Since oxygen is the principal mobile component of swimbladder gas of most physoclists, the following description is

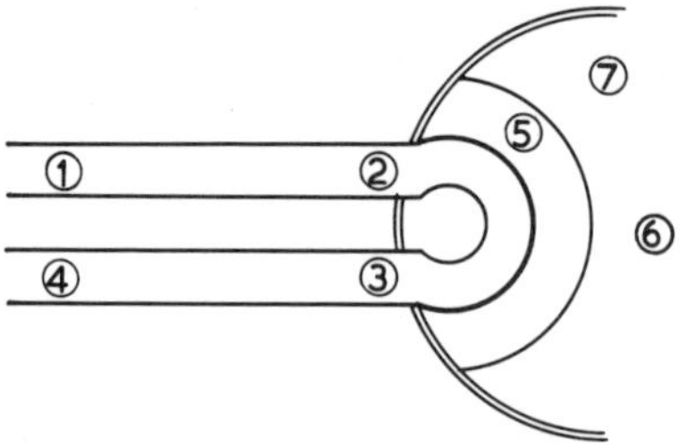

Fig. 18.2. The countercurrent multiplier system in the rete mirabile. The condition of the blood within the rete and the composition of the swimbladder gas during re-inflation of the swimbladder of the eel *Anguilla vulgaris*. (1) pre-rete artery pH = 7·53, P_{O_2} = 0·2 atm, P_{CO_2} = <0·01 atm, lactate concentration = 14 mg%. (2) post-rete artery pH = 7·05, P_{O_2} = 1·00 atm, P_{CO_2} = 0·03 atm, lactate concentration = 45 mg%. (3) pre-rete vein pH = 6·65, P_{O_2} = 1·00 atm, P_{CO_2} = 0·08 atm, lactate concentration 92 mg%. (4) post-rete vein pH = 7·43, P_{O_2} = 0·07 atm, P_{CO_2} = <0·01, lactate concentration 60 mg%. During these changes in the blood, oxygen and carbon dioxide diffuses (6) from the gas gland epithelium (5) into the lumen of the swimbladder (7). The P_{O_2} and P_{CO_2} in (7) at the time of measurement were 0·70 atm and 0·08 atm respectively. From Steen (1963), *Acta. Physiol. Scand.* **50,** 221–41.

confined to the multiplication of P_{O_2} but the principle also holds for nitrogen [45]. The countercurrent multiplier system depends on the establishment of a P_{O_2} gradient between the afferent and efferent capillaries along the length of the rete. The secretion of lactic acid by the glandular epithelium into the loops of the rete capillaries produces substantial arteriovenous P_{O_2} differences which persist along the efferent capillaries by virtue of the retention of hydrogen and lactate ions. Part of the excess oxygen thus produced will diffuse into the swimbladder but sufficient is retained within the rete to maintain the P_{O_2} gradient. As the efferent blood passes down the rete, oxygen will diffuse outwards with the gradient into the afferent system (Fig. 18.2). The afferent blood now entering the gas gland will have a P_{O_2} greater than the initial atmospheric level. Continued acidification of the blood in the gas gland together with the excess oxygen absorbed by the afferent blood will tend to increase the P_{O_2} in the efferent capillaries still further. This process of accumulation of oxygen retained within the rete by the countercurrent arrangement of capillaries will reach a maximum when the physical limits of the system are reached. A quantitative evaluation of the potential of the rete and the physical limitations imposed on it can be made using the following equation [53]:

$$P = \frac{DQ}{\alpha^2 V}$$

where P = excess Po_2 of the swimbladder gas
Q = transrete diffusion (which is proportional to the rete diffusion area)
α = solubility coefficient of oxygen
V = blood flow
D = volume of gas which diffuses into the swimbladder lumen

Thus by altering these physical factors the effectiveness of the rete can be changed. In deep-sea fish, for example, the length of the rete, the number of capillaries and consequently the value for Q is directly related to their depth distribution [38]. By introducing plausible values for the components of the equation Scholander [45] showed that P could be 4060 atm assuming no losses from respiration or diffusion through the swimbladder wall. Clearly the rete has the potential to create values of Po_2 in excess of that required even by bentho-pelagic species. For a more detailed treatment see [25] and [33].

The original assumption that the hydrogen ions and lactic ions do not diffuse across the rete from efferent to afferent blood flows is now known to be incorrect [46]. It has been shown instead that the rates of association and dissociation of oxygen for fish haemoglobin are substantially different [51]. The half-time for association is 10–20 seconds while the reverse process of dissociation is 0·05 seconds. This means that all the oxygen dissociated by acidification does not have time to recombine with the haemoglobin during the short time the blood flows through the efferent capillaries. A high Po_2, therefore, persists in the efferent capillaries and consequently a Po_2 difference is maintained between efferent and afferent blood systems.

In addition to multiplying the Po_2 the rete also acts as a barrier to diffusion from the high Po_2 within the swimbladder to the surrounding tissues and body fluids since the efferent retial blood will have unloaded almost all of the excess gas to the afferent capillaries within the rete. The blood in the gas gland vein will have a partial pressure of dissolved gas, at the most, slightly higher than the arterial partial pressures. The loss of gas by transverse diffusion across the rete is probably very small since the ratio of the surface area of the outer wall of the rete to the total diffusion area of the rete is minute.

The maintenance of high Po_2 values is also dependent upon the swimbladder wall acting as a barrier to diffusion. In fact it has been shown that the swimbladder wall in the conger eel *Conger conger* is about 100 times less permeable to O_2, N_2 and CO_2 than connective tissue [20]. The impermeability appears to arise from the presence of many layers of overlapping crystals of guanine imbedded in the tunica externa of the swimbladder wall. The rate of gas loss from the swimbladder of the conger was found to be 0·001 and 0·03 ml (cm^2 min atm)

μM[1] at STP. In a 2 kg conger eel with a swimbladder area of 143 cm^2 and a thickness of 200 μ, containing oxygen with a Po_2 of 10 atm the total loss of oxygen by diffusion would be 0·22 ml kg^{-1} h^{-1} at STP which is small in relation to the capacity for gas production (see below). Clearly the presence of guanine crystals in the tunica externa provides a formidable barrier to diffusion of oxygen.

The intracellular processes within the glandular epithelium used to release gas into the lumen are not known. It has been suggested that the secretion of phospholipids which have a low surface tension may facilitate in the formation of gas bubbles [12]. The pressure required to maintain a bubble is directly proportional to the surface tension of the enveloping liquid and inversely proportional to the radius of the bubble. By using lecithin as an example it was calculated that the pressure required to form a bubble was 14% less than that required in water. This process would greatly improve the diffusion of gas from liquid-cytoplasm phase to the gaseous phase of the swimbladder lumen.

In many deep living fresh-water physostomous salmonids the PN_2 of swimbladder gas was found to be higher than the Po_2. It has been suggested that the initial filling of the swimbladder involves the formation of bubbles of oxygen on the glandular epithelium as previously described. Into this bubble nitrogen diffuses passively from the surrounding tissues and fluids. At a later stage, as neutral buoyancy is reached, oxygen is probably removed by some means or other so that the gas in the swimbladder is finally predominately nitrogen [54]. However the observed increase in PN_2 with the release of nitrogen from red cells by the addition of lactic acid and the counter-current multiplication of the rete may be sufficient explanation [1].

The rates of gas production in several epipelagic physoclists have been found to be between 1·0 and 2·5 ml kg^{-1} h^{-1} at STP depending on ambient pressure and temperature [37, 52]. Unfortunately there are no values for deep-sea fish which may have a greater capacity for gas production due to longer retes and more than one gas-producing apparatus in their swimbladder [38]. However, since deep-sea fish have to secrete more gas molecules to compensate for the same relative pressure change than epipelagic fish it is generally assumed that their ability to compensate for buoyancy changes is the same as the epipelagic fish [38]. In these case a reduction in volume of the swimbladder of 50% equivalent to a relative pressure change of 150% would require 24 hours with a gas production rate of 1·65 ml kg h^{-1} at STP to restore the swimbladder to a neutral buoyancy level [52]. Since many vertically migrating species of mesopelagic fish experience relative pressure changes of between 120 and 193% in 3–4 h it is unlikely that they can maintain neutral buoyancy throughout their vertical range especially those experiencing relative pressure changes greater than 125%. It is significant that many species of mesopelagic fish which have the most extensive vertical movements have modified swimbladders in which the gas has been wholly or partly replaced by lipids [7, 9] and have assumed many of the static buoyancy mechanisms previously described.

The deflatory or gas reabsorption mechanism necessary to compensate for exposure to reduction in pressure during upward movements in the water column is relatively simple compared with the complex gas-production apparatus. In the true physoclists the gas reabsorption occurs in the posterior dorsal wall of the swimbladder [26, 43]. The inner epithelium and muscularis mucosal layer of the tunica interna form a muscular sphincter, *the oval*, which apparently opens during reabsorption to expose an extensive capillary bed which lies within the submucosal layer. The capillary bed is formed by capillary tufts connecting the dorsal aorta and the posterior cardinal veins. The capillary tufts pass through tiny apertures in the impervious tunica externa. During gas resorption swimbladder gas appears to diffuse into the capillaries and thence by way of the posterior cardinal veins to the heart and gills. The excess gas produced by a 50% reduction in pressure can be reabsorbed in three to five hours which is about eight times faster than gas secretion [52]. During gas production the oval sphincter is apparently closed, the capillary bed constricted and possibly the elastic tissue of the tunica externa closes the apertures during vasoconstriction sealing the impervious layer [42].

Hyperbaric oxygen is extremely toxic to aerobic organisms by inhibiting many enzymes of glycolysis and the citric acid cycle. Fish are no exception to the rule. Experiments with the rockfish *Sebastodes miniatus* have shown that exposure to P_{O_2} values greater than 3 atm causes convulsions and death within 24 hours [11]. Thus during gas reabsorption the P_{O_2} in the efferent oval blood vessels must not be allowed to exceed toxic levels since diffusion to other sensitive tissues would be extremely harmful. Also rapid diffusion through the swimbladder wall would have similar effects.

The control of the inflatory and deflatory mechanisms appears to be autonomic. Electrical stimulation of the swimbladder branch of the vagus and pharmacological studies suggest that gas production may be controlled by the parasympathetic system [13, 51]. Epinephrine appears to cause vasodilatation of the reabsorbant capillary bed and opening of the oval and pneumatic duct sphincters suggesting sympathetic control of the gas reabsorption mechanism.

The sensory input for controlling the buoyancy has not been fully investigated although inflatory and deflatory reflexes can be produced by deflating and inflating the swimbladder artificially, suggesting the presence of proprioceptors within the swimbladder wall [26].

It would appear that although the swimbladder can produce neutral buoyancy in fish exposed to extremely high ambient hydrostatic pressures it is only capable of complete compensation when exposed to short term, small, relative pressure changes.

18.3 RIGID BUOYANCY CHAMBERS

18.3.1 Cephalopod chambered shell

Nautilus, *Spirula* and *Sepia* are the only living cephalopods which have retained buoyancy mechanisms in the form of a chambered shell. Although the shells of

Spirula and *Nautilus* are external and coiled they are functionally similar to the internal cuttlebone of *Sepia* [18, 14, 15]. In all three, the shells are rigid and consist of many chambers each of which is an independent functional unit. Buoyancy is altered by regulating the proportions of fluid and gas in chambers.

In Sepia, for which most information [15] is available, each main chamber is subdivided by about six thin sublamellae which run parallel with the thicker walls or lamellae of the chambers (Fig. 18.3). The sublamellae are supported by

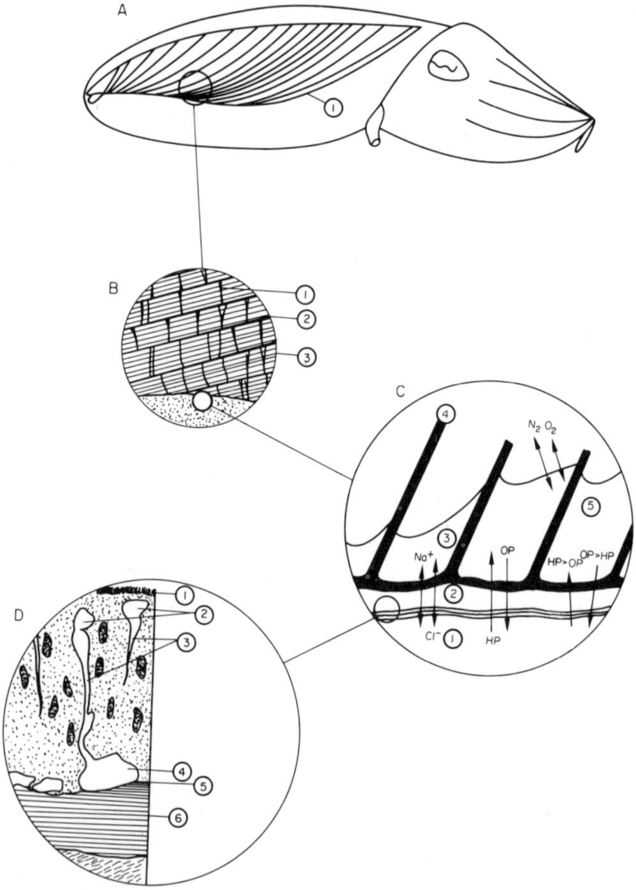

Fig. 18.3. The cuttlebone of *Sepia officianalis*. (A) A diagram of internal location of the cuttlebone and its multi-chamber structure. (B) A detailed diagram of the arrangement of the lamellae (2), sublamellae (3) and the pillars (1). (C) A diagram showing the control of water flow (5) by the balance between hydrostatic pressure (HP) and the osmotic pressure gradient (OP) between the blood (1) and the cuttlebone fluid (3). The osmotic pressure gradient is altered or maintained by the transfer of Na^+ and Cl^- ions between blood and fluid by the siphuncular epithelium (2). The gas contained within the sublamellae (4) is composed of nitrogen and oxygen which diffuses into or from the cuttlebone fluid. (D) A detailed diagram showing the characteristic features of siphuncular epithelium: (1) brush border, (2) ampullae, (3) intracellular ducts, (4) channels, (5) basement membrane, (6) underlying tissue containing blood vessels. From [14] and [15].

many calcified pillars which originate and insert on adjacent lamellae and greatly strengthen the fragile structure. The chambers are sealed laterally and anteriorly by the thick calcified layer forming the curved dorsal surface of the cuttlebone. Ventrally the tips of the lamellae are turned posteriorly so that they touch and fuse with adjacent lamellae and close the chambers. The ventral surface formed in this way is homologous with the siphuncular tube of *Nautilus* and *Spirula*. The lamellar surfaces exposed ventrally are permeable to water and are in the intimate contact with a layer of epithelial cells of the siphuncular membrane (Fig. 18.3C & D). As in the other species, *Sepia* adds new chambers

Table 18.2. The approximate initial composition of the bone per 100 ml of cuttlebone of *Sepia* [17].

	Weight (g)	Volume (ml)
Dry matter	36	16
Liquid	32	31
Gas space	trivial	53

(several in each year) as it grows to compensate for the increased mass of the animal. The upthrust produced by the cuttlebone of any individual animal ranged from 2·62–6·64% of the whole animal's weight in air while the downthrust remained constant at 3·96%. Analysis of the composition of the main constituents of the cuttlebone are shown in Table 18.2. The combined liquid and gas space represents 84% of the volume but less than half of the weight of the cuttlebone. If it is assumed that the liquid in the cuttlebone has the same relative density as sea water and that the liquid and gas contents are interchangeable then the density of the cuttlebone can be altered between 0·36 and 0·68 which is close to the measured values. Thus by altering proportions of fluid and gas in the cuttlebone the cuttlefish can change its overall relative density so that the buoyancy will change from +2·68 to −1·34% of the weight of the whole animal in air. The gas contained within the chambers is at a pressure less than atmospheric pressure. It is clear, therefore, that gas pressure is not responsible for the movement of the fluid across the siphuncular membrane.

The siphuncular membrane which lies immediately below the ventral surface of the cuttlebone consists of columnar epithelium with a brush border on the cell membrane close to the porous lamellar caps of the ventral surface. Within the siphuncular epithelium are ampullae and intracellular ducts. The ducts are connected to channels which run between the epithelium and the thick impervious basement membrane (Fig. 18.3D). The blood vessels in this area appear to anastomose with these channels, although injection techniques have failed to show a direct connection between them [15]. The cuttlefish, therefore, has the necessary equipment for the transport of fluids to or from the chambers of the cuttlebone.

The role of osmosis in the adjustment of buoyancy of *Sepia* was demonstrated by measurement of the osmotic concentration of blood and cuttlebone fluid of individuals at intervals after capture at 73 metres by bottom trawling [17]. It was assumed that they were all neutrally buoyant at the pressure at the depth of capture (7·3 atm). After decompression to atmospheric pressure, the osmotic pressure of the blood remained constant and identical to that of sea water. The cuttlebone fluid on the other hand was initially hyposmotic to sea water but gradually, over a period of six hours, became isosmotic with sea water. Extrapolation from the relationship between osmotic concentration and time gave an osmotic pressure of the fluid at the time of capture equal to 69% sea water and equivalent to an osmotic pressure gradient of 7·3 atmospheres. Thus the body fluids which tend to penetrate the chambers of the cuttlebone under the influence of an excess hydrostatic pressure of 7·3 atmospheres are resisted by the osmotic pressure difference between the cuttlebone fluid and blood. Moreover the gas volume in the cuttlebone will be unaffected by the hydrostatic pressure of the surrounding medium. The osmotic pressure difference between blood and cuttlebone fluid is created by the unselective active absorption of salts by the siphuncular membrane [17].

The degree of compensation for changes in ambient hydrostatic pressure by the cuttlefish is limited by the strength of the cuttlebone and the maximum osmotic pressure differential which can be created across the siphuncular membrane. The cuttlebone can tolerate hydrostatic pressures up to 24 atm but implodes at about 25 atm [29]. Thus the extreme limit of downward movement is about 240 metres which is much less than that for *Nautilus* and many species of fish. The maximum osmotic gradient will be achieved when all the salts are removed from the cuttlebone fluid which would then be equivalent to pure water. It has been calculated that the osmotic pressure created between distilled water and sea water of 35‰ and at 10°C is 24·0 atmospheres which means that at ambient pressures above 25 atm the system would not be able to compensate [17]. Thus, on both counts, the maximum depth of distribution is less than 240 metres. In *Nautilus* and *Spirula* similar osmotic limitations to the depth distribution also apply, but the implosion pressures are 45 and 170 atm respectively [29]. A more complicated osmotic device as found in the vertebrate kidney could however sustain a higher osmotic gradient being limited ultimately by the solubility of the solutes employed. It is also possible that in *Nautilus* the depth distribution may be greater than that set by the maximum osmotic gradient if the fluid in the chamber is isolated from the blood and fluids of the siphuncular area. In fact some such explanation is necessary to explain the capture of specimens at depths of 570 m. If uncoupling occurs during rapid vertical movements within the depth limit set by the shell strength then no change in internal gas volume or buoyancy such as experienced by fish and siphonophores will result. Even allowing for the osmotic work required to maintain neutral buoyancy during vertical migration the energy cost will be much less than for fish or siphonophores exposed to similar rates of change in relative pressure.

Young cuttlefish appear to perform diurnal changes in buoyancy which is linked to light intensity [16]. Under natural conditions they spend the day negatively buoyant buried in the gravel or sand of the sea bed, become positively buoyant at dusk and move off the bottom towards the surface. At dawn they lose their positive buoyancy and return to the sea bed. The rate of change in buoyancy in *Sepia* is between 0·2 and 0·4 g h^{-1} (100 g weight in air) which is within the range of buoyancy changes measured in fish (loc cit. p. 380). Thus *Sepia* can increase its buoyancy faster than fish, but fish appear to be able to eliminate excess gas faster and thus decrease buoyancy faster.

18.4 CONCLUSIONS

18.4.1 Static buoyancy mechanisms

The obvious advantage of such mechanisms arises from the generation of an upthrust which is virtually independent of pressure and will therefore remain constant during vertical movements within the aquatic environment. There is evidence however to suggest that the upthrust is dependent upon the nutritional status of the organism and may vary in the long term [4, 36].

Many species develop neutral buoyancy by laying down large reservoirs of high energy content lipids within the body. In some species the lipids are available as an energy store for metabolism while in others they are isolated from the normal metabolic processes [36]. The size of lipid depots may be as high as 25% of the total body weight [4, 8] which results in a substantial increase in resistance to locomotion [2].

In other aquatic organisms the static buoyancy involves a reduction in the concentration of relatively dense components such as muscle protein, calcareous skeletal inclusions and 'heavy' ions with a reciprocal increase in the water content of tissues and fluids [21]. Such modifications, although reducing the downthrust, may cause a reduction in structural strength and locomotor power.

The development of the large coelomic sac containing high concentrations of 'ammonia' in oceanic squids results in neutral buoyancy but with a 70% increase in body size and reduction in motility [19].

18.4.2 Adjustable buoyancy mechanisms

All the examples described have gas-filled buoyancy chambers which provide greater upthrust per unit of volume than any of the static mechanisms. However the gas is compressible and, in order to maintain the upthrust at depth each type of gas-filled chamber is equipped with a mechanism for adjusting its volume. In all the animals with adjustable gas bladders, except those living near the surface, the major component gases are maintained at partial pressures higher than in the surrounding water.

Although the energetic cost of maintaining buoyancy in flexible gas chambers is small in relation to the total cost of maintaining other vital processes [3] it does appear to become of significant disadvantage when the ambient hydrostatic pressure is high and the availability of food is low, as in the case of bathypelagic fish [38]. In addition to the hydrostatic function, flexible buoyancy chambers such as the swimbladder have important secondary functions such as pressure and sound discrimination and sound production which complicate any evaluation of their selective disadvantage simply on the basis of energy cost of maintaining buoyancy.

There is insufficient experimental evidence to demonstrate unequivocally that the adjustable buoyancy mechanisms described here have the capacity to compensate completely for the large short-term reduction in relative pressure changes experienced by vertical migrants known to possess such mechanisms. There is theoretical and experimental evidence, however, which suggests that many of these organisms are able to compensate for relative pressure changes of less than 25% of their adaptation pressure within 24 h [3, 37, 49, 55].

Perhaps the rigid buoyancy mechanism of the cuttlefish represents the most effective mechanism for rapid buoyancy adjustment. In this animal, controlled ascent and descent appears to be produced by quite simply adjusting the fluid gas ratio within a rigid incompressible chamber. However the depth range is limited by the strength of the cuttlebone and the osmotic pressure gradient.

18.5 REFERENCES

1 Adernethy J.D. (1972) The mechanism of secretion of inert gases into the swimbladder. *Aust. J. exp. Biol. med. Sci.* **50** (3), 365–74.

2 Alexander R.McN. (1966) Physical aspects of swimbladder function. *Biol. Rev.* **41,** 141–76.

3 Alexander R.McN. (1972) The energetics of vertical migration by fishes. In *The Effects of Pressure on Organisms* (eds M. A. Sleigh & A. G. MacDonald). Symposia of the Society for experimental biology No. 26, pp. 273–94. Cambridge University Press, London.

4 Baldridge N.D. (1970) Sinking factors and average densities of Florida sharks as functions of liver buoyancy. *Copeia* **4,** 744–54.

5 Barham E.G. (1966) Deep scattering layer migration and composition observations from a diving saucer. *Science, N.Y.* **151,** 1399–1403.

6 Bilinski E. (1974) Biochemical aspects of fish swimming. In *Biochemical and Biophysical Perspectives in Marine Biology* (eds Malins & Sargent). Academic Press, New York & London.

7 Bone Q. (1973) A note on the buoyancy of some Lantern fishes (Myctophoidei). *J. mar. biol. ass. U.K.* **53,** 619–33.

8 Brawn V. (1969) Buoyancy of Atlantic and Pacific herring. *J. Fish. Res. Bd Can.* **26,** 2077–91.

9 Butler J.L. and Pearcy W.G. (1972) Swimbladder morphology and specific gravity of Myctophids off Oregon. *J. Fish. Res. Bd Can.* **29,** 1145–50.

10 Copeland E.D. (1968) Fine structure of the carbon monoxide secreting tissue in the float of Portuguese-Man-of-War (*Physalia physalis*). *Biol. Bull. mar. biol. Lab., Woods Hole* **135,** 486–500.

11 D'Aoust B.G. (1969) Hyperbaric oxygen: Toxicity to fish at pressures present in their swimbladders. *Science, N.Y.* **163,** 576–8.

12 D'Aoust B.G. (1970) The role of lactic acid in gas secretion in the teleost swimbladder. *Comp. Biochem. Physiol.* **32,** 637–68.

13 Deck J.E. (1970) Lactic acid production by the swimbladder gas gland in vitro as influenced by glucagon and epinephrine. *Comp. Biochem. Physiol.* **34** (1), 317–24.

14 Denton E.J. (1964) The buoyancy of marine molluscs. In *Physiology of Mollusca 1* (eds K. M. Wilbur & C. M. Yonge). Academic Press, New York & London.

15 Denton E.J. & Gilpin-Brown J.B. (1961) The buoyancy of the cuttlefish, *Sepia officianalis* (L). *J. mar. biol. Ass. U.K.* **41,** 319–42.

16 Denton E.J. & Gilpin-Brown J.B. (1961) The effect of light on the buoyancy of the cuttlefish. *J. mar. biol. Ass. U.K.* **41,** 343–50.

17 Denton E.J., Gilpin-Brown J.B. & Howarth J.V. (1961) The osmotic mechanism of the cuttlebone. *J. mar. biol. Ass. U.K.* **41,** 351–64.

18 Denton E.J. & Gilpin-Brown J.B. (1966) On the buoyancy of the Pearly Nautilus. *J. mar. Biol. Ass. U.K.* **46,** 723–59.

19 Denton E.J., Gilpin-Brown J.B. & Shaw T.I. (1969) A buoyancy mechanism found in cranchid squid. *Proc. R. Soc.* B **174,** 271–8.

20 Denton E.J., Liddicoat J.D. & Taylor D.W. (1972) The permeability to gasses of the swimbladder of the Conger eel, *Conger conger. J. mar. biol. Ass. U.K.* **52,** 727–46.

21 Denton E.J. & Marshall N.B. (1958) The buoyancy of bathypelagic fishes without a gas-filled swimbladder. *J. mar. biol. Ass. U.K.* **37,** 753–67.

22 Denton E.J., Shaw T.I. & Gilpin-Brown J.B. (1958) Bathyscaphoid squid. *Nature* **182,** 1810–11.

23 Denton E.J. & Shaw T.I. (1961) The buoyancy of gelatinous marine animals. *J. Physiol., Lond.* **161,** 14–15.

24 Dorn E.von (1961) Über den Feinbau der Schwimmblase von *Anguilla vulgaris* L. *Zeitschrift für Zellforschung* **55,** 849–912.

25 Enns T., Douglas E. & Scholander P.F. (1967) Role of the swimbladder rete of fish in secretion of inert gas and oxygen. *Adv. biol. med. Physics* **11,** 231–44.

26 Fange R. (1953) The mechanisms of gas transport in the euphysoclist swimbladder. *Acta physiol. scand.* **30** (110), 7–133.

27 Forster R.E. & Steen J.B. (1969) The rate of the root shift of eel red cells and haemoglobin solution. *J. Physiol., Lond.* **204,** 259–82.

28 Gee J.H. *et al.* (1974) Adjustment of buoyancy and excess internal pressure of swimbladder gases in some North American freshwater fishes. *J. Fish. Res. Bd Can.* **31** (1) 35–41.

29 Gilpin-Brown J.B. (1972) Buoyancy mechanisms of cephalopods in relation to pressure. In *The Effects of Pressure on Organisms* (eds M. A. Sleigh & A. G. MacDonald). Symposia of the society for experimental biology No. 26, pp. 251–9. Cambridge University Press, London.

30 Haeckel E. (1888) Siphonophorae of the *Challenger. Reports of the Scientific Results, HMS Challenger* **28,** 1–380.

31 Hahn W.E. & Copeland D.E. (1966) Carbon monoxide concentrations and the effect of aminopterin on its production in the Gas Bladder of *Physalia physalis. Comp. Biochem. Physiol.* **18,** 201–7.

32 Jones F.R.H. & Marshall N.B. (1953) The structure and function of the teleostean swimbladder. *Biol. Rev.* **28,** 16–83.

33 Kuhn W., Ramel A., Kuhn H.J. & Marti E. (1963) The filling mechanism of the swimbladder. *Experientia* **19,** 497–552.

34 Kutchai H. & Steen J.B. (1971) The permeability of the swimbladder. *Comp. Biochem. Physiol.* **39**A, 119–23.

35 Lane C.E. (1960) The Portuguese Man-of-War. *Scient. Am.* **202,** 158–68.

36 Lewis R.W. (1970) The densities of three classes of marine lipids in relation to their possible role as hydrostatic agents. *Lipids* **5** (1), 151–3.

37 McNabb R.A. & Mechan J.A. (1971) The effects of different acclimation temperatures on gas secretion in the swimbladder of the blue gill sunfish *Lepomis macrochirus*. *Comp. Biochem. Physiol.* **40**A, 609–16.

38 Marshall N.B. (1972) Swimbladder organisation and depth ranges of deep-sea teleosts. In *The Effects of Pressure on Organisms* (eds M. A. Sleigh & A. G. McDonald). Symposia of the Society for Experimental Biology No. 26, pp. 261–72.

39 Moreau A. (1876) Recherche experimentale sur les fonctions de la vessie natatoire. *Ann. Sci. Nat. Zool. Palaentol.* **4,** (8), 1–85.

40 Muller J. (1840) Ueber Nebenkiemen und Wundernetze. *Arch. Anat. Physiol. Wisschaftl. Med.* 101–42.

41 Pickwell G.W., Barham E.G. & Wilton J.W. (1964) Carbon monoxide production by a bathypelagic siphonophore. *Science, N.Y.* **144,** 860–2.

42 Ross L.G. (1974) Personal communication.

43 Rostorfor H.H. (1942) The gas content of the swimbladder of the rock bass, *Ambloplites rupestris*, in relation to hydrostatic pressure. *Biol. Bull. mar. biol. Lab., Woods Hole* **82,** 138–53.

44 Sand G. & Hawkins A.D. (1970) Movements of swimbladder volume and pressure in cod. *Norwegian Journal of Zoology.*

45 Scholander P.F. (1954) Secretion of gases against high pressures in the swimbladder of deep sea fishes. II. Rete Mirabile. *Biol. Bull. mar. biol. Lab., Woods Hole* **107,** 260–77.

46 Scholander P.F. (1956) Observations on the gas gland in living fish. *J. cell. comp. Physiol.* **48,** 523–8.

47 Scholander P.F. & Van Dam L. (1953) Composition of the swimbladder gas in deep-sea fishes. *Biol. Bull. mar. biol. Lab., Woods Hole* **104,** 75–86.

48 Scholander P.F. & Van Dam L. (1954) Secretion of gases against high pressures in the swimbladder of deep sea fishes. I. Oxygen dissociation in blood. *Biol. Bull. mar. biol. Lab., Woods Hole* **107,** 247–59.

49 Scholander P.F., Van Dam L. & Enns T. (1956) Nitrogen secretion in the swimbladder of white fish. *Science, N.Y.* **123,** 59–60.

50 Stasko A.B. & Rommel S.A. (1974) Swimming depth of adult American eels (*Anguilla rostrata*) in a salt water bay as determined by ultrasonic tracking. *J. Fish. Res. Bd Can.* **31** (6), 1148–50.

51 Steen J.B. (1970) The swimbladder as a hydrostatic organ. In *Fish Physiology*, Vol. 4 (eds W. S. Hoar & D. J. Randall) pp. 414–43. Academic Press, New York & London.

52 Tytler P. & Blaxter J.H.S. (1973) Adaptations by Cod and Saithe to pressure changes. *Netherlands Journal of Sea Research* **7,** 31–45.

53 Wilson D.P. & Wilson M.A. (1956) A contribution to the Biology of *Ianthina janthina* L. *J. mar. biol. Ass. U.K.* **35,** 291–305.

54 Wittenberg J.B. (1958) The secretion of inert gas into the swimbladder of fishes. *J. gen. Physiol.* **44,** 783–804.

55 Wittenberg J.B. (1958) Carbon monoxide in the float of Physalia. *Biol. Bull. mar. biol. Lab., Woods Hole* **115,** 371–82.

56 Wittenberg J.B. (1960) The source of carbon monoxide in the float of the Portuguese Man-of-War, *Physalia physalis*. *J. exp. Biol.* **37,** 698–705.

Prelude to Chapter 19

Many animals respond to environmental challenge by altering the colour of their bodies. In the following chapter, colour change is considered chiefly in relation to predation in which it is clearly of great importance in natural selection. Colour change may, however, also be triggered by thermal and other physical stimuli. Many amphibians and reptiles, for example, become lighter in colour when the temperature rises. This change in *albedo*, may lessen the heat load on their bodies by reflecting more of the incoming solar radiation. At the same time, it has been suggested that changes in pigment distribution may serve to protect internal body organs from excess radiation. In some animals, too, colour changes are related to mating behaviour. There is no doubt, however, that predation is the main selective influence leading to the evolution of mechanism of colour change in animals.

Rhythmic colour change, whatever its function, is often under control of the 'biological clock', as in the fiddler crabs cited below. Rhythmicity is characteristic of many environmental phenomena; both physical and biological. Since it permeates every aspect of physiology, we have not allotted a separate chapter to it in this book. Nevertheless, it should be remembered that the whole field of biological rhythms is an inter-disciplinary one. Claude Bernard's concept of homeostasis must therefore be modified: the internal environment of an animal alters rhythmically to mirror the cyclical changes that are taking place in the environment. Fiddler crabs must surely benefit from the preadaptation by which appropriate colour changes take place before the animals emerge from their burrows, and not afterwards.

Chapter 19
Colour changes

H. E. HINTON

19.1 INTRODUCTION

The colours of animals that are normally visible to others are determined either by the requirements of deception or advertisement. Most animals resort to deception for protection. Many have patterns of colours and tones that so match the background that they are indistinguishable even when plainly in view. Concealment may be effected by countershading so that the normal visual clues by means of which solid objects are recognized as such are lost. In others, strongly contrasting colours break up the continuity of surface and recognizable outline so that the appearance of form is destroyed. Sometimes both colour and form so exactly resemble common inedible objects in the environment—leaves, twigs, stones—that they pass unnoticed by predators. A goodly few are distasteful or poisonous, and they advertise their presence by bright colours so that predators recognize them for what they are. Some harmless animals escape attack because they mimic the bright colour patterns of dangerous species and so falsely trade upon an evil reputation.

Animals that pass their entire existence concealed from view in the soil, or as parasites in plants and animals, are more or less colourless. If not colourless, such colour as they have may be determined by the natural colour of compounds used in hardening the skin or by the colour of the materials they eat that can be seen through the skin. The really important point which is often overlooked is that there is no long-term neutrality in nature: colour, like any other feature, will be selected against and in time disappear when it ceases to have a selective advantage.

Speaking generally, animals change colour during development simply because at different times during development they are subjected to different selective pressures. This is particularly evident in animals that have a marked metamorphosis and different stages that live in quite different environments. The same stage of the animal may move from one environment to another and back again. When this kind of thing happens there is pressure to develop the capacity for reversible change, which may be slow like the change in seasons that results in distinct summer and winter coats. But the change may be a very rapid one. For instance, a squid has dark and pale stripes when swimming, but when it comes to rest on a sandy bottom, pebbles, or some other kind of background it can adjust its colour and tone to match in less than a second.

In the following pages attention is drawn to the many and very different ways in which animals change colour. The selective advantages of the colour changes are noted even when sometimes we can do no more than speculate about these. It is usual to think of rapid and reversible colour changes as 'physiological', but many animals can change their colour rapidly and reversibly in other ways, and some of these are included at the end of the chapter. Much is now known about the biochemistry [22] of animals' pigments and about their structural colours [7, 8], but all this and much else has been omitted for lack of space.

19.2 MORPHOLOGICAL COLOUR CHANGES

19.2.1 Obligatory colour changes

Most animals change colour during development. Such changes usually take place slowly, are not reversible, and are known as morphological colour changes. Differences in colour between young and old are often spectacular, especially in animals that have a more or less drastic metamorphosis such as insects and amphibia. Many such changes are referred to in later sections but here a few examples, chosen from insects, are given of obligatory colour changes between different stages in the life cycle and those that occur during development within the same stage.

Obligatory colour changes between different stages

The aquatic larvae of the Thaumaleidae, Simuliidae, and several other families of flies have a transparent body-wall cuticle. In these families the colour pattern of the body depends entirely upon pigmented mesodermal cells. In *Thaumalea* the pigmented mesodermal cells or chromatocytes are part of the peripheral fat body [11]. In *Simulium* they may be derived from fat body cells in the embryo, but during larval growth increases in their number occur by division and not by recruitment from the fat body [12]. The selective value of forming cryptic and disruptive patterns in this way seems clear enough: the process of shedding the cuticle can occur without even a temporary change in body colour.

Chromatocytes are beneath the basement membrane and therefore cannot exist between a muscle and its insertion. Thus in these larvae all muscle insertions are colourless spots. The head is full of the muscles of the mouthparts, and so little of the cranial area is free of muscle insertions in the basement membrane that colour has to be retained in the cuticle. Simuliids often undergo their moulting cycles in exposed places in streams, and then only the head changes colour for a few minutes. One of the characteristics of small streams is their sudden and drastic change in water level. Thus a simuliid may expect to be caught occasionally out of water in the middle of a moulting cycle. At such times one might have expected that they would be particularly damaged by ultra-violet. However, the pigment in the chromatocytes strongly absorbs U-V. That one of its functions is to shield against U-V is suggested by the fact that the brain, larger nerves, gonads, and larger muscles are partly or entirely enclosed in a sheath of chromatocytes.

At metamorphosis in both *Thaumalea* and *Simulium* the chromatocytes dissociate, round up, migrate to other parts of the body, and there form new aggregation patterns. For instance, in *Thaumalea* there are no chromatocytes in the head of the larva, pupa, or very young adult, but during the pharate adult stage 500 to 700, or a little more than a third of the chromatocytes of the prothorax, invade the head, a few even entering the labial palpi [11]. It is necessary for the chromatocytes to leave the dorsal part of the prothorax to allow room for the enlargement of the insertions of the indirect flight muscles. During their migration from the prothorax they travel at rates of 10 to 20 microns per hour for prolonged periods. This kind of colour change in some ways resembles the kind of colour pattern formation that occurs in the early stages of some urodeles, e.g. *Triturus torosus*. In this amphibian the melanophores form new aggregation patterns shortly after their dispersal from the neural crest.

Obligatory colour changes within the same stage

It is among insects that some of the most interesting and instructive examples of obligatory colour changes occur during development. An increase in size may of itself necessitate a complete change in appearance. This happens if the animal or object mimicked when the larva is small is itself always small. For instance, young larvae of a number of kinds of moths and butterflies resemble fresh bird droppings so closely that they are indistinguishable from them unless actually touched. Now bird droppings up to an inch or so long are common enough on leaves and twigs, but droppings that greatly exceed this sort of size are rare and in some regions absent. Thus, before the larvae become too large to render the resemblance to a bird dropping ludicrous, selective pressures will result in a change of colour and often also of form. Most of the swallowtail butterflies of the genus *Papillo* (e.g. *cenea*, *demoleus*, *pammon*, *ophidicephalus*, *echerioides*, *demodocus*, *dardanus*, *cresphontes*, *memnon*, *aegeus*, *polytes*) resemble bird droppings in the first few instars, but in the last instar, which is usually the fourth or fifth, they are cryptic. This change of colour and appearance is usually accompanied by a marked change in habits: they no longer rest on the upper surface of the leaf but stay on the underside of the leaf or on twigs. Sometimes the switch is not to a cryptic form but to an aposematic one, as in the alder moth, *Apatele alni*, in which the first three instars resemble bird droppings and the last is a bright yellow with black bands, has long hairs with flatted tips, and can smell badly. We might imagine that if the caterpillar is exceptionally large the switch from a bird-dropping mimic would have to be made well before the final instar.

The African bombycid moth, *Trilocha kolga*, is unusual in that the young are gregarious and suggest a bird roosting just above the leaf. They are unusual in another way too: the last instar continues to rest on the upper surface of the leaf but it is now brown and mimics the dropping of another kind of bird, a very large one without a conspicuously white uric acid part, or even the dropping of a large lizard [5].

Striking colour changes also occur during larval growth in other insects. In a number of praying mantids, e.g. *Sphodromantis lineola*, *Miomantis paykullii*, *Oxypilus hamatus*, and *Tarachodes afzellii*, the first instar larva closely resembles an ant, but the later stages are cryptic green or brown, although often with bright patches that are exposed when danger threatens. The first instar of *Spodromantis* looks like the dangerous *Oecophylla longinoda*, and both *Oxypilus* and *Tarachodes* resemble a local carpenter ant, *Camponotus acvapimensis* [5]. Similar changes from a first instar that resembles an ant to later instars that are cryptic occur in the Queensland stick insect, *Extatosoma tiratum*, and they occur in other orders, especially the Hemiptera.

Change from one type of cryptic colour to another or to a warning colour

Birds and mammals that nest in the open or lack a well-defined nest have young that can walk or run from birth. These young are spotted or striped. When danger approaches they freeze, and their spots and stripes help make them invisible to enemies. As they grow older and faster, most species moult and assume another kind of cryptic colour or even a warning colour. For instance, some deer are conspicuously spotted when young, and these spots make them difficult to see among leaves on which odd patches of sunlight fall. As the deer grow older they lose their bold spots and become all fawn-coloured with the belly countershaded. In sharp contrast are most birds and mammals that are at first helpless and unable to move effectively. These are born in nests in the ground, in wood, in cliffs, in trees, or nests protected in some other way. The young of most such species begin life naked. Their first plumage or coat of hair tends to be a uniform brown or black.

The distinctions I have mentioned hold even between related species. The sand-grouse is a relative of pigeons but unlike them nests on the ground like a game bird. Its young are not naked and helpless as are those of pigeons but are very active and have a cryptic plumage like that of a game bird.

Some deer that live in savannahs or forests in warm countries live in surroundings where sunlight makes bright patches that contrast sharply with shade. They may, like the African bush buck (*Tragelaphus s. sylvaticus*) keep their juvenile spots. Adults of others, e.g. the Japanese deer (*Sika nippon*), have spots in summer and a uniform coat in winter if they live in deciduous forests, but races of this deer that live in evergreen forests tend to keep their spots in winter [3].

A number of Carnivora—civets and mongooses to the larger cats—may have spotted or striped young even though the young are hidden in nests or dens. However, in all of these species the mother is apt to leave the young unattended for long periods while she is out hunting. This is particularly dangerous during the time when the young begin to venture out of the nest by themselves: it is then that a cryptic coat may have an especially high selective value.

Change from one kind of aposematic colour to another or to a cryptic colour

Most aposematic colours are bright. They are often patterns of red, yellow, or white, frequently with black spots or stripes. They may contrast strongly with uniform black, which is sometimes also aposematic. It is not often that black is thought of as aposematic. Whether a black animal is aposematic or not depends upon how it contrasts with a particular background and also upon how often casual predators encounter conspicuous black animals that harm them in some way. Assain bugs (Reduviidae) have very painful bites. In a recent study of these bugs in central Mexico, I found that a species that was almost entirely black was about as conspicuous on green vegetation as the species with the usual bright aposematic patterns.

Leaf-feeding larvae that are black when they are young often undergo a gradual or a sudden change to a typical bright aposematic colour or pattern when they grow larger. For instance, the young larvae of the leaf-beetle, *Chrysomela tremula*, are dark brown or nearly black and remain together in groups that are very conspicuous. After each ecdysis the cuticle between the dark brown plates and tubercles of the skin becomes paler. By the time that the skin has been shed four or five times, the cuticle is a dirty white or yellowish, and the plates and tubercles are black or nearly so and very conspicuous as separate spots. Here then there is a change from a black aposematic animal to one with a typical bright aposematic pattern that coincides with a change from gregarious to solitary habits.

If some of the larval instars of an insect are an aposematic black, it is almost invariably the smaller and not the larger. This change in aposematic garb is normally accompanied by a marked change in habits: when larvae are dark or black they are gregarious and stay close to one another. With a change to a bright aposematic pattern they tend to become solitary. This suggests that (1) if an aposematic effect is to be made against a green background, to be black and effective requires a greater area than a single small larva, or (2) that gregarious young are black because individual movements of larvae of uniform colour do not break up the visual effect of a single object as much as such movements would if each of the individual units had two or more colours.

A change from an aposematic black or very dark brown to a bright aposematic colour is common in other groups of insects, e.g. some sawflies and caterpillars. It is also fairly common among tree hoppers, e.g. the Mexican *Anthianthe foliacea.* The adults of this species stay with the young and appear to protect them. Young larvae are conspicuously black and are gregarious, remaining close to parents and other young larvae. However, larvae in their final instar have a bright aposematic pattern, mostly reddish with some black markings. These larvae tend to wander off to the edge of the leaf away from the rest of the group. But there is still another colour change to come: the adults are green and cryptic, and, at least for a time, are solitary. In *Antianthe*, as in many other Membracidae, the sequence of colour change is: black aposematic→bright aposematic→green and cryptic. Young larvae of lady birds are often aposematic black but later have a more or less bright aposematic pattern. But both pupae and adults of these beetles may be conspicuously red and black. Many kinds of toads and frogs that have very black young tadpoles are highly cryptic as adults.

19.2.2 Facultative morphological colour changes

According to season

Many birds and mammals that live where there is snow on the ground for part of the year are white in the winter and difficult to see against the snow, but when the snow melts away they become brownish and difficult to see against the earth and sparse vegetation. This switch from one kind of cryptic colouration to another according to season is usually triggered by the length of the day. It always involves a moult and the appearance of new feathers or hair.

The fact that some birds and mammals change colour with the season and others do not has misled some into thinking that colour changes are without significance: because winter or summer the raven remains boldly and impudently black and the snowy owl a constant white, it is held that a colour change in others must be of small import. But the significance of any colour, or change of colour, can only be fully understood in the light of the actual conditions of existence of the animal and not just in respect of one facet of its relations with its biological or physical environment. The polar bear is white throughout the year. It is more or less restricted to the southernmost limits of ice flows and is generally found where there is open water and seals. Its white is therefore nearly always cryptic.

The raven is an omnivorous scavenger with relatively few predators. Other subarctic and arctic animals like the sable, glutton, musk ox, moose, and reindeer likewise have no special need of concealment and do not become white in winter. However, willow grouse, ptarmigan, and mountain hare become white in winter and more difficult to detect by their predators—stoats, weasels, and foxes—which themselves become white and so more difficult for their prey to detect. Some of these species may change to white in the more northern parts of their range but retain their summer coat in warmer climates. For instance, the arctic fox becomes white in winter in the northern part of its range, but in Iceland with its less severe winters it retains it summer brown. Arctic foxes from the extreme north will change to white even when kept in zoos in much warmer climates. The weasel becomes white in winter in northern Europe, but in England it nearly always keeps its summer brown.

The ptarmigan (*Lagopus*) provides support for my theory that sexual dimorphism has little to do with sexual selection but is primarily a response to predators. The males of some species retain their winter plumage until the female in her cryptic summer plumage has hatched the eggs. During this time the males in their winter plumage are very conspicuous and tend to deflect predators away from the females.

According to density

Individuals of a cryptic species are generally widely spaced in nature, and their predators tend to forget about them between encounters: if a predator accidentally encounters one, it is not likely quickly to encounter others and so it does not form a 'searching image' of the species that might result in a systematic search for it. The relation of crypsis to density is particularly clear in a few insects that are cryptic when few and have bright aposematic colours when many. Some locusts (*Locusta* [26], *Schistocerca*), stick insects (*Podocanthus*, *Didymuria* [18]), and caterpillars (*Laphygma*, *Spodoptera*, *etc.*) [17, 20, 23, 24] are cryptic when the population density is low but are aposematic when the population density is high. That is, a mechanism has been evolved that effects a switch-over from a cryptic to an aposematic colour according to the population density at which each of these colours has the most survival value. The significance of the colour differences between the solitary and gregarious phases of some insects was first clearly noted by Key [18], who was at the time working with stick insects in which the effects of high and low population densities could be examined uncomplicated by gregarious and migratory behaviour.

19.3 PHYSIOLOGICAL COLOUR CHANGES

Rapidly reversible colour changes are generally described as physiological colour changes, but there are many other kinds of rapidly reversible colour changes, and a few of these other kinds of quick colour changes are briefly referred to later.

In most animals rapid colour changes are brought about by rapid changes in the concentration of pigment granules or pigment vesicles in cells that are commonly called chromatophores. There are four rather distinct kinds of chromatophores: (1) ectodermal cells that are beneath the epidermis and are often branched; (2) unbranched ectodermal cells of insects that are always part of the epidermis and are never beneath the basement membrane; (3) muscled cells confined to the cephalopods; and (4) mesodermal chromatocytes of insects always beneath the epidermis and basement membrane.

Although there are more kinds of insects than all other animals put together, few are known to exhibit physiological colour changes. However, these few effect reversible colour changes in more different ways than all other animals combined: in no other group are colour changes effected by mesodermal cells that change their shape or by epidermal cells that hydrate and dehydrate thin films or spongy layers. When we say that reversible colour changes are rare in insects, we except the iris cells because the changes brought about in these cells by migrating pigment granules do not really affect the colour of the animal.

19.3.1 Subepidermal chromatophores

These are the common cells concerned in colour change in both invertebrates and vertebrates, but, oddly enough, they are quite unknown among insects although they are common enough in other groups of arthropods, e.g. Crustacea. They are ectodermal cells but they lie beneath the epidermis and are sometimes associated with internal organs even in the Crustacea. The branched chromatophores may be single cells or a close association of cells sometimes called a chromatosome. In mono- or polychromatic chromatosomes contraction or dispersion of the pigment granules in one chromatophore may occur while the pigment granules of other chromatophores are stationary [29]. Chromatophores have received many names according to the chemical nature of the pigment, e.g. melanophores contain melanins, or their precise function, e.g. iridiophores have the organelles orientated to reflect light. Reflecting iridiophores are commonly intimately associated with xanthophores and melanophores (Fig. 19.1).

Among vertebrates chromatophores are not innervated in elasmobranchs but are innervated in many teleosts, in which melanophore concentration is controlled by adrenergic neurons that either directly mediate their effects or release catecholamine near the chromatophores. There is no evidence of nervous regulation of chromatophores in the Amphibia. In these the presence of a circulating hormone from the pituitary, intermedin, is adequate to account for colour change in response to background. However, it has been claimed that in some anurans the chromatophores forming the spots and stripes may be innervated and therefore separately controlled [1].

Among lizards it is chiefly the arboreal chameleons, agamids, and iguanids that exhibit spectacular colour changes. In some iguanids, e.g. *Anolis*, the chromatophores are not innervated, and the change of colour from brown to brilliant green or pale green is triggered by hormones and is not impaired by

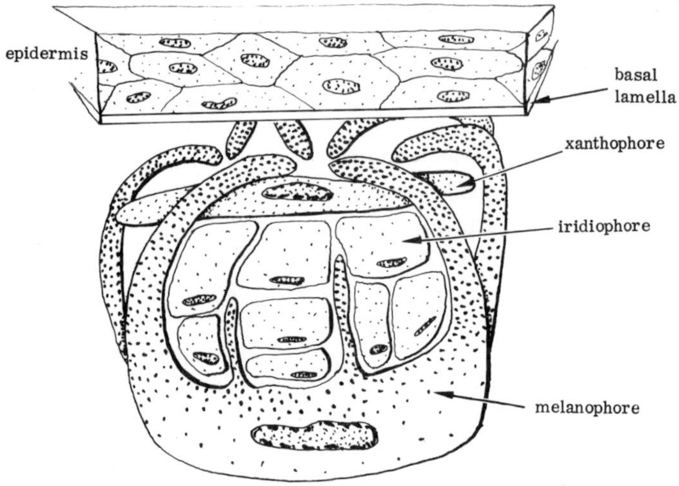

Fig. 19.1. Branched subepidermal melanophore of the lizard, *Anolis*, showing associated xanthophore and iridophore cells. The melanin granules in the melanophore are concentrated in the distal parts of the cell branches. In some amphibia branched melanophores may also be present among the epidermal cells. (Based on [26a]).

cutting the spinal cord or the peripheral nerves. In chameleons, on the contrary, the chromatophores are innervated, and preparations (*Lophosaura*) with the head and viscera removed continue to give skin responses to light and dark providing that the spinal cord and peripheral nerves are intact. It thus appears that in chameleons there is a spinal reflex initiated by light receptors in the skin, but such light receptors have not yet been identified [1]. Chameleons tend to become pale on a background that scatters light and dark on one that absorbs light. If an object is held against the flank of a chameleon for a couple of minutes, its shape will appear as a pale print on the darker skin. The really vivid colours of both sexes appear during inter- and intrasexual encounters and in defence against other animals. Chromatophore control in chameleons may not be entirely nervous. For instance, injections of intermedin (MSH) darken *Chameleon jacksoni*, which suggests that hormones may play a part in the colour change of at least some chameleons [1].

Persistent diurnal and tidal rhythms of colour change

The fiddler crab, *Uca pugilator*, is dark by day and pale by night. This colour change has an endogenous rhythm that persists for several weeks when the crab is kept under constant conditions. The rhythm is unaffected by changes of temperature within the range 6° to 26°C, but it is inhibited at lower temperatures. If the crab is kept at 0° to 3°C for several hours, the onset of the next change of colour is delayed by a period roughly equal to that of the chilling. But changes brought about in this way do not affect the 24-hour periodicity of the rhythm. If the lengths of the light and dark periods in a 24-hour cycle are altered there is a corresponding shift in the form of the rhythm without a change in its 24-hour periodicity: it has so far not been possible to impose upon the crabs a rhythm other than a 24-hour one [2]. Clearly the phases of the rhythm can be efficiently reset or otherwise environmental changes, such as exceptionally cold weather, would soon alter the relation of the rhythm to the tides. When there are local differences in tidal changes, the rhythms of the fiddler crabs of each locality are adjusted accordingly.

The tidal cycle itself progresses daily so that low tide is about 50 minutes later each day in cycles of 14·76 days. The cycle in pigment movement exactly parallels this. Thus, on each day any particular condition of melanin dispersion is reached about 50 minutes later than it was the day before. A tidal rhythm of colour change (Fig. 19.2) that parallels the 12·4-hour ocean tides modulates the daily

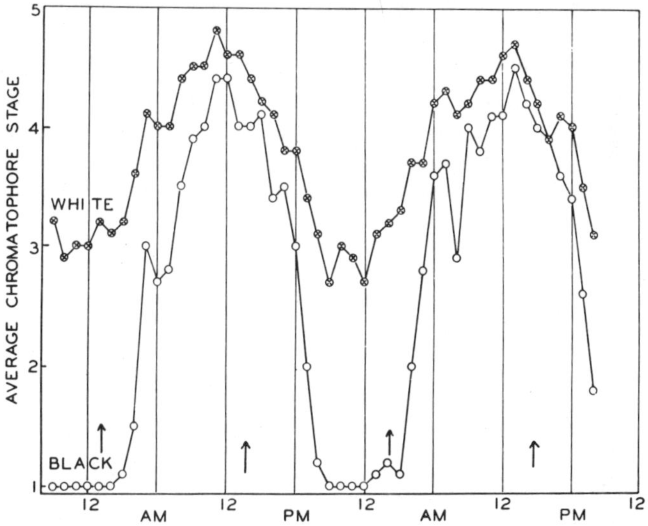

Fig. 19.2. Changes in the degree of dispersion of the black and white pigment of the fiddler crab during a 48 hour period in darkness. The stages are 1 = pigment fully concentrated to 5 = pigment fully dispersed. The arrows indicate the times of low tide in the native habitat of the crabs. From [2].

rhythm and therefore produces patterns of fluctuations in the daily colour rhythm with a periodicity of 14·8 days. The 14·8 days is the average expected interval between days on which low tides occur at the same time of day. Because the fiddler crab has a rhythm with both 12·4- and 24-hour cycles, it also has a 14·8-day cycle, which is the interval between the days on which these rhythms repeat similar relations with one another.

The fiddler crab has three kinds of monochromatic chromatophores (iridiophores) that contain white, red, or black pigment respectively. The granular organelles within the chromatophores resemble the reflecting platelets of vertebrate iridiophores, but we do not know if they contain purines as do the vertebrate platelets. The most evident change in colour is the result of the movement of black melanin granules. The melanin-dispersing hormone is a polypeptide secreted in part at least by the sinus gland. There must be a nightly release of a melanin-contracting substance into the blood from some tissue other than the sinus gland. Extracts of the sinus gland are less effective in dispersing the black pigment when injected at night than when injected during the day. Surprisingly little attention has been paid to the selective value of the colour change of the fiddler crab: it is sometimes even implied that the change has no selective value, which is absurd.

19.3.2 Unbranched epidermal chromatophores

Epidermal cells containing pigment granules that can be displaced from one part of the cell to another are the only kind of ectodermal chromatophores found in insects. Little is known about the occurrence of this kind of chromatophore in other groups of arthropods.

Among insects physiological colour changes have been most studied in the common stick insect, *Carausius morosus*. *Carausius* has polychromatic chromatophores: the cells contain yellow, orange, and red lipochromes, insectoveridins, and various brownish ommochromes. The stick insect is normally dark at night and pale by day (Fig. 19.3), an endogenous rhythm that continues for several

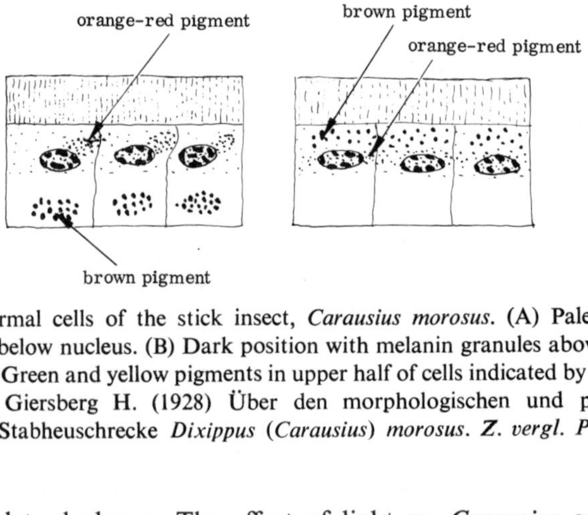

Fig. 19.3. Epidermal cells of the stick insect, *Carausius morosus*. (A) Pale position with melanin granules below nucleus. (B) Dark position with melanin granules above nucleus near upper wall of cell. Green and yellow pigments in upper half of cells indicated by lightly stippled area. (Based on Giersberg H. (1928) Über den morphologischen und physiologischen Farbwechsel der Stabheuschrecke *Dixippus* (*Carausius*) *morosus*. *Z. vergl. Physiol.* **7,** 657–95).

weeks in complete darkness. The effect of light on *Carausius* appears to be mediated only by the eyes and can be eliminated by cutting the optic nerves or by blackening the eyes. It seems to be determined by the amount of contrast in the background. The effect of light is absent in individuals kept in the dark from hatching but a colour change rhythm can be induced by periodic illumination. The hormone that triggers the darkening response is liberated from the suboesophageal ganglion. *Carausius* and other phasmids [25] exhibit both physiological and slow 'morphological' colour changes.

Kosciuscola tristis of the Australian Alps is the only grasshopper that changes colour rapidly and reversibly [6]. The colour change of the male is particularly striking. When it is cold it is nearly black, but if it is warmed it changes to a bright sky blue within minutes. The cuticle is more or less transparent, and the epidermal cells contain dark brown or blackish granules about 1 micron wide and small granules about 0·17 μm wide. The small granules are white when isolated. They consist of a mixture of uric acid and pteridine, probably leucopterin [6].

The blue colour is produced by Tyndall scattering of light by the small granules, and the blue is intensified by being seen against a dark background. When the insect is warmed, the small granules migrate to the distal (outer) part of the cells, whereas the dark granules migrate to the proximal or inner part of the cell. When the insect is cooled, the change to a dark colour is produced by the large granules migrating distally, mingling with the small granules, and 'quenching' the light scattering. The epidermal cells contain numerous microtubules that are more or less normal to the surface, and, because their major axes are orientated in the direction of movement of the granules, they may play a part in this movement. The cells act as independent effectors. Changes of colour occur without central nervous control, and epidermal cells in pieces of integument isolated in saline change from nearly black to bright blue as do those in the intact insect.

Many dragonflies change colour rapidly and reversibly as does the grasshopper *Kosciuscola*. Many Australian dragonflies in the suborders Zygoptera and Anisoptera are known to change the colour of some areas of the epidermis from bright blue to dark purple or brown by migration of granules [27, 28]. The epidermal cells of the different species are essentially alike. Each contains reversible layers of light-scattering granules and pigment vesicles, both of which respond to changes of temperature in such a way that the patches are dark at night and bright blue during the day. It has been shown that the temperature threshold of species from warmer regions are higher than those of species from colder regions.

After sunset there is a gradual change in colour so that before dawn the transition to the dark phase is complete. At day break the insects are covered with dew, and it is usually not until the dew has evaporated later in the morning that the dragonflies begin to assume positions with respect to the incident sunlight that enable them to warm up as quickly as possible. The average rise in body temperature of some species simply because of the dark colour is about 0·2°C. but a gain of about 15°C may accrue to individuals that are correctly orientated with respect to the sun. By using a filter opaque to infra red it was possible without reducing the visible light intensity to reduce the amount of radiant energy to which two species of *Austrolestes* dragonflies were exposed. When this was done, the amount of colour change was greatly reduced. Thus colour change is primarily a response to a change in temperature and not light intensity.

Most believe that the selective advantage of colour change lies in (1) the slightly greater speed with which the dark phase warms up in the early morning and so is able to use a greater part of the day for hunting, and (2) the greater resistance to overheating in the bright phase [28]. The idea that colour change is chiefly to do with thermoregulation is very firmly held, but I think that it is more likely that the chief selective value of the change is that at night it is more difficult for predators to see the dark phase, whereas by day they find the bright phase more difficult to see, especially as in some circumstances the bright patches have a disruptive effect that makes the outline of the insect more difficult to apprehend. In other words, I think that both in the dragonflies and *Kosciuscola* the selective value of the colour change lies chiefly in its effect on predators. But this is not, of course, to deny that thermoregulation may be of minor importance. In dragonflies, as in the Hercules beetle (see below) colour changes in the integument are autonomous in some circumstances but are under central nervous control in others.

19.3.3 Muscled chromatophores of cephalopods

Each chromatophore of a cephalopod is an organ that includes five kinds of cells: (1) the chromatophore that contains brown, red, or yellow pigment; (2) radial muscle fibres; (3) axons of nerve cells; (4) glial cells; and (5) sheath cells. When the muscles contract, the diameter of the sac containing the pigment increases about seven times.

Squids, cuttlefish, and octopuses have long been known for the speed with which their skin takes on the colour of the background. However, things are not quite what they seem: cephalopods (*Loligo*, *Sepia*, *Octopus*) do not change colour. All that happens is that local areas become paler or darker. Pigment in the chromatophores is concentrated or dispersed by muscular action so that it matches the tones of the background [21]. Colour changes, as in the chameleons, do not involve integration of sensory input in the brain. Cephalopods are probably colour blind. The skin has iridiophores and leucophores below the chromatophores [21]. These reflect the wavelengths of the incident light. Thus, when the chromatophores are retracted in a particular area, the colour of that area of skin is determined by the colour of the background, which is reflected without change of wavelength by the iridiophores and leucophores. In cephalopods the innervated and muscled chromatophores are also used for intraspecific signals and in deimatic displays, and both of these involve central nervous control.

19.3.4 Chromatocytes

As we have already seen, the obligatory morphological colour changes of some fly larvae are effected by rearrangement of pigmented mesodermal cells that I have called chromatocytes. It is only in mosquitoes of the genus *Chaoborus* (= *Corethra*) that chromatocytes are responsible for reversible colour changes, and the way they do it is without parallel in the animal kingdom. These mosquito larvae, sometimes called phantom midges, have two large tracheal air sacs in the metathorax and two somewhat smaller ones in the seventh abdominal segment. By varying the size of these air sacs the larva can vary its buoyancy and so the depth at which it floats in the water. But the air sacs present a real difficulty. The larva itself is transparent and while it is over a bright sandy bottom reflections from the liquid–air interface of the air sacs do not make it conspicuous. However, as soon as the larva swims over a dark bottom, for instance of earth or rotting vegetation, the two pairs of air sacs will make it extremely conspicuous. What happens should the larva swim over such a bottom is that the darkly pigmented chromatocytes on the air sacs move over the surface and each chromatocyte becomes a flattened polygon so that very quickly a pavement of flattened polygonal cells is formed over the dorsal and lateral sides of the air sacs as shown in Fig. 19.4. This covering of darkly pigmented chromatocytes prevents the

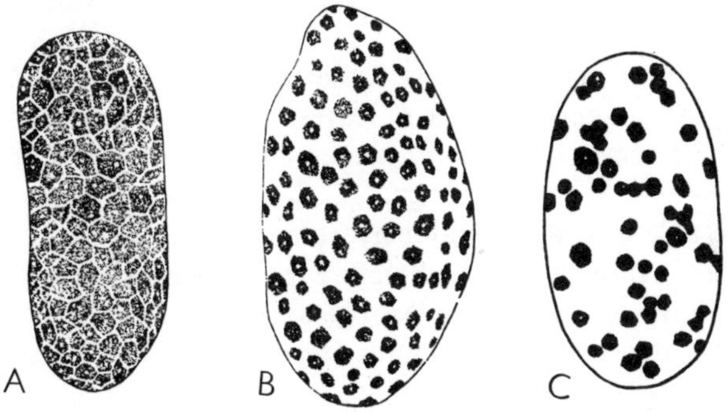

Fig. 19.4. A tracheal sac of *Chaoborus crystallinus* with (A) chromatocytes in the dark-adapted condition, (B) partly light-adapted, and (C) light-adapted. After [4].

transparent larva from being made conspicuous on a dark background by light reflected from the air sacs. When the larva then moves back again over a light background, the chromatocytes round up and move away from one another, many of them migrating on to the sides and ventral surface of the air sacs (Fig. 19.4) [4]. Thus, on a light background the larva is no longer made conspicuous by four large blackish bodies that look solid. The change in colour shown in Fig. 19.4 can occur in 10 to 30 minutes. Should the larva once more move over a dark background the cells migrate and change shape and eventually reform a pavement covering the dorsal and lateral sides of the air sacs.

The movements of the chromatocytes are under endocrine control [4]: the change from the light-adapted to the dark-adapted condition can be invoked by injections of extracts from the brain, corpora allata, and ventral ganglia: in the absence of hormone, the light-adapted condition is maintained. As the larva grows the number of chromatocytes increases with an increase in the surface area of the air sacs. In a newly hatched larva of *Chaoborus crystallinus* there are only 4 to 6 chromatocytes on each sac, whereas in the fully grown larva there may be over 100.

Thin film interference

The irridescent colours of butterflies and birds, like almost all other irridescent colours of animals, are produced by thin-layer interference. Indeed, the only notable exceptions are some beetles in which the irridescence is produced by diffraction gratings. A thin-film system consists of layers of high refractive index alternating with layers of a lower refractive index. I have previously pointed out that when the mean refractive index is low the colour changes with small differences in angle of viewing, but when the mean refractive index is high, say, 1·5 or a little more, irridescence may not be evident through a wide change of angles. For instance, in butterfly scales layers of cuticle alternate with layers of air so that the mean refractive index is about 1·3 and there is a large change of colour with angle of viewing. In the tortoise beetles the mean refractive index must be about 1·5 or more because irridescence is not evident until grazing incidence.

In tropical and warm temperate climates tortoise beetles (Cassidinae) are often common on the upper surface of leaves. The colours of some are produced entirely by interference, whereas in others pigments modify structural colours. In *Aspidomorpha*, and many other genera, the epidermal cells of the pronotum and elytra are able to hydrate and dehydrate the cuticle and so alter the thickness of the interference layers and therefore the colours produced [14]. No other animals are known to be able reversibly to alter interference colours. These beetles are also unusual in the complexity of their thin-film system: *Aspidomorpha tecta* has 88 or more interference layers in the elytra.

If *Aspidomorpha tecta* is poked or abused in any way, it changes from gold to red. The change usually requires two or more minutes. Because it is so slow, its selective value is not clear to me. It could be of value in some circumstances, say, when the disturbance caused by a small flock of birds hopping about a plant is enough to cause some of the beetles to turn red. In such an instance, a few beetles might escape attack because they had become red before they were discovered by a bird.

Spongy layers

The Hercules beetle (*Dynastes hercules*) is the second heaviest insect in the world, and because of its size and spectacular appearance has attracted much attention. It has been known for some considerable time that the beetle could change the colour of its elytra from black to greenish-yellow and back again to black. However, it is only since 1972 that we have known how it manages to achieve this. A diagram of the upper part of the elytra is shown in Fig. 19.5. The outer layer or epicuticle of the elytra is transparent and about 3 μm thick. Below this is a yellowish spongy layer about 5 μm thick. The cuticle below the yellow sponge is black. When the spongy layer is full of air it is optically heterogenous and reflects yellow light back through the transparent layer. However, when the yellow sponge is filled with liquid it becomes optically homogenous and the light, instead of being reflected back, passes through it and is absorbed by the layer below so that the elytra now appear black. As we have shown, it is quite easy to change the colour of the elytra of museum specimens from yellow to black by

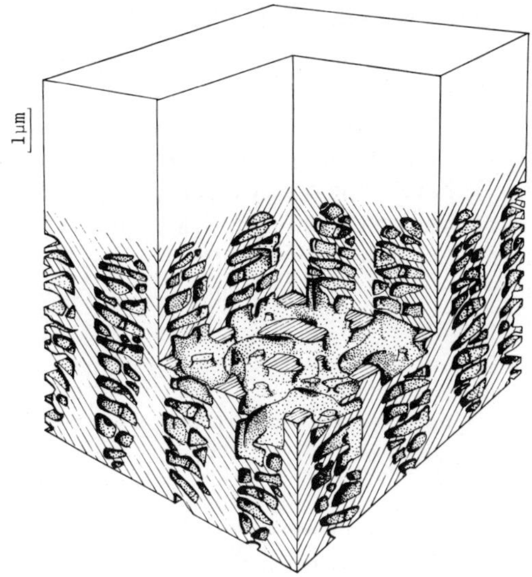

Fig. 19.5. Diagram of the structure of the yellow spongy layer of the elytra of *Dynastes hercules*. The outer transparent layer is unshaded. After [16].

filling the layer of sponge with water or other liquids. As soon as these liquids evaporate the elytra become yellowish once again [16].

If a drop of liquid nitrogen is placed on the black elytra of a live beetle, a yellow spot immediately appears as the liquid in the spongy layer is frozen and the layer made optically heterogenous. As soon as the nitrogen has evaporated the spongy layer once again becomes optically homogenous and the yellow spot becomes black.

We are not yet sure about the nature of the liquid used by the live beetle to flood the layer but it would seem to be largely or entirely water. The movement of liquid in and out of the spongy layer of a live beetle must be under the direct control of the epidermal cells, which are a long way below the yellow sponge.

We have shown that the elytra changes colour according to the ambient relative humidity: they are black when the humidity is high and become yellowish when the humidity falls sufficiently. Laboratory experiments indicate that the elytra are normally black at night when the humidity is high and yellow during the day when the humidity is lower. The advantage of this appears to lie in the fact that at night there is usually enough light so that the beetle with yellow wing cases will be more easily seen by predators than one with black wing cases. However, during the day this is reversed: a beetle with yellow elytra, especially if it is feeding on fruit, will be less conspicuous than an entirely black one.

Sometimes the elytra change colour very rapidly: when the beetle is transferred from about 100% relative humidity to 80% or less yellow patches sometimes appear on the elytra within 30 seconds. Colour change can be local and autonomous [16]. When we removed one elytron from a live beetle and kept it with the beetle the changes in the colour of the attached and the amputated elytra were exactly the same for more than half a day. Local areas of the elytra can be exposed to quite different humidities from the rest of the elytron by attaching cells containing silica gel or moist filter paper. Thus it was possible to cause the area under the filter paper to be black while the rest of the elytron was yellow or *vice versa*. On a few occasions the beetle would become yellow when exposed to high humidities that should have made it stay black. It seems that the colour change of the beetle, like the colour change of some dragonflies, is local and autonomous in some circumstances and under central nervous control in others. Several other species of the genus *Dynastes* change colour in the same way, and in a few the pronotum also changes colour [16].

19.4 SPECIAL CASES OF RAPIDLY REVERSIBLE COLOUR CHANGES

Animals may undergo rapid and reversible colour changes in a number of quite different ways none of which is normally thought of as belonging to the category of physiological colour change. A few of these 'non-physiological' rapid colour changes are noted below.

19.4.1 By special movements

Sudden exposure of previously concealed warning signal

When attacked many animals adopt postures or engage in displays that are sometimes effective in intimidating the attacker. This kind of behaviour is called deimatic or frightening behaviour. Among vertebrates deimatic displays that involve rapid changes of colour effected by chromatophores can be very dramatic, as in some fish and chameleons. It is perhaps not stretching a point too much to say that flushing in some birds (turkeys, vultures) and man and some monkeys is a kind of deimatic display. Flushing pink or red depends upon increasing the amount of haemoglobin close to the surface of the skin by forcing blood into superficial capillaries.

Deimatic displays commonly involve the sudden exposure of bright markings normally concealed [4]. This kind of sudden and reversible change in colour is not what is meant by physiological colour change. For instance, in the iguanid lizard *Anolis carolinensis* the sudden display of the red throat fan does not involve a colour change in the throat but only a dilation so that the red skin between the whitish or buff scales is exposed. Deimatic displays of this kind are perhaps best known in mantids, moths, butterflies, and many other kinds of insects that when attacked suddenly reveal a brightly coloured pair of eyes. Other 'flash' colours in animals that do not stand their ground but flee may be very effective: the predator pursues a bright colour that very suddenly and inexplicably disappears when the pursued animal stops. For instance, a moth may have a brightly coloured hind wing that 'catches' the eye but as soon as it lands the hind wing is covered by the cryptically coloured fore wings and the moth effectively disappears [5].

Disruptive colour pattern altered to a mimetic one

One of the most unusual instances of reversible colour change concerns the spider, *Cyclosa tremula* of Guyana. This spider is an orb-weaver. The spider, which has a striking white and black disruptive pattern, rests in the centre of the hub. The spider uses the remains of insects it has sucked to make four imitation spiders in its web, one in front of it and three behind. Around each fake spider is a wavy thread that mimics the hub of a web (Fig. 19.6). These four imitation

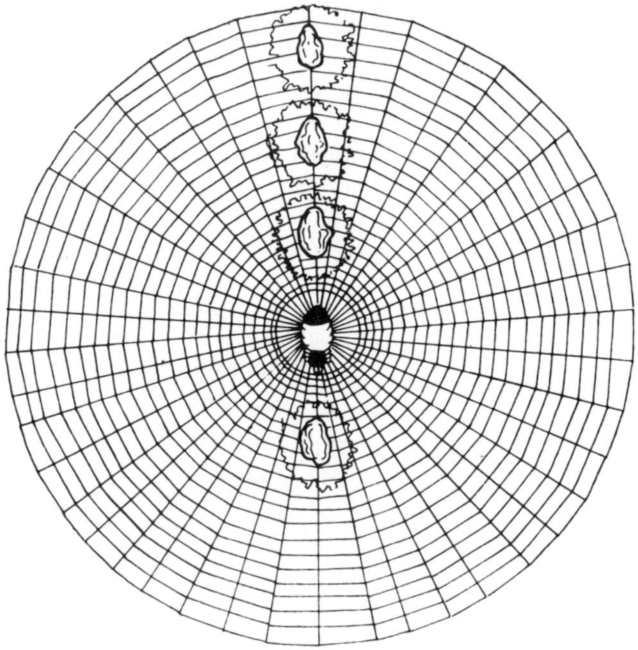

Fig. 19.6. Web of *Cyclosa tremula* of Guyana.

spiders are of course greyish. If for one reason or another the spider, despite its disruptive markings, attracts attention from a predator and is threatened, it raises itself a little from the surface of the hub and vibrates its body sufficiently rapidly so that the black and white patches cannot be resolved and the spider therefore appears grey like the fake spiders above and below it.

Ultra-violet flashing

Insects see far into the ultra-violet: some can be trained to distinguish wavelengths that neither they nor their ancestors have ever seen, that is, much shorter than 300 nanometres, which are the shortest waves that can penetrate the ozone layer. The visible spectrum for vertebrates, including man, ranges from about 400 nm to about 780 nm. Insects, on the other hand, usually do not see into the red, but as we have seen are sensitive to wavelengths shorter than any reaching the surface of the earth [14]. A few insects do see into the red, for instance some butterflies, and they have a visible spectrum wider than that of man or any other known animal, i.e. from 800 to far below 300 nm. Most insects have a peak of spectral sensitivity at about 350 nm and another between 490 and 500 nm.

There are many assemblages of quite different insects that have the same pattern of warning colours. In these assemblages there can be (1) many different poisonous or distasteful insects that resemble each other (Müllerian mimicry) or (2) there may be harmless insects resembling poisonous ones and so trading on the dangerous reputation of others (Batesian mimicry). The fact that all insects can see into the ultra-violet means that there is a part of the spectrum invisible to vertebrates that they can exploit (14). If different insects are to look alike in the part of the spectrum visible to vertebrates, one would have thought that there must be some means by which they can distinguish not only their own species but also the opposite sex. Now we know that insects usually recognize their own species and the opposite sex by odour. However,

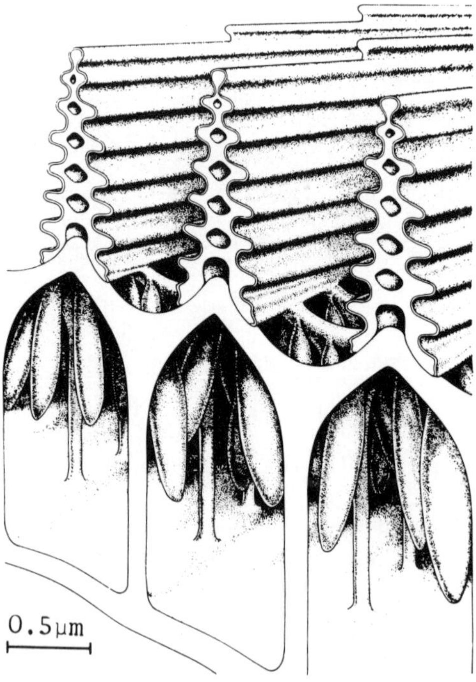

Fig. 19.7. Diagram of part of a wing scale of the pierid butterfly *Eurema lisa*. The laminate ridges projecting upwards are the interference films responsible for the ultra-violet reflection. The pigment granules responsible for the yellowish colour of the scale project downwards into the air space within the main body of the scale. After [10].

many diurnal insects have patterns in the ultraviolet which enable them to recognize not only their own species but also the opposite sex.

Many butterflies of the family Pieridae have ultra-violet patterns that differ between the sexes and many of these also belong to groups of unrelated insects that are warningly coloured. The Pieridae are, so far as we know, unique among animals in having a thin film interference in the ultra-violet part of the spectrum. Most will have seen the brilliant iridescent colours of the species of *Morpho*, the large tropical American butterflies that change colour rapidly as the angle of viewing is changed. In the Pieridae (10) the thin film interference is produced precisely as in other butterflies (Fig. 19.7) but in the ultra-violet part of the spectrum and therefore visible to other insects but not to us or other vertebrates. When a Pierid butterfly with structural ultra-violet is flying, bright flashes will be continually emitted as the wings beat through the appropriate angle. There is some evidence for the view that the ultra-violet pattern of the male Pierid butterfly plays a part in successful courtship. The Pieridae are particularly interesting among butterflies because the ultra-violet reflection is sometimes structural in both sexes, but more often it is either structural in the male and pigmentary in the female or produced by pigments in both sexes. No species is yet known in which the female produces ultra-violet by thin film interference and the male by pigment.

19.4.2 According to incident light

We have already seen how thin-film interference may be used in the ultra-violet part of the spectrum. The iridescent colours of birds and insects, with the exception of some beetles, are interference colours in the visible part of the spectrum. When the mean refractive index is as low as about 1·3, colour changes dramatically with changes in the angle of viewing. In recent years much attention has been paid to the iridescence produced by a very different kind of structure, the diffraction grating [13, 15]. Diffraction gratings have been independently evolved more than a hundred times among beetles. The gratings are usually on the elytra and pronotum, but in some species they are on the underside and legs. In the shade, or in diffuse light when the sky is overcast, the spectra from different parts of the grating may overlap so much that little if any colour can be seen. However, bright spectra are formed when the grating is illuminated by parallel light such as is produced by a small distant source like the sun.

Many ground beetles of the family Carabidae have diffraction gratings. These beetles live among grass roots or concealed in other places. In their normal environment the brown or black colour of their cuticle harmonizes with the background. However, from time to time they have to cross open patches of ground where they are exposed to sunlight, and it is at such times that the bright warning colours produced by their diffraction gratings are advantageous. Insects with diffraction grating have an 'all or none' warning colour. In dim diffuse light the colour of the cuticle may be procryptic but as soon as it is exposed to the sun, warning colours appear. These ground beetles could not solve their particular problem so well by evolving interference colours because these would still be brilliant in diffuse light and so would make them conspicuous even when they were not fully exposed to the sun. A pattern of warning colours formed by pigments in the cuticle would also render them conspicuous even in the dim light around grass roots.

19.4.3 Bioluminescence

Many kinds of marine animals—crustacea, cephalopods, fish—have light-producing organs called photophores by means of which they can rapidly alter their appearance. For instance, spots of light from the photophores of some break up the outline and the appearance of solidity of the body so that it becomes more difficult for predators to recognize them. In some fish, light from the photophores is directed by a system of mirrors and/or lenses in the direction in which the shadow of the fish would naturally fall. By eliminating shadow the fish becomes less visible to predators. It has been shown that light produced by the photophores of some fish passes through colour filters so that it exactly matches the wavelengths of the sunlight that penetrates to the depth at which the fish live. Some fish, such as the hatchet fish, *Argyropelecus affinis*, are able rapidly to alter the intensity of light produced from the photophores to take account of differences in depth or differences in sunlight caused by clouds passing overhead.

Light produced by fireflies has long been known to subserve a variety of functions. The males of many kinds of fireflies emit a flash pattern that is simple and constant at short, fairly regular intervals. The females of many species remain on the ground and respond to the flash pattern of their particular males by flashing. This exchange of flashes enables the males to find the females. But other functions for the flashes of light are known. For instance, they enable females to attract others to suitable oviposition sites. Some carnivorous fireflies attract their prey by flashing, and it has been suggested that in some species flashing is used to intimidate potential predators. Perhaps it is not surprising that flashing is sometimes used simply to light up the landing ground. For instance, in one species of *Photuris* that lives in Florida, females that are about to land fly towards the ground at a slight angle and increase their rate of flashing until the flashes fuse into a continuous flickering emission. It may be that this prevents them from landing on unsuitable places such as spider webs or puddles. Females of species of *Photuris* are indeed remarkable among fireflies. Not only do they eat other beetles but the females of some species mimic the flash pattern of the females of another genus of firefles, *Photinus*. They can thus entice males of *Photinus* to them, which they promptly eat. Some species of *Photuris* can mimic the female flash patterns of two species of *Photinus* and thus their repertoire includes one flash pattern to attract their own males for mating, and two other kinds of flash patterns to attract males of two different species of *Photinus* for eating [19].

19.5 REFERENCES

1 Bagnara J.T. & Hadley MacE. (1973) *Chromatophores and Color Change*. Prentice-Hall, New Jersey.

2 Brown F.A. Jr., Fingerman M., Sandeen M.I. & Webb H.M. (1953) Persistent diurnal and tidal rhythms of colour change in the fiddler crab, *Uca pugnax*. *J. exp. Zool.* **123,** 29–60.

3 Cott H.B. (1966) *Adaptive Coloration in Animals*. Methuen, London.

4 Dupont-Raabe M. (1957) Les méchanismes de l'adaptation chromatique chez les insectes. *Arch. Zool. exp. gén., Paris* **94,** 61–293.

5 Edmunds M. (1974) *Defence in Animals*. Longman, London.

6 Filshie B.K., Day M.F. & Mercer E.H. (1975) Colour and colour change in the grasshopper, *Kosciuscola tristis*. *J. Insect Physiol.* **21,** 1763–70.

7 Fox D.L. (1953) *Animal Biochromes and Structural Colours*. Cambridge University Press, London.

8 Fox H.M. & Vevers G. (1960) *The Nature of Animal Colours*. Sidgwick & Jackson, London.

9 Fufii R. (1969) Chromatophores and pigments. *Fish Physiology* (eds W. S. Hoar & D. J. Randall) **3,** 307–53. Academic Press, New York & London.

10 Ghiradella H., Aneshansley D., Eisner T., Silberglied R.E. & Hinton H.E. (1972) Ultraviolet reflection of a male butterfly: interference color caused by thin-layer elaboration of wing scales. *Science, Wash.* **178,** 1214–17.

11 Hinton H.E. (1958) On the nature and metamorphosis of the colour pattern of *Thaumalea* (Diptera, Thaumaleidae). *J. Insect Physiol.* **2,** 249–60.

12 Hinton H.E. (1960) The ways in which insects change colour. *Sci. Progr., Lond.* **48,** 341–50.

13 Hinton H.E. (1970) Some little known surface structures. *Symp. R. ent. Soc. Lond.* **5,** 41–58.

14 Hinton H.E. (1973) Natural deception. In *Illusion in Nature and Art* (eds R. L. Gregory & E. H. Gombrich), pp. 96–159. Duckworth, London.

15 Hinton H.E. & Gibbs D.F. (1971) Diffraction gratings in gyrinid beetles. *J. Insect Physiol.* **17,** 1023–35.

16 Hinton H.E. & Jarman G.M. (1973) Physiological colour change in the elytra of the Hercules beetle, *Dynastes hercules*. *J. Insect Physiol.* **19,** 533–49.

17 Iwao S. (1962) Studies on the phase variation and related phenomena in some Lepidopterous insects. *Mem. Coll. Agric. Kyoto* **84** (Ent. Ser. no. 12), 1–80.

18 Key K.H.L. (1957) Kentromorphic phases in three species of Phasmatodea. *Aust. J. Zool.* **5,** 247–84.

19 Lloyd J.E. (1969) Flashes of *Photuris* fireflies: their value and use in recognizing species. *Florida Ent.* **52,** 29–35.

20 Matthee J.J. (1946) A study of the phases of the army worm (*Laphygma exempta* Walk.) *J. ent. Soc. sthn Afr.* **9,** 60–77.

21 Messenger J.B. (1974) Reflecting elements in cephalopod skin and their importance for camouflage. *J. Zool., Lond.* **174,** 387–95.

22 Needham A.E. (1974) *The Significance of Zoochromes*. Springer-Verlag, Berlin, Heidelberg & New York.

23 Ogura N. & Saito T. (1972) Hormonal function controlling pigmentation of the integument in the common army worm larva, *Leucania separata* Walker. *Appl. Ent. Zool.* **7,** 239–42.

24 Ogura N., Yagi S. & Fukaya M. (1971) Hormonal control of larval coloration in the common armyworm, *Leucania separata* Walker. *Appl. Ent. Zool.* **6,** 93–5.

25 Raabe M. (1966) Étude des phénomènes de neurosécrétion au niveau de la chaîne nerveuse ventrale des phasmides. *Bull Soc. zool. Fr.* **90,** 631–54.

26 Staal G.B. (1961) Studies on the physiology of phase induction in *Locusta migratoria migratorioides* R. & F. *Meded. Lab. Ent., Wageningen* **72,** 1–125.

26a Taylor J.D. & Hadley M.E. (1970) Chromatophores and color change in the lizard, *Anolis carolinensis*. *Z. Zellforsch. mikrosc. Anat.* **104,** 282–94.

27 Veron J.E.N. (1973) Physiological control of the chromatophores of *Austrolestes annulosus* (Odonata). *J. Insect Physiol.* **19,** 1689–703.
28 Veron J.E.N. (1976) Responses of Odonata chromatophores to environmental stimuli. *J. Insect Physiol.* **22,** 19–30.
29 Waring H. (1963) *Color Change Mechanisms of Cold-blooded Vertebrates.* Academic Press, New York & London.
30 Wickler W. (1968) *Mimicry in Plants and Animals.* Weidenfeld & Nicolson, London.

Prelude to Chapter 20

Thermoregulation deserves consideration first because of the biological significance of the emergence of species that can maintain a high and stable internal thermal environment largely independent of variations in the external thermal environment; and secondly, because it can be treated as a representative, and fairly well understood, example of a homeostatic function.

The merit of thermoregulation as an example of homeostasis is that thermal stimuli are easily applied, the responses are fairly easily measured, and the relations observed between disturbance and response are expressible in terms of physical models based on engineering theory and practice. On the other hand, the homeothermy of the mammals and birds is a relatively recent biological innovation which seems to have evolved separately in the two lines no more than 200 million years ago. All other forms of life are usually described as poikilothermic, and for the most part the temperature of their internal environment is largely dependent on environmental thermal influences.

Clearly, then, temperature is not one of the fundamental and essential environmental conditions which must be kept within narrow limits for the survival of the constituent cells of an organism, yet its fine control in the birds and mammals depends on the integrity of hypothalamic structures which lie close to those concerned with other, and presumably much older, homeostatic functions. Whether this is because some kind of thermoregulation existed long before the separate evolution of the birds and mammals from different reptilian lines, or because a relatively new homeostatic function adopted the central nervous machinery already existing for autonomic homeostasis, remains unclear. Since the hypothalamus controls blood pressure and thermoregulatory salivation in tortoises, however, it is probable that the first of these postulations is the correct one.

Recent evidence of the occurrence of thermoresponsive structures in the central nervous systems of fishes, amphibians and reptiles, as well as in mammals and birds, and the widespread occurrence of behavioural responses to ambient temperature in both poikilothermic and homeothermic animals, is proof of the existence of some control over the thermal relations between organism and environment long before the evolution of mammalian and avian homeothermy.

The chemical processes of life involve the redistribution of energy at rates which are temperature dependent. Thus all biological processes are greatly influenced by the ambient temperature, and with the increasing complexity of organisms, the emergence of means of exerting some degree of control over the internal thermal environment of the constituent cells might well be expected.

Indeed, it is now evident that few, if any, poikilothermic organisms are true thermal conformers (which, by definition, are totally unreactive to variations in ambient temperature); most use some tropic or behavioural means of selecting the thermal environment and therefore the temperatures of their tissues, or employ some autonomic means of modulating tissue temperature in relation to that of the environment. For example, diurnally active butterflies may bask in the sun to absorb exogenous heat before flight, while nocturnally active moths raise tissue temperature by pre-flight muscular activity akin to shivering. The flight muscles of insects are in the thorax, and it is only this part of the body which requires an elevated temperature for flight. The bumble bee has, in addition to the hairy insulation of the thorax, an intriguing system of heat exchange whereby the heat can be retained in the thorax despite the continuous transfer of blood between the thorax and the abdomen.

The pre-occupation with mammalian homeothermy, and the teaching of a thermoregulatory dichotomy between poikolothermic and homeothermic organisms, has long obscured the fact that temperature has always been an important component of the environment of animals, and that most animals respond in one way or another so as to exert some control over the changes in the temperature of their own tissues.

Chapter 20
Temperature regulation

J. BLIGH

20.1 THE TEMPERATURE-BOUNDED NATURE OF ANIMAL LIFE

'La respiration est donc une combustion'

This dramatic description of the essential sameness of biological and non-biological processes of oxidation and degradation [30] was colourfully translated by Kleiber [29] as a fire. In both cases chemically stored energy (fuel) is converted into chemically unbonded kinetic energy (heat) which ultimately flows down a thermal gradient to the environment to increase entropy. But there is a crucial difference between the controlled low-temperature combustion of fuel by animals and the relatively uncontrolled high-temperature combustion of a fire.

In the animal the complex and well-modulated steps from fuel and oxygen to heat and carbon dioxide include the temporary conversion of some fuel into other forms of chemically bound energy which play essential roles in the structures and functions of the organism. The delicate feats of anabolism (synthetic change) which occur concurrently with the controlled katabolism (degradative change), and which are the characteristics of self-repairing and reproducing organisms, would not be possible at the temperature of a fire.

There are, however, even more restrictive influences of temperature. Except where specialized cellular adaptations permit the tolerance of temperature below 0°C and above 45°C, these are the thermal limits of viability. The *lower temperature limit* is that at which water, the universal biological solvent, crystallizes and causes cellular dehydration. This results in the collapse of the cellular structure, the concentration of the solutes, and irreversible damage [22, 34]. The *upper temperature limit* is that at which the chemical components of cells become unstable and suffer irreversible changes. Heat-induced death is largely due to the 'denaturing' of intracellular proteins, but changes in membrane phospholipids may also be contributory [22].

20.2 THE TEMPERATURE-DEPENDENCE OF METABOLISM AND ACTIVITY

Within the range of temperature compatible with life, the rates at which metabolic processes proceed are temperature dependent. The change in the rate of reaction with temperature is described by the temperature coefficient (Q_{10} value) of van't Hoff [45]. This expresses the factor by which the reaction rate is increased when the temperature of the system is raised by 10°C, and for most biological functions is of the order of 2–3. For some functions, however, the Q_{10} may be much greater or may be unity or less than unity.

The rate of heat production of the so-called 'cold-blooded' organisms is too low to have very much influence on tissue temperatures, which vary passively with that of the environment. Because of the van't Hoff effect of temperature on tissue functions, activities as well as temperatures rise and fall with daily and seasonal variations in ambient thermal conditions.

It has been argued that in a 'cold-blooded' world these effects of temperature on activity would provide no competitive advantage. In an aqueous environment this may be a valid proposition, at least to some extent, but it is a considerably less valid comment on organisms in atmospheric environments. The proposition ignores the fact that small organisms with large surface areas relative to mass will warm up and cool down much more rapidly than will larger organisms with a smaller surface area relative to mass. Thus in the morning, when ambient temperatures are rising, the smallest organisms will be warmed-up and have the advantage of being active before the larger animals, but in the evening, they will suffer the disadvantage of cooling down more rapidly. This phase differential in the daily periods of high activity in organisms of different sizes is of undoubted ecological significance, and has provided a selective pressure for the evolution of behavioural characteristics by which organisms can optimize the periods of high body temperature and high activity.

20.3 THE OPTIMUM TEMPERATURE OF LIVING ORGANISMS

It is evident, from the above considerations, that terrestrial organisms must keep their tissue temperature within the limits of the lower and upper lethal temperature. They can gain competitive advantage in the search for food and the avoidance of predators if they can maintain body temperature somewhere in the upper half of this thermal range compatible with life.

One might therefore suppose that the nearer the tissue temperature can be held to the upper lethal temperature, the more efficient and more competitive the organism will be in these vital activities. However, activities themselves can cause rises in tissue temperature. In cold-blooded animals there is the risk of prolonged exposure to solar radiation, with the uptake of excessive heat from the environment, and in warm-blooded animals, activity may itself generate sufficient additional heat to cause fatal hyperthermia. Thus there is likely to have been pressure for genetic selection of a preference for a behaviourally regulated temperature sufficiently below the upper lethal temperature to allow for the inevitable periods of activity and the concomitant temporary storage of heat within the body.

The behaviourally regulated (preferred) body temperatures of many species of tropical reptiles [14], and the autonomically and behaviourally regulated body temperature of many species of mammals [24, 44] and birds [17, 44] are, indeed, in the upper part of the range of physiologically tolerable temperatures, yet sufficiently below the upper lethal temperature to permit the storage of heat during exposure to solar radiation and activity.

Obviously, since the thermoregulating reptiles are ectotherms which derive most of the tissue heat from the environment, the evolution of species with preferred temperatures above 30°C must have occurred in environments in which solar radiation was sufficient for the regular (daily) achievement of tissue temperatures of between 30° and 40°C.

20.4 BODY HEAT—CONFORMITY OR CONTROL

If an organism exerts no control whatever over its rate of heat production and over the flow of heat between itself and its environment, it is a **thermal conformer**. This does not mean that tissue temperatures are equal to that of the environment, but that they will fluctuate passively with changes in heat production, or with changes in environmental temperatures.

If an organism does *anything* to modulate either its heat production or the flow of heat between itself and its environment in a way that seems to have the object of raising, lowering, or stabilizing tissue temperatures, the organism is a **thermal regulator** [35]. This description implies nothing about the form of the thermal regulation, or of its effectiveness.

20.5 PROCESSES OF THERMAL REGULATION—BEHAVIOURAL AND AUTONOMIC

A distinction is frequently made between *behavioural* and *physiological* thermal regulation, but as there is nothing unphysiological about behaviour, a now preferred distinction is between **behavioural** and **autonomic** processes [10]. A behavioural thermoregulatory action is one which involves the whole organism and is readily observable (in animals large enough to be observed). In large multicellular organisms it involves complex sequences of integrated muscle movements and, in the higher vertebrates at least, these require the integrity of the cerebral cortex. In man, behavioural thermal regulation is apparently motivated and triggered by the conscious experience of thermal comfort and discomfort [13].

These readily observable responses of whole organisms to their thermal environments occur at all levels of animal life, and extend from the thermotropism (tropism = movement) of unicellular aquatic organisms, through, for example, the pre-flight wing spreading of the butterfly for the absorption of solar energy, to the elaborate nest-building activities of mammals and birds. It must be conceded that few forms of animal life (apart from those which are sessile) show the total indifference to their thermal environments attributed to *thermal conformers*. The linear relation between body temperature and environmental temperature characteristic of thermal conformity can be readily demonstrated in the so-called lower vertebrates when exposed to different temperatures under laboratory conditions. In these circumstances the natural behavioural responses to the thermal environment are frustrated and such experiments can demonstrate only the absence, or the feeble development, of autonomic control over heat production and heat flow.

Autonomic thermal regulation, like behavioural regulation, is concerned with the modulation of heat production within the body, or with the rate of heat exchange between the organism and its environment, but unlike behavioural regulation it acts through changes in the functions of particular organs and systems rather than of the whole organism; and their operation may not be immediately apparent without the aid of sensing instruments. The term *autonomic* means self-governing, and describes those thermoregulatory functions of organs and tissue of higher vertebrates which can still operate after the removal of the cerebral cortex, and after the animal has been deprived of the ability to respond to stimuli with integrated muscular activity. These thermoregulatory responses can, therefore, be grouped together with those other functions which operate automatically, which are controlled subconsciously and sub-cortically, and which serve to maintain the homeostasis of the internal environments of organisms.

20.6 EXOGENOUS HEAT

Animals other than the birds and mammals yield insufficient heat to sustain an appreciable temperature difference between organism and environment, and body temperature is determined by environmental thermal influences. The flow of heat is sometimes from the body to the environment and at other times from the environment to the body. During the night heat generally flows away from the organism, and during the day, heat flows into the organism. Many cold-blooded organisms (e.g. butterflies and lizards) and some warm blooded animals (e.g. the hyrax) use behavioural means to maximize the heat uptake from the environment at the beginning of the day. Thereafter they may keep their body

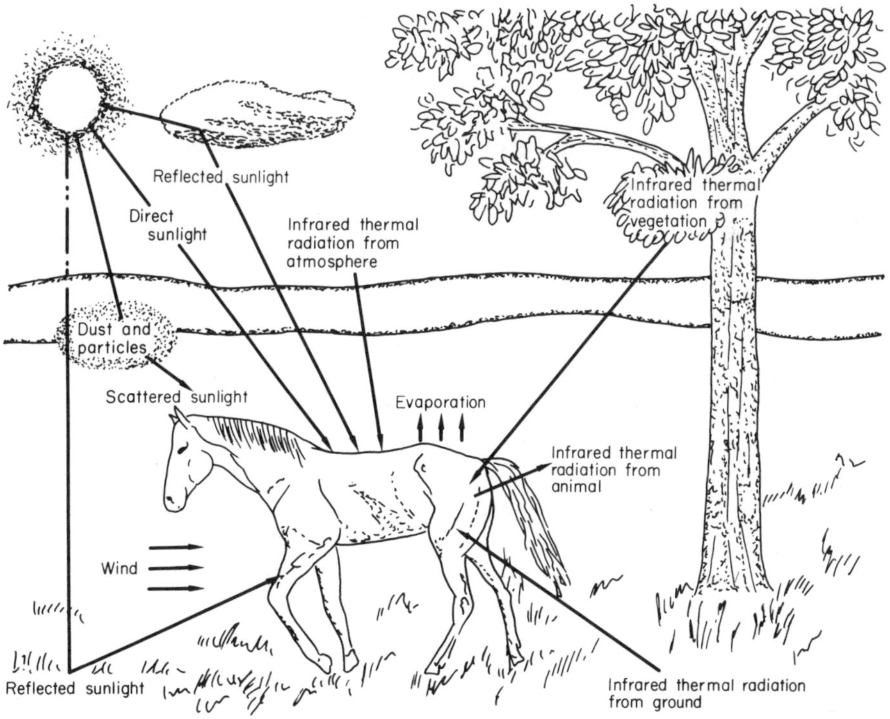

Fig. 20.1. Channels of heat transfer for an animal exposed to an outdoor environment. From [33].

temperature within a *preferred zone* by variations in posture, and by movements into and out of conditions which cause high rates of heat absorption. This control over the uptake of heat from the environment as a means of optimizing the rates of metabolism and activity is termed **ectothermy**. It can be sub-divided into (a) **heliothermy**, which is the direct absorption of solar energy, together with the orientation of the body in relation to the sun so as to regulate the rate of absorption; and (b) **thigmothermy**, which is the conductive uptake of heat from solar-heated surfaces, and the adjustment of body posture to control the rate of uptake. In reality the exchange of heat between organism and environment is physically complex (Fig. 20.1).

20.7 ENDOGENOUS HEAT

The energy content of the fuel used by animals is, of course, of solar origin, but although both plants and animals may absorb solar heat, and thereby raise their tissue temperatures, only plants can convert the electro-magnetic energy radiated from the sun into chemically-bonded energy within their tissues. Directly or indirectly, all animals depend on plant matter for fuel and its energy is ultimately released as heat inside or outside the organism.

Apart from relatively minor amounts of heat released during digestive processes in the gut, and by the frictional conversion of kinetic energy within the circulatory system, endogenous heat is released intracellularly.

Current evidence indicates that more than half of it is liberated within the mitochondria, and relates largely to the synthesis of ATP, the efficiency of which is of the order of 25% [25]. A smaller, but quite considerable proportion is liberated in the cell membrane [43], and relates to such membrane pumping functions as the active transport of charged and uncharged molecules across the membrane against concentration gradients.

20.8 METABOLIC RATE IN RELATION TO BODY SIZE AND SURFACE AREA

The rate of metabolism, and therefore of heat production increases with body size, but not in direct proportion to body size. As with most other biological functions [11, 27], when the logarithm of metabolic rate (MR) is plotted against the logarithm of body weight (BW) a straight line relation is obtained [11] (Fig. 20.2). The slope of this line indicates that MR is a function of $BW^{3/4}$ and since the surface area of a sphere varies with $mass^{2/3}$, this relation is interpreted as an indication of large but not exclusive influence of surface area on metabolic rate. This relation was first observed in mammals and birds [11] and the plot of log. MR against log. BW is known as Benedict's mouse-elephant curve since the data were derived from Benedict [2]. When a double-logarithmic plot is made of MR

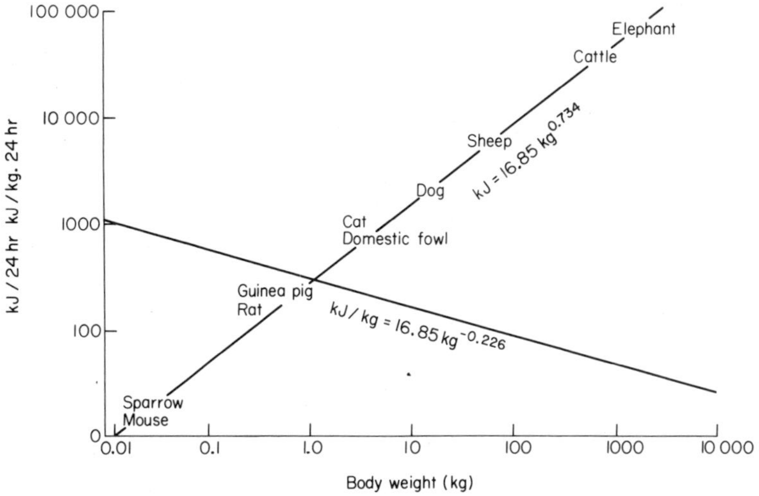

Fig. 20.2. A simplified reconstruction in S.I. units of a figure from [11] in which the basal metabolism of mature animals is plotted against body weight on a double logarithmic grid. The rising curve represents metabolism per animal per day; the declining curve represents the metabolism per kg body weight per day. The slope of the rising curve, 0·73, means that an increase in body weight of 100% is associated with an increase in basal metabolism of about 73%.

per unit mass (e.g. W kg^{-1}) against BW, the resultant straight line is negative (Fig. 20.2). This means that the metabolic rate per unit mass declines as total mass increases, but of course, this slope still expresses the strong influence of surface area.

Since the rate of total heat flow into or out of a body along a thermal gradient is a function of surface area relative to mass, the maintenance of a body temperature above that of the environment and at more-or-less the same level irrespective of body size requires rates of heat production proportional to the rates of heat loss. If the rate of heat production per unit mass of the tissues of an elephant equalled that of the mouse, the elephant would cook. Conversely, if the mouse had the rate of heat production per unit mass of tissue equal to that of the elephant it could not sustain a body temperature anywhere near to that of most mammals (36°–38°C). Thus mammalian homeothermy at core temperatures which are similar in animals of vastly differing body sizes is only possible because of this particular relation between the rate of heat production and body mass. Contrary to earlier assumptions, however, this relation did not evolve with mammalian homeothermy: the same relation exists in cold-blooded (= bradymetabolic—see below) poikilothermic organisms from the largest of reptiles and fishes to the smallest marine organism [23] (bradymetabolic line in Fig. 20.3). Precisely to what this relation between metabolic rate and mass is to be attributed, how it is influenced by surface area, and what changes produce the decline in metabolic rate per unit mass of tissue as an organism grows, remains enigmatic.

20.9 METABOLIC RATES—BRADYMETABOLISM AND TACHYMETABOLISM

There is a fundamental difference in the rates of metabolism of the 'cold-blooded' and 'warm-blooded' animals. When the double logarithmic plot is used to describe the relations between metabolic rates and body weight of a variety of animals, it becomes apparent that there are two distinct but parallel lines (Fig. 20.3). The lower one relates to the 'cold-blooded' animals, and the upper one

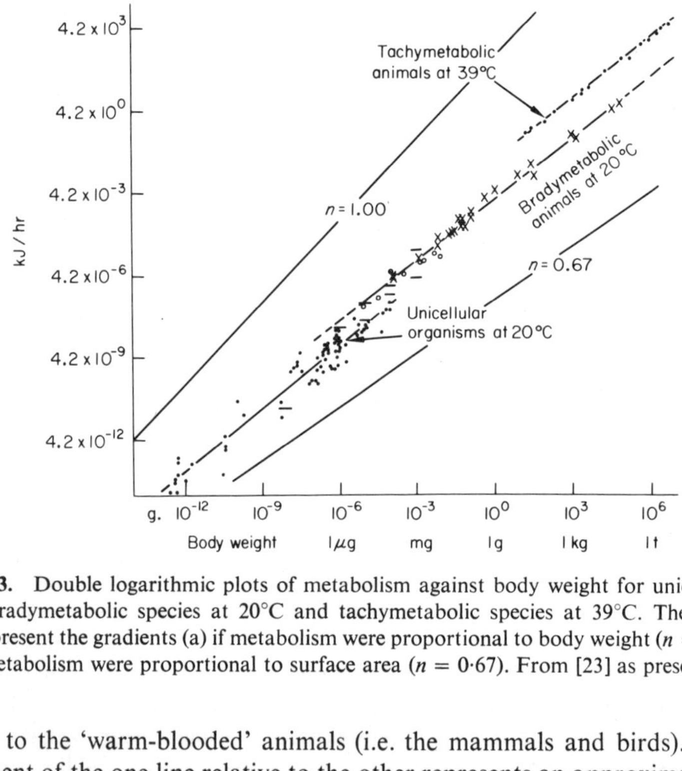

Fig. 20.3. Double logarithmic plots of metabolism against body weight for unicellular and larger bradymetabolic species at 20°C and tachymetabolic species at 39°C. The two outer lines represent the gradients (a) if metabolism were proportional to body weight ($n = 1{\cdot}00$) and (b) if metabolism were proportional to surface area ($n = 0{\cdot}67$). From [23] as presented in [5].

relates to the 'warm-blooded' animals (i.e. the mammals and birds). This displacement of the one line relative to the other represents an approximately fourfold increase in the metabolic rates of mammals and birds over that of cold-blooded animals of the same body size, after corrections have been made for differences in their controlled or 'preferred' levels of body temperature (Q_{10} effects). It is, of course, these differences in metabolic rates which form the basis of the distinction between cold-bloodedness and warm-bloodedness, but these terms are poetic rather than precise, as many reptiles maintain their tissue temperatures in the same range as those of the mammals by behavioural means. There is now growing support for the terms **bradymetabolic** (= slow rate of chemical change) and **tachymetabolic** (= fast rate of chemical change) to describe these two categories of animals [10].

Two abiding problems lie behind this apparently neat classification: one is the biochemical or biophysical explanation for the higher rate of metabolism in mammals and birds; the other is why the birds and mammals which evolved quite independently from distinctly different and, presumably, bradymetabolic reptilian ancestors should have effected the same order of increase in their metabolic rates. It is generally presumed that particular thermal conditions of the environment influenced both the evolution of this elevated metabolic capacity of the tissues, and of the similar level at which body temperature is regulated in the mammals and birds. Various speculative efforts have been made to account for these evolutionary progressions [19, 23, 43].

20.10 TEMPERATURE REGULATION

The regulation of any variable quantity requires the presence of all the essential components of a regulatory system. Basically these are fourfold (Fig. 20.4):

Sensors of disturbances (or of threats of disturbances) to the variable quantity.

Correction effectors which can respond to and correct for a signalled disturbance.

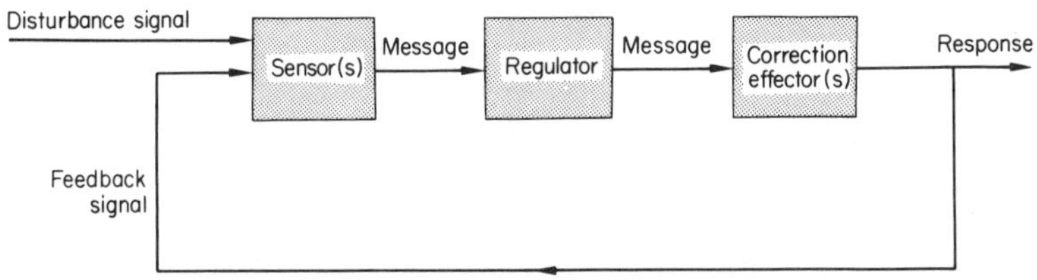

Fig. 20.4. A simple feedback scheme. Taken from [3].

Central regulator which receives the information from the sensors and directs the operation of correction effectors.

Feedback of the consequences of the effector functions onto the sensors, so that when the effectors have carried out the necessary correction the disturbance signals will be withdrawn.

All these components of a regulatory system are readily identifiable in the mammals, and there is growing evidence of their existence in birds [36, 37] and reptiles [32] and possibly also in amphibia and fishes [15]. The more detailed description which follows, however, relates with certainty only to the mammals.

20.10.1 Disturbance sensors

Specific warm-sensitive and cold-sensitive nerve-endings in the skin contribute immediate information of a change in the thermal relation between organism and environment which, if uncorrected, will cause a change in the rate of heat flux, and therefore in body temperature. Temperature-sensitive structures also exist in the central nervous system—the brain and the spinal cord, and possibly in other deep tissues [41]. These contribute information relative to changes in heat production and in heat storage. Between them therefore, the peripheral and central sensors provide information about changes in heat production, in the rate of heat exchange with the environment, and in the resultant heat content of the body.

20.10.2 Correction effectors

(*a*) *Heat production*

Thermoregulatory effector processes which modify heat production can be classified as *behavioural*, *autonomic* or *adaptive* as follows:

Behavioural—co-ordinated movements of the whole body, e.g. exercise

Autonomic—immediately effective thermogenic response to cold stress. Generally this is by shivering, but in some small mammals there may also be a response known as non-shivering thermoregulatory thermogenesis which is entirely or largely a function of brown adipose tissue [28, 42].

Adaptive—hormonally effected changes in the basal rate of tissue metabolism.

(*b*) *Heat exchange*

Thermoregulatory effector processes which modify heat exchange with the environment can be similarly classified:

Behavioural—These are manifold [12] and extend from changes in conformation which vary the ratio of surface area to mass, and therefore the rate of heat flow into or out of the animal, to the elaborate endeavours to modify the immediate environment—e.g. the nest-building of insects, birds and mammals including man. Retiring to burrows or rock crevices to avoid nocturnal cooling, and the emergence into sunshine in the morning to absorb solar heat are most characteristic of the reptiles and other bradymetabolic animals, but are by no means exclusive to these classes of animal.

Autonomic—Immediate variations in the thermal gradient from organism to environment are effected by changes in the tone of the skin blood vessels and other vascular changes. These vary the extent of the blood flow through the skin, and so vary skin temperature relative to core temperature and ambient temperature. The activation of piloerector muscles causes fur and feather fluffing with resultant changes in the insulative property of the pelage. Variations in the rate of evaporative heat loss from the body are mostly by panting or sweating.

Adaptive—These include long-acting variations in the degree of the supra- or sub-dermal insulation by changes in, respectively, the extent and structure of the pelage or in the extent of fat-layers. Long-acting variations may also be induced in the efficiency and/or capacity of the autonomic processes of evaporative heat loss.

The above is an illustrative, not a complete, summary of the means by which organisms can modify the rates of heat production and heat exchange.

20.10.3 The thermoregulator

The nature and location of the central nervous control processes by which appropriate activator signals are sent to the thermoregulatory effectors in response to information signals received from thermosensors, remains equivocal. The hypothalamic region of the brain is important, both as an area of temperature sensitivity, and as a thermoregulatory centre, but is not the exclusive location of deep body sensors, or of thermoregulatory processes. Interaction of thermosensors and thermoregulatory effectors occur at the level of the medulla and perhaps also in the spinal cord [41]. There is little doubt, however, that the principle 'centres' of thermoregulation are in the hypothalamus, and it is noteworthy that hypothalamic structures in fishes, amphibians and reptiles, as well as in birds and mammals seem to have thermosensory and thermoregulatory roles.

Just how a complex of neurones lying between the afferent pathways from sensors and the efferent pathways to effectors can relate the one to the other so as to effect regulation remains undetermined.

The similarities between the thermodynamics of animals and machines have stimulated analyses of the relations between thermal disturbances and thermoregulatory responses of the possible regulatory functions in the central nervous system and have permitted descriptions of mammalian thermoregulation in terms of the physical control processes employed by engineers [20, 31].

When the intensity of the effector functions are plotted against deep body temperature, the pattern of the responses can be expressed as in Fig. 20.5. Within the normal range of body temperature, which varies between species, fine adjustments in heat flow are effected by peripheral vasomotor tone and by behavioural responses which are less readily quantifiable. The onset of thermoregulatory heat production by shivering occurs only when core temperature has fallen to some threshold or 'set-point' temperature, and then increases in proportion to further decreases in core temperature. Similarly, evaporative heat loss by panting or sweating occurs only when core temperature has risen to some threshold or 'set-point' temperature, and increases in proportion to further rises in core temperature. This general pattern of relations between body temperature and thermoregulatory effector functions is the basis of the view that the thermoregulatory nerve complexes in the brain function in a manner closely analogous to that of a *proportional controller*, in which the intensity of the drive to a correction effector is proportional to the extent by which the controlled variable has deviated from a set-point. Concepts of how the interrelating neurones lying between sensor and effector pathways could achieve this are emerging from these disturbance/response analyses and from studies of temperature-dependent electrical activities of hypothalamic neurones and of the thermoregulatory effects of chemical

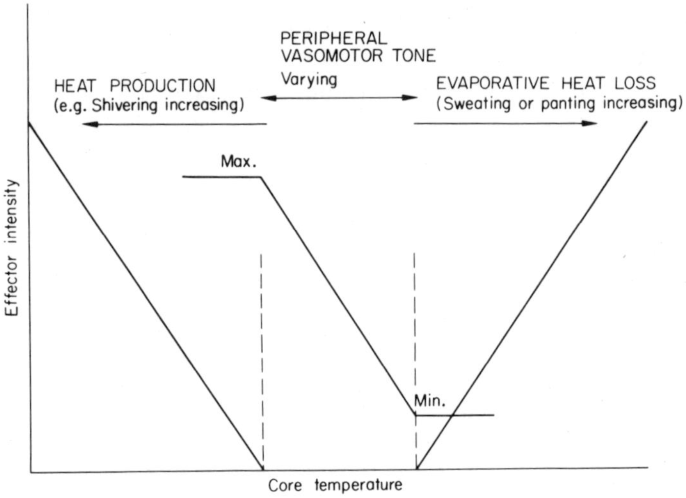

Fig. 20.5. A general representation of the relation between thermoregulatory effector intensity and body temperature in mammals.

interference with hypothalamic synapses [4, 6]. If this promise of a true understanding of how the central nervous system relates thermoregulatory responses to thermal disturbances is fulfilled it could be the beginning of an understanding of how the brain performs its many similar tasks of organizing appropriate physiological responses to changes in the environment which effect the organisms.

20.10.4 Feedback

The feedback from thermoregulatory effects to temperature sensors is, as illustrated diagrammatically in Fig. 20.6, via the circulating blood.

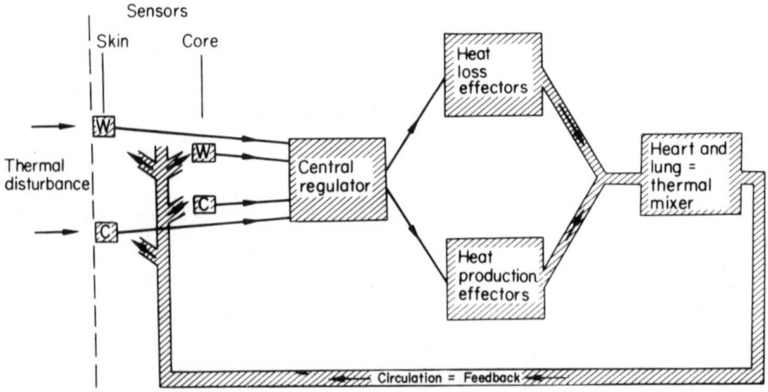

Fig. 20.6. A schematic representation of the components of the mammalian thermoregulatory system to illustrate the essential similarity between a simple physical feedback scheme (Fig. 20.4) and the physiological system. Based on a figure in [16].

20.11 HOMEOTHERMY AND HETEROTHERMY

The advantage, in a competitive environment, of an animal with a regulated body temperature over one whose temperature conforms with that of the environment, is obvious. The advantage of a fine regulation of body temperature, as in the sheep [9], over a somewhat coarser regulation, as in the camel [39], is not so obvious. A stable body temperature is an advantage because of the animal's ability to respond immediately and at all times to environmental hazards and opportunities, but it limits the range of climatic conditions which the animal can tolerate. Sustained homeothermy requires a constant supply of food which may not be available in either very cold or in very hot and arid seasons or environments, and in hot arid environments the water needed to dissipate heat by evaporation may be in short supply.

Seasonal migration is one behavioural means of averting such environmental threats to homeothermy. The harvesting and hoarding of food during seasons of plenty is another. The retreat into burrows is a third behavioural means of avoiding the extreme heat or the extreme cold of the macroclimate. A thick insulating coat may eliminate the need to increase metabolic rate even in the extreme cold: the arctic fox, for example, can endure an air temperature of -40° without elevating its metabolic rate [40]. Some species store energy as fat during the seasons of plenty, and draw on this to maintain tachymetabolism during periods of food shortage. However, such behavioural and other physiological means of avoiding or combating heat and cold cannot succeed in all circumstances. The smaller mammals, with their relatively high metabolic rates per unit mass of tissue, and with large surface areas relative to mass, are physically unable to provide themselves with sufficient insulation and sufficient fat reserves to survive long periods of extreme cold and famine. The larger mammals, though unable to escape from a stressful macroclimate by burrowing carry a coat thick enough to insulate them against the cold. However, they may be physically unable to obtain enough water to maintain thermostability in hot arid environments by evaporation.

A means of escape used by some mammals which would otherwise be unable to cope with the thermal conditions of their habitats is to revert seasonally from homeothermy to poikilothermy (or heterothermy). Such seasonal torpidity, of which hibernation is the most studied example, involves the temporary abandonment of the fine control of body temperature. As body temperature falls passively, so does metabolism, thus effecting an economy of fuel. Despite this temporary absence of thermoregulation, hibernating mammals can switch-on thermogenesis and return towards their normal high level of body temperature when tissue temperatures fall to below 0°C, and towards the point at which tissue water would begin to crystallize.

The one-humped camel which naturally inhabits hot and arid regions, together with some other mammals in similar environments, has a somewhat greater 24-hourly variation in body temperature than that of most other mammalian species [8, 39]. This apparently passive diurnal rise and nocturnal fall in body temperature is well suited to an animal in such a habitat, because it greatly reduces the dissipation of the body water for evaporative heat loss. These species use their bodies as heat sinks, storing up generated or absorbed heat during the day time, and later shedding this thermal load by radiation to the cold night sky.

All the available evidence indicates that the various kinds of seasonal and nychthemeral heterothermy in mammals are environmental adaptations of erstwhile fully established homeotherms [5]. The hibernators, for example, occur in several mammalian orders, all of which contain permanently stable homeothermic species. Furthermore a hibernating species may be well capable of maintaining a stable body temperature during its seasons of activity. The thermolability of the one-humped camel is not shared by the South American camelidae [7], and this has been interpreted as possible evidence of the acquisition of the thermolability of the camels by natural selection when they were forced by some ecological pressure to inhabit desert terrain.

20.12 SUMMARY

Life and the environment which has shaped it and which sustains it, are inseparable components of a whole. Temperature—the index of molecular motion resulting from the amount of free energy within a chemical structure—is so fundamental to the nature of both the environment and life that its many influences on the functions of animals (physiology) has only been touched on in this chapter. More detailed texts are available [5, 18, 21, 29, 38, 44].

At the cellular level all forms of animal life have much in common [26], and the chemical basis of life imposes quite sharply defined limits on the range of temperatures within which life can be sustained. Because chemical reactions are temperature dependent (Q_{10} effect), there is an evolutionary tendency towards physiological systems which enable animals to keep tissue temperatures in the upper part of this range of viability. This is achieved largely by behavioural control of the uptake of heat from the environment, but the high metabolic rates of mammals and birds relative to those of reptiles and lower forms of animal life, permit body temperature to be maintained at a fairly steady level which is generally above that of the environment. This is achieved by the regulation of the rates of both heat production and of heat loss to the environment, by both behavioural and autonomic processes.

The permanency of a high and stable temperature, while generally advantageous, is a disadvantage in some environments where there are seasonal variations in the availability of food and water as well as in the environmental temperature. The temporary abandonment of homeothermy (e.g. hibernation and estivation) are further adaptations of established homeothermic animals to the seasonal changes in the environment.

20.13 REFERENCES

1 Baumann I.R. & Bligh J. (1975) The influence of ambient temperature on drug-induced disturbances of body temperature. In *Temperature Regulation and Drug Action* (eds J. Lomax, E. Schonbaum & J. Jacob) pp. 241–51. Karger, Basel.

2 Benedict F.G. (1938) *Vital Energetics, a study in comparative basal metabolism.* Carnegie Inst., Washington. Pub. 503.

3 Bertalanffy L. von (1971) *General System Theory.* Allen Lane, Harmondsworth.

4 Bligh J. (1972) Neuronal models of mammalian temperature regulation. In *Essays on Temperature Regulation* (eds J. Bligh & R. E. Moore) pp. 105–20. North Holland, Amsterdam.

5 Bligh J. (1973) *Temperature Regulation in Mammals and other Vertebrates.* North Holland, Amsterdam.

6 Bligh J. (1974) Neuronal models of hypothalamic temperature regulation. In *Recent Studies of Hypothalamic Function* (eds K. Lederis & K. E. Cooper) pp. 315–27. Karger. Basel.

7 Bligh J., Baumann I., Sumar J. & Pocco F. (1975) Studies of body temperature patterns in South American camelidae. *Comp. Biochem. Physiol.* **50A**, 701–8.

8 Bligh J. & Harthoorn A.M. (1965) Continuous radiotelemetric records of the deep body temperature of some unrestrained African mammals under near-natural conditions. *J. Physiol., Lond.* **176,** 145–62.

9 Bligh J., Ingram D.L., Keynes R.D. & Robinson S.G. (1965) The deep body temperature of an unrestrained Welsh Mountain Sheep recorded by a radiotelemetric technique during a 12-month period. *J. Physiol., Lond.* **176,** 136–44.

10 Bligh J. & Johnson K.G. (1973) Glossary of terms for thermal physiology. *J. appl. Physiol.* **35,** 941–61.

11 Brody S. (1945) *Bioenergetics and Growth.* Rheinhold, New York.

12 Cabanac M. (1974) Thermoregulatory behaviour. In *Environmental Physiology* (ed. D. Robertshaw). MTP Intl. Rev. Sci. Series 1, Vol. 7. pp. 231–69. Butterworth, London.

13 Chatonnet J. & Cabanac M. (1965) The perception of thermal comfort. *Int. J. Biometeor.* **9,** 183–93.

14 Cloudsley-Thompson J.L. (1971) *The Temperature and Water Relations of Reptiles,* p. 13. Merrow, Watford.

15 Crawshaw L.I. & Hammel H.T. (1973) The regulation of internal body temperature in the Brown Bullhead *Ameiurus nebulosus.* In *The Pharmacology of Thermoregulation* (eds E. Schonbaum & P. Lomax) pp. 142–5. Karger, Basel.

16 Cremer J.E. & Bligh J. (1969) Body temperature and responses to drugs. *Br. med. Bull.* **25,** 299–306.

17 Dawson W.R. & Hudson J.W. (1970) In *Comparative Physiology of Thermoregulation* (eds G. F. Whittow) Academic Press, New York & London.

18 Dill D.B. & Adolph E.F. (eds) (1964) *Adaptation to the Environment, Handbook of Physiology,* Section 4. Amer. Physiol. Soc., Washington.

19 Hammel H.T. (1976) On the origin of endothermy in mammals. *Israel J. Med. Sci.* (in press).

20 Hardy J.D. (1965) The 'set-point' concept in physiological temperature regulation. In *Physiological Controls and Regulation* (eds W. S. Yamamoto & J. R. Brobeck) pp. 98–116. Saunders, Philadelphia.

21 Hardy J.D., Gagge A.P. & Stolwijk J.A.J. (eds) (1970) *Physiological and Behavioural Temperature Regulation.* Thomas, Springfield.

22 Heber U. & Santarius L.A. (1973) Cell death by cold and heat and resistance to extreme temperatures. Mechanisms of hardening and dehardening. In *Temperature and Life* (eds H. Precht, J. Christopherson, H. Hensel & W. Larcher) pp. 232–63. Springer-Verlag, Berlin, Heidelberg & New York.

23 Hemmingsen A.M. (1960) Energy metabolism as related to body size and respiratory surfaces, and its evolution. *Rep. Steno. Memo. Hosp. Nord. Insulin Lab.* 9, part 2, 1–110.
24 Hensel H., Brück K. & Paths P. (1973) In *Temperature and Life* (eds H. Precht, J. Christopherson, H. Hensel & W. Larcher) p. 514. Springer-Verlag, Berlin, Heidelberg & New York.
25 Hochachka P.W. (1974) Regulation of heat production at the cellular level. *Fed. Proc.* **33,** 2162–9.
26 Hochachka P.W. & Somero G.N. (1973) *Strategies of Biochemical Adaptation*. Saunders, Philadelphia.
27 Huxley J.S. (1932) *Problems of Relative Growth*. Methuen, London.
28 Jansky L. (1973) Non-shivering thermogenesis and its thermoregulatory significance. *Biol. Rev.* **48,** 85–132.
29 Kleiber M. (1961) *The Fire of Life*. Wiley, New York.
30 Lavoisier A.L. (1780) *Memoire sur la chaleur. Histoire de l'Académie Royale des Sciences* **85,** p 355.
31 Mitchell D., Atkins A.R. & Wyndham C.H. (1972) Mathematical and physical models of thermoregulation. In *Essays on Temperature Regulation* (eds J. Bligh & R. E. Moore) pp. 37–54. North Holland, Amsterdam.
32 Myhre K. & Hammel H.T. (1969) Behavioural regulation of internal temperature in the lizard *Tiliqua scincoides*. *Am. J. Physiol.* **217,** 1490–5.
33 Porter W.P. & Gates D.M. (1969) Thermodynamic equilibria of animals with environment. *Ecol. Monographs* **39,** 227–44.
34 Precht H. (1973) Limiting temperatures of life function. In *Temperature and Life* (eds H. Precht, J. Christopherson, H. Hensel & W. Larcher) pp. 400–40. Springer-Verlag, Berlin, Heidelberg & New York.
35 Prosser C.L. & Brown F.A. Jr. (1961) *Comparative Animal Physiology*. Saunders, Philadelphia.
36 Rautenberg W., Necker R. & May B. (1972) Thermoregulatory responses of the pigeon to changes of the brain and spinal cord temperatures. *Pflügers Arch.* **338,** 31–42.
37 Richards S.A. (1970) Physiology of thermal panting in birds. *Ann. Biol. anim. Biophys.* 10 (series 2), 151–68.
38 Robertshaw D. (ed.) (1974) *Environmental Physiology*. MTP Intnl. Rev. Sci. Ser. 1, Vol. 7. Butterworth, London.
39 Schmidt-Nielsen K., Schmidt-Nielsen B., Jarnum S.A. & Houpt T.R. (1957) Body temperature of the camel and its relation to water economy. *Am. J. Physiol.* **188,** 103–12.
40 Scholander P.F., Hock R., Walters V., Johnson F. & Irving L. (1950) Heat regulation in some arctic and tropical mammals and birds. *Biol. Bull.* **99,** 237–58.
41 Simon E. (1974) Temperature regulation: the spinal cord as a site of extrahypothalamic thermoregulatory functions. *Rev. Physiol. Biochem. Pharmacol.* **71,** 1–76. Springer-Verlag, Berlin, Heidelberg & New York.
42 Smith R.E. & Horwitz B.A. (1969) Brown fat and thermogenesis. *Physiol. Rev.* **49,** 330–425.
43 Stephens E.D. (1973) The evolution of endothermy. *J. Theor. Biol.* **38,** 597–611.
44 Swan H. (1974) *Thermoregulation and Bioenergetics*, pp. 330–1. Elsevier, Amsterdam.
45 Van't Hoff J. (1884) *Etudes sur la Dynamique Chimique*. Muller, Amsterdam.

PART VI
POSTSCRIPT

Chapter 21
Postscript: some concepts central to the study of environmental physiology

By now it must be evident to the reader that the range of animal functions that relate directly or less directly to the total environment in which organisms now live, or in which their ancestors once lived, is so great that virtually *all aspects of physiology are relevant to the theme of this book*. Of necessity, the complex interrelating and environmentally interacting processes of life have to be examined under artificially stabilized conditions in which the precise actions, and sequences of actions, of component systems can be analysed. However, to study the details of function in permanent isolation from either the whole organism or its environment is to run the risk of missing much of the significance of the resultant observations. Resynthesis must follow analysis and ultimately every aspect of function will be seen to be involved in the interrelations of life and the environment in which it occurs.

The potential subject matter of a treatise on environmental physiology is thus enormous. This single volume could only be illustrative of the theme, and could not be encyclopaedic in its cover. Thus the editors do not claim to have directed the reader to all he ought to know about environmental physiology, but only to the general pattern of the relations of organism to environment.

Can any general or unifying principles be derived from a study of environmental physiology? Certainly within specific functions, general patterns or 'rules' are discernible—for example in gas exchange processes in aquatic animals, or in temperature control or locomotion. But much larger generalizations can be made, and it would seem that three concepts are central to environmental physiology.

The first is the concept of '*fitness*'. Evolution is opportunist and can only work on the raw materials to hand. At the molecular and biochemical levels there is a large but finite number of mechanisms which could, in principle, be used for certain tasks. As a rule, however, nature has settled for one or two mechanisms which, for one reason or another, afforded to different evolutionary lines some marginally greater chance of surviving to maturity and of reproducing in their particular environments. Thus the fish gill, amphibian skin and crustacean gland each perform a variety of regulatory processes, the 'fitness' of which can only be seen in their natural contexts. Generally speaking, 'fitness' can only be appreciated in terms of 'being' or 'not being' through evolutionary time, and in the context of contemporary environments. It may be possible to measure effectiveness of particular adaptations by experimental means, but at present the only way we seem to have of measuring adaptation is by observing natural selection. Adaptations are frequently discussed in terms of 'strategies' or 'solutions to problems', and an attempt might be made to compare adaptations by using some common currency such as energy. Unfortunately, design criteria such as 'versatility' or 'efficiency' are fraught with quantitative difficulties, and this may be why the experimental measurement of efficacy of physiological adaptations—that is of 'fitness'—remains a largely unexplored territory.

A second concept of importance in the study of environmental physiology is that of the *hierarchical structure of biological systems*: cells are components of organs, which are components of organisms, which are parts of populations (or communities), which are parts of ecosystems (Fig. 21.1). Between a mutation and the resultant marginal benefit detectable in a population there lies an enormously complicated drama acted out by individual organisms in an environment which is certainly indifferent and is often hostile. Environmental physiology *is* this drama, and is thus the central subject of biology. It embraces the intracellular molecular biology which accounts for the occurrence of mutations, as well as classical unicellular and multicellular morphology, physiology, biochemistry and ecology. It demands the ability to think at different levels of analysis—at those of molecules, of cells, of organs, of organisms and of populations, because organisms adapt in different ways at these different levels.

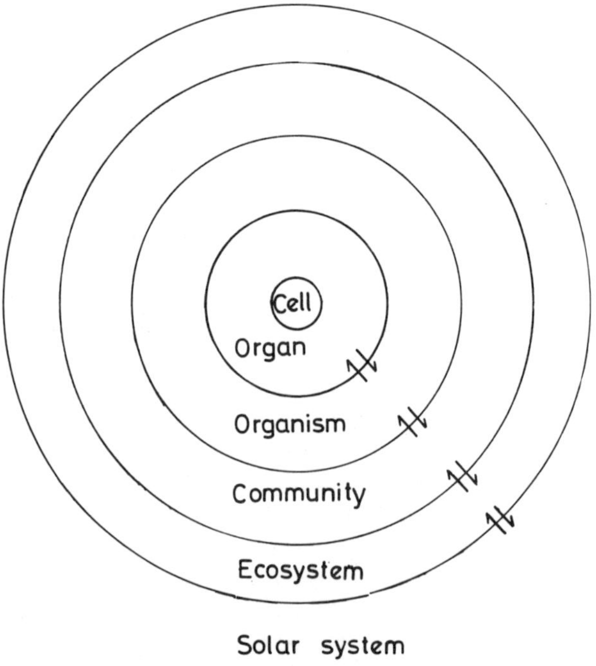

Fig. 21.1 A representation of the relations of cells, organs, organisms, communities (populations) and ecosystems with their respective environments (see text).

A third concept central to environmental physiology is the *responsiveness* of cells, organisms and populations to environmental influences, and the *integration* which this property brings about. This must be considered in some detail, and must start at the level of the cell. Indeed, the environment of every single living cell of unicellular and multicellular organisms alike is by far the most important aspect of environmental physiology, for life and death are essentially cellular phenomena, determined by whether or not the extracellular environment is such that the intracellular chemistry can remain organized and able to work against the energy flow towards entropy of the inorganic world.

The fluid environment of multicellular organisms may be the sea, fresh water or the atmosphere, but the component cells have apparently been unable to divorce themselves from the salt water environment in which they evolved. Thus the environment of each living cell remains essentially a sea, and the fundamental role of homeostatic processes is to maintain the saline environment of the individual cells within the narrow physical and chemical limits compatible with life. The lungs, the heart and circulation, the kidneys and the digestive processes of any animal are principally concerned with maintaining an internal environment in which the constituent cells can thrive. With the exception of the reproductive system and processes such as sweating which are involved in countering physical stresses imposed on the organism by the habitat, almost all the other systems of a multicellular organism relate in some way to locomotor processes used in the search for food, avoidance of predators and mating.

Thus, virtually all physiology relates to the means whereby the individual constituent cells, and the organism as a whole, remain in harmony with their environments.

It is argued in this book that, in the final analysis, not only is all physiology environmental physiology but also that all, or almost all, the variations in form and function are the result of the success of random mutations which have afforded improved chances of survival and reproduction in particular environments. This, it would seem, is the basis of the evolution of systems of biological engineering by which the structures and functions of each organism is so well matched to the features of its particular habitat.

Although each cell of a multicellular organism behaves as part of the whole and executes particular functions which are meaningful only in terms of the physiology of the entire organism, each constituent cell remains basically an autonomous unit of life: tissue-culture studies amply demonstrate this. How essential, then, are the other cells of the whole organism to the individual cell? The answer seems to be that the existence and the influence of the other cells is of significance only while the cell is behaving as part of a whole organism. For this its shape must be restrained and its activity synchronized and disciplined to serve the larger entity. But what shapes it and instructs it when and what to do for the good of the whole organism?

The embryological partition of cellular function and the organization of the structural and functional relations of cells to each other, and of organs to each other, seems to depend on the influence of the chemical environment on the rapidly dividing cells. At an early stage of this development, cells appear to be uncommitted to a particular function and can give rise to different structures according to different environmental circumstances. The neural and humoral (endocrine) actions of one cell on another are brought about by the discharge of a substance from one type of cell, and the specialized responsiveness of another cell to that particular substance in its environment. This suggests that the ability of cells to discharge substances (e.g. metabolites or hormones) into the environment of other cells, and the selective responsiveness of cells to the constituents of their immediate environments, is not only the basis of the mechanisms by which multicellular organisms are formed but also the means by which the individual units subsequently function as parts of a whole.

The consequences of a mutational change in a cell—whether spontaneous or induced environmentally—such that it is no longer subject to the restraining influences of its neighbours, are disastrous to the integrity of cellular interaction. We call this insurrection *cancer* because, crablike in its spread, its lawless progeny infiltrate and ultimately destroy the community of cells of which they are an unconforming part.

The immediate responses of the whole organism to a change in its external or internal environment depends on a well-rehearsed chain of events, by which cells sensing an environmental disturbance, release a substance into the intercellular environment, and so activate other cells, until finally effector cells are similarly activated and effect the appropriate responses to the initial environmental stimulus. This is, of course, a gross oversimplification, but the principle expressed here would seem to be the basis of all the organizational complexity of the sensor, the central nervous system and the effectors by which all organisms harmonize with their particular environments, and by which they respond immediately and appropriately to environmental changes.

The slower acclimatory changes are also largely induced by chemical substances which are liberated by one class of cell, and which act on another class of cell. These substances, which usually travel through the circulation from the discharging cell to the responding cell, are by custom, referred to as *hormones*. It is noteworthy, however, that the word merely means that the discharged substance has an urging or *excitatory** influence somewhere else (*hormaein* (Gk) = urging). Strictly speaking, synaptic transmitters also merit this description. There is, however, a difference between synaptic transmitters and 'hormones' which relates not so much to the distance between the discharging cell and the responding cell, as to the effect of the substance on the responding cell. This is dangerous ground, because we have still a great deal to learn about the actions of synaptic *detonator* transmitters and humoral *facilitatory* transmitters (hormones) on the 'target' cells, but it seems that whereas the action of a synaptic transmitter is on the cell membrane, and has an immediate effect on the state of the permeability and electrical polarization, the hormones cause changes in the internal functions of the cells which take longer to effect, and which persist for longer once effected.

* The *excitatory influence* of a hormone, as used here, must now embrace the inhibitory influences of hormones which were unrecognized when the term 'hormone' was coined.

In this way, cells may be aroused from a state of inactivity to perform a particular function at a particular phase in the life of an organism. The hormonal control of reproduction fits this description. In some processes of acclimatization, the effect of an activating hormone is to change the immediate responsiveness of an effector cell to neural excitation.

We can now see that both the immediate 'reflex' responses of organisms to external or internal environmental changes, and the more slowly developing acclimatory responses to the environment, are effected by the specialized responsiveness of cells to changes in their immediate environments, and in specializations in the substances cells emit into the immediate environments of other cells.

In Chapter 12 (on cellular adaptation to the environment) an interesting comparison is made between the division of labour within the individual cell, and the division of labour within the whole organism (Fig. 12.5): knowledge of the specialized functions of the whole organism is used to describe the way each individual unit of life operates on the basis of similar intracellular division of functions. Evolution actually worked the other way round, of course, and the multicellular organism is doing on a grander scale all the things which the individual cell has to accomplish by itself.

The multicellular organism is described here as a community of cells each of which is potentially autonomous, but restrained by other cells to behave as an integral and essential part of the community. It is tempting to extend the model and suggest that the same holds for the individual organism as part of a society—the nest of ants, the hive of bees or a city of humans—and for a society as part of an ecosystem. The individual animal, and the particular microcosm, might appear to be potentially autonomous and capable of functioning independently, but in fact each individual organism, and each microcosm, is restrained by the environmental influences of the ecosystem of which they are part.

This thesis might be represented by a series of concentric rings (Fig. 21.1). Inside each ring is the unit: first the cell, then the organ, then the organism, then the microcosm and finally the ecosystem. Outside each circle is the environment to which the unit of life must be suitably adapted and responsive, and which limits the autonomy of the unit. Life at all levels of organization, is environmentally fixed and environmentally ordered. But for the influences of environments on life, and the capacity of life to adapt to these influences, there would be no life as we now know it, and the earth might have been as barren as its moon.

The absence of any detailed discussion on immunoresponses results from the initial design of the volume which might not be quite the same were the editors able to start again with hindsight. Immunology has become so complex and places such heavy emphasis on biochemistry and biophysics, that many researchers in the field would scarcely consider their subject as a branch of physiology, and certainly not of environmental physiology. Nevertheless, immunoresponses are the results of environmental changes, and the survival of the individual until it can reproduce may depend as much on this particular kind of phenotypic adaptation to the environment as on anything else.

The common ancestry and common machinery of living cells makes the internal environment of a multicellular organism an acceptable habitat for other smaller organisms. Such intruding bodies, however, are not part of the integral community of cells, and may demonstrate an indifference to those environmental influences by which the endogenous cells are constrained to function as part of a system. As the cancer cell can be likened to an anarchist born of a society whose rules he later rejects, so can the intruding cell be likened to an invader who pays no heed to the established social order of the land he invades. If unrepelled, he would ravage the land and finally destroy it.

The recognition of the cells of the individual organism as 'self', and the recognition of invading cells as 'not self' is achieved by intercellular signalling effected through changes in cellular environments. The invaders are uninfluenced by the 'normal' signals which regulate legitimate members of the cellular community, but what they discharge, the *antigen*, is detected by specialized cells as a pollution of the environment by a foreign cell. These specialized cells respond by producing and secreting specific antibodies, which react on the foreigners in a destructive way.

There may be danger in this simple-minded view of the way a family of cells behaves as a single organism; of the concept that the responses of the whole organism to changes in its external and internal environment are effected by a chain of local changes in the chemical environments of cells as a result of the secretions of other cells; of cancer as the occurrence of native cells which no longer respond appropriately to intercellular signals; and of infections as the invasion of the internal environment by foreign cells that are no part of the organized community. There is equal danger, however, in assuming, as many people do, that the fundamental principles of biology are so infinitely complex that no simply expressed pattern could be a valid generalization. We have offered this pattern, not for blind acceptance, but for critical consideration.

The challenge which environmental physiology poses is in the quantitative study of 'fitness' at all levels of analysis. This would surely lead to a more penetrating understanding of life and its adaptations. One way to meet this challenge is to consider the different time scales into which adaptations may be conveniently classified.

We have considered environmental physiology, not in terms of the hierarchical structure of cells and organs and whole animal homeostatic systems indicated in Fig. 21.1, but according to the different time scales in which adaptations may be conveniently classified. In this way we have sought to emphasize the multiple levels of organization at which responsiveness and integration are achieved in the struggle for survival.

APPENDICES AND INDEX

Appendix 1
Units of measurement

So far as has been considered practicable the *International System of Units for Measurement* (S.I.) [1] has been used in this text. It has been recognized that difficulties exist in the use of strict S.I. in the biological sciences and recommendations have, indeed, been made for adaptations of S.I. for physiology [2]. Here we have allowed deviations from S.I. in expressions of time, pressure and temperature, as follows:

Time

The S.I. unit for time is the SECOND (s). This is an unnatural interval and even when raised to the power of 3 or multiples of 3, as S.I. allows, this remains a meaningless way of expressing either the time scale of life or of the natural periodicities related to the rotation of the earth on its axis (a nychthemeron), the moon round the earth (a lunar month) and the earth round the sun (a year). The interval since life began is considered to be of the order of three thousand million years, which is about 10^{17} seconds. Even if we had decided to use this unthinkable form of expression, we would have encountered the difficulty that S.I. runs out of prefixes and symbols after *tera* (T) for 10^{12}. Clearly life relates to natural and meaningful periodicities. Thus we are compelled to accept the nychthemeron, the lunar month and the year as time intervals beyond the jurisdiction of man. It is sensible to accept the fact that hours and minutes are universally understood and convenient divisions of the nychthemeron.

Pressure

The S.I. unit for pressure is the PASCAL (Pa) which is the pressure exerted by a force of one NEWTON (N) on an area of one square metre. Many other units of pressure are still in use, e.g. the bar, the atmosphere, the torr, pounds per square inch, mm Hg, cm H_2O. There can be little doubt that the only way out of this confusion is to accept the Pascal, and not to argue special cases. However, there can also be little doubt that the expression here in Pascals of pressures familiar to physiologists in terms of mm Hg or cm H_2O would detract from the heuristic intention of this volume. The editors have therefore accepted the recommendation [2] that in physiology mm Hg and cm H_2O continue to be used. The relations between these forms of expression and S.I. are:

$$1 \text{ mm Hg} = 133{\cdot}322387415\ (133)\ \text{Pa}\ (\text{N}\,.\,\text{m}^{-2})$$
$$1 \text{ cm } H_2O = 98{\cdot}0665\ (98)\ \text{Pa}\ (\text{N}\,.\,\text{m}^{-2})$$

Temperature

The S.I. unit for temperature is the KELVIN (K). Opinion is divided whether the very limited range of tissue and ambient temperatures biologically tolerated are best expressed on the Kelvin (absolute) scale or the Celsius scale. Except where, for physical formulation, K is the necessary scale, the Celsius scale is used here.

Energy

The S.I. unit for energy is the JOULE (J), and there is no reason why this should not be accepted as the unit of measurement and expression of biological energetics. The use of the calorie has therefore been disallowed. For those who still find difficulty in relating Joules and calories the conversions are:

$$1 \text{ cal} = 4{\cdot}1868\ (4{\cdot}2)\ \text{J}$$
$$1 \text{ J} = 0{\cdot}2388\ (0{\cdot}24)\ \text{cal}$$

Power

The S.I. unit is the WATT (W).

$$1 \text{ W} = 1 \text{ J}\,.\,\text{s}^{-1}$$
$$1 \text{ kcal}\,.\,\text{hr}^{-1} = 1{\cdot}16 \text{ W} = 1{\cdot}16 \text{ J}\,.\,\text{s}^{-1}$$

REFERENCES

1 Lowe D.A. (1975) *Progress in standardization*: **2.** A guide to international recommendations on names and symbols for quantities and on units of measurement. World Health Organization, Geneva.

2 Assendelft O.W. van Mook G.A. & Zijlstra W.G. (1973) International System of Units (SI) in physiology. *Pflügers Arch.* **339,** 265–72.

Appendix 2
The geological time scale

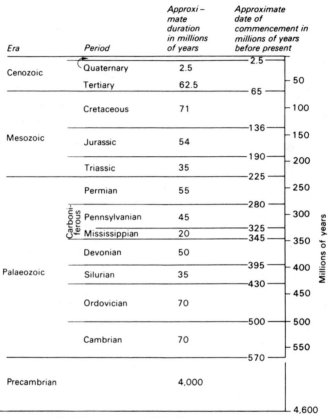

Era	*Period*	*Approxi-mate duration in millions of years*	*Approximate date of commencement in millions of years before present*
Cenozoic	Quaternary	2.5	2.5
	Tertiary	62.5	65
Mesozoic	Cretaceous	71	136
	Jurassic	54	190
	Triassic	35	225
Palaeozoic	Permian	55	280
	Carboni-ferous: Pennsylvanian	45	325
	Carboni-ferous: Mississippian	20	345
	Devonian	50	395
	Silurian	35	430
	Ordovician	70	500
	Cambrian	70	570
Precambrian		4,000	4,600

Formation of Earth's crust about 4,600 million years ago

Ages of the Epochs of the Cenozoic Era

Pleistocene Epoch	1.8— 0	million years ago
Pliocene Epoch	5.0— 2.5	" " "
Miocene Epoch	22.5— 5.0	" " "
Oligocene Epoch	37.5—22.5	" " "
Eocene Epoch	53.5—37.5	" " "
Paleocene Epoch	65.0—53.5	" " "

Index